Introduction to Audiologic Rehabilitation

Third Edition

Ronald L. Schow

Idaho State University

Michael A. Nerbonne

Central Michigan University

Allyn and Bacon

Boston   London   Toronto   Sydney   Tokyo   Singapore

> **To our colleagues, for their expertise, new ideas, patience, and enduring friendship.**

Vice President, Education: Nancy Forsyth
Executive Editor: Kris Farnsworth
Editorial Assistant: Christine Shaw
Manufacturing Buyer: Megan Cochran
Marketing Manager: Kathy Hunter
Editorial-Production Service: Electronic Publishing Services Inc.
Cover Administrator: Suzanne Harbison

Copyright © 1996, 1989 by Allyn & Bacon
A Simon & Schuster Company
Needham Heights, Massachusetts 02194

Library of Congress Cataloging-in-Publication Data

Introduction to audiological rehabilitation / [edited by] Ronald L.
    Schow & Michael A. Nerbonne. — 3rd ed.
        p. cm.
    Previously published under the title: Introduction to aural
rehabilitation.
    Includes bibliographical references and indexes.
    ISBN 0-205-16069-7
    1. Deaf—Rehabilitation.   2. Audiology.   I. Schow, Ronald L.
II. Nerbonne, Michael A.   III. Introduction to aural rehabilitation.
RF297.I57   1995
617.8'03—dc20   95-23683
                                                                CIP

Printed in the United States of America

10 9 8 7 6 5 4   00 99 98 97

Contents

Preface

Using the feedback from our colleagues and students, we have made extensive updates and revisions to *Introduction to Audiologic Rehabilitation*. Even the title reflects improvement by incorporating the now more preferred term *audiologic*. As a result, we believe this third edition is well-suited for preparing current undergraduate or graduate students in rehabilitative audiology. Included are the same features that have prompted many professors to adopt this book in speech and hearing programs for over 15 years. Seven chapters introduce the fundamentals. Three more chapters cover comprehensive methods and procedures that focus on each age group—children, adults, and elderly adults. We have continued the tradition of thorough documentation and ample illustration. Finally, the text concludes with two case-study chapters and a resource chapter. Included in the updating is a reference to the changing state of audiology wherein a new degree, the Doctor of Audiology, is gradually emerging to revitalize our profession.

We expect that others who teach in this area will find this a readable, current, and practical textbook that will be easily understood by students. Working professionals and students will find a complete listing of resources, with ample appendices containing tests, self-report questionnaires, and other updated materials useful in their clinical rehabilitative work. Recent surveys and position statements by professional organizations are included to make this a valuable compendium of information.

We have included a broad array of case studies to help students understand the variety of audiologic rehabilitation procedures and how they may be applied. Students can learn how today's audiologists are providing complete service—from the use of cochlear implants for deaf youngsters, to the application of the latest programmable hearing aids and assistive devices for adults—in a vast array of commercial, health, and traditional clinical settings.

It goes without saying that the completion of this textbook is the result of efforts made by many contributors who should be commended for their willingness to share their expertise and time in writing major portions of the book. We also appreciate the flexibility and cooperative spirit they had when we requested revisions and imposed deadlines. All are true professionals in every sense of the word. In the final stages of editing, we were saddened by the sudden death of one of our contributors, Carl Binnie. His case study in Chapter 12 exemplifies the commitment Carl had to providing quality audiologic rehabilitation to his clients and a quality education to his students as well.

Once again, our university colleagues have been both helpful and supportive to us throughout the project. In particular, we would like to single out Diana Hughes, Jerry Church, Linda Seestedt-Standford, Mike Arsenault, Thayne Smedley, Dave Sorensen, Ken Medley, Jeff Brockett, David Mercaldo and Barry Griffing for their suggestions and support, which helped immeasurably as we worked to update the book. We also thank Tracie Radford, Nancy O'Brien and Rob Shaw for the much-appreciated word processing and cheerful assistance they have rendered. Our thanks also to the folks at Allyn and Bacon for their expertise throughout. Users of the second edition, both professors and students, who have offered insightful comments and suggestions to us and thus had a major influence on the content of this third edition are likewise appreciated.

Finally, we want to express love and appreciation once again to our respective families for their continued support and understanding throughout the time we were engaged in writing and editing this edition.

Contributors

Jerome G. Alpiner, Ph.D.
Chief of Audiology/Speech Pathology Services "126"
VA Medical Center
1055 Clermont St.
Denver, CO 80220

Carl A. Binnie, Ph.D. (Deceased)
Former Professor of Audiology
Department of Audiology and Speech Sciences
Purdue University
West Lafayette, IN 47907

Dean G. Garstecki, Ph.D.
Professor and Program Head: Audiology and Hearing Impairment
Communication Sciences and Disorders
Northwestern University
Evanston, IL 60208-3550

Thomas G. Giolas, Ph.D.
Dean of the Graduate School, Director of the Research Foundation, and Professor of Communication Disorders
University of Connecticut
Storrs, CT 06268

Nicholas M. Hipskind, Ph.D.
Associate Professor and Director of Clinical Audiology
Department of Speech and Hearing Sciences
Indiana University
Bloomington, IN 47401

Alice E. Holmes, Ph.D.
Associate Professor of Audiology
Department of Communicative Disorders
University of Florida
Gainesville, FL 32610-0174

Adrienne Karp, M.A.
Audiologist
New York Association for the Blind
111 East 59th St.
New York, NY 10022

Patricia B. Kricos, Ph.D.
Professor of Audiology
Department of Communication Processes and Disorders
University of Florida
Gainesville, FL 32611

James F. Maurer, Ph.D.
Professor Emeritus of Audiology
Speech and Hearing Sciences
Portland State University
Portland, OR 97207

Mary Pat Moeller, M.S.
Coordinator: Center for Childhood Deafness
Boys Town National Research Hospital
Omaha, NE 68181

Donald F. Moores, Ph.D.
Director: Center for Studies in Education and
    Human Development
Gallaudet Research Institute
Gallaudet University
Washington, DC 20002

H. Gustav Mueller, Ph.D.
Senior Audiology Consultant: Siemens Hear-
    ing Instruments, USA
Faculty Appointments: Vanderbilt University,
    Nashville, TN; University of Northern
    Colorado, Greeley, CO; University of Col-
    orado, Boulder, CO

Michael A. Nerbonne, Ph.D.
Professor of Audiology
Department of Communication Disorders
Central Michigan University
Mt. Pleasant, MI 48859

Ronald L. Schow, Ph.D.
Professor of Audiology
Department of Speech Pathology and Audiol-
    ogy
Idaho State University
Pocatello, ID 83209

Deborah Noall Seyfried, Ph.D.
Assistant Professor of Audiology
Department of Communication Sciences and
    Disorders
Radford University
Radford, VA 24142

Thayne C. Smedley, Ph.D.
Professor of Audiology
Department of Speech Pathology and Audiol-
    ogy
Idaho State University
Pocatello, ID 83209

Anne L. Strouse, M.A.
Division of Hearing and Speech Sciences
Vanderbilt University School of Medicine
Nashville, TN 37212

Nancy Tye-Murray, Ph.D.
Associate Professor
Department of Otolaryngology-Head and
    Neck Surgery
University of Iowa Hospitals
Iowa City, IA 52242

McCay Vernon, Ph.D.
Professor Emeritus
Department of Psychology
Western Maryland College
Westminster, MD 21157

Susan Watkins, Ed.D
SKI-HI Institute
Department of Communicative Disorders
Utah State University
Logan, UT 84321-9605

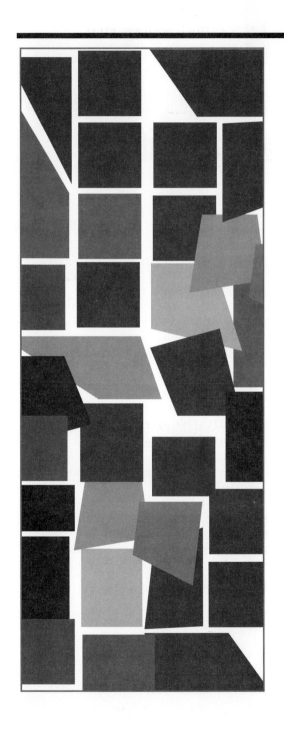

PART ONE

Fundamentals of Audiologic Rehabilitation

1

Overview of Audiologic Rehabilitation

Ronald L. Schow
Michael A. Nerbonne

Contents

INTRODUCTION

Most of us have had occasion to converse with someone who has a hearing problem. Unless the person had received proper help for the hearing difficulties it probably was a frustrating experience for both parties. When the person with hearing loss is a family member or close friend we become aware that the emotional and social ramifications of this communication barrier can be substantial as well. Providing help to address all of these hearing problems is the focus of this book. Help is possible, but often not utilized. This chapter gives an overview of a process that is crucial for the welfare of persons who suffer from hearing impairment and, in turn, for those who communicate with them.

Definitions—Synonyms

Simply stated, we may define *audiologic habilitation/rehabilitation* as those professional efforts designed to help a person with hearing loss. These include services and procedures for lessening or compensating for a hearing impairment, and specifically involve facilitating adequate receptive and expressive communication (ASHA, 1984; ASHA, 1992). A key consideration in this rehabilitation process involves assisting the person with hearing impairment to attain full potential by using personal resources to overcome difficulties resulting from the hearing loss. Two kinds of important service that are closely related but distinct from the audiologic habilitation/rehabilitation process are *medical intervention* and *teaching academic subjects to the deaf.*

Several terms have been used to describe this helping process. *Audiologic habilitation* refers to remedial efforts with children having a hearing loss at birth, since technically it is not possible to restore (rehabilitate) something that has never existed. *Audiologic rehabilitation*, then, refers to efforts designed to restore a lost state or function. In the interest of simplicity, the terms *habilitation* and *rehabilitation* are used interchangeably in this text, technicalities notwithstanding. Variations of the *audiologic rehabilitation* term include *auditory and aural rehabilitation, hearing rehabilitation*, and *rehabilitative audiology.* Terms used to refer to rehabilitative efforts with the very young child include *parent advising/counseling/tutoring* and *pediatric auditory habilitation. Educational* (or *school*) *audiology* is sometimes used to refer to auditory rehabilitative efforts performed in the school setting.

Providers of Audiologic Rehabilitation

Audiologic rehabilitation (AR), then, is referred to by different names, and is performed in a number of different settings. All aspects of assisting the client in the audiologic rehabilitation process are not performed by one person. In fact, professionals from several different disciplines are often involved, including educators, psychologists, social workers, and rehabilitation counselors. Nevertheless, the audiologist in particular, and in some circumstances the speech-language pathologist or the educator of those with impaired hearing, will assume a major AR role. These professionals provide overall coordination of the process or act as advocates for the person with impaired hearing. Audiologic rehabilitation is not something we *do* to a person following a strict "doctor-knows-best" medical model. It is a process designed to counsel and work with persons who are deaf and hard of hearing so they can actualize their own resources in order to meet their unique life situations. This text has been written with the hope of orienting and preparing such "counselors" or "advocates for the hearing-impaired."

Education Needs of Providers

Recently, much discussion has centered around establishing a professional doctorate in audiology as the minimum educational requirement to practice as an audiologist. The Academy of Rehabilitative Audiology (ARA) recently adopted a position statement which emphasizes the need for future Au.D. students to be well prepared in audiologic rehabilitation. The ARA provides a list of relevant content areas in AR which should be incorporated into any Au.D. program to insure adequate preparation in this all-important area of audiology. This statement and an earlier document along similar lines are available as a resource in this text (see ARA, 1993 and ASHA, 1984, statements on competencies for AR in Chapter 13).

Regardless of academic background, those from the different professions mentioned in the previous section who successfully perform AR must, like competent audiologists, possess an understanding of and familiarity with several areas of knowledge. These include (a) characteristics of hearing impairment, (b) effect of hearing loss on persons, and (c) the previously noted competencies needed for providing audiologic rehabilitation. For purposes of the present treatment, it is assumed that other coursework or study has brought the reader familiarity with the various forms of hearing impairment, as well as procedures used in the measurement of hearing loss. These procedures, referred to as *diagnostic audiology*, serve as a preliminary step towards rehabilitative audiology. The task at hand, then, is to review briefly some characteristics of hearing loss, to explore the major consequences of hearing impairment, and finally to discuss the methods and competencies needed to help with this condition.

HEARING-LOSS CHARACTERISTICS

Important characteristics of hearing loss as they relate to audiologic rehabilitation include (a) degree of impairment, (b) time of onset, (c) type of loss, and (d) auditory speech recognition ability.

Hearing-Impairment Degree

One major aspect of hearing impairment or loss is the person's hearing sensitivity or degree of loss (see Table 1.1). The category of hearing impairment includes both the hard of hearing and the deaf. Persons with limited amounts of hearing loss are referred to as being *hard of hearing*. Those with an extensive loss of hearing are considered deaf. Generally, when hearing losses, measured by pure tone average (PTA) or speech recognition threshold (SRT), are poorer than 80–90 dB HL, a person is considered to be *audiometrically deaf*. However, deafness can also be described as the inability to use hearing to any meaningful extent for the ordinary purposes of life, especially for verbal communication. This latter way of defining deafness is independent of the findings from audiometric test results.

The prevalence of hearing impairment may be considered for all persons combined and for children and adults separately. In the United States the prevalence of hearing impairment is estimated to be from 14 to 40 million, depending on whether conservative or liberal figures are used (Goldstein, 1984; Ries, 1994; Schow, et al., 1994). These estimates vary depending on the definition of loss; the loss may be self defined or involve different dB fence levels, some as low as 15 dB HL, but most are higher, commonly 20–25 dB HL. Authorities have suggested that a different definition of loss should be applied for children because in a younger person the consequences are greater for the same amount of loss (Roeser, 1988). The prevalence of loss also varies depending on whether the conventional pure-tone average (500, 1000, 2000 Hz) is used or whether some additional upper frequencies (like 3000 and 4000 Hz) are included. In this book we recommend that different pure-tone average fences be used for children and adults at the "slight-to-mild" degree of loss level, although the degree designation is similar at most levels. In addition, we recommend that either 3000 or 4000 Hz be used in evaluating loss, although the usual three-frequency pure-tone average will typically be used in analyzing audiograms. Table 1.1 indicates that a hearing loss is found in children at a lower (better) dB level than in adults; this is consistent with ASHA screening levels for school children that define normal hearing up to and including 20 dB HL (ASHA, 1985). A reasonable estimate from recent prevalence studies would be that at least 10% of the population have permanent, significant impairment of hearing (25 million in the U.S.). Approximately ⅓ of 1% of the total U.S. population is deaf (about .7 million). Thus, the remaining 24.3 million are in the hard-of-hearing group (Schow, et al., 1994).

Children form a subpopulation of the total group of 25 million individuals with impaired hearing. It is estimated that about 3 million children in the United States are

TABLE 1.1 *Degree of Hearing Impairment Descriptions, Based on Pure-Tone Findings*[a]

Degrees of Hearing Impairment	PTA in dB based on .5, 1, 2, 4 K[b] Hz	
	Children	*Adults*
Slight to Mild	21–40	26–40
Mild to Moderate	—— 41–55 ——	
Moderate	—— 56–70 ——	
Severe	—— 71–90 ——	
Profound	—— 91 plus ——	

[a]Based on levels advocated by the Committee on Hearing of the American Academy of Ophthalmology and Otolaryngology (adapted from AAOO, 1965).

[b]K = 1000.

deaf and hard of hearing, and even more fit in this category if high-frequency and conductive losses are included (Shepherd, Davis, Gorga, & Stelmachowicz, 1981; see Chapter 8). Of this total 3 million, about 50,000 school-age youngsters are classified as deaf (American Annals of the Deaf, 1994; Schein & Delk, 1974). As with children, most adults with impaired hearing are considered to be hard of hearing and only a small minority are deaf (Ries, 1994, Schow, et al., 1994; Davis, 1994).

Degree (sensitivity), however, is only one of several important dimensions of a hearing loss. Even though it is often the first measure available and provides useful evidence of the impact of the loss, there are exceptions to this generalization. Some children with a profound impairment of 90 dB HL outperform—in language and academic areas, average children who have a loss of only 70 dB HL.

Table 1.2 contains a description of deafness and hard-of-hearing categories in terms of typical hearing aspects, use of hearing, use of vision, language development, use of language, speech, and educational needs. Prevalence estimates are also shown.

Time of Onset

Most hard-of-hearing youngsters are thought to have hearing loss beginning early in life, but mild losses may not be detected, so prevalence data on young children are scarce and somewhat uncertain (Lundeen, 1991). With youngsters who are deaf or have more severe impairment, the time when a hearing loss is acquired will determine, in part, the extent to which normal speech and language will be present. Severe hearing loss (deafness) may be divided into three categories (*prelingual*, *postlingual*, *deafened*) depending on the person's age when the loss occurs (Department of Labor, 1971; see Tables 1.2 and 1.3). *Prelingual deafness* refers to impairment present at birth or prior to the development of speech and language. The longer during the crucial language development years (up to age five) a person has normal hearing, the less chance there is that language development will be profoundly affected. *Postlingual deafness* means loss occurs after about age five; its overall effects are therefore usually less serious. However, even though language may be less affected, speech and education will be affected substantially (see Chapters 5 and 7). *Deafened* persons are those who lose hearing after their schooling is completed (i.e., sometime in their late teen years, or thereafter). Normal speech, language, and education can be acquired by these individuals, but difficulty in verbal communication and other social, emotional, and vocational problems may occur (see Table 1.3).

Type of Loss

The type of loss may be *conductive* (damage in the outer or middle ear), *sensorineural* (impairment in the inner ear or nerve of hearing), or *mixed* (a combination of conductive and sensorineural). Generally, conductive losses are amenable to medical intervention whereas sensorineural losses are primarily aided through audiologic rehabilitation. Other less common types of loss are possible as well, such as *functional* (nonorganic) problems and *central auditory processing* (CAP) *disorders*

TABLE 1.2 Categories and Characteristics of Hearing Impairment

Characteristic	Hard of Hearing (24,333,000)[a]	Category of Deafness		
		Prelingual (75,000)[a]	Postlingual (150,000)[a]	Deafened (442,000)[a]
Hearing impairment	Sensitivity: mild, moderate, or severe; Recognition: fair to good (70%–90%)	Sensitivity: severe or profound degree of loss; Recognition: fair to poor		
Use (level) of hearing	Functional speech understanding (lead sense)	Functional signal-warning/environmental awareness (hearing minimized)		
Use of vision	Increased dependence		Increased dependence	
Language and speech development	Dependent on rehabilitation measures (e.g., amplification)	Dependent on amplification and early intervention	Dependent on amplification and school rehabilitation	Normal
Use of language	May be affected	Almost always affected	May be affected	Usually not affected
Use of speech	May be affected	Always affected	Usually affected	May be affected
Educational needs	Some special education	Considerable special education	Some special education	Education complete

[a]United States prevalence data for these categories, based on Schow, et al. (1994); Davis (1994); and Goldstein (1984) incidence figures

TABLE 1.3 *Definitions of Hearing Impairment*

Persons with hearing impairment have been divided into the following groups:

Prelingually Deaf persons were either born without hearing (congenitally deaf) or lost hearing before the development of speech and language: 3–5 years (adventitiously deaf). Both speech and language are affected to varying degrees and—because they usually are acquired formally instead of naturally—may be stilted, mechanical, and difficult to understand. The pre-lingually deaf person communicates primarily through fingerspelling, signs, and writing, but may possess enough speech and speechreading ability for basic social expression.

Postlingually Deaf persons are those who became profoundly deaf after the age of 5–10 years and, although possessing no hearing for practical purposes, had normal hearing long enough to establish fairly well developed speech and language patterns. While speech generally is affected (more for the 5- than for the 10-year-old), communication may be through speech, signs, fingerspelling, and writing. Once the counselor becomes accustomed to their speech, it may be quite understandable. Speechreading, however, may be more haphazard and not always dependable.

Deafened refers to those people who suffer hearing loss after completing their education—generally in their late teens or early twenties and upward. Such people usually have fairly comprehensible, nearly normal speech and language, but they need instruction to acquire useful speechreading. Quite frequently they face problems of adjustment because of the late onset of their hearing loss.

Hard-of-Hearing persons may have been born thus or subsequently experienced a partial loss of hearing. While they have acquired speech normally through hearing and communicate by speaking, speech may be affected to some extent; for example, the voice may be too soft or too loud. They understand others by speechreading, by using a hearing aid, or by asking the speaker to raise his or her voice or enunciate more distinctly.

Source: Interviewing Guides (pp. 1–2) by U.S. Dept. of Labor, 1971, Washington DC: Author; as adapted from Moores, 1996 and Vernon and Andrews, 1990.

(which arise from the processing centers in the brainstem or the brain) In the latter type of loss the symptoms may be very subtle. In cases of sensorineural loss, auditory speech recognition or hearing clarity is usually affected. This is also the case in difficult listening situations for those with CAP problems.

Auditory Speech Recognition Ability

Auditory speech recognition or identification ability (clarity of hearing) is another important dimension of hearing loss. The terms *speech recognition, speech identification, speech discrimination* and *speech intelligibility* will be used interchangeably throughout this text, and all are included under the general category of speech perception or comprehension (see Chapter 3). *Speech discrimination* has been used for many years to describe clarity of hearing as measured in typical word intelligibility tests, but *speech recognition* and *identification* have now replaced *discrimination* since they more precisely describe what is being measured. *Discrimination* technically implies only the ability involved in a same—different judgment, whereas *recognition* and *identification* indicate an ability to repeat or identify the stimulus. *Recognition* is commonly used by diagnostic audiologists, but *identification* meshes nicely with the nomenclature of audiologic rehabilitation procedures as discussed further in Chapter 3. *Intelligibility* is a more generic term. All four terms will at times be used due to historical precedents and evolving nomenclature.

The speech recognition ability in an individual who is hard of hearing typically is better than in a person who is deaf. Persons who are deaf are generally considered unable to comprehend conversational speech with hearing alone whereas those who are hard of hearing can use their hearing to a significant extent for speech perception. As Ramsdell (1978) pointed out, however, some minimal auditory recognition may be present in persons who are deaf even if verbal speech reception is limited, since a person may use hearing for signal-warning purposes or simply to maintain contact with the auditory environment (see Table 1.2). Nevertheless, auditory recognition ability and degree of loss are somewhat independent.

In a person of advanced age, a mild degree of loss sometimes may be accompanied by very poor speech recognition. This is referred to as *phonemic regression* and is not unusual in hearing losses among elderly persons who evidence some degree of central degeneration. Disparity in degree of loss and speech-recognition ability is also possible in young persons with hearing impairment. For example, a child may be considered deaf in terms of sensitivity but not in terms of auditory recognition or educational placement. Some children with a degree of loss that classifies them as audiometrically deaf (e.g., PTA = 90 + dB) may have unexpectedly good speech recognition. Thus, speech recognition also is an important variable in describing a hearing loss.

CONSEQUENCES OF HEARING LOSS: PRIMARY AND SECONDARY

Communication Difficulties

The primary and most devastating effect of hearing loss is its impact on verbal communication. Children with severe to profound hearing loss do not generally develop speech and language normally, because they are not exposed to the sounds of language in daily living. In instances of a lesser degree of loss or if the loss occurs in adult years, the influence on speech and language expression tends to be less severe. Nevertheless, affected individuals still experience varying degrees of difficulty in receiving the auditory speech and environmental stimuli which allow us to communicate and interact with other humans and with our environment. For children, the choice of a communication (educational) system relates directly to this area of concern. If the educational setting and methods are chosen and implemented appropriately, according to the abilities of the child, the negative impact of the loss can be minimized. Secondary consequences and side effects of hearing loss include educational, vocational, psychological, and social implications (see Chapters 4 and 6 for a discussion of communication systems and their psychosocial implications).

Variable Hearing Disability/Handicap

Disability is a term that expresses the *effects* of a hearing loss, as opposed to the *characteristics* of the loss as measured by the loss degree and speech identification ability. A similar term, *handicap*, may be thought of as a related descriptor since both *disability* and *handicap* concern the effect of the loss, but since the emergence of the American Disabilities Act (1990), *disability* has been the more popular term—in the U.S. at least. Europeans use both *disability* and *handicap*, following a scheme promoted by the World Health Organization (WHO, 1980). In that system, *disability* refers to the primary communication effects of loss, and *handicap* is the name for secondary consequences (including vocational). Nevertheless, in the USA *disability* has a very long and entrenched pattern of use in the context of vocational and employment compensation issues. Until uniform terminology is finally accepted by most international and American sources we will refer to these consequences from hearing loss as *primary* and *secondary* as a way to resolve the uncertainty surrounding these expressions.

A useful method for measuring the impact of hearing loss is through self-assessment of hearing, wherein persons make personal estimates about their hearing difficulties. This procedure has been applied with children and adults. Both the person with impaired hearing and other significant individuals can respond on questionnaires to provide a more complete picture of the communication, psychosocial, and other effects from the loss (see Chapter 9; Schow & Smedley, 1990; Erdman, 1994).

In preparing to deal with the broad consequences of hearing loss, we must recognize that the impact of a hearing impairment will vary considerably depending on a number of factors. Several of the most important of these factors are presented in Table 1.2. Although not included there, other variables were also important. For example, certain basic characteristics of the individual may have considerable impact on the primary consequences in verbal communication and the secondary effects in education, social, emotional, and vocational areas. The presence of other serious disabilities like blindness, physical limitations, or mental retardation will complicate the situation. A person's native intelligence can also have a tremendous impact in conjunction with a hearing loss. Naturally, basic intelligence will vary from person to person regardless of whether or not he/she is hearing impaired. However, Vernon (1968; 1985) reported on 50 years of research showing that, as a group, persons with hereditary deafness demonstrate a normal range of IQs as measured by performance scales. Whatever the native intellectual ability, it will influence the resultant primary and secondary consequences of hearing loss.

REHABILITATIVE ALTERNATIVES

Little can be done to change basic, innate IQ or native abilities. Nevertheless, a number of AR procedures may have a profound effect on the personal consequences resulting from a hearing loss. For example, it is estimated that more than 80% of Americans who could benefit from hearing aids are not using amplification (Smith,

1991). In addition, there are: babies and young children who have hearing loss requiring amplification, but whose losses have not been identified; school children whose aids are not in good condition (Elfenbein, et al., 1988; Smedley and Plapinger, 1988); teenagers and young adults who, because of vanity or unfortunate experiences with hearing aids, are not getting the necessary help; adults and elderly individuals who have not acquired hearing aids because of pride or ignorance; and others whose instruments are not properly fitted or oriented to regular hearing-aid use. Adults also have been found to be using many poorly functioning hearing aids (Schow, et al., 1993a). All of these cases represent a need for audiologic rehabilitation. Identifying those who need amplification, persuading them to obtain and use hearing aids, adjusting them for maximum benefit, orienting the new user to the instrument, are all tasks in the province of AR that may reduce the negative effects of a hearing loss.

Audiologic rehabilitation also includes efforts to improve communication, as well as addressing a variety of other concerns for the hearing-impaired person. Before discussing procedures and the current status of audiologic rehabilitation, however, a brief review of the history of AR is in order.

Historical Background

Although audiologic rehabilitative procedures are common today, they have not always been utilized for individuals with hearing loss. For centuries it was assumed that prelingual deafness and the resultant language development delay and inability to learn were inevitable aspects of the impairment. The deaf were thought to be retarded, so for many years no efforts were made to try to teach them. The first known teacher of persons with severe to profound hearing loss was Pedro Ponce de León of Spain, who in the mid- to late 1500s demonstrated that persons who are deaf can be taught to speak and are capable of learning. Other teachers, including Bonet and de Carrion in Spain and Bulwer in England, arose in the 1600s, and their methods gained some prominence. During the 1700s, Pereira (Pereire) introduced education of the deaf to France, and the Abbé de L'Epée founded a school there. Schools were also established by Thomas Braidwood in Great Britain and by Heinicke in Germany. De L'Epée employed fingerspelling and sign language in addition to speechreading, whereas Heinicke and Braidwood stressed oral speech. Beginning in 1813, John Braidwood, a grandson of Thomas Braidwood, tried to establish this oral method in America, but he was unsuccessful because of his own ineptness and poor health. Thomas Gallaudet went to England in 1815 to learn the Braidwood oral method, but was refused help because it was feared that he would interfere with John Braidwood's efforts. Consequently, Gallaudet learned de L'Epée's manual method in Paris through contact with Sicard and Laurent Clerc. He returned to the United States and opened his own successful school. (See additional details in Chapter 7; and in Moores, 1996.)

The manual approach to teaching persons who were deaf remained the major force in America until the mid-1800s, when speechreading and oral methods were promoted and popularized by Horace Mann, Alexander Graham Bell, and others. The stress on the use of residual hearing had been suggested earlier, but it began to receive strong emphasis with the oral methods used during the 1700s and 1800s. Until electric amplification was developed in the early 1900s, the use of residual hearing required ear trumpets and *ad concham* (speaking directly in the ear) stimulation. More vigorous efforts in the use of hearing followed the introduction of electronic hearing aids in the 1920s (Berger, 1988).

Also in the early 1900s—between 1900 and 1930, several schools of lipreading were started and became quite prominent. Although these institutions were directed principally toward teaching adults with hearing impairment how to speechread, considerable public recognition also was gained for this method of rehabilitating the hearing impaired. (*Speechreading* and *lipreading* will be used interchangeably in this text although *speechreading* is the more technically accurate term; see Chapter 4 for details.)

Birth of Audiology. During World War II, the need to rehabilitate servicemen with impaired hearing resulted in the birth of the audiology profession. The cumulative effect of electronic amplification developments, adult lipreading courses, and the World War II hearing rehabilitation efforts gradually led to the recognition of audiologic rehabilitation as separate from education for persons who are deaf. Eventually, audiologists were recognized as the professionals responsible for providing such services to adults, and soon it was also realized that audiologists could provide crucial help to youngsters who are deaf or hard of hearing.

In the military rehabilitation centers a number of methods were developed to help those with impaired hearing, including procedures for selecting hearing aids (Carhart, 1946). Hearing aid orientation methods requiring up to 3 months of coursework were developed. Considerable emphasis was also placed on speechreading and auditory training (Northern, Ciliax, Roth, & Johnson, 1969).

In the late 1940s and 1950s, as audiology moved into the private sector, the approach to hearing aids changed. Whereas hearing aids were freely dispensed in government facilities, in civilian life people bought amplification exclusively from hearing-aid dealers. Methods evolved wherein audiologists would perform tests and recommend hearing aids, but dealers would sell and service the instruments. At that time, the American Speech-Language-Hearing Association (ASHA) maintained that audiologists could not sell hearing aids because this would compromise their professional objectivity. Thus, strict rules were written into the ASHA Code of Ethics, and, except in military facilities, audiologists were excluded from hearing aid sales and follow-up (ASHA, 1967).

In audiologic rehabilitation, audiologists performed preliminary hearing-aid work (hearing aid evaluations), but concentrated on providing speechreading and auditory training. These two methods were promoted and used in certain places. For example, speech and hearing centers often set up speechreading and auditory training classes, and adult community education programs using these methods were sponsored (Mussen, 1977). With newer and better hearing aids, however, the magic and motivation of the lipreading schools dissipated, and the ideas worked out in the leisurely 3-month military rehabilitation programs were found to be economically unfeasible in the "real world." In one center it was reported that everything had been tried to attract clients for audiologic rehabilitation therapy except "dancing girls" (Alpiner, 1973).

Difficulties in Acceptance of Audiologic Rehabilitation. Because of these setbacks, the 1960s and 1970s were years of examination and reflection for audiologists committed to AR. Such self-examination revealed that the potential clientele for auditory rehabilitation is large and most are not receiving help.

INFANTS. Beginning in the 1960s many audiologists recognized the need for early identification of hearing loss so that management could be initiated during the critical language-development years (Downs & Sterrit, 1964). The incidence of hearing loss in newborns was found to be about 1 per 1000 children, a higher prevalence than for other disabilities screened routinely in the newborn. Identification methods were subsequently developed and recommended during this time (Cunningham, 1971; Mencher, 1974), and programs evolved to provide early auditory rehabilitation (Clark, Watkins, Reese, & Berg, 1975; Horton, 1972; Northcott, 1972; John Tracy Clinic Correspondence Course, 1983). The advent of cochlear implantation in young children who are deaf during the past decade has provided another important avenue for management of these youngsters.

CHILDREN. School-age youngsters with hearing impairment were also found to be in need of assistance. Many children who were hard of hearing were (and still are) educated in the regular schools, and several studies indicated that these children were not receiving the specialized support they needed (Quigley, 1970). Compared to youngsters with normal hearing, children with 15 to 45 dB losses showed delays of 15 to 19 months in reading skills and arithmetic (Ling, 1972). In addition, educational lags of 1 to 2 years were common with children with hearing impairment, and many of them repeated grades (Kodman, 1963). Even children with mild temporary losses from otitis media showed serious delays in academic progress (Holm & Kunze, 1969). As of 1972–73 it was estimated that only 21% of the 440,000 hard-of-hearing school-age youngsters (40–90 dB) in the United States received any of the special education assistance they needed (Marge, 1977). The actual number of school children who are hard of hearing is probably much greater; these are only the ones identified (see Chapter 8). Recent reports indicate these children are still being underserved (Bess, 1986; Blair, et al., 1985). Hearing-aid procurement for these children has been deficient since an estimated 15–75% (depending on degree of loss) do not use hearing aids (Matkin, 1984; Shepherd et al., 1981). There is little reason to believe this has changed in the last few years and, in fact, there is some evidence that the prevalence of high-frequency loss is increasing due to noise exposure (Chermak & Peters-McCarthy, 1991). Even with the advent of promising sound-field amplification in classrooms, recent progress reports indicate we are still in the early stages of implementation (Flexer, 1992). Thus, rehabilitation for school-age children has become an important priority and there is an acute need for the rehabilitative or educational audiologist.

ADULTS. Among adults, the needs for hearing rehabilitation are also apparent. Ries' (1994) data revealed that hearing problems are reported by 4% of the population from 25 to 34 years of age. This figure rises dramatically with age, so that for those 75 years and older, 38% of the population report problems. In addition, it is estimated that there are between 5 and 6 million hearing-aid users in this country, but conservative estimates suggest that another 15 to 20 million should be using hearing aids (Goldstein, 1984; Kochkin, 1991; Strom, 1994). Further, about ¼ of the aids being used by adults have been shown to be in poor working condition (Schow et al., 1993a).

Difficulties in Acceptance of Audiologic Rehabilitation. When audiologists reflected on the limited acceptance of audiologic rehabilitation, it became apparent that, despite the subject's importance, many in the profession lacked interest. In 1966, the Academy of Rehabilitative Audiology was organized to help audiologists with rehabilitative interests direct their efforts toward reversing these trends (Oyer, 1983). This organization and its members have had an important influence on the emergence of AR as a viable part of audiology.

One reason for the noted neglect of rehabilitation in the past is the hearing aid situation. Primarily because of the success of aggressive sales practices by hearing aid dealers and the ASHA policy which prevented heavy audiologic involvement, 70–90% of all hearing aids in this country were for many years being sold without active involvement of medical or audiological consultants (DHEW, 1975). Because audiologists did not, until the 1970s, dispense hearing aids, they were for many years deprived of close contact with clients during the post-fitting period. In contrast, the hearing aid dealers were intimately involved in the most crucial rehabilitation process. This situation began to change in the mid- to late 1970s because of relaxation in the ASHA policy prohibiting audiologists from dispensing hearing aids. Finally, due to a Supreme Court decision, ASHA removed these restrictions in 1979 (ASHA, 1978, 1979). This decision has had a profound effect on AR and the role of the audiologist in working with persons who are deaf and hard of hearing.

Current Status

Fortunately, audiologists generally have begun to recognize the opportunities for rehabilitation through early intervention and the provision of services in schools and in neglected adult and geriatric settings. This awareness has been reflected within ASHA, as evidenced in a series of policy statements on rehabilitative audiology issued by special ASHA subcommittees (ASHA, 1972, 1974, 1984, 1992). Recently, similar supportive statements on rehabilitation issues have emerged from a new professional organization for audiologists called the American Academy of Audiology (AAA, 1988, 1993).

In the past 25 years, a number of alternate audiologic rehabilitation approaches have been developed and have gradually moved away from an emphasis on speechreading and auditory training toward a major focus on hearing-aid fitting and orientation, with considerable attention on communication patterns and the environment (Alpiner, 1971; Tannahill, 1973; Giolas, 1982). This change in emphasis has continued and become more widespread, as documented in a recent survey (Schow, et al., 1993b).

A common factor in all new approaches is the recognition that hearing-aid orientation and general communication help are the central issues in most audiologic rehabilitation. In most cases now, the focus in AR is on amplification, whereas extensive speechreading and auditory training have become occasional, ancillary procedures. Heavy emphasis on these methods is needed only in certain instances.

The 1980s and 1990s have seen the emergence of a new breed of audiologists, more aware of the millions of children and adults in need of audiologic rehabilitation. Results of recent surveys show that approximately 75–80% of all ASHA audiologists are involved in direct dispensing of hearing aids (ASHA, 1991; Schow, et al., 1993b). According to one survey conducted in 1990, 86–88% of all audiologists are involved in hearing-aid evaluation, hearing-aid orientation, and rehabilitation counseling. A smaller number (23%) reported being involved in communication rehabilitation, including speechreading and auditory training (Schow, et al., 1993b).

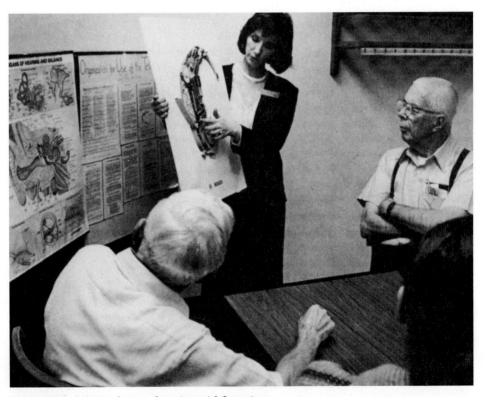

Orienting adults to how a hearing aid functions.

Procedures in Audiologic Rehabilitation: An AR Model

This section will describe important procedures and elements of audiologic rehabilitation in order to provide a framework for the remainder of this text.

The audiologic rehabilitation model used here emerged in 1980 when the first edition of this text appeared. It has been slightly revised, with each new edition of the text based on the work of Goldstein and Stephens (1981) and trends in audiology, and in its current form is in harmony with the statement on AR competencies from the ASHA Committee on Rehabilitative Audiology (ASHA, 1984). The model is intended to encompass all types and degrees of hearing impairment as well as all age groups.

Entry and discharge are considered peripheral to the central aspects of the model. The model consists of two major components: assessment and management. Each component has four divisions and associated subsections. The model is shown in Table 1.4.

Rehabilitation Assessment Procedures. Following the initial auditory diagnostic tests that indicate the need for audiologic rehabilitation, it is necessary to perform more in-depth workups to determine the feasibility of various forms of audiologic rehabilitation. These assessment procedures should focus on Communication status, Associated variables, Related conditions, and Attitude (which are collectively abbreviated as CARA).

COMMUNICATION STATUS. Within the area of communication status, both traditional audiometric tests and questionnaires may be used to assess auditory abilities and self-reported consequences of hearing loss. Visual abilities assessment should include a simple screening and measurement of speechreading abilities. Any evaluation of communication must also consider language, since it is at the heart of verbal communication. If the patient understands a manual/gesture system, this needs to be evaluated as does any prior treatment. Included in *overall communication* are combined sensory abilities, such as audiovisual and tactile-kinesthetic capacities. Expressive and receptive communication skills should both be considered.

ASSOCIATED VARIABLES. Included in this area are secondary consequences of hearing loss including psychological, sociological, vocational, and educational factors. Personality and intelligence are major psychological factors, along with motivation, emotional stability, conformity, and assertiveness. Sociological factors such as family and significant others, social class, and lifestyle are also relevant according to the Goldstein and Stephens model. The vocational domain includes position, responsibility, and competence. In addition, the patient's level and form of education must be considered.

RELATED CONDITIONS. In this area, physical conditions like visual acuity and physical mobility are evaluated, along with upper-limb movement, sensation, and control, due to their bearing on hearing-aid use. In addition, symptoms of tinnitus, vertigo, pres-

TABLE 1.4 *Audiologic Rehabilitation Model Used in This Text*

		(Enter through Diagnostic-Identification Process)	
Assessment (CARA)	Communication Status	(I-A, B)	Auditory Visual Language Manual Communication Strategies Previous Rehabilitation Overall
	Associated Variables	(II-B)	Psychological Sociological Vocational Educational
	Related Conditions		Mobility Upper Limb Audiologic Pathology
	Attitude	(II-D)	Type I Type II Type III Type IV
Management (PACO)	Psychosocial/Counseling	(II-A, B, D)	Interpretation Information Counseling/Guidance Acceptance Understanding Expectation

	Amplification (Instrumental)	(I-C)	Hearing Aid Fitting
			Cochlear Implants
			Assistive Devices
			    Assistive Listening
			    Alerting/Warning
			    Tactile
			    Communication
			Instruction/Orientation

	Communication Training	(II-B, C; III-A, V)	Goals Philosophy Tactics Skill Building
	Overall Coordination (Ancillary)	(II-B, C, E; III-C, IV)	Vocational Educational Social Work Medicine
		(Discharge)	

Note: This model is consistent with the Goldstein/Stephens (1981) model and the ASHA position statement on definitions and competencies in Audiologic rehabilitation (ASHA, 1984). The numbers and letters in parentheses refer to the ASHA statement related to the procedures listed.

sure, and otitis media should be considered. Finally, the acoustic environmental conditions confronted by the hearing-impaired person should be evaluated.

ATTITUDE. The person's attitude is considered a crucial aspect of rehabilitation. Goldstein and Stephens (1981) suggested that rehabilitation candidates can be categorized into four types according to attitude. Type I candidates have a strongly positive attitude toward management and are thought to comprise ⅔ or ¾ of all patients. Most of the remaining candidates fit into Type II: Their expectations are essentially positive, but slight complications are present such as hearing loss that is difficult to fit with amplification. Persons with Type III attitudes are negative about rehabilitation, but show some willingness to cooperate, while those in Type IV reject hearing aids and the rehabilitation process altogether. In the latter two categories management cannot proceed in the usual fashion until some modification of attitude is achieved. For these reasons, we consider it important to evaluate attitude prior to rehabilitation; However, Goldstein and Stephens include it as the first phase in the management process.

Management Procedures. Once a thorough, rehabilitation-oriented assessment has been completed, management efforts should be initiated. These may take the form of short- or long-term therapy, and may involve individual or group sessions. The four aspects of management included here are those detailed in the previous edition of this book. They are also prominently featured in the Goldstein/Stephens model as well as in the ASHA position statement (ASHA, 1984). These include (a) Psychosocial and counseling aspects, (b) Amplification aspects, (c) Communication management, and (d) Overall coordinative functions (abbreviated as PACO).

Though all four management components are listed sequentially, they may occur simultaneously or in a duplicative and interactive fashion. For example, information about communication is generally introduced early in the counseling phase. However, additional information on how we hear, basics of speech acoustics, visible dimensions of speech, and how to maximize the use of conversational cues may be further emphasized in the communication training phase.

PSYCHOSOCIAL/COUNSELING. Psychosocial/counseling includes interpretation of audiologic findings to the client and other significant persons. In addition, pertinent information, counseling, and guidance are needed to help these individuals understand the educational, vocational, psychosocial, and communicative effects of hearing impairment. Considerable understanding and support are necessary in dealing with children who are deaf and hard of hearing, their parents, adults of all ages with hearing impairment, and their families. It is hoped that this process will bring acceptance and understanding of the conditions along with appropriate expectations for management. It is at this stage that good-attitude—Type I and II patients can be moved into amplification, whereas clients with poor attitudes (Types III and IV), if not modified toward acceptance and understanding, can be given ideas for modifying communicative behavior, attitudes, and strategies rather than being confronted with amplification fitting which they may resist.

AMPLIFICATION/ASSISTIVE DEVICES. *Amplification fitting.* This phase is sometimes referred to as *hearing-aid evaluation*, but it needs to be broader in scope. Here we must consider all forms of amplification, not just hearing aids. For example, cochlear implants, signal warning devices, and other assistive devices like telephone amplifiers should be considered in this phase. In many cases, accurate fitting of these devices will go a considerable way toward resolution of the hearing problem. In most cases, the fitting of hearing devices should be followed by adjustment, modification, and alteration of the basic controls and coupler arrangement until satisfactory amplification is achieved. Effort should be made to insure that no other amplification arrangements are substantially superior to the ones being used. (This is called *instrumental II* by Goldstein and Stephens.)

Amplification orientation. Individuals need to learn about the purpose, function, and maintenance of hearing aids and other assistive devices used by themselves or their child or other family member to avoid misunderstanding and misuse. Amplification units are relatively complex and this instruction must be given more emphasis than a 5-minute explanation or a pamphlet. (This is referred to as *instruction* by Goldstein and Stephens.)

COMMUNICATION TRAINING. As previously indicated, the major impact of hearing loss lies in the area of communication. Communication deficits often manifest themselves in educational difficulties for children and in vocational difficulties for adults. While, in most cases, amplification is considered the most important tool in combating this problem, communication training and related strategies still remain central to audiologic rehabilitation.

The first phase here consists of joint planning, with the client developing overall plans, goals, and tactics that suit the patient's lifestyle, philosophy, and attitudes. An "expert-dictated" medical model, wherein the client's desires and feelings are ignored, should be avoided. As Goldstein and Stephens suggested (1981), assertiveness may be a good tactic for overcoming hearing impairment unless it is contrary to the patient's personality. With children the educational philosophy carefully selected in family-centered therapy will help dictate the methods and tactics used.

Skill building involves helping the patient acquire skills that facilitate effective communication. Speechreading and improvement of auditory listening strategies are included here as are related speech- and language-rehabilitation efforts. Specific communication difficulties are identified in this phase of therapy, and then through assertiveness training and incorporation of anticipatory and repair strategies clients may learn to cope better with these problems.

OVERALL COORDINATION: REFERRAL AND ASSESSMENT (ANCILLARY). This refers to referral and coordination rather than direct service. While referrals in all areas are not always necessary, they should be considered. Liaison among client, family, and other agencies is included as are reassessment and modification of the intervention program.

Coordination and teamwork are a useful concept in audiologic rehabilitation. Particularly in the case of the hearing-impaired youngster, many persons may work with or need to work with the child. The parents should be at the center of the rehabilitative process. Also, physicians, social workers, hearing-aid dispensers, teachers, school psychologists, and other school personnel need to be coordinated to assist the child and family. For adults, much depends on the particular setting in which the rehabilitation occurs. Sometimes physicians, psychologists or social workers function in the same clinical setting. In these cases, involvement of another professional may occur naturally and easily. In other situations, the AR therapist can make referrals, when indicated, and encourage the adult to follow up. Sometimes persons are resistant to obtaining medical care or seeing a rehabilitation counselor. Often, parents or adults resist social services, psychiatric assistance, or hearing-aid devices. When a client refuses to accept advice, the audiologist must provide whatever insight and help possible, based on the audiologist's background and training, but must respect the rights of the client or the parents. Nevertheless, the audiologic rehabilitation process demands that referrals be made when indicated, and overall coordination and assessment of progress are important dimensions which should not be neglected.

Additional clarification and details on this AR model can be found in Goldstein and Stephens (1981).

Settings For Audiologic Rehabilitation

Audiologic rehabilitation may be conducted in a variety of settings with children, adults, or the elderly who are either deaf or hard of hearing. A review of these settings may help to demonstrate the many applications of AR (see Table 1.5).

Children. Very young children with hearing impairment and their parents may be recipients of early intervention efforts through home visits or clinic programs. Parent groups are also an important rehabilitation option. As children enter preschool and other school settings, audiologic rehabilitation takes on a supportive, coordinative function with teachers of youngsters with impaired hearing managing the classroom learning. Specifically, children in resource rooms, in residential deaf school classrooms, and in regular classrooms can be helped with amplification (both group and individual), communication therapy, and academic subjects. Important help and insights can also be given to the child's parents and teachers, and other professionals may be involved as needed. Hearing-conservation follow-up for youngsters who fail traditional school screenings represents another type of rehabilitative work carried out with children.

Adults. Adult AR services are needed for individuals with long-standing hearing loss as well as for persons who acquire loss during adulthood. Such traumatic or progressive hearing disorders may be brought on by accident, heredity, disease, or noise.

Adults may be served in university or technical school settings, through vocational rehabilitation programs, in military-related facilities, in the office of an ear specialist, or in the private practice of an audiologist. In addition, many adults are served in community, hospital, or university hearing clinics or through hearing-aid dealers/dispensers. A variety of rehabilitative services may be provided in all of these settings.

TABLE 1.5 *Summary of Audiologic Rehabilitation Settings for Children, Adults, and Elderly Persons*

Children	Adults	Elderly Adult
Early Intervention	University and Technical Schools	(Most settings listed under Adults)
Pre-school	Vocational Rehabilitation	Community Programs
Parent Groups	Military-Related Facilities	Nursing Homes/Long-Term Care Facilities
Regular Classrooms	ENT Clinic-Private Practice	
School Conservation Program Followup	Community, Hospital, and University Hearing Clinics	
School Resource Rooms	Hearing Aid Specialists/Dispensers	
Residential School Classrooms		

Adult Elderly. The vast majority of elderly clients are served through the conventional programs previously described for adults. A substantial proportion of clients seen in these settings for hearing-aid evaluations and related services are 65 years of age or older.

The full array of hearing-aid and communication rehabilitation services may be provided for the elderly in these clinics, including hearing-aid evaluation, orientation, and group and individual therapy. Aside from conventional clinical service, rehabilitation may be provided to the elderly in community screening and rehabilitation programs in well-elderly clinics, retirement apartment houses, senior citizen centers, churches, and a variety of other places where senior citizens congregate. Nursing homes or long-term care facilities also provide opportunities for audiologic rehabilitation since so many residents in these settings have substantial hearing loss and are required to have hearing screening under Medicare law (Bebout, 1991). Nevertheless, rehabilitation personnel should be realistic and anticipate less than 100% success with the elderly who are residents in health care facilities (Schow, 1992). Audiologic rehabilitation will be better accepted if it can be applied before persons enter such a facility.

SUMMARY

Audiologic habilitation/rehabilitation involves a variety of assessment and management efforts for the person who is deaf or hard of hearing, coordinated by a professional with audiologic training. Audiology's commitment to this endeavor has waxed and waned during the past 50 years, but recently a resurgence of interest has been spurred by a variety of factors.

A model of rehabilitation has been presented here to provide a framework for assessment and management procedures in audiologic rehabilitation. Professionals who intend to engage in AR must be familiar with the ramifications of hearing loss if they are to perform effective rehabilitation assessments. They also need to be aware of AR management procedures rendered through amplification, communication rehabilitation, counseling, and other ancillary services such as the educational alternatives available for the hearing impaired. The ASHA position statement on audiologic rehabilitation lists a number of minimal competencies required by those involved (ASHA, 1984; see Chapter 13). Consistent with this model and ASHA & AAA guidelines, the present text is designed to introduce basic information pertaining to amplification (Chapter 2), communication (Chapters 3, 4, 5), psychosocial aspects (Chapter 6), and educational alternatives (Chapter 7). These chapters are followed by a thorough discussion of audiologic rehabilitation for children (Chapter 8), adults (Chapter 9), and the elderly (Chapter 10). The next two chapters (11, 12) contain case examples, while Chapter 13 includes resource options to assist readers as they carry out their efforts in AR.

RECOMMENDED READINGS

Alpiner, J. G., & McCarthy, P. A. (1993). *Rehabilitative audiology: Children and adults* (2nd ed.). Baltimore: Williams & Wilkins.

Berg, F. S., Blair, I. C., Viehweg, S. H., & Wilson-Vlotman, A. (1986). *Educational audiology for the hard of hearing child.* New York: Grune and Stratton.

Katz, J. (Ed.). (1994). *Handbook of clinical audiology* (4th ed., pp. 587–801). Baltimore: Williams & Wilkins.

Ripich, D. (Ed.). (1991). *Handbook of geriatric communication disorders.* Austin, TX: Pro Ed.

Ross, M., Brackett, D., & Maxon, A. B. (1991). *Assessment and management of mainstreamed hearing-impaired children: Principles and practices.* Austin, TX: Pro-Ed.

Spitzer, J. B., Leder, S. B, & Giolas, T. G. (1993). *Rehabilitation of late-deafened adults.* St. Louis: Mosby.

Tyler, R. (1992) *Cochlear implants: Audiologic foundations.* San Diego: Singular Publishing Group.

REFERENCES

Alpiner, J. G. (1971). Planning a strategy of aural rehabilitation for the adult. *Hearing and Speech News, 39,* 21–26.

Alpiner, J. G. (1973). The hearing aid in rehabilitation planning for adults. *Journal of the Academy of Rehabilitative Audiology, 6,* 55–57.

American Academy of Audiology (AAA). (1988). Early identification of hearing loss in infants and children. *Audiology Today. 2,* 8–9.

American Academy of Audiology (AAA). (1993). Audiology: Scope of practice. *Audiology Today, 5*(1).

American Academy of Ophthalmology and Otolaryngology (AAOO). (1965). *Guide for the classification and evaluation of hearing handicap.* Committee on Conservation for Hearing. Transact, *AAOO, 69,* 740–751.

American Annals of the Deaf. (1994). Annual survey of hearing-impaired children and youth. *American Annals of the Deaf, 139*(2), 239–243.

Americans with Disabilities Act of 1990 (Public Law 101-336), 42 USC Sec. 12101.

ASHA-American Speech and Hearing Association. (1967). A conference on hearing aid evaluation procedures. *Asha, 7*(2), 57–66.

ASHA-American Speech and Hearing Association. (1972). Comprehensive audiologic services for the public. *Asha, 14,* 204–206.

ASHA-American Speech and Hearing Association. (1974). The audiologist: Responsibilities in the habilitation of the auditorily handicapped. *Asha, 16,* 68–70.

ASHA-American Speech and Hearing Association. (1978). Board moves to change dispensing rules. *Asha, 20,* 491–493.

ASHA-American Speech-Language-Hearing Association. (1979). Legislative council changes ASHA's name, ratifies ERA motion, adopts code changes. *Asha, 21,* 33–35.

ASHA-American Speech-Language-Hearing Association. (1981). On the definition of hearing handicap: A report of the American Speech-Language-Hearing Association task force. *Asha, 23,* 293–297.

ASHA-American Speech-Language-Hearing Association. (1984). Definition of and competencies for aural rehabilitation. A report from the committee on rehabilitative audiology. *Asha, 26,* 37–41.

ASHA-American Speech-Language-Hearing Association. (1985). Guidelines for identification audiometry. *Asha, 27,* 49–52.

ASHA-American Speech-Language-Hearing Association. (1991). Results of 1989 ASHA audiology opinion survey. *Asha, 33*(1), 9–11.

ASHA-American Speech-Language-Hearing Association. (1992). Spotlight on special interest division 7: Audiologic Rehabilitation. *Asha, 34,* 18.

Bebout, J. M. ((1991). Long term care facilities: A new window of opportunity opens for hearing health care services. *Hearing Journal, 44*(11), 11–17.

Berger, K. W. (1972). *Speechreading: Principles and methods.* Baltimore: National Educational Press, Inc.

Berger, K. W. (1988). History and development of hearing aids. In M. C. Pollack (Ed.), *Amplification for the hearing-impaired* (3rd ed., pp. 1–20). New York: Grune & Stratton.

Bess, F. H. (1977). Condition of hearing aids worn by children in a public school setting. In *The condition of hearing aids worn by children in a public school program.* DHEW Publication N. (OE) 7705002. Washington, DC: U.S. Printing Office.

Bess, F. H. (1986). Unilateral sensorineural hearing loss in children. Special issue. *Ear and Hearing, 7*(1), 3–54.

Blair, J. C., Peterson, M., & Viehweg, S. H. (1985). The effects of mild hearing loss on academic performance among school-age children. *The Volta Review, 87,* 87–94.

Carhart, R. (1946). Selection of hearing aids. *Archives of Otolaryngology, 44,* 10–18.

Chermak G. & Peters-McCarthy, E. (1991). The effectiveness of an educational hearing conservation program for elementary school children. *Language, Speech, and Hearing Services in Schools, 22,* 308-312.

Clark, T. C., Watkins, S., Reese, R., & Berg, F. (1975). *A state-wide program for identification and language facilitation for hearing handicapped children through home management.* Unpublished progress performance report for Handicapped Children's Early Education Program. Washington, DC: DHEW Office of Education, Bureau of Education for the Handicapped.

Cunningham, G. C. (1971). *Conference on newborn hearing screening.* Berkeley: California Department of Public Health. Rockville, MD: Public Health Service, DHEW.

Davis, A. (1994). *Public health perspectives in audiology.* 22nd International Congress of Audiology. Halifax, NS, Canada.

Department of Health Education and Welfare (DHEW). (1975). *Final report to the secretary on hearing aid health care.* Springfield, VA: U.S. Department of Commerce.

Department of Labor (1971). *Interviewing guides.* Washington, DC: Department of Labor.

Downs, M. P., & Sterrit, G. M. (1964). Identification audiometry for neonates: A preliminary report. *Journal of Auditory Research, 4,* 69-80.

Elfenbein, J. L., Bentler, R. A., Davis, J. M., and Nielbuhr, D. P. (1988). Status of school children's hearing aids relative to monitoring practices. *Ear and Hearing, 9,* 212-217.

Erdman, S. A. (1994). Self-Assessment: From research focus to research tool [Monograph]. In J. P. Gagne and N. Tye-Murray (Eds.) *Research in Audiological Rehabilitation.* Journal Academy of Rehabilitative Audiology.

Fleming, M. (1972). A total approach to communication therapy. *Journal of the Academy of Rehabilitative Audiology, 5,* 28-31.

Flexer, C. (1992). FM classroom public address systems. In M. Ross (Ed.), *FM auditory training systems: Characteristics, selection and use.* Parkton, MD: York Press.

Giolas, T. G. (1982). *Hearing-handicapped adults.* Englewood Cliffs, NJ: Prentice Hall, Inc.

Glorig, A., & Roberts, J. (1965). *Hearing level of adults by age and sex: United States* (1960-62). National Center for Health Statistics, Series 11, No. 11. Washington, DC: U.S. Department of Health, Education and Welfare.

Goldstein, D. P. (1984). Hearing impairment, hearing aids, and audiology. *Asha, 25*(9), 24-38.

Goldstein, D. P., & Stephens, S. D. G, (1981). Audiological rehabilitation: Management Model I. *Audiology, 20,* 432-452,

Hardick, E. G. (1977). Audiologic rehabilitational programs for the aged can be successful. *Journal of the Academy of Rehabilitative Audiology, 10,* 51-66.

Holm, V. A., & Kunze, L. H. (1969). Effect of chronic otitis media on language and speech development. *Pediatrics, 43,* 833-839.

Horton, K. B. (1972). Early amplification and language learning—Or sounds should be heard and not seen. *Journal of the Academy of Rehabilitative Audiology*, *5*, 15–23.

John Tracy Clinic Correspondence (1983). *For parents of young deaf children. Parts A and B.* John Tracy Clinic, 806 West Adams Blvd. Los Angeles, CA 90007.

Kochkin, S. (1991). MarkeTrak II: More MD's give hearing tests, yet hearing aid sales remain flat. *The Hearing Journal*, *44*(2), 24–35.

Kodman, F., Jr. (1963). Educational status of hard-of-hearing children in the classroom. *Journal of Speech and Hearing Disorders*, *28*, 297–299.

Ling, D. (1972). Rehabilitation of cases with deafness secondary to otitis media. In A. Glorig & K. S. Gerwin (Eds.), *Otitis media* (pp. 249-253). Springfield, IL: Charles C. Thomas Publisher.

Lundeen, C. (1991). Prevalence of hearing impairment among school children. *Language, Speech and Hearing Services in Schools*, *22*, 269–271.

Marge, M. (1977). The current status of service delivery systems for the hearing impaired. *Asha*, *19*, 403–409.

Matkin, N. D. (1984). Wearable amplification. A litany of persisting problems. In J. Jerger (Ed.), *Pediatric audiology: Current trends* (pp. 125-145). San Diego, CA: College Hill Press.

Mencher, G. T. (1974). Infant hearing screening: The state of the art. *Malco Audiological Library Series*, *12*, 7.

Moores, D. (1996). *Educating the deaf—psychology, principles, practices* (4th ed.). Boston: Houghton Mifflin.

Mussen, E. F. (1977). Problems of rehabilitative audiology in the retirement community setting. *Journal of the Academy of Rehabilitative Audiology*, *10*, 68–70.

Northcott, W. H. (Ed.). (1972). *Curriculum guide: Hearing impaired children–birth to three years—and their parents.* Washington, DC: Alexander Graham Bell Association for the Deaf.

Northern, J. L., Ciliax, D. R., Roth, D., & Johnson, R. (1969). Military patient attitudes toward audiologic rehabilitation. *Asha*, *11*, 391–395.

Oyer, H. J. (1983). Founding philosophy of the Academy of Rehabilitative Audiology. *Journal of Academy of Rehabilitative Audiology*, *16*, 9–11.

Quigley, S. F. (1970). *Some effects of impairment upon school performance.* Manuscript prepared for the Division of Special Education Services. Springfield, IL: Office of the Superintendent of Public Instruction for the State of Illinois.

Ramsdell, D. (1978). The psychology of the hard-of-hearing and the deafened adult. In H. Davis & R. Silverman (Eds.), *Hearing and deafness* (4th ed., pp. 499–510). New York: Holt, Rinehart & Winston.

Ries, P. W. (1994). *Prevalence and characteristics of persons with hearing trouble: United States.* National Center for Health Statistics, *Vital Stat*, *24*, 188.

Roeser, R. (1988). Audiometric and immittance measures: Principles and interpretation. In R. Roeser and M. Downs (Eds.) *Auditory disorders in school children* (2nd ed.) New York: Thieme.

Schein, J., & Delk, M. (1974). *The deaf population of the United States.* Silver Spring, MD: National Association of the Deaf.

Schow, R. L. (1992). Hearing assessment and treatment in nursing homes. *Hearing Instruments, 43*(7), 7-11.

Schow, R. L. & Smedley, T. C. (1990). (*Special Issue) Self assessment of hearing. Ear and Hearing, 11*(5) (Suppl.), 1-65.

Schow, R. L., Maxwell, S., Crookston, G., & Newman, M. (1993a). How well do adults take care of their hearing instruments? *Hearing Instruments, 44*(3), 16-20.

Schow, R. L., Balsara, N. R., Smedley, T. C., & Whitcomb, C. J. (1993b). Aural rehabilitation by ASHA audiologists: 1980-1990. *American Journal of Audiology, 2*(3), 28-37.

Schow, R. L., Mercaldo, D., & Smedley, T. C. (1994). *The Idaho hearing survey.* Pocatello, ID: Idaho State University Press.

Shepherd, N., Davis, J., Gorga, M., & Stelmachowics, P. (1981). Characteristics of hearing impaired children in the public schools: Part I—Demographic data. *Journal of Speech and Hearing Disorders, 46*, 123-129.

Smedley, T. C., & Plapinger, D. (1988). The non-functioning hearing aid: A case of double jeopardy. *Volta Review, 90*, 77-88.

Smith, M. The role of age and ageism in the "80% barrier." *Asha, 33*(11), 36-37.

Strom, K. (1994). Review of the 1993 hearing instruments market. *The Hearing Review, 1*(3), 6-8.

Tannahill, J. C. (1973). Hearing aids: Trial and adjustment by new users. *Audecibel, 22*, 90-97.

Vernon, M. (1968). Fifty years of research on the intelligence of the deaf and hard-of-hearing. A survey of literature and discussion of implications. *Journal of Rehabilitation of the Deaf, 1*, 1-11.

Vernon, M. (1985). The relationship of language and thought, bilingualism and critical stage theory to reading. In M. Douglass (Ed.), Proceedings of Claremont reading conference, *985* (pp. 21-30). Claremont, CA: Claremont Graduate School.

Vernon, M., & Andrews, J. (1990). *The psychology of deafness.* White Plains, NY: Longman Press.

WHO (1980). *International classification of impairments, disabilities and handicaps: A manual of classification relating to the consequences of disease.* Geneva: World Health Organization.

2

Amplification/Assistive Devices for the Deaf and Hard of Hearing

H. GUSTAV MUELLER
ANNE L. STROUSE

Contents

INTRODUCTION

In nearly all cases, audiologic rehabilitation involves working with individuals who can benefit from the use of hearing aids or other assistive listening devices. While all forms of auditory rehabilitation are important, reliance on visual and situational cues is inversely related to the quality of the hearing aid fitting. A critical first step for most patients, therefore, is to provide amplification that, whenever possible, makes soft speech audible, average speech comfortable, and loud speech and environmental sounds tolerable, without introducing distortion. This might sound like a fairly simple philosophy, and it is. Unfortunately, hearing aids are sometimes fitted in a haphazard manner, without careful consideration of these underlying principles. Getting the right hearing aids on a patient, and adjusting them precisely for that patient's listening needs, can facilitate significantly many of the other aspects of auditory rehabilitation.

Fifteen or twenty years ago many master's degree training programs in audiology lumped the study of hearing aids together with speech audiometry (and other assorted topics) to create a single three–credit-hour course. Today, at many universities, two or more courses are devoted solely to the selection and fitting of hearing aids. Why the change? Hearing-aid fitting has become increasingly complex, and dispensing hearing aids has become an integral part of the scope of practice of audiology. To do it right, extensive training is necessary.

In recent years, several factors have had a significant impact on the way we select and fit hearing aids, which indirectly has influenced the amount of training required for proficiency. As you are reading this chapter, it is important to keep these issues in mind, as they are shaping the way hearing aids are currently being fit. The following, adapted from Mueller and Grimes (1993), is a summary of some of the major factors:

- *Advanced circuit design.* Each year, new hearing-aid circuits are introduced that provide a variety of new signal processing formulas. It is the audiologist's responsibility to determine if these circuits are beneficial, and which type are best for what patient.
- *Programmable hearing aids.* An increasing number of hearing aids available from different manufacturers are programmable either by a dedicated system or through the use of a personal computer. The more sophisticated programmable hearing aids have two or three channels, multiple memories, and compression and frequency adjustments that allow for as many as 15,000 to 20,000 different fitting options. How do we select the correct program during the time frame of a routine hearing aid fitting?
- *Probe-microphone measurements.* The ability to measure reliably the output of hearing aids at the patient's tympanic membrane allows for the use of precise verification protocols. Additionally, the performance of many other hearing aid features can be evaluated and quantified. The equipment is available today that would allow us to do all our testing and fitting in ear canal SPL.
- *Computerization.* Hearing-aid specifications, prescriptive fitting methods, automated testing procedures, and hearing-aid selection formulas are now all

available from computer software. Combine this with programmable hearing aids and PC-based probe-microphone measurements, and the personal computer becomes the work station for audiometric testing, hearing-aid selection, adjustment, and fitting.

- *Miniaturization.* Hearing aids continue to be made smaller and placed deeper in the ear canal. Evaluation and fitting techniques need to be modified for these smaller instruments. This trend also encourages more individuals with mild hearing loss to use amplification.
- *Delivery system.* Twenty years ago it was considered unethical for audiologists to sell hearing aids for profit. Today, approximately half of all hearing aids are dispensed by audiologists, and this percentage increases annually.

In this chapter, we will cover a wide range of information about hearing aids, beginning with a simple description of how they work and how they are tested, and eventually leading to the latest details concerning automated fitting procedures and programmable instruments. We will also discuss some other important assistive listening and rehabilitative devices that can be used as an alternative to hearing aids.

HEARING AIDS

A successful hearing-aid fitting, which should lead to a happy hearing aid user, is dependent upon the audiologist's understanding of hearing aid technology, and how to apply this technology to different types of hearing losses and loudness growth functions. Some say that hearing aid fitting is both a science and an art.

To get things started, the following is a simplified description of what makes a hearing aid work. Later in this chapter we'll provide a more detailed description of some of these components.

Basic Components

The purpose of a hearing aid is to amplify, or make sounds louder. You don't have to be an electrical engineer to understand how a hearing aid works. There are certain basic components, common to all types of hearing aids (see block diagram in Figure 2.1). Here's a step-by-step walk-through of how things work:

1. Sound waves enter the hearing aid through the *microphone*.
2. The *microphone* converts the sound waves into an electrical signal.
3. The *amplifier* increases the strength of the electrical signal.
4. A smaller loudspeaker called a *receiver* functions to convert the amplified signals back into sound waves.
5. The amplified sound is channeled from the *receiver* directly to the ear canal. For hearing aids that fit behind the ear, the receiver sends the amplified sound into a clear plastic tube attached to a custom-made earmold. For

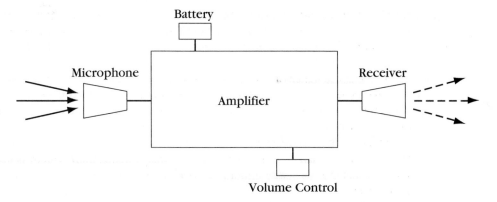

Figure 2.1 Basic components of a hearing aid.

From M. Pollack (1988). Electroacoustic characteristics. In M. Pollack (Ed.), *Amplification for the Hearing Impaired* (3rd ed.). Orlando, FL: Grune & Stratton.

those hearing aids that fit into the ear, the amplified sound is channeled into the ear canal by a small piece of tubing within the instrument.

6. The *battery* provides electrical energy to power the hearing aid and enable the amplification process to occur.

Pretty simple, isn't it? But that's just the start. As we go on you will see that there are variations of each one of these basic components. It is these variations, along with other controls and features, that allow us to customize each hearing aid for the individual patient.

Controls and Features

In addition to the basic components that we've just discussed, many hearing aids include additional controls or circuits. The following is a listing of the most common of these features:

1. *On-Off Switch*   Allows the user to turn the hearing aid off when not in use. In some hearing aids, this switch also activates the telecoil (see below). Generally, the "M" position indicates that the microphone is on, "O" turns the aid off, and "T" (if present) activates the telecoil. For custom instruments, the on-off switch (if present) usually is part of the volume control wheel.

2. *Telecoil*   A special circuit designed to enhance use of the hearing aid with the telephone. A telecoil switch may be incorporated into a toggle on-off switch, or exist as a separate control. Electromagnetic signals are picked up by the telecoil from the receiver of the telephone (leakage), amplified, and transduced to acoustic energy before entering the ear. Thus, the telecoil takes the place of the hearing-aid microphone as the input component of the hearing-aid system. While proven beneficial for many users, the telecoil shows substantial variability in performance within each indi-

vidual hearing aid, particularly custom instruments, due to size and placement restrictions, making it necessary to carefully evaluate performance characteristics of each device. Telecoils are not available on smaller custom hearing aids due to space limitations.

3. *Volume Control*   A rotating wheel that allows the user to select a preferred listening level for a specific listening situation. The volume control functions by adjusting the amount of amplification of the input signal. As mentioned earlier, in some smaller hearing aids, the volume control also acts as an on-off switch. For older individuals with poor dexterity, the volume control wheel can be raised for ease of use. For the very small completely-in-the-canal instruments, there usually is no volume control wheel due to space limitations. For these instruments, the volume is screwset by the audiologist.

4. *Tone Control*   A circuit designed to provide high- or low-frequency reduction, such as treble and bass adjustments on a stereo. Using a screwdriver-controlled potentiometer, or a digitally controlled programmable system, the audiologist can make an adjustment so that there is greater or lesser amplification in certain frequency regions. For example, a patient's hearing loss may involve only the frequencies above 2000 Hz. The hearing aid, by manipulation of the tone control, can be adjusted so that it will not amplify substantially any frequencies below 2000 Hz. Conversely, a patient with an upward-sloping hearing loss might need some reduction of amplification in the higher frequencies.

5. *Output Limiting*   All hearing aids use some form of output limiting. Output limiting potentiometers allow the audiologist to control the maximum output of the hearing aid; the purpose of this adjustment is to assure that loud sounds are not uncomfortably loud to the user. If a hearing aid is not limited using compression (see below), peak clipping is the method utilized.

In a *peak-clipping* linear system, increases in input level result in an equivalent increase in output. There is a limit, however, to the maximum output level that can be produced. When this point is reached, the output will not increase with further increases in input level, the system is forced into non-linearity when peak-clipping occurs, and the hearing aid is said to be in saturation. As the name implies, peaks of the signal which exceed a given voltage within the circuit are "clipped off." Thus, hearing-aid output is limited by means of distorting the signal and can result in poor sound quality and lack of clarity; hence, it is nearly always wise to use hearing aids that employ some type of compression. As with peak clipping hearing aids, the audiologist adjusts the maximum output for compression instruments as well, so that it does not exceed the patient's loudness discomfort level (LDL) (LDL measurements will be discussed in a later section).

Given that most individuals fitted with hearing aids have a nonlinear hearing loss, and need the output of the hearing aid limited with minimal distortion, some form of *compression* is usually an appropriate feature. Compression circuits limit the maximum output that the hearing aid can deliver by automatically reducing the amplification of sounds that reach a preselected level. Compression can be *input*- or *output*-controlled (see comparative block diagrams in Figure 2.2). If compression is input-controlled, monitoring of the signal level takes place

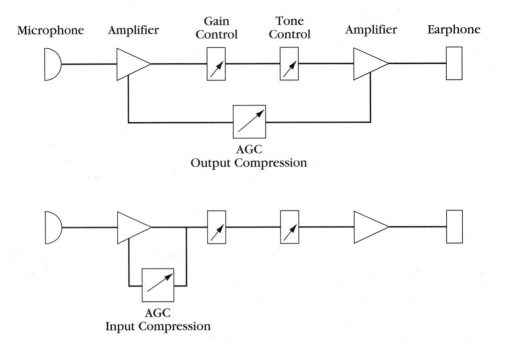

Figure 2.2 Block diagram of output compression hearing aid and input compression hearing aid.

From W. Olsen (1986). Physical characteristics of hearing aids. In W. Hodgson (Ed.), *Hearing Aid Assessment and Use in Audiologic Habilitation* (3rd ed.). Baltimore: Williams & Wilkins.

before the volume control. In this case, volume control adjustments do affect output levels and the user has direct control over maximum output levels. If compression is output-controlled, monitoring of the signal level occurs *after* the volume control. Thus, changes in the position of the volume control will not affect maximum output of the hearing aid and the audiologist has direct control of output levels. For both types of compression, however, precise adjustments of compression parameters can be made by the audiologist at the time of the fitting to tailor the compression activation to the loudness growth function of the individual patient.

As we stated earlier, all types of hearing aids include the microphone, amplifier, receiver, and power source. The additional controls and circuitry that we have discussed may or may not be a part of the hearing aid system. It should be noted that the basic features described thus far are not the only options available. We will consider more specialized features, including five different types of compression and digitally programmable instruments, later in this chapter.

Optional controls and circuitry must be selected depending on the needs of the user. As an example, for the patient who wants a very small hearing aid and seldom uses the telephone, it might not be necessary to include a telecoil in the hearing aid. Similarly, for a person being fitted with a hearing aid with no gain in the lower frequencies, a low-frequency tone control might not serve any meaningful purpose.

On smaller instruments it is not always possible to obtain several features because of space limitations. If a person needs several of the features we have discussed, there might need to be a trade-off: a larger instrument for more features. Thus, in selecting the appropriate device for a patient, we must consider the type of hearing loss, as well as the special needs of the user. This information will then guide the audiologist in choosing the most appropriate style of hearing aid, so we will consider that topic next.

Hearing-Aid Styles

There are currently six major styles of hearing aids available. These include: (1) body aid; (2) eyeglass aid; (3) behind-the-ear (BTE) aid; (4) in-the-ear (ITE) aid; (5) in-the-canal (ITC) aid; and (6) completely-in-the-canal (CIC) aid. (Examples for five of the different hearing aid styles are illustrated in Figure 2.3; Figure 2.4 shows the newest addition to the family, the CIC.)

Why so many choices? First, technological advances have resulted in the increased sophistication and miniaturization of hearing-aid components, which was not possible when the large body style aid was developed several decades ago. Market statistics show that smaller hearing aids become more popular each year. Second, a certain style of hearing aid may not be appropriate for the degree and configuration of the patient's hearing loss. Larger-style hearing aids are capable of providing a greater amount of amplification as compared to smaller devices. Third, as you will recall from the previous section, the need for additional controls and/or circuit types may influence the style of hearing aid selected. Before we go any further, let's take a look at each style individually, to give you a better idea of the need for different styles of hearing aids and reasons why each style may or may not be selected for a particular patient.

The Body Aid. Body style hearing aids have larger microphones, amplifiers, and power supplies enclosed in cases that can be carried in a pocket, attached to clothing, or placed on the body in a harness. The external receiver attaches directly to a custom earmold and is powered through a flexible wire from the amplifier. Although not as popular as other hearing aid styles because of their size and poor microphone placement (off-the-ear), body aids are very powerful and can be beneficial for those with very severe hearing losses. Due to the larger controls, they may also be indicated for small children or patients with dexterity problems. Because of the importance of placing the hearing aid microphone at the ear, and the importance of binaural amplification, body hearing aids usually are only used when behind- or in-the-ear models are not practical. Today, a popular alternative to a body hearing aid is some type of *assistive listening device*, which in many cases is simply a body hearing aid

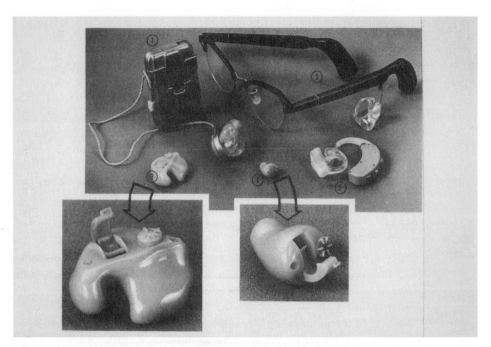

Figure 2.3 The different types of hearing aids. (1) body aid; (2) eyeglass; (3) in-the-ear; (4) in-the-canal; and (5) behind-the-ear.

From F. Bess and L. Hume (1995). *Audiology: The Fundamentals* (2nd ed.). Baltimore: Williams & Wilkins.

with a new name. We will discuss the different types and applications of assistive devices later in this chapter.

Who is a candidate for the body style hearing aid? We have already mentioned two or three examples. The following is a summary of reasons why the audiologist may or may not choose the body-style hearing aid for a particular patient.

Why?
- High levels of amplification are available without feedback as compared to ear-level hearing aids, since there is more distance between the microphone and receiver.
- Larger size controls and battery are easier to manipulate for small children or patients with dexterity problems.
- Due to its size, and possibility of secure placement, there may be less chance of loss or damage, particularly for small children.

Why Not?
- Binaural amplification is important; it is difficult to place two body aids on small children.

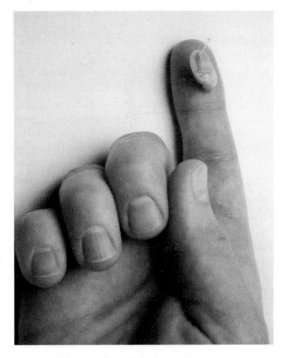

Figure 2.4 A completely-in-the-canal (CIC) hearing aid.
Courtesy of Siemens Hearing Instruments, Inc.

- There are acoustic advantages of having the microphone of hearing aids at ear level.
- Body aids are subject to clothing noise.
- The frequency response of a body aid is influenced by the baffle effect produced by the body, which reduces high-frequency amplification.
- Many special circuits are not available for this style.
- There is a lack of cosmetic appeal.

The Eyeglass Aid. Once someone thought that it would be a good idea to combine hearing aids and eyeglasses (since many people who need hearing aids already wear eyeglasses). While this style sounds logical, it is rarely selected today.

In the eyeglass-style hearing aid, the microphone, amplifier, and receiver are built into the temple portion of the eyeglass. Sound is channeled into the ear from the hearing aid through plastic tubing connected to a custom earmold. Eyeglass hearing aids can be fit monaurally or binaurally and can generally accommodate mild to moderately-severe hearing losses. Once occupying a 20% or more market share, the popularity of the eyeglass style hearing aid has dramatically decreased (less than .5% of 1994 total sales). Even if the user needs to wear glasses and a hearing aid, it is rather impractical to have these two sensory devices tied together. Let's look at some reasons why the audiologist may, or in most cases, will not, choose the eyeglass hearing aid:

Why?
- Some previous eyeglass–hearing-aid users might prefer to be fitted with the same style of hearing aid they have been using for the past 30 years.
- Some special applications of CROS and BICROS fittings (see following section) are easily accomplished using eyeglasses.

Why Not?
- They tend to be heavy, uncomfortable, and difficult to fit, adjust, and repair.
- Unless the user wears eyeglasses at all times, there is a loss of amplification every time the glasses are removed. A hearing-aid repair means loss of eyeglasses.
- It is difficult to find manufacturers who build and repair eyeglass hearing aids; because of limited demand, sophisticated circuitry is not available in this style.

The BTE. Behind-the-ear (BTE) hearing aids are housed in small curved cases which, as the name implies, fit behind the ear. The microphone, amplifier, and receiver are all housed in the hearing-aid case, connected to a custom earmold by a flexible plastic tube. This hearing-aid style can be worn monaurally or binaurally, and has about a 20% market share of total hearing-aid sales. BTE hearing aids usually are larger in size than the small in-the-ear custom instruments, and thus can accommodate a greater range of additional controls and circuitry. Figure 2.5 shows a modern BTE that is digitally programmable, and also has multiple memories (storage of different electroacoustic settings for different listening conditions). The button shown in the middle of the back of the instrument is for changing memories. The opening between the button and the volume control wheel is for the computer adapter for programming the settings. The screw driver adjustment (potentiometer) located between the button and the M-T-O toggle switch is for adjusting the maximum output.

Because of their flexibility, BTE aids can be used successfully by most hearing-aid users. Why aren't they? Let's discuss the "why's" and "why not's" of selecting a BTE model hearing aid:

Why?
- User can achieve greater gain and maximum output than with a custom instrument.
- Telecoil circuitry is more powerful than can be obtained with smaller custom instruments.
- For children with rapidly growing ears, only the earmold needs to be replaced when fitting becomes loose; with custom hearing aids the hearing aid needs to be re-cased.
- Direct audio input is available.

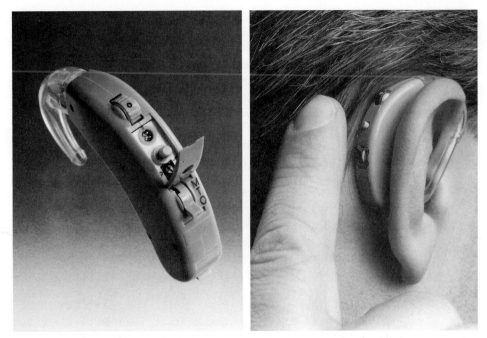

Figure 2.5 A digitally programmable behind-the-ear (BTE) hearing aid.
Courtesy of Siemens Hearing Instruments, Inc.

- There is increased flexibility and range of adjustment of features due to larger size casing.
- If there is a medical reason why the ear canal should not be occluded, BTE hearing aids can be fit with open earmolds.
- Digitally programmable circuitry is available to enhance flexibility.

Why Not?
- The smaller custom hearing aids are less noticeable.
- Some consumers consider BTE instruments to be "old fashioned".
- BTE hearing aids tend to be less secure than custom instruments (e.g., tend to fall off ear during strenuous work or recreation).
- More difficult to insert, remove, and adjust volume control than a custom instrument.

The ITE. In-the-ear (ITE) hearing aids fit directly in the external ear. The circuitry is housed primarily in the concha area, and thus this model has no external wires or tubes. Because of its larger size, as compared to the ITC or CIC discussed below, the ITE can accommodate additional controls and larger circuitry when indicated. The ITE is the most commonly dispensed hearing aid in the U.S., as its flexibility makes this style useful for all but the most severe cases of hearing loss. As discussed earlier, we'd probably fit these severely hearing-impaired patients with BTE hearing aids. Let's summarize additional reasons why we may or may not select the ITE style aid:

Why?
ADVANTAGES OF ITEs COMPARED TO BTEs:
- Considered more modern and cosmetically acceptable.
- Better microphone placement for obtaining high frequency gain.
- More secure fit.
- Easier to insert and remove, and to adjust volume control.

ADVANTAGES OF ITEs COMPARED TO ITCs:
- More gain and output can be attained.
- Telecoil and direct audio input are available.
- More sophisticated circuitry (e.g., multi-channel compression) and greater circuit flexibility are available.
- Volume control and battery are larger in size, and therefore easier to manipulate.
- ITEs are less expensive.

Why Not?
DISADVANTAGES OF ITEs COMPARED TO BTEs:
- For very severe losses, ITE hearing aids are more prone to feedback due to the closer proximity of the microphone and receiver.
- User might require the greater power of BTE telecoil.
- For younger children, rapidly changing size of ear might make use of custom instrument impractical.

DISADVANTAGE OF ITEs COMPARED TO ITCs:
- If all necessary features and functions can be placed in a more cosmetically acceptable hearing aid, then why not do it?

The ITC. In-the-canal (ITC) hearing aids are a variation of the ITE, only smaller in size. Importantly, this style of hearing aid is not really totally "in-the-canal," but is partially "in-the-concha." The ITC hearing aids, in contrast to the ITE style, occupy the ear canal but only part of the concha, leaving a portion free for natural resonance and diffraction effects. Because of its smaller size, the device may or may not have room for several controls or switches, depending on the size of the user's ear canal. ITC hearing aids can generally accommodate mild to moderate, and some severe hearing losses. The following summarizes reasons why we would or would not select the ITC style hearing aid for a particular patient.

Why?
- It is more cosmetically appealing than the ITE.
- A portion of the concha is left free, allowing for natural resonance and diffraction effects, resulting in an increase in high-frequency amplification.
- Users often experience less difficulty with feedback when using the telephone, compared to the larger ITE style.

- Users experience less wind noise due to a more deeply seated micro-phone.

Why Not?
- Instrument is unable to provide necessary gain and output.
- Telecoil is typically not available.
- Several types of sophisticated circuitry will not fit in a shell this small.
- Because of the smaller size, there often is not room for more than one screw-driver-controlled adjustment (potentiometer).
- Smaller battery size and volume control may be difficult for individuals with dexterity problems.
- If the patient's ear is very small, there might not be room to place the circu-ity in an ITC shell.
- It is more expensive than an ITE.

The CIC. Completely-in-the-canal (CIC) hearing aids are the smallest type of hearing aid available to date. In addition to the obvious cosmetic appeal, they offer many acoustic advantages (see Mueller, 1994 for review). As the name implies, these devices fit completely within the ear canal and thus are practically invisible when worn (see Figure 2.4). In general, these hearing aids also fit deeper in the ear canal than do the ITE or ITC styles. This hearing aid, however, is easily inserted if the ear canal is rela-tively straight. It is removed using a short transparent cord. Because of its small size, volume control wheels, tone controls, and other features are not an option on the CIC. CIC hearing aids generally are suitable for patients with mild to moderate hear-ing losses. The pros and cons of selecting the CIC style hearing aid are similar to those listed for ITC aids. Let's take a look.

Why?
- There is an obvious cosmetic advantage over other custom instruments.
- Deep microphone placement and reduced residual ear canal volume (deep-er fit) result in a significantly increased output, and in high-frequency ampli-fication.
- Deep fitting helps to reduce the occlusion effect (unnatural sound quality related to the ear being plugged).
- It is easy to insert and remove.
- There is a reduction in wind noise since the microphone is seated within the ear canal.
- Feedback problems are reduced, including during phone use.

Why Not?
- Enough gain cannot be achieved, especially when substantial low-frequency gain is necessary.
- Limited circuits and adjustments are available.
- Limited models are available in programmable versions.

- The small battery and hearing-aid size require reasonably good dexterity.
- The hearing aid cannot be built for some individuals because of the size or geography of the ear canal.
- It is more expensive than the ITC hearing aid.

Matching the right hearing aid style to the patient is an important first step in the hearing-aid fitting procedure, although it is not always easy. Sometimes a little trial and error must be applied. We listed several "whys" and "why nots" for the various devices, but we probably missed some. In most situations, one of these six styles will be fitted binaurally, or in some instances in a monaural arrangement. There will be, however, some cases in which more specialized types of hearing-aid fittings may be more appropriate.

SPECIALIZED FITTING OPTIONS

CROS/BICROS

For the individual with an unaidable hearing loss in one ear, and normal hearing or an aidable hearing loss in the other ear, Contralateral Routing of Signal (CROS) or Bilateral Contralateral Routing of Signal (BICROS) amplification may be the most appropriate hearing-aid arrangement. A CROS hearing aid is used when there is good hearing in one ear and the opposite ear cannot benefit from amplification. This device places a microphone on the side of the poor ear and its receiver directed to the normal ear, so the good ear can receive sound from the opposite side of the head. We have made the person a "two-sided" listener, but importantly, *not* a "two-eared" listener.

Somewhat different from the CROS fitting, BICROS hearing aids are used in cases where one ear is unaidable but there is some degree of aidable hearing loss in the other. This device has two microphones, one near the better ear and the other near the poorer ear. The acoustic signals from both sides are delivered to a single amplifier and receiver, and the output is then directed into the better ear.

There are two basic types of CROS or BICROS fittings:

- Hardwired

    ITE

    BTE

    Eyeglass

- Frequency-modulated (FM)

In the *hardwire* system, the signal is carried from one side of the head to the other by wires concealed within the eyeglass frame or by a tube or cord around the back of the neck as in the ITE and BTE styles. If an *FM system* is utilized, signals are transferred across the head by an FM transmitter and picked up by an FM receiver positioned near the better ear. The signal is then converted back to acoustic energy and presented to the better ear. A more detailed description of FM systems is provided later in this chapter when we discuss assistive listening devices.

Bone-Conduction Hearing Aids

In traditional bone-conduction devices, amplified sound is delivered through a vibrator placed behind the ear and over the mastoid bone. These devices are most commonly integrated into body- or eyeglass-style hearing aids. In the body aid, a vibrating device is held against the mastoid process by a metal headband. In the eyeglass hearing aid, the vibrator is mounted into the stem of the eyeglass that extends behind the ear. This type of hearing aid usually is selected when some type of middle-ear pathology prohibits the use of standard hearing aids.

Implantable bone-conduction devices are also available. As summarized by Hough, et al. (1986) the basic components include:

1. A microphone for receiving acoustic energy and converting it to electric energy.
2. A sound processor to energize the coil.
3. An external processor to energize the coil, magnetically held in place on the skin behind the ear adjacent to the internally implanted device.
4. A magnet-screw assembly implanted subcutaneously in the temporal bone.

When sound is picked up by the microphone and amplified, it is directed to the coil, which is attached to the magnetic implant in the mastoid. The magnetic forces from the coil set the implant into vibration. This action then sets the skull into vibration. Skull vibrations are transmitted to both cochleas. Once in place, the bone-anchored system works similarly to traditional bone-conduction devices.

Bone-conduction hearing aids are not widely used, but if the outer ear is not fully formed, if there is a severe ear infection with drainage problems, or if a surgical procedure prevents the use of a conventional instrument, bone-conduction hearing aids can be the most practical solution.

THE EARMOLD

Remember the description of the BTE hearing aid style? How is the signal delivered from the hearing aid to the ear canal? We've mentioned the term *earmold* numerous times, so now let's take a closer look at its characteristics. The earmold serves a variety of important functions. As you may recall, the earmold couples the hearing aid to the user's ear via a tube, as in the case of the BTE and eyeglass-style hearing aids (or a wire cord and external receiver, as in the body-style hearing aid). As such, the earmold provides support for the BTE hearing aid, and most importantly, directs and modifies the amplified sound that reaches the ear canal. For ITE, ITC and CIC instru-

BTE AND EYEGLASS

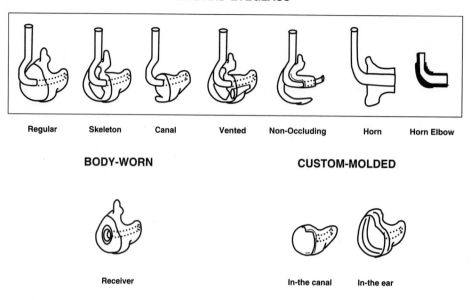

| Regular | Skeleton | Canal | Vented | Non-Occluding | Horn | Horn Elbow |

BODY-WORN   **CUSTOM-MOLDED**

Receiver   In-the canal   In-the ear

Figure 2.6 Basic types of earmolds.

From W. Staab & S. Lybarger (1994). Characteristics and use of hearing aids. In J. Katz (Ed.), *Handbook of Clinical Audiology* (4th ed.). Baltimore: Williams & Wilkins.

ments, the earmold is actually the shell of the hearing aid itself, where all of the components are housed.

As with custom hearing aids, custom earmolds come in various styles, ranging from large models which fill the entire concha of the outer ear, to models in which only a small piece of tubing extends into the ear canal. In general, the greater the hearing loss, the larger the earmold needed. Figure 2.6 shows samples of many of the available earmold styles.

Once the earmold is coupled to the hearing aid, the properties of the sound reaching the user's ear are changed. The acoustic properties of the earmold itself, and the length and diameter of the connecting tube, play an important part in the final acoustical characteristics of the hearing aid system.

Acoustic Effects of Earmolds

The most important characteristic of the earmold is that it can be modified to alter the amplified signal delivered to the user's ear. As we'll discuss later, it is important that the real-ear frequency response is tailored to each patient. By utilizing the fol-

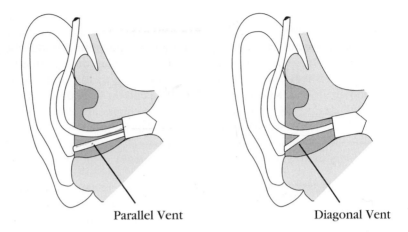

Parallel Vent   Diagonal Vent

Figure 2.7 Diagrams of parallel and diagonal vents.

From S. Lybarger (1985). Earmolds. In J. Katz (Ed.), *Handbook of Clinical Audiology* (3rd ed.). Baltimore, Williams & Wilkins.

lowing techniques, the audiologist can modify one or more portions of the frequency response of the hearing aid in order to deliver the acoustic signal more appropriately. While this section concerns earmolds, it is important to remember that many of the same damping and, in particular, venting principles and techniques applied to earmolds also can be used with custom hearing aids.

Low-Frequency Modification. THE VENT. The most common modification is called a *vent*, which is a small hole drilled into the canal portion of the earmold. The vent is usually parallel to the sound bore, although in some instances a diagonal vent is used (see Figure 2.7 for examples of the two different types of earmold vents). Earmolds (and custom hearing aids) are vented for three primary reasons:

- To allow unwanted amplified low frequencies to escape from the ear canal.
- To release pressure, preventing a "plugged ear" sensation.
- To allow the normal input of unamplified sound.

Vents can be drilled to various diameters, depending on the results desired. The diameter of an earmold vent may vary from a small pressure equalization vent to an "open earmold" where the vent has been enlarged until nothing remains of the earmold but its outermost portion. In general, the larger the vent, the greater the low-frequency attenuation. Variable vents are also available. These use small plastic plugs or different sizes of tubing that can totally occlude an existing vent or provide smaller openings of various diameters.

Mid-Frequency Modification. THE DAMPER. Acoustic dampers are placed within the tubing or earhook of BTE style hearing aids and in the receiver tubing of custom instruments. They are small inserts that act as resistors, altering the acoustic dimensions of the hearing-aid system. In general, dampers will smooth out peaks of the frequency response and reduce the overall output. Metal pellets, mesh screens, cotton, and lamb's wool have all been used for this purpose. Without the use of dampers, some hearing aids produce a strong output peak in the mid-frequency range, typically near 1500 Hz, which can cause discomfort to the user. The effects of acoustic dampers on the hearing aid response depend on the value of the acoustic resistance of the dampers. Commercially available dampers are color coded (e.g., grey = 330 ohms, white = 680 ohms, etc.). Higher ohm values (acoustic resistance) cause more flattening of peaks and reduction in overall output. The location and number of dampers used will also influence the frequency response of the hearing aid.

High-Frequency Modification. THE ACOUSTIC HORN. An acoustic horn is produced by progressively increasing the internal diameter of the earmold tubing (e.g., 2mm to 3mm to 4mm). The effect is an enhancement of high-frequency gain, especially in the important 3000–4000 Hz region. Not all ear canals are large enough to accommodate 4mm diameter tubing, and the use of a 3mm diameter horn is common (see Figure 2.8). The use of horn tubing was advanced by Killion and Libby in the 1970s—see Mueller and Grimes (1987) for a review of this work.

Through the use of venting, damping, and horning it is possible to shape the hearing aid's frequency response to a variety of different desired gain characteristics. It is important to remember that any modification to the hearing aid-earmold system can change the output delivered in the ear canal, and many of these alterations cannot be predicted from 2cc-coupler measurements. We recommend measuring real-ear output (using probe-microphone measurements), therefore, whenever alterations in the earmold are made.

The Earmold Impression

No matter which type of earmold is chosen, all must be made from an impression of the user's ear, so that the exact shape can be replicated to ensure a proper fit. To make the ear impression, the audiologist follows these general steps:

1. A thorough inspection of the patient's ear canal, using an otoscope.
2. Careful insertion of a cotton or foam-rubber eardam to a point beyond the second bend of the ear canal. The eardam allows the impression material to fill the entire canal area and at the same time helps protect the eardrum from injury.
3. Mixing and injection into the ear of impression material, once the eardam is in place. Material is injected with a syringe into the ear canal, starting from the position of the eardam and working outward until the entire concha and helix areas are filled.
4. After the material hardens, removal of the material by gently pulling outward and upward. If imperfections are observed, the ear impression must be remade.
5. Following removal, another inspection of the ear canal, this time for remnants of impression material.

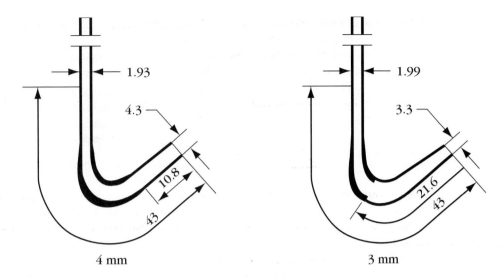

Figure 2.8 Libby 4- and 3-mm one-piece tapered horns.

From S. Lybarger (1985). Earmolds. In J. Katz (Ed.), *Handbook of Clinical Audiology* (3rd ed.). Baltimore, Williams & Wilkins.

6. Mailing of the finished impression to an earmold laboratory for fabrication of the earmold.

BATTERIES

Hearing-aid batteries are of two main types, mercury and zinc-air. Rechargeable batteries are also available. These can be removable batteries, or built-in types that cannot be removed except by the manufacturer. Rechargeable batteries are not commonly used because of the need for frequent recharging, and the relatively low cost of the replaceable batteries. Zinc-air batteries have an advantage over mercury cells in that they have a longer shelf life, since they are not activated until an adhesive strip is removed from the face of the battery. Although the zinc-air battery will last longer than the mercury battery in most hearing aids, they are also more costly. Consequently, cost per hour of operation is similar for zinc-air versus mercury type batteries.

In general, body hearing aids use a common AA battery, such as that used in a Walkman-type pocket radio. BTE and eyeglass hearing aids usually require a size 675 hearing aid battery; however, smaller models will use size 13. ITE hearing aids will use either the 13 battery or the next smaller size (312), depending on the size of the aid itself. Most ITC hearing aids use a size 312, and CIC hearing aids require a size 10 battery.

Hearing-aid batteries typically produce 1.3 to 1.5 volts. Battery life varies considerably from hearing aid to hearing aid, although manufacturers usually specify the expected battery performance for a given hearing aid. Battery life may vary depending on (1) type of battery; (2) type of hearing aid; (3) hours per day of continuous use;

TABLE 2.1 *Electroacoustic Properties Describing Hearing Aid Function*

Gain	The difference between the output sound pressure level (SPL) in the earphone coupler and the input SPL; describes how much the input signal is amplified. Maximum or "full-on gain" is measured with the volume control full on.
Reference or "use gain"	Usually is measured with the volume control set at approximately half on, which generally represents the typical user setting.
Frequency Response	Describes the available gain at each frequency; obtained by changing the frequency of the input signal and holding the input level constant.
Frequency Range	Describes the useful range of the frequency response. It is expressed by two numbers which represent the low and high frequency limit of amplification.
Saturation Sound Pressure Level (SSPL90)	Sound pressure level developed in a 2cc coupler when the input SPL is 90 dB and the volume control is in the full-on position; describes the maximum output the hearing aid is capable of producing.
Harmonic Distortion	The percentage of total output SPL which is a result of harmonics generated by the hearing aid. Total harmonic distortion is typically reported for 500, 800, and 1600 Hz.
Equivalent Input Noise	The level of internal noise generated by the hearing aid.

(4) circuitry contained within the hearing aid; and (5) volume-control setting during use. Generally, batteries may last anywhere from several days for high-output BTE hearing aids to several weeks for the some of the low-gain instruments.

ELECTROACOUSTIC PROPERTIES

Electroacoustic properties are used to describe hearing-aid characteristics and are important when selecting the appropriate hearing aid for a particular patient. This applies when the hearing aid is ordered, and again during the initial verification procedure. Hearing-aid manufacturers also rely heavily on standardized electroacoustic testing for promotional specifications, quality control, and repair, and to satisfy many FDA regulations.

Commonly considered electroacoustic characteristics are defined in Table 2.1. Typically, such measures are made within acoustical isolation boxes where the input and output levels can be reliably measured and controlled. Thus, these electroacoustic measures are basically measures of input/output functions. (Test systems are available from several different manufacturers; Figure 2.9 is an example of one type.)

In a hearing-aid test box, a regulating microphone monitors the input level and determines the appropriate compensation to maintain a constant sound level. Either a continuously variable sweep-frequency tone or a series of discrete frequencies is generated, generally ranging from 100 to 10,000 Hz. The input level can be selected from 50 to 100 dB SPL, depending on the specific parameter being measured.

Hearing-aid output is measured within a standard *2cc coupler* that attempts to imitate some of the acoustic conditions of the aided ear. While we know that the

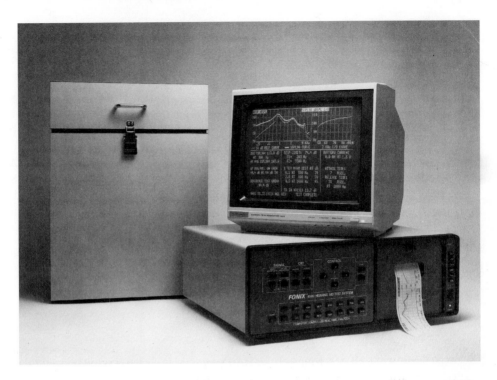

Figure 2.9 A hearing-aid analyzer for making electroacoustic measures of hearing-aid performance.

Courtesy of Frye Electronics.

residual volume (after the hearing aid or earmold has been inserted) of the human ear canal (after the hearing aid or earmold has been inserted) is not 2cc, this standard has been in place for many years, and it is unlikely that it will change soon. For quality-control purposes, it is not really a disadvantage that the volume is larger than the volume of the real ear.

There are different coupler types for the various hearing aid styles (Figure 2.10). The *HA-1 coupler* has a large opening into which any tubing, earmold, or custom instrument can be mounted using a putty-like substance to ensure a tight acoustic seal. The original form of the *HA-2 coupler* was designed to test button-type receivers on body aids. A second type of HA-2 coupler includes an earmold simulator via entrance through a tube, and is designed to test BTE aids when an earmold is not included. The hearing-aid coupler is attached to a measuring microphone, allowing input/output measures to be made and graphically displayed.

Although not typically used in clinics, another common tool used by manufac-turers (or in research) is the Knowles Electronics Manikin for Acoustic Research (KEMAR) (see Figure 2.11). Use of the KEMAR allows for hearing-aid measurements that are more representative of how a hearing aid would perform on a real person. In addition to the body baffle and head diffraction effects that can be measured, the

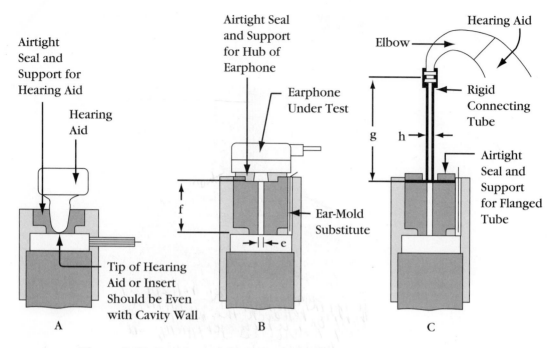

Figure 2.10 Drawings of the HA-1 (A) and HA-2 (B-c) couplers used in analyzing hearing-aid performance.

From R. Kasten & J. Franks (1986). Electroacoustic characteristics of hearing aids. In W. Hodgson (Ed.), *Hearing Aid Assessment and Use in Audiologic Habilitation* (3rd ed.). Baltimore: Williams & Wilkins.

KEMAR uses a Zwislocki coupler (rather than the 2cc), which is closer to the real-ear volume.

The various hearing-aid measurements, as described in Table 2.1, are specified by the American National Standards Institute (ANSI) in their 1992 ANSI Standard S3.22, and provide a standardized system for comparing different hearing aids between manufacturers. As mentioned earlier, in accordance with these standards, hearing-aid manufacturers provide specification sheets for each hearing aid to describe how the device is designed to operate. Let's take a specific example, and discuss the information shown in Figure 2.12.

1.   As you will recall, SSPL90 is the maximum output that the hearing aid is capable of producing. The upper-left graph of Figure 2.12 shows the maximum output available for this hearing aid across frequencies—the upper curve for a 90 dB input. Observe that in general the maximum output is around 110 dB SPL. Because the real-ear is smaller than the 2-cc coupler, the hearing aid output will be greater than 110 dB SPL when placed in the ear. In selecting an appropriate hearing aid, the audiologist must ensure that this output level does not exceed the patient's loudness discomfort level. This is extremely important in assuring that the hearing aid will not

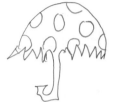

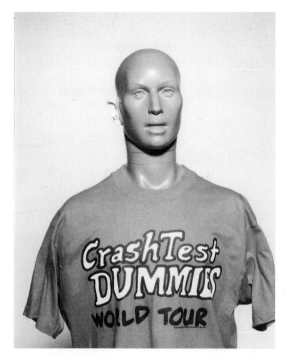

Figure 2.11 The Knowles Electronics Mannequin for Acoustic Research (KEMAR).

produce uncomfortably loud sounds and still be able to provide enough output to amplify sound adequately for the user.

2. The upper-right chart of Figure 2.12 shows the available gain at each specific frequency for this particular hearing aid, referred to as the frequency-response curve. As described in Table 2.1, gain is the difference, in decibels, between the input level to the microphone of the hearing aid and the output at the level of the receiver, as measured in the hearing-aid test box. This testing was conducted with a 50 dB input; hence, the gain for a given frequency is the value shown on the chart, minus 50 dB. For example, observing the upper curve (solid line), the coupler output for 2000 Hz is 88 dB—the gain for this frequency would be 38 dB (88 dB output minus the input of 50 dB). Notice that this hearing aid is designed to produce more gain in the higher frequencies than in the low. This is a common design, as most hearing losses are downward-sloping.

3. The two bottom panels of Figure 2.12 show the changes in the frequency response for this hearing aid that the audiologist can make at the time of the fitting (either using screwdriver controls or through a computerized programmable feature). Notice that the original frequency response can be altered to accommodate a wide variety of hearing losses and amplification needs. Prescriptive formula fitting methods, which we'll discuss a little later, provide guidance regarding what setting is best for a given patient.

Saturated Output
SSPL 90 / Full-On Gain 40/06/110

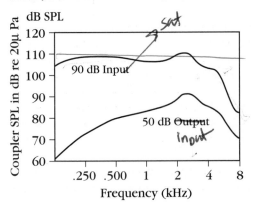

Frequency Response and Effect
of Full-On Gain (50 dB Input)

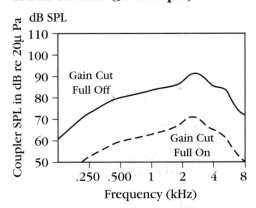

Frequency Response and Effect
of the N-H Control (50 dB Input)

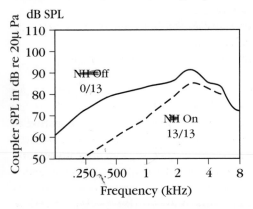

Frequency Response and Effect
of the N-L Control (50 dB Input)

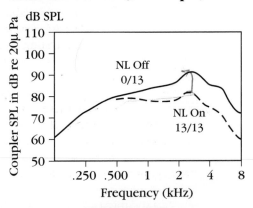

Figure 2.12 Hearing-aid performance specifications from the manufacturer.
Courtesy of Siemens Hearing Instruments, Inc.

THE SELECTION AND FITTING OF HEARING AIDS

Up to this point, we have provided some general information concerning how hearing aids are constructed, how they work, the variety of styles that are available, and how we can measure their performance on a standard coupler. Now comes the hard part: getting the right hearing aids on the right person! There is not a clear consensus today, nor has there ever been, regarding how hearing aids are selected and fitted. In the 1930s and 1940s, many hearing aids were chosen based on "selective amplification." That is, a belief that pure-tone thresholds, or a patient's maximum comfort level (MCL) could be used to predict gain-by-frequency. A major change occurred following Raymond Carhart's (1946) publication of his recommended hearing-aid selection procedure, which was based on his extensive work in the military. Carhart's procedure, sometimes referred to as the comparative approach, advocated the use of clinical speech testing to help determine the "best" hearing aid. This approach suggested that there might be a patient/hearing-aid interaction, and therefore, the best frequency response could not always be predicted from pure-tone test results. For many years (e.g., 1950s, 1960s) it was common practice for audiologists to conduct speech testing (e.g., monosyllable words) with different BTE instruments (coupled to the patient's custom earmold). The audiologist would then recommend that the patient purchase the hearing aid that he or she was wearing when the best test score was obtained.

The comparative hearing-aid selection procedure remained popular among audiologists until the mid-1970s. At this time several contributing factors caused most audiologists to abandon this selection method:

- Custom ITE hearing aids were becoming popular.
- Audiologists began direct dispensing in private practice, and they needed a more efficient and reliable selection method.
- Additional research was published showing the poor reliability of comparative hearing-aid testing with speech material.
- New prescriptive fitting approaches were published and promoted.

In the past 15 to 20 years there has been a shift back to prescriptive fitting approaches. Some of these are, in fact, very similar to the fitting methods of the 1930s. This shift has been fueled by two factors: first, the popularity of custom instruments, which has forced manufacturers to "individualize" hearing aids, using primarily pure-tone threshold data; and second, the development of probe-microphone measurements, which provide the audiologist the ability to verify gain-by-frequency in the real ear.

Many prescriptive fitting methods are available today, with no specific procedure identified as superior. Whatever method is used, however, we believe that it must be approached systematically, and we have outlined a five-step protocol for selecting and fitting hearing aids. While it is tempting to grab a couple of hearing aids out of a box and go directly to Step 4, you will find that the key to successful fittings is directly related to the time and thought that is expended during Steps 1, 2, and 3.

Step 1: Selecting the Hearing-Aid Candidate

Several issues must be considered when an individual is selected as a hearing-aid candidate. Three of the most important factors are degree of hearing loss, amount of communication difficulty, and motivation to use hearing aids. Quite frequently, these three factors interrelate, and it is difficult to make a fitting decision based on information from only one or two of these categories.

Degree of Hearing Loss. Usually, the first step in determining hearing-aid candidacy is to examine the patient's pure-tone thresholds. If the patient has a profound hearing loss (with accompanying poor word recognition), it might be that the hearing impairment is too severe to be helped with conventional hearing aids. It is then appropriate to consider the alternative amplification devices that we discuss later in the chapter.

A more basic decision that needs to be made is determining if the hearing loss is severe enough to warrant amplification. There are no strict rules for this determination, but most audiologists agree that if hearing is normal (thresholds of 20 dB or better) for 4000 Hz and below, it is unlikely that hearing aids will be beneficial. As hearing loss starts to affect the higher speech frequencies of 3000 and 4000 Hz (this is the typical loss pattern), the patient will need to be considered for amplification. Many successful hearing aid users today have normal, or near normal hearing through 2000 or 3000 Hz.

One method to assess the effects of the pure-tone impairment is to calculate an audibility index; that is, the percent of average speech that is audible to the patient. The chart shown in Figure 2.13, developed by Mueller and Killion (1990), can be used for this purpose. Simply plot the audiogram on the chart and count the dots that are not audible (above the threshold line). Subtract this from 100% and you have the audibility index. Anyone with an audibility index below 85% could probably benefit from hearing aids, but only if the criteria of the next two categories are met.

Degree of Communication Disability. A patient can have a significant hearing loss based on pure-tone findings, yet might not believe that he or she has a hearing disability (or at least a hearing disability that needs to be treated). This attitude can be influenced by the patient's lifestyle, occupation, and the amount of time spent communicating with others. In some cases it is denial, or simply a lack of awareness of the problem—"I can hear fine, it's just that my family members mumble."

A standardized self-assessment inventory is an excellent way to survey each individual's communication problems. While much of the same information could be gleaned from an extensive case history, a standard inventory is a more reliable and efficient method of collecting this information (see McCarthy, 1994). There are several self-assessment inventories available, some specific to communication, others related to social and emotional issues (see Chapter 9 for a review). We will discuss three abbreviated inventories that are well researched, can be easily adapted for routine clinical use, and can be used as pre- and post-testing to determine efficacy of the hearing aid fitting.

SELF-ASSESSMENT OF COMMUNICATION (SAC). Developed by Schow and Nerbonne (1982), this easy-to-administer 10-item inventory poses questions for the hearing-impaired person's response. These questions are related to how the subject is able to communicate in various situations. Additionally, the subject's feelings about the hearing problem and the reactions of others with whom he or she interacts are assessed. Responses for each of the items on the SAC range from 1 (never) to 5 (always), and an overall total score is derived for interpretation (see Chapter 9).

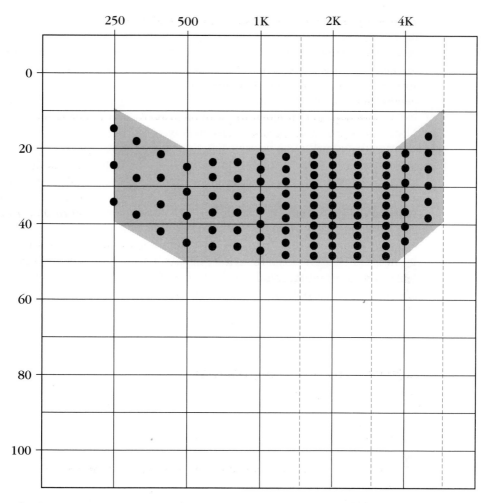

Figure 2.13 The count-the-dot audiogram form for calculation of the Articulation Index.

From G. Mueller & M. Killion (1990). An easy method for calculating the Articulation Index. *The Hearing Journal*, 45 (9), 14–17.

HEARING HANDICAP INVENTORY FOR THE ELDERLY-SCREENING (HHIE-S). This inventory (Ventry and Weinstein, 1983) consists of 10 items that are answered on a three-point scale: yes, sometimes, and no. Four points are scored for a *yes* answer, two points for a *sometimes* answer, and no points are scored for a *no* answer. Five of the ten questions are categorized as social, the other five as emotional (see Chapter 10).

Both the SAC and the HHIE-S are brief self-assessment inventories that have been shown to be successful tools in assessing hearing-aid candidacy and for quantifying the benefits of hearing-aid use (Schow and Gatehouse, 1990; Weinstein, 1993). They were endorsed in a recent ASHA report (ASHA, 1992).

ABBREVIATED PROFILE OF HEARING AID BENEFIT (APHAB). A third brief self-assessment inventory that can be used in conjunction with hearing-aid fittings is the newly developed APHAB (Cox and Alexander, 1994). The APHAB is a 24-item questionnaire, with a 7-point scale for answers: always (99%), almost always (87%), generally (75%), half the time (50%), occasionally (25%), seldom (12%), and never (1%). The 24 items are divided equally into 4 subscales: ease of communication (listening in quiet), reverberation, background noise, and aversiveness (annoyance from loud or harsh sounds). The APHAB can be used to quantify hearing-related problems experienced by the client with and without a hearing aid(s), as well as hearing-aid benefit. The APHAB is recommended for use by the Independent Hearing Aid Fitting Form (IHAFF) protocol (see Chapter Nine).

Motivation to Use Hearing Aids. A final area concerning hearing-aid candidacy is related to the motivation of the patient to use hearing aids. A person might have a significant hearing loss, admit that he or she has communication problems, yet not be willing to use hearing aids. Logic suggests that these patients probably won't be happy hearing-aid users, and it is tempting simply to tell them, "Come back when you're ready." There is some evidence to suggest, however, that if we somehow can get these people to start using hearing aids, they might become very successful hearing-aid users (see Mueller and Grimes, 1993)—sort of a "Try it, you'll like it" approach.

Certainly, as with other health care providers, we have a responsibility to tell the patient firmly what we believe is the best treatment for him or her. Given that no one *really* wants to use hearing aids, a lukewarm recommendation is often viewed as no recommendation. Obviously, the final decision to purchase lies in the patient's hands.

Step 2: Pre-Selection Measurements

Once it has been established that the patient meets the criteria for hearing-aid candidacy, it is time to conduct pre-selection testing (some of this testing might have been conducted previously as part of the audiologic diagnostic assessment).

Before describing some specific audiologic measurements, it is important to first discuss prescriptive fitting procedures. This is because the prescriptive method that you select will determine what pre-fitting testing is necessary. It is important to formalize the method we are using so that we have a gold standard for our hearing-aid ordering and verification procedures. Several formalized methods are already available, and recently Hawkins (1992) has reviewed what most audiologists would consider to be the six most popular methods.

Does it matter what prescriptive fitting method we use? It certainly does, and this is illustrated in Figure 2.14, taken from the comparative study by Hawkins (1992). Notice that the chart is labeled *Prescribed REIR.* This is the real-ear gain of the hearing aid for each frequency called for by the respective prescriptive method. Observe that differences among methods are as great as 20 dB for the higher frequencies. Would a patient notice a 20-dB difference in the gain of a hearing aid? We think so.

Prescribed REIR

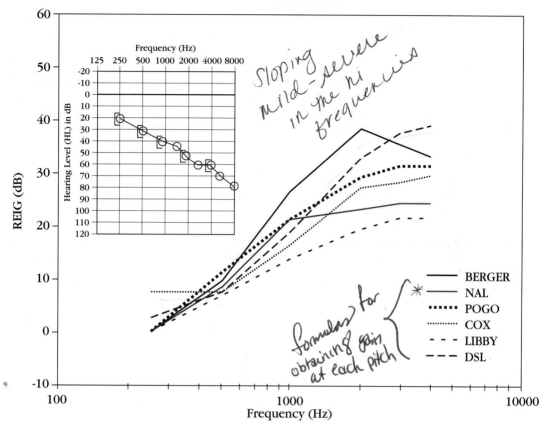

Figure 2.14 Prescribed REIRs for the audiogram shown in the inset using Berger, NAL, POGO, Cox, Libby, and DSL procedures. A monaural ITE hearing aid has been assumed.

D. Hawkins (1992). Prescriptive approach to selection of gain and frequency response. In G. Mueller, D. Hawkins, & J. Northern (Eds.), *Probe Microphone Measurement*. San Diego, CA: Singular Press.

Once you have selected the prescriptive method that you believe is best, which might be different for different patients, the necessary pre-fitting testing can be conducted. Some methods require only pure-tone thresholds; other methods require more extensive testing.

Pure-Tone Thresholds. You might already have the pure-tone thresholds available from the auditory diagnostic testing. If not, thresholds must be determined for all frequencies of interest (e.g., 250 to 6000 Hz, including 1500 and 3000 Hz.) For many prescriptive methods, these thresholds will be used to calculate the hearing-aid gain requirements. It is also important to know if there is a conductive component to the hearing loss, as this might alter your gain requirements.

Important note: It is *not* possible to calculate reliably a patient's loudness discomfort level (LDL) based on pure-tone thresholds, which is why we recommend measuring the LDL.

Loudness Discomfort Level (LDL). One of the leading reasons that hearing aids are rejected is that the maximum output is placed too high. Obtaining the data that will assist in getting the output right, therefore, is one of the most important pre-selection measurements. This measurement, sometimes referred to as uncomfortable level (UCL) or threshold of discomfort (TD) rather than LDL, is conducted using pure tones (or very narrow bands of noise) at two or three key frequencies (e.g., 500; 1500; and 3000 Hz). We recommend using the chart shown in Table 2.2; a rating of "Loud, But O.K." is the value used for specifying the hearing aid's maximum output (see Mueller and Bright, 1994 for a review).

Loudness Contour Testing. Rather than viewing only thresholds and LDLs, it is sometimes helpful to establish an entire loudness growth function. This can be especially useful when selecting different types of compression and automatic signal processing parameters. Loudness contour testing, using the chart shown in Table 2.2, is part of the protocol of the IHAFF. This testing is automated through the use of the IHAFF software, using a personal computer in conjunction with your audiometer. At the completion of testing, values are obtained from the patient for all seven categories of the loudness growth chart.

Step 3: Hearing-Aid Selection

There are several important aspects of the hearing-aid selection procedure, ranging from the style of the hearing aid, to the type of signal processing, to whether the hearing aid should be remote-controlled. Many of these decisions require input from the patient, as a mistake in any one area could lead to hearing-aid rejection.

TABLE 2.2 *Categories of Loudness*

Uncomfortably Loud

Loud, but O.K.

Comfortable, but slightly loud

Comfortable

Comfortable, but slightly soft

Soft

Very Soft

Source: From Independent Hearing Aid Fitting Forum (IHAFF). A Complete Hearing Aid Fitting Protocol. Presented in Jackson Hole, WY. August 1994. Based on Hawkins et al., CT. (1987).

Hearing Aid Style. Earlier in this chapter we summarized the pros and cons of different hearing-aid styles. Using the information obtained from the pre-selection testing, it is now time to find the best style for your patient. You must consider, in addition to the audiometric information available, such aspects as the patient's dexterity, the pinna and ear canal geography, and the need for a cosmetically acceptable product. Financial resources cannot be overlooked, as the small CIC hearing aids can be two to three times the cost of the larger ITE models.

It is important to note that some patients seem reluctant to admit that they want a hearing aid that is small ("invisible" is often what they are thinking!). For this reason, it might be best to assume that nearly everyone has cosmetic concerns, even though they might not be interested in discussing them with you.

Gain and Frequency Response. Hearing-aid specifications are based on measurements in a 2-cc coupler. Hence, it is important that the pre-selection measurements are converted to this standard when the hearing aids are ordered. The precise values that are selected, for the most part, are based on the prescriptive method that is utilized. After desired real-ear gain is calculated, reserve gain and coupler corrections are applied to derive desired 2-cc coupler values. This information then can be used to select a hearing aid that matches these specifications.

Maximum Output. Recall that LDL testing was part of the pre-selection assessment. These pure-tone LDL values also need to be converted to 2-cc coupler values (see Mueller and Bright, 1994, for specific procedures). A hearing aid that matches these derived 2-cc coupler output specifications then can be selected.

Automatic Signal Processing. Several specialized types of non-linear gain/output limiting circuits, termed automatic signal processing (ASP) circuits, are available in today's hearing aid. For many fittings, one of the following five types of ASP will be selected (modified from Killion, Staab, & Preves, 1990):

- *Limiting compression.* This type of ASP has linear processing for the majority of inputs. It differs from peak-clipping in that there is less saturation-induced distortion.
- *Dynamic range compression.* Using AGC-I circuitry, this type of ASP is based on the notion that someone with a non-linear loudness growth function should be fitted with a hearing aid that also is non-linear. The hearing aid usually begins compression for inputs of 50–70 dB.
- *Wide dynamic range compression.* A variation of dynamic range compression instruments, this designator suggests that the hearing aid has a low kneepoint (e.g., around 40 dB SPL). The design is based on the philosophy that speech should always, or nearly always, be in compression.
- *Bass increase for low levels (BILL).* A special type of AGC-I is referred to as BILL processing. It is based on the theory that background noise is primarily

low frequency, and that it should only be minimally amplified when it reaches high inputs.

- *Treble increase for low levels (TILL).* Somewhat the opposite of BILL processing, TILL circuits vary high frequency gain as a function of the input; the softer the input, the greater the high frequency gain (low frequencies also increase, but not by as much).

We have described five different types of ASP, each of which has advantages. Selection of the "best" type of ASP for a given patient must be carefully considered.

Programmable Hearing Aids. How would you like to use a typewriter rather than computerized word processing for your next 20-page report? No way, you say. Well, audiologists who have become accustomed to fitting programmable hearing aids feel the same when they have to go find a screw driver to adjust a potentiometer. In a few years, programmable hearing aids will be the standard fitting, just as word processing is the standard way to write a report today. At present, however, programmable hearing aids only have an 8–10% market share.

Programmable hearing aids can have one, two, or three channels (discrete regions for adjustment of gain, output, and signal processing), and can have multiple memories (each memory can be programmed with different fitting parameters).

Programmable hearing aids that have two or three channels can be adjusted to provide any one of the ASP strategies that we discussed earlier. They can be programmed with small handheld devices, remote controls, or personal computers. The different memories can be accessed by a remote device or by a button on the hearing aid.

There are several advantages of programmable hearing aids, as summarized by the following (modified from Mueller, 1994):

- Greater flexibility and more precise adjustments than a non-programmable product; the equivalent of four or more conventional adjustment trim-pots.
- Ability to make fine-tuning adjustments for compression parameters to control and shape the maximum output.
- Ability to make precise adjustments for shaping the frequency response.
- Ease of adjustments, and a greater fitting range for a fluctuating or progressive hearing loss.
- Range of signal processing and maximum output for different frequency regions (requires multichannel instrument).
- Different frequency response and/or signal processing strategy for different listening conditions (requires multiple memory instrument).

Binaural Hearing Aids. Like shoes, gloves, and eyeglasses, hearing aids are usually fitted in pairs. It was once thought that a single hearing aid was satisfactory for someone with an aidable hearing impairment in both ears, but fortunately few professionals continue to hold this outdated belief. There are many advantages of a binaural fitting over a monaural one, and the following summarizes several of the most significant reasons (from Mueller and Grimes, 1993):

- *Elimination of head shadow.* The patient's head attenuates the important high frequencies of speech by as much as 12–16 dB to the ear on the side farther away from a speaker. With binaural fittings, a talker on either side of the head is always speaking into the microphone of a hearing aid.
- *Loudness summation.* Binaural summation results in thresholds that are approximately 3 dB better than monaural; the summing effect can be several decibels greater than this for supra-threshold signals.
- *Binaural squelch.* When a patient is listening to speech in background noise, binaural hearing aids provide an improvement in the signal/noise ratio of 2–3 dB when compared to a monaural fitting.
- *Localization.* Localization of sound in the horizontal plane is dependent on interaural differences in intensity, time, and phase, and hence requires that information throughout the important frequencies be available from both sides of the head. It is unlikely that a monaural fitting will improve localization, and in fact, it might make it worse than if the person were unaided.
- *Wider dynamic range.* Binaural summation lowers thresholds, but does not lower the patient's LDL. The result is a wider dynamic range available in which to place the aided speech signal.
- *Other Considerations.* We have discussed many of the most important features of hearing-aid selection. Some other decisions which might need to be made include the need for a telecoil, direct audio input, directional microphone, or other special circuits. It is important to review all the features that we mentioned earlier in this chapter to assure that everything has been considered when the hearing aids are ordered.

Step 4: Verification

The first verification procedure is to measure the performance of the hearing aids in the 2-cc coupler, as discussed earlier in this chapter. The gain, frequency response, SSPL90, and distortion of the hearing aid are checked to assure that they match specifications, and are consistent with the electroacoustic characteristics that were ordered. Additionally, an input/output function is conducted to evaluate the automatic signal processing that was requested.

If the hearing aid is programmable, or even if it has the more traditional screwdriver-controlled adjustments, the audiologist can make changes during the 2cc-coupler testing to facilitate the verification measurements that will be conducted when the patient arrives. For example, if pre-selection testing revealed that the patient's LDL was 105 dB SPL when corrected to the 2-cc coupler, then adjustments to the output can be made at this time to obtain this value. Likewise, the audiologist can adjust compression parameters to match the patient's loudness growth characteristics.

The most important verification procedures are conducted when the patient is wearing the hearing aids (if pre-fitting testing and coupler verification were conducted carefully, there should be few surprises).

In general, four different methods are used to verify if the hearing aids being fitted have the correct gain, frequency response, and signal-processing characteristics. Some audiologists might use different methods for different patients, or combine methods for a single patient.

User Feedback/Self-Report. "So, how does that sound?" is perhaps the most common question posed to a new hearing aid user. While this question is frequently asked, opinions vary concerning how much emphasis should be placed on the patient's answer. Can a patient reliably select what is best? Can he or she hear the difference between small but important changes in the frequency response? Is the frequency response that *sounds the best* necessarily the one that will result in the *best understanding of speech*? It is, of course, always important to listen to the comments from the patient. Pre-Post self-report, which compares previous unaided scores to the aided ones, is a more formalized, but valuable, form of feedback. We believe that user feedback, along with self-report and the three other approaches described below, are all needed to verify hearing-aid fitting.

Speech-Recognition or Intelligibility Testing. Because the patient usually sought amplification because of difficulty understanding speech, it seems logical that the verification procedure should measure his or her ability to understand aided speech. A speech-testing approach can be used fairly successfully to compare *unaided* to *aided* speech; however, it is difficult to use speech testing for selecting the best frequency response or signal processing strategy. Why? Because of the inherent unreliability of available speech material, and the time constraints of the hearing-aid fitting procedure (patients do not like to sit in a booth while you deliver thousands of words). So, clinical speech testing can be used successfully to determine if hearing aids are better than no hearing aids, but not for determining which set of hearing aids is best.

Functional Gain. If, as part of your pre-selection testing and ordering procedure, you used a gain-based prescriptive fitting procedure (such as the NAL or POGO), then it is necessary to verify that the patient is receiving the appropriate gain for the frequencies of interest. Functional gain is established by first obtaining the patient's unaided hearing thresholds in the sound field, then placing the hearing aid in the ear, setting the gain of the instrument to the patient's maximum comfort level, and then obtaining aided hearing thresholds. The difference between the aided and unaided thresholds is the functional gain.

Ideally, aided thresholds will fall in the 20–30-dB HL range. Aided versus unaided audibility scores (using the chart shown in Figure 2.13) can be used for patient counseling.

Probe-Microphone Measurements. Perhaps the most reliable method to verify the performance of hearing aids is to measure the output at the tympanic membrane of the hearing-aid user. This is accomplished by placing in the ear canal a small silicone tube that is attached to a measurement microphone. A loudspeaker is used to present a variety of test signals, and the output from the hearing aid is analyzed using computerized equipment. The results are displayed on a monitor, and can be printed for the patient's file. Figure 2.15 shows a typical probe-microphone system.

There are few reasons *not* to use probe-microphone measurements as part of the verification procedure. Although there is an initial outlay of funds to purchase this equipment ($5000 to $12,000), the long-term payoff is well worth the investment. In addition to verification of gain and frequency response, this equipment has a variety of other uses in the assessment of hearing aids and assistive listening devices. Probe-microphone measurements come with their own terminology, and a review of the key terms is shown in Table 2.3.

Using probe-microphone measurements, the real-ear gain of the hearing aid can be compared to the gain specified by a prescriptive fitting protocol. Additionally, var-

TABLE 2.3 *Common Terminology Used for the Real-Ear Measurement of Hearing Aid Performance*

Real-ear unaided response	The real-ear unaided response (REUR) is the SPL, as a function of frequency, at a specified point in the unoccluded ear canal for a specified soundfield. This can be expressed either in SPL or a gain in decibels relative to the stimulus level.
Real-ear occluded response	The real-ear occluded response (REOR) is the SPL, as a function of frequency, at a specified point in the ear canal for a specified soundfield, with the hearing aid in place and turned off. This can be expressed either in SPL or as gain in decibels relative to the stimulus level.
Real-ear aided response	The real-ear aided response (REAR) is the SPL, as a function of frequency, at a specified measurement point in the ear canal for a specified soundfield with the hearing aid in place and turned on. This can be expressed either in SPL or as gain in decibels relative to the stimulus level.
Real-ear saturation response	The real-ear saturation response (RESR) is the SPL, as a function of frequency, at a specified measurement point in the ear canal with the hearing aid in place and turned on. The measurement is obtained with the stimulus level sufficiently intense as to operate the hearing aid at its maximum output level.
Real-ear insertion response	The real-ear insertion response (REIR) is the difference, in decibels as a function of frequency, between the REUR and the REAR measurements taken at the same measurement point in the same soundfield.
	The real-ear insertion gain (REIG) is the value, in decibels, of the REIR at a specific frequency.
Real-ear coupler difference	The real-ear coupler difference (RECD) is the difference, in decibels, as a function of frequency, between the outputs of a hearing aid measured in a real-ear versus a 2-cm³ coupler.

Source: Mueller, H., Terminology and procedures. In H. Mueller, D. Hawkins, and J. Northern (Eds.), *Probe Microphone Measurements.* San Diego, CA: Singular Publishing Group (1992b).

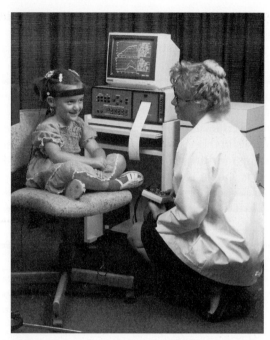

Figure 2.15 A probe-microphone system for making real-ear measurements of hearing-aid output.

Courtesy of Frye Electronics.

ied inputs can be presented to the hearing aid to evaluate the effects of different automatic signal processing strategies. The hearing aid's telephone coil and other special features also can be reliably assessed using this equipment.

The preceding was a brief review of the various methods to determine if the gain and frequency response of the hearing aids meet your gold standard. In addition, it is also critical to conduct aided LDL testing to verify the maximum output of the instrument is set correctly. Mueller and Bright (1994) have outlined a step-by-step protocol for conducting these measures. In general, they recommend using the chart shown in Table 2.2 to assure that both pure tones and speech signals of 90 dB SPL do not cause a patient rating of "Uncomfortably Loud". Using probe-microphone measurements, the real ear saturation response (RESR, see Table 2.3) can be used as a cross-check, and can also be used to quantify the ear canal SPL (a very important measurement for young children, who have small ear canals).

A final loudness verification is to produce loud obnoxious environmental sounds, both transient and sustained, outside the test booth (e.g., slamming doors, rattling keys, clanging spoons in glass jar). Because too much output is one of the leading reasons for hearing aid rejection, it is important to conduct a variety of aided LDL tests so that you can make changes before the patient leaves the office. If your imagination is lacking, you can use CD recordings of various signals provided by hearing-aid manufacturers.

Step 5: Post-Fitting Counseling, Orientation and Follow-up

Even the best hearing aid, with the best circuitry, adjusted precisely for the patient's hearing loss, can be a failed fitting if appropriate counseling and follow-up are not conducted.

Post-Fitting Counseling and Orientation. After the verification procedure is completed, it's time to sit down with the patient and walk through the use and care of the instruments. This is not something that can be rushed through. If possible, include significant others who spend time with the hearing-aid user. It is good to have a hand-out that includes all the information that you will be presenting orally (the user guide furnished by the manufacturer will have some of the information). Here is a brief list of some of the things that you might want to discuss at the time of the hearing-aid orientation (but there are many more; see Chapters 8, 9 and 10):

- *Realistic expectations*: Unfortunately, hearing aids do not work just like eyeglasses. Everything will not be perfectly clear once they are put in place. The patient needs to know this.
- *Acoustic feedback*: Demonstrate what it sounds like (if the patient can hear it), what causes it, when it is O.K. and when it is not O.K.
- *Occlusion effect*: Have the patient talk with the hearing aids in place, but *turned off*—see if an occlusion effect is present. If so, and if it is bothersome, explain why you can't make it go away (assuming that you can't).
- *Batteries*: Discuss different battery types and sizes, what batteries the hearing aids use, how the patient can obtain batteries, how long a battery lasts, and what to do with the sticky tabs (don't put them back on the battery!). Have the patient demonstrate proficiency in opening and closing the battery door, and inserting and removing the battery.
- *Operation*: The patient should be able to turn the hearing aid on and off, use the telecoil (if present), adjust the volume.
- *Telephone*: Demonstrate use of the hearing aid on the telephone, discuss assistive telephone listening devices.
- *Maintenance*: Talk about taking the battery out when storing the instrument; use of a dry-aid kit if moisture is a problem; keeping the instrument away from water; excessive heat; hair spray; avoidance of dropping the hearing aid on a hard surface.
- *Cleaning*: Show the patient where wax accumulates in the receiver tubing, demonstrate a wax-cleaning tool, show how the hearing aid itself can be wiped clean.
- *Insertion and removal*: Demonstrate on an artificial ear, then have the patient practice in front of a mirror.
- *Trouble-shooting*: Provide the patient with a trouble-shooting chart (see Table 2.4).

TABLE 2.4 *Troubleshooting of Common Problems with Hearing Aids*

Problem	Cause	Possible Solution
Instrument has no sound or sound is weak	Battery polarity reversed	Make sure battery is inserted correctly
	Low or dead battery	Replace with fresh battery
	Instrument not turned on	Rotate volume control
	Clogged wax guard	Clean wax guard
	Volume turned down	Turn up volume control
Instrument whistles	Improper seating in ear	Reinsert the instrument until it fits securely
	Volume control too high	Turn down volume control
	Clogged wax guard	Clean wax guard
	Excessive wax in your ears	Consult your hearing health care professional
Sound is distorted or intermittent	Low battery	Replace battery
	Battery compartment is not completely closed	Gently close the battery compartment
"Buzzing" sound	Low battery	Replace battery
Swelling or discharge in ear		Check with your physician

- *Warranty and repairs:* Explain warranty and repair policies, give the patient a warranty card, explain how repairs are handled in your office (e.g., do you allow walk-ins?).

Follow-Up Visits. On follow-up visits, it is useful to recheck some of the verification procedures that were conducted at the time of the fitting. Some general post-fitting verification procedures might be:

- Present average conversational speech (e.g., 65 dB SPL) and note where the patient sets the volume control wheel—it should be somewhere between a $\frac{1}{3}$ and $\frac{2}{3}$ rotation (neither all the way up nor barely turned on).
- With the volume-control wheel set for speech at MCL, present loud speech (e.g., 80–90 dB SPL) to assure that it is not uncomfortably loud (you can use the chart shown in Table 2.2).
- Repeat the obnoxious loud sounds test that you conducted on the day of the fitting; the patient should judge these sounds as loud and annoying, but not uncomfortable.

This is also a good time to repeat the SAC, HHIE-S, or APHAB self-assessment inventory that you gave the patient before the hearing aids were fitted. The patient can now respond to the questions relative to his or her performance with hearing aids, and you can determine if hearing-aid benefit is present. At this time it is also appropriate to consider providing, in addition to hearing aids, additional audiologic rehabilitation which is designed further to facilitate communication for the patient. Both short- and long-term forms of AR are discussed in detail in the chapters to follow.

A few things to consider during your post-fitting testing, adjustments, and counseling are:

- *Acclimatization:* Some research has suggested that it takes several weeks or even months for the brain to adjust to a new acoustic input, that is, the new speech spectrum delivered by the hearing aid. It is possible, therefore, that maximum performance, or improvement in performance from a previous hearing aid, will not occur until acclimatization is complete.
- *Auditory Deprivation:* Research has suggested that an ear (or ears) that has not been stimulated appropriately for a period of time will possibly show a decline in performance for understanding speech. Can this decline be reversed? Possibly. If it can, speech understanding after some hearing-aid use might be better than predicted based on standard testing prior to the fitting of the hearing aids.

CONSIDERATIONS FOR THE PEDIATRIC PATIENT

In many respects, fitting hearing aids to infants and young children is the same as for adults; the goals of making soft speech audible, average speech comfortable, and loud speech loud, but not too loud, are equally important for this population. There are some additional factors, however, which must be considered, and some procedural variations as well.

Pre-Fitting Testing

For infants and young children, it often is not possible to obtain precise pure-tone thresholds or loudness growth functions. In many cases, however, pure-tone thresholds for different frequency regions can be estimated from auditory electrophysiologic testing. Methods are available to estimate loudness discomfort levels for children based only on thresholds data (see Bentler, 1994, for review). Because precise threshold and loudness data often are not available, two factors are important: (1) the child should be re-evaluated frequently so that changes in the fitting can be made as additional audiometric information becomes available; and (2) the child should be fitted with hearing aids that are highly adjustable (digitally programmable when appropriate) so that alterations in the gain or output can be made easily.

Fitting Considerations

As we have discussed previously, different types of assistive listening technology rely on by-passing the hearing aid's microphone, either through direct auditory input (DAI) or through the hearing aid's telecoil. For children who are developing speech and language, this technology becomes even more critical. This reason alone might dictate which hearing-aid style is selected; for example, the telecoil of an ITE might not provide enough gain and output. As with adults, binaural amplification should be the standard fitting whenever there are two aidable ears.

Prescriptive fitting approaches specifically designed for children are available. The most commonly used today is the Desired Sensation Level (DSL) method (Seewald and Ross, 1988). In particular, this selection procedure takes into account the need to deliver extended high-frequency information to the child, and to limit the output to "safe levels." Also available is a computerized version of this procedure, which aids the audiologist in efficiently selecting the best hearing aid for a given child.

Verification of Fitting

Because the infant or young child cannot provide subjective reports of the hearing aid's performance, objective verification strategies are essential. The DSL method discussed above can be verified easily using probe-microphone measurements. With even the somewhat uncooperative child, this testing can be reliably conducted. Many times young children are sedated for the electrophysiology measures; some audiologists also conduct their probe-microphone measurements at this opportune moment.

Probe-microphone measurements will reveal the amount of gain present throughout the frequency range. Importantly, this testing will also determine the maximum output delivered in the child's ear canal. Because the child's ear canal is much smaller than an adult's, the real-ear output often is 10–15 dB higher than shown in the 2-cc coupler. Too high a hearing-aid output can result in a noise-induced hearing loss. As the child becomes older (e.g., three to four years of age) it is possible to conduct reliable loudness behavioral testing, using specially designed charts (see Mueller and Bright, 1994). Just because a child says that sounds are not uncomfortably loud, however, does not guarantee that the hearing-aid output is not damaging the ear—this is why objective ear-canal SPL measurements are essential.

Post-Fitting Procedures

Extensive parent counseling following the fitting is very important. The parents must know how to adjust and care for the hearing aid (see Chapter 8). Several practical accessories for children's hearing aids are available (e.g., "huggies"—devices to help hold BTE hearing aids on the ear); a list of these accessories can be reviewed with the parents.

Follow-up visits for children need to be scheduled more frequently than for adults because:

1. The hearing loss needs to be monitored to assure that it is not progressive, to verify previous findings, and to obtain additional information for hearing-aid adjustment.

2. The fit of the hearing aid or earmold in the ear must be monitored. Because of children's rapid ear growth, an earmold might become loose in a few months, causing acoustic feedback (see Chapter 8, Table 8.2).

3. The electroacoustic characteristics of the hearing aids should be monitored. Children's hearing aids are subject to many bumps and bruises; it is important to ensure that the hearing aid maintains its appropriate gain and frequency response, and that excessive distortion is not present.

4. Parent counseling and training must be on-going.

ASSISTIVE/ALTERNATIVE REHABILITATION DEVICES

While hearing aids are designed to assist the hearing-impaired individual in almost all listening environments, some patients, because of their age, degree of hearing loss, or other factors, might not derive significant benefit from hearing aids. Additionally, many hearing-aid users will encounter difficult situations in which hearing aids may not provide optimal speech intelligibility. For instance, it might be difficult to listen in a noisy restaurant or in a business meeting where the speaker is at a distance from the listener. A hearing-impaired child may have difficulty hearing the teacher when extraneous noise is present in the classroom, or other children are talking in the hallways or on the playground outside. When the telephone is being used, a hearing aid may not provide necessary amplification. Hearing doorbells or safety alarms is another area where special assistance might be helpful, especially for the patient with severe hearing impairment.

You will recall that the microphone of the conventional hearing aid is located at the listener's ear. We have previously enumerated the advantages of this arrangement; however, in one respect this is a disadvantage to the hearing impaired listener. The reason is that since all incoming signals, both speech and noise, are amplified before being sent to the user's ear, an unfavorable signal-to-noise ratio remains unfavorable. Assistive listening devices can help to overcome this problem by increasing the loudness of the primary signal without significantly amplifying the background noise. This is accomplished by placing the microphone of the system close to the sound source, and the receiver at the listener's ears so that the signal is transferred directly to the ear canal.

Several categories of assistive devices are available. These include:

- Personal and group amplification devices
- Telephone devices
- Radio/television amplifiers
- Signaling devices
- Cochlear Implants
- Tactile Devices
- Tinnitus Maskers

We will take a look at each category throughout the following section. For a more detailed discussion of assistive devices, the reader is referred to Compton (1989).

Personal and Group Amplification Devices

Listening in groups, meetings, theaters, or classrooms can be adversely affected by interference from noise, room reverberation, and the distance from the speaker. Even individuals with only a mild degree of hearing loss may find it difficult to understand speech in such environments. Assistive listening devices increase the loudness of the person talking without significantly amplifying the background noise, and can be used for listening one-to-one as well as in large groups.

A simple version of a personal or group amplification device comprises an amplifier with a microphone input, with a wire leading to an earphone. More elaborate systems are wireless, in which the signal is transmitted from the microphone/amplifier directly to the receiver (listener) by wireless transmission. Such transmission is via either infrared lightwave, or FM radio wave signals. Another assistive listening system is the induction loop, in which an electromagnetic or induction signal is picked up by the telecoil in the user's hearing aids.

There are several important factors in examining how these systems work, where they may be used, and the advantages and disadvantages of each system type.

Hardwire Systems. Hardwire systems were among the earliest assistive systems developed for use by the hearing impaired. These systems consist of a direct wire connection from a microphone, to an amplifier, and finally to a receiver. The receiver can be either the personal hearing aids, receiving the signal by direct audio input, or earphones. Since hardwire systems physically tether the listener to the sound source, there is typically a short distance between the listener and the sound source. A hardwire system, like all assistive listening devices, allows a favorable signal-to-noise ratio due to the proximity of the microphone to the sound source. Although hardwire systems can provide high-fidelity sound, an obvious disadvantage of this type of setup is limited mobility. For this reason, hardwire systems for group communication are used less frequently today than in the past.

Induction Loop Systems. Induction loop systems offer an advantage over hardwire systems in that they are wireless, thus avoiding the need for a cord between the sound source and listener. This system consists of a microphone, an amplifier, and a length of wire that surrounds a designated area, such as a theater or a classroom. A pick-up microphone is placed near the sound source, transmitting the signal via hard-wire coupling or FM radio waves to a receiver/amplifier that transforms the signal into electrical energy. This electric current flows through the wire loop, creating a magnetic field that can be picked up by the telecoil of a conventional hearing aid or a specially designed induction receiver (see Figure 2.16 for an example of induction loop for a large area listening system). Induction loop systems are sometimes used as classroom amplification devices, as an alternative to the more restrictive hardwired systems previously in use. A number of limitations have been identified with induction loop systems, however, predominantly because of their dependence on the hearing-aid telecoil. Induction loop systems typically require use of a hearing aid with a strong telecoil. Even with a strong telecoil, however, the distance and

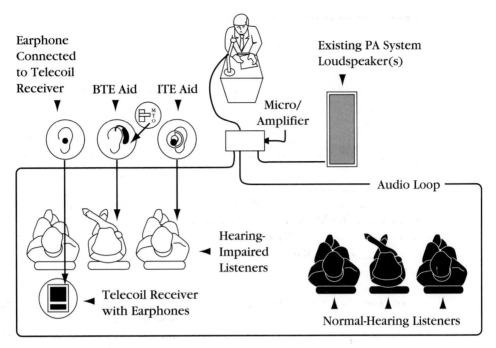

Figure 2.16 Use of an induction-loop large-area listening system. A coil of wire (loop) is added to existing sound system. Listeners with hearing impairment pick up sound using telecoil circuits contained in hearing aids or special receivers.

Reprinted with permission from C. Compton (1991). *Assistive devices: Doorways to independence.* Annapolis, MD: Van Comp Associates.

orientation of the hearing-aid telecoil from the loop can significantly affect the gain and frequency response of the signal. Moreover, as you will recall from an earlier discussion, placement of the telecoil within the hearing aid itself varies substantially, making performance characteristics within the induction loop even more variable. An additional disadvantage of the induction loop system is the possibility of electromagnetic interference. Any device that produces a magnetic field, such as a television or fluorescent light, may interfere with signal reception. Many of these drawbacks have been overcome with the emergence of the 3-D loop system. Induction loop systems are inexpensive, require little maintenance, and work relatively well in the home and in small meeting rooms where the listeners have telecoil-equipped hearing aids. Their use in classroom amplification, however, has generally been replaced by FM listening systems.

Infrared Systems. In the infrared system, a microphone picks up acoustic energy from the sound source, converts it to electrical energy and transmits it to an infrared converter. The converter changes the electrical energy to light energy and transmits it on a infrared carrier beam. The listener wears a receiver which picks up the light energy and converts it back to acoustic energy. The receiver consists of lightweight earphones with an adjustable volume control, although an induction neckloop coupled to personal hearing aid telecoils can also be employed (see Figure 2.17 for examples of different infrared use with the television). Infrared systems are moderately priced, provide a high quality signal, and generally require little maintenance. Moreover, they have the advantage of increased mobility since they do not require physical hardwiring or positioning within a designated loop, and are relatively easy to install and use. There are, however, several limitations to infrared systems. For maximum sound quality, the receiver must be in direct line with the transmitter. Unfortunately, in many applications the infrared signal is subject to reflection by walls, ceiling, and room furnishings, so the reception of the signal may not be completely directional, thus limiting the quality of the signal received by the listener. In addition, infrared systems cannot be used outside because they are subject to interference from sunlight. Like the induction loop system, infrared systems are seldom used in classroom settings, but remain relatively popular in large areas such as theaters and churches, as well as for personal use in the home.

FM Systems. The function of an FM system is similar to that of the infrared system, except that FM radio waves, rather than infrared light waves, are used to transmit the signal. With this system, a microphone/transmitter is placed at the sound source and the signal is transmitted via FM radio waves to an FM receiver worn by the listener. This receiver may be earphones, or may be a neckloop which generates an electromagnetic signal which is picked up by the hearing aid telecoils.

There are many advantages to using FM systems. FM systems are easily portable, making them useful for situations that take place outside, or where multiple rooms are being utilized. Electromagnetic interference is generally not a problem with FM systems. FM signals are transmitted easily without having to maintain the line-of-sight orientation necessary with the infra-red transmitter. In addition, FM systems are flexible enough to fit a variety of hearing losses and may be coupled to the user's ear in a number of ways, depending on the needs of the listener (see Figure 2.18). A disadvantage of FM-system use is the potential for interference from a variety of sources, such as cellular telephones, police band radios, and paging systems. Because of their increased flexibility as compared with other systems, FM systems can be used successfully in practically any listening environment, and are the most common assistive listening devices used in classrooms by students with hearing loss.

A recent addition to personal FM system amplification is the ear-level (BTE) FM receiver/hearing aid combination. This unit provides the user with a personal hearing aid and allows FM reception while eliminating the cords, neckloops, and body-worn receivers inherent in conventional FM systems.

FM technology is also available for use in soundfield amplification. In such systems, the audio signal is transmitted through a wireless FM microphone to several

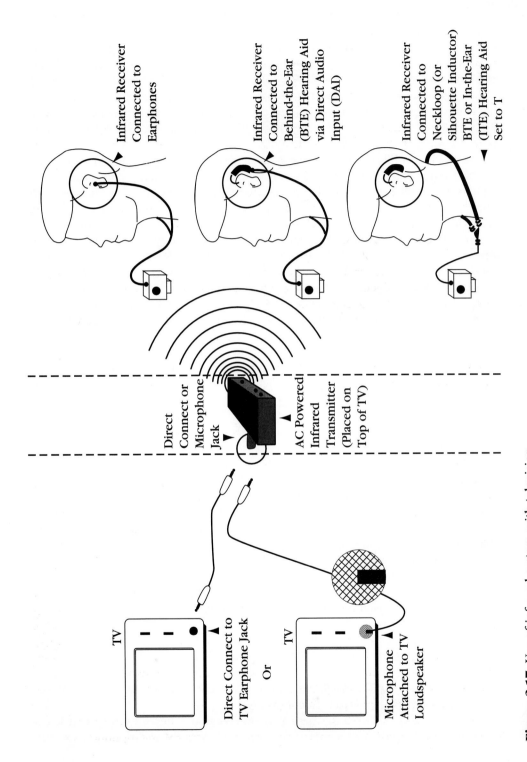

Figure 2.17 Use of infrared system with television.

Reprinted from C. Compton (1991). *Assistive devices: Doorways to independence.* Annapolis, MD: Van Comp Associates.

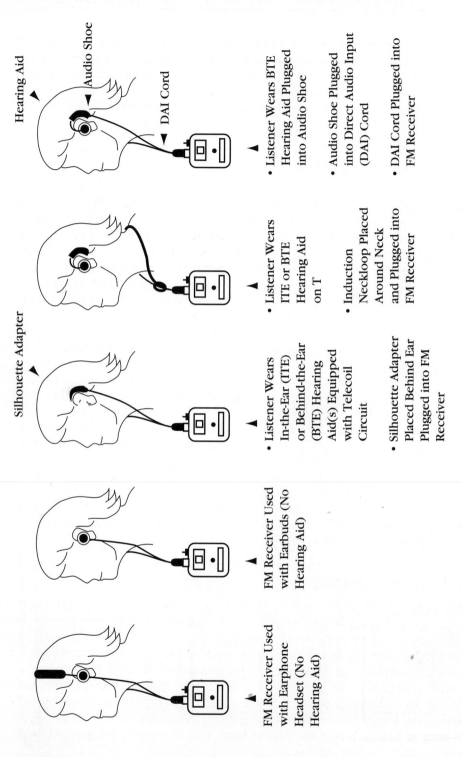

Figure 2.18 Methods of sound pickup from an FM receiver.

Reprinted with permission from C. Compton (1991). *Assistive devices: Doorways to independence.* Annapolis, MD: Van Comp Associates.

FM Receiver Used with Earphone Headset (No Hearing Aid)

FM Receiver Used with Earbuds (No Hearing Aid)

Silhouette Adapter

- Listener Wears In-the-Ear (ITE) or Behind-the-Ear (BTE) Hearing Aid(s) Equipped with Telecoil Circuit

- Silhouette Adapter Placed Behind Ear Plugged into FM Receiver

- Hearing Aid Set to Telecoil

- Listener Wears ITE or BTE Hearing Aid on T

- Induction Neckloop Placed Around Neck and Plugged into FM Receiver

Hearing Aid

Audio Shoe

DAI Cord

- Listener Wears BTE Hearing Aid Plugged into Audio Shoe

- Audio Shoe Plugged into Direct Audio Input (DAI) Cord

- DAI Cord Plugged into FM Receiver

loudspeakers mounted on the walls or ceiling. Soundfield FM systems are typically utilized in the classroom, and offer an advantage over personal FM systems in that they provide an improved signal for all students in the classroom without requiring use of a specialized receiver. They are also lower in cost and easier to maintain as compared to personal FM systems. Their use is generally limited to milder degrees of hearing loss.

Telephone Devices

People with hearing impairments often complain about problems using the telephone. As discussed earlier in this chapter, many hearing aids have a built-in telecoil which, when activated, helps to eliminate background noise and the acoustic feedback that occurs when the telephone receiver is held near the hearing-aid microphone. Unfortunately, telecoils are not available on all hearing aids and are not equally efficient with all telephones. Moreover, performance characteristics of hearing aid telecoils often vary substantially, depending on the type of hearing aid and its manufacturer. As an alternative, telephone amplifiers that increase the loudness of the telephone signal are available. These units may be portable and attach directly over the earpiece of the telephone, or they can be built into the receiver of the telephone. Most models have a volume control so the user can adjust the signal to a comfortable listening level.

Individuals who are deaf and profoundly hearing impaired must rely on nonauditory means of telephone communication via the TDD, or Telecommunication Device for the Deaf. This device is also referred to as a "text telephone." TDDs are computerized systems which allow the user to directly call another person having similar equipment. Messages are typed and transmitted to the other individual's telephone/TDD and the typed message is visually displayed on a screen. Some TDDs have a paper printout for a permanent record of the conversation. Calls from a TDD user also can be placed indirectly with individuals not having a TDD through a recently introduced relay system, available throughout the United States (see Chapter 6). Although TDDs are used mostly by people who are deaf, they are also used by individuals with less severe hearing losses and by speech-impaired people who experience difficulty communicating over the telephone.

Radio/Television Devices

Listening to the television or radio in the presence of background noise may also be frustrating for the person with hearing impairment. With the use of an assistive listening device, however, the user can maintain control over the loudness he or she receives, while the volume on the radio or television is set to a level comfortable for others. As described earlier, devices may be connected via direct wiring from the TV or radio to earphones, or may couple to the listener's hearing aid via direct audio input or by induction neckloop (for use with the telecoil on a hearing aid). Transmission may be accomplished through direct wiring from the amplifier to the earphone or hearing aid, or via wireless infrared or FM devices that send the audio signal directly to a compatible receiver worn by the listener.

Closed-captioned decoders provide television access to individuals with deafness as well as severe hearing impairment. These units inset subtitles onto the screen of the television, allowing the user to understand the audio portion of the television program by reading the subtitles. Closed-captioned capability is now required on all new televisions with screens larger than 13 inches, in accordance with the Television Decoder Circuitry Act of 1993.

Signaling Devices

A hearing aid generally enables a person to hear most sounds, but if a person is not wearing the hearing aid, is in another room from the sound, or is using an assistive device to listen to the television, some sounds may go unnoticed. To address these situations, signaling devices can be set up to monitor the telephone, alarm clock, doorbell, smoke alarm, and even a crying baby. Most of these devices automatically flash a light or activate a wrist-worn vibrator to alert the person to the sound source. Others increase the intensity of the sound source, or change its frequency, to make it audible to the hearing impaired listener. Still other types of alerting devices are capable of activating a bed vibrator or fan to awaken a sleeping person. These devices can be very important for individuals with hearing impairment as they carry out their daily routines.

Cochlear Implants

When the ear cannot be stimulated acoustically, as with a conventional hearing aid, it is sometimes possible to stimulate electrically whatever nerve fibers may remain. Cochlear implants are used for direct stimulation of the auditory nerve via electrode(s) placed within the cochlea. The number of electrodes may range from 1 to 22. Several cochlear implant systems are commercially available. Although each system differs in design, all consist of the same basic components. You should notice that cochlear implants function in a manner somewhat similar to that of a conventional hearing aid, although they are more complex (Figure 2.19):

1. An external microphone picks up sound waves, converts them to an electrical signal, and transmits them to an external processor.
2. The processor amplifies and filters the electrical signal and then transmits it to the external receiver located behind the pinna.
3. From the external receiver, the signal is magnetically induced across the skin barrier to the internal receiver, which is surgically implanted under the skin behind the pinna.
4. The internal receiver converts the magnetic signal into an electrical signal which is directed to the electrodes leading to the cochlea.
5. The electrodes stimulate available nerve fibers within the cochlea, producing a sensation of sound.

Approximately four to six weeks following surgical placement of the cochlear implant, an audiologist can program the external speech processor. Using customized

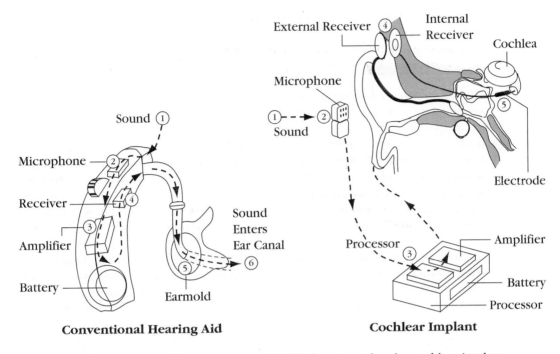

Figure 2.19 Basic components of a BTE hearing aid and a cochlear implant.

From F. Bess and L. Hume (1995). *Audiology: The Fundamentals* (2nd ed.). Baltimore: Williams & Wilkins.

software, each electrode is programmed to respond to a specific frequency and amplitude range. Generally, more basally located electrodes will respond to high frequencies and more apically located electrodes will respond best to lower frequencies, following the normal tonotopic organization of the cochlea. Although the implant will not restore hearing, it is capable of providing sound awareness and timing cues such as rate and rhythm, which can assist the listener in speechreading. In recent years, an increasing number of implant patients also are able to realize some *auditory-only* speech perception, even for open set material—some are able to conduct conversations on the telephone. The implant also allows the user to monitor vocal pitch and loudness more effectively and thus aid in speech production.

Not all individuals with profound hearing loss will benefit from implantation. A potential user must undergo complete medical, psychological, and audiological assessment as well as assessments by other professionals such as speech-language pathologists. Potential adult implant candidates can be categorized according to three protocols: profound, severe, or pre/perilinguistic (see Skinner, Holden, & Binzer, 1994 for review). Implant patients must be psychologically motivated to undergo the necessary surgery and subsequent aural rehabilitation following implantation, and be motivated to use hearing for communication and other purposes. Consequently, only a small portion of individuals with hearing impairment are viable candidates for cochlear implantation at present. However, this device has been improved dramatically in the past three decades, and its use will likely increase in the future.

Tactile Devices

Like the cochlear implant, the purpose of the tactile device is to provide cues for speech and environmental sounds to persons with profound hearing impairment, to aid in speech reception and production. Tactile devices have been shown to significantly enhance speechreading abilities and can be used in conjunction with conventional hearing aids in patients for whom cochlear implants are contraindicated. Tactile devices receive sound waves through a microphone, and convert the sound waves into electrical signals. These electrical signals are transmitted directly to small vibrators which are worn on the surface of the skin, and stimulate the sense of touch. The number, size, and spacing of the vibrators depends on the body site where they will be used. Vibrators may be placed on the hand, wrist, arm, thigh, or chest. There are currently 6 commercially available tactile devices, which range in price from $400 to approximately $1500, depending on the complexity of the system. Devices range from simple one-channel units to complex multichannel systems. Single-channel devices vibrate the skin at a constant rate. The strength of vibration is proportional to the intensity of the signal. For speech, the single channel device is somewhat limited and capable of displaying only rudimentary fundamental frequency information. Multiple channel aids can present tactile information along two dimensions. Signals of different frequency result in stimulation at different places on the skin, and the strength of stimulation at each location is proportional to the intensity of the signal.

Tinnitus Maskers

A relatively high percentage of the hearing impaired experience tinnitus along with their hearing loss. In some cases where the degree of tinnitus is excessive, it may be very disruptive for the individual; so much so, for example, that it may cause them to lose sleep. In these instances, it may be adviseable to consider the use of a device termed *tinnitus masker*. The tinnitus masker produces a band of noise composed of frequencies at or near those of the patient's tinnitus, thereby masking it. The circuitry needed to produce the masking noise for the tinnitus is often built into a conventional BTE hearing aid, thus providing help for the person's hearing difficulties as well. When this is done, the unit is referred to as a *tinnitus instrument*. Of course, other methods of relieving the effects of tinnitus also exist, and patients are encouraged to discuss their individual circumstances with their physicians and audiologist.

SUMMARY

We know that the hearing aid (or assistive listening device) is a crucial portion, but certainly not the only part of the audiologic rehabilitation process. It is, however, an important early step! Identifying the candidate and selecting the most appropriate style of amplification is a necessary starting point. Choosing the best circuitry, and adjusting this circuitry to the individual's hearing loss and listening needs is also essential. Valid and reliable verification techniques must be chosen. Appropriate post-fitting adjustments, counseling, and hearing aid orientation are also critical. Is all this easy? No. Does it take time? Yes. But with some effort, the pay-off is a patient with improved speech intelligibility and communication skills, who is appropriately equipped to hone these skills through the other facets of the audiology rehabilitative process.

SUGGESTED READINGS

Bentler, R. A. (1993). Amplification for the hearing-impaired child. In J. G. Alpiner & P. A. McCarthy (Eds.), *Rehabilitative audiology: Children and adults* (pp. 72–105). Baltimore: Williams & Wilkins.

Compton, C. L. (1989). *Assistive devices: Doorways to independence.* Washington, DC: Assistive Device Center, Gallaudet University.

Hawkins, D. B. (1992). Prescriptive approaches to selection of gain and frequency response. In Mueller, H.G., Hawkins, D. B., & Northern, J. L. (Eds.), *Probe microphone measurements* (pp. 91–112). San Diego: Singular Publishing Group.

Mueller, H. G. (1992). Terminology and procedures. In Mueller, H.G., Hawkins, D. B., & Northern, J. L. (Eds.), *Probe microphone measurements* (pp. 41–66). San Diego: Singular Publishing Group.

Mueller, H. G. & Bright, K. E. (1994). Selection and verification of maximum output. In Valente, M. (Ed.), *Strategies for selecting and verifying hearing aid fittings* (pp. 38–63). New York: Thieme Medical Publishers, Inc.

Mueller, H. G. & Grimes, A. M. (1993). Hearing aid selection and assessment. In Alpiner, J. G. & McCarthy, P.A. (Eds.), *Rehabilitative audiology: Children and adults* (pp. 284–310). Baltimore: Williams & Wilkins.

Pascoe, D. P. (1990). Post-fitting and rehabilitative management of the adult hearing aid user. In Sandlin, R. E. (Ed.), *Handbook of hearing aid amplification* (Vol. 2, pp. 61–86). Boston: College Hill Press.

REFERENCES

American Speech-Language-Hearing Association (1992, August). Report: Considerations in screening adults/elderly persons for handicapping hearing impairment. *Asha, 34,* pp. 81–87.

Bentler, R. A. (1993). Amplification for the hearing-impaired child. In J. G. Alpiner & P. A. McCarthy (Eds.), *Rehabilitative audiology: Children and adults* (pp. 72–105). Baltimore: Williams & Wilkins.

Carhart, R. (1946). Selection of hearing aids. *Archives of Otolaryngology, 44,* 1–18.

Compton, C. L. (1989). *Assistive devices: Doorways to independence.* Washington, DC: Assistive Device Center, Gallaudet University.

Cox, R. M., & Alexander, G. C. (1984, April). *The abbreviated profile of hearing aid benefit (APHAB).* Paper presented at the annual meeting of the American Academy of Audiology, Richmond, VA.

Hawkins, D. B. (1992). Prescriptive approaches to selection of gain and frequency response. In Mueller, H.G., Hawkins, D. B., & Northern, J. L. (Eds.), *Probe microphone measurements* (pp. 91–112). San Diego: Singular Publishing Group.

Killion, M., Staab, W., & Preves, D. (1990). Classifying automatic signal processors. *Hearing Instruments, 41*(8), 24–26.

McCarthy, P.A. (1994). Self-assessment inventories: They're not just for aural rehab anymore. *The Hearing Journal, 47*(5), 10, 41–43.

Mueller, H. G. (1994). Small can be good too! *The Hearing Journal, 47*(10), 11.

Mueller, H. G. (1994). Update on programmable hearing aids. *The Hearing Journal, 47*(5), 13–20.

Mueller, H. G. (1992). Terminology and procedures. In Mueller, H.G., Hawkins, D. B., & Northern, J. L. (Eds.), *Probe microphone measurements* (pp. 41–66). San Diego: Singular Publishing Group.

Mueller, H. G., & Bright, K.W. (1994). Selection and verification of maximum output. In Valente, M. (Ed.), *Strategies for selecting and verifying hearing aid fittings* (pp. 38–63). New York: Thieme Medical Publishers, Inc.

Mueller, H. G., & Grimes, A. M. (1987). Amplification systems for the hearing impaired. In J. G. Alpiner & P.A. McCarthy (Eds.), *Rehabilitative audiology: Children and adults* (pp. 115–160). Baltimore: Williams & Wilkins.

Mueller, H. G., & Grimes, A. M. (1993). Hearing aid selection and assessment. In J. G. Alpiner & P.A. McCarthy (Eds.), *Rehabilitative audiology: Children and adults* (pp. 284–310). Baltimore: Williams & Wilkins.

Mueller, H. G., & Killion, M. C. (1990). An easy method for calculating the articulation index. *The Hearing Journal, 45*(9), 14–17.

Pascoe, D. P. (1990). Post-fitting and rehabilitative management of the adult hearing aid user. In Sandlin, R. E. (Ed.), *Handbook of hearing aid amplification* (Vol. 2, pp. 61–86). Boston: College Hill Press.

Seewald, R. C. & Ross, M. (1988). Amplification for young hearing impaired children. In M. C. Pollack (Ed.), *Amplification for the hearing impaired* (3rd ed.). New York: Grune and Stratton.

Schow, R. L., & Nerbonne, M. A. (1982). Communication screening profile: Use with elderly clients. *Ear and Hearing, 3,* 135–147.

Schow, R. L., & Gatehouse, S. (1990). Fundamental issues in self-assessment of hearing. *Ear and Hearing, 11,* 6S–16S.

Skinner, M. W., Holden, L. K., & Binzer, S. M. (1994). Aural rehabilitation for individuals with severe and profound hearing impairment: Hearing aids, cochlear implants, counseling, and training. In Valente, M. (Ed.), *Strategies for selecting and verifying hearing aid fittings* (pp. 267-299). New York: Thieme Medical Publishers, Inc.

Ventry, I. & Weinstein, B. (1983). Identification of elderly people with hearing problems. *American Speech and Hearing Association Journal*, 25, 37-42.

Weinstein, B. E. (1993). Needs of the geriatric population. In J. G. Alpiner & P. A. McCarthy (Eds.), *Rehabilitative audiology: Children and adults* (pp. 489-499). Baltimore: Williams & Wilkins.

Weinstein, B. E. & Ventry, I. (1983). Audiometric correlates of the hearing handicap inventory for the elderly. *Journal of Speech and Hearing Disorders*, 48, 379-384.

3

READ!

Auditory Stimuli in Communication

MICHAEL A. NERBONNE
RONALD L. SCHOW

Contents

INTRODUCTION

Traditionally, the ability to communicate meaningfully has been considered a prime factor in differentiating humans from other forms of life. A human act of communication can take a variety of forms, involving the conveyance of various stimuli to one or more of our sensory modalities. The form of communication most often used to express oneself, oral communication, involves utilization of speech. This creates an extraordinary dependence on the sense of hearing in order to receive and perceive adequately the complex network of auditory stimuli which comprise speech. The sense of hearing, therefore, is crucial to the process of oral communication.

The onset of a significant auditory impairment in an individual can seriously impede the ability to communicate. Although a hearing loss may trigger other difficulties of a psychosocial, educational, or vocational nature, the inability of the person with hearing impairment to communicate normally serves as a fundamental cause of these other problems. Based on the critical role of audition in communication, audiologic rehabilitation represents an extremely important process whereby an individual's diminished ability to communicate as the result of a hearing loss can, it is hoped, be sharpened and improved. One of the areas of audiologic rehabilitation which has traditionally been included in this process is auditory training. This procedure generally involves an attempt to assist the child or adult with a hearing impairment in maximizing the use of whatever degree of residual hearing remains.

This chapter will provide information regarding auditory training with patients with hearing impairment, including objectives and applications, assessment of auditory skills prior to therapy, and exposure to some of the past and present approaches to providing auditory training. Because of the conviction that the professional providing auditory training must be familiar with the basic aspects of oral communication, information is also provided about the oral communication process. This includes the introduction of a communication model, information regarding auditory perception and the acoustics of speech, and a discussion of the possible effects of hearing loss on speech perception.

A COMMUNICATION MODEL

Although a portion of the communication that normally takes place between individuals is nonverbal, we remain heavily dependent on our ability to receive and interpret auditory stimuli presented during oral communication. Successful oral communication involves a number of key components that deserve elaboration so that the reader may gain an appreciation of the basic process. All oral communication must originate with a source or speaker who has both a purpose for engaging in communication and the ability to properly encode and articulate the thought to be conveyed. The actual thought to be expressed is termed the *message*. The message is made up of auditory stimuli organized in meaningful linguistic units. Visual cues are also provided by the speaker in conjunction with the production of the auditory message. A critical component of the encoding process is the feedback mechanism, made up primarily of the auditory system of the speaker, which makes it possible to monitor, and if need be, correct the accuracy of the intended message. The communication situation in which the message is conveyed is referred to as the *environment*. Factors associated with the environment, such as the presence of competing background noise, can drastically alter the amount and quality of the communication that takes place. The final major component of the communication process is the *receiver* or *listener*, who is charged with the responsibility of receiving and properly decoding and interpreting the speaker's intended thought.

These basic components of the oral communication process and their sequence are found in Figure 3.1. All the major components are equally important in accomplishing the desired end—communication. Disruption or elimination of any one part may result in partial or complete failure of the communication process. Proper application of this communication model is of concern to us throughout the chapter and the entire book.

AUDITORY PERCEPTION

Our ability to communicate verbally with others depends to a great extent on the quality of our auditory perception of the various segmental (individual speech sounds) and suprasegmental (rate, rhythm, intonation) elements that comprise speech. The following sections will focus on the auditory perception of nonspeech stimuli; the intensity, frequency, and duration components of speech; and transitional cues. The impact of hearing loss on speech perception is also discussed.

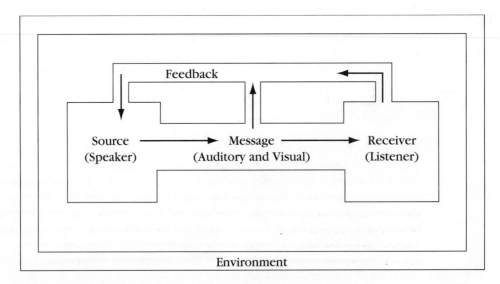

Figure 3.1 A simple model of the oral communication process.

Development of Auditory Skills

Substantial evidence exists to support the fact that the unborn infant possesses a functional auditory system that allows the child to perceive auditory stimuli several weeks prior to birth (Bench, 1968; Eisenberg, 1965a, 1965b). Further development and refinement in the neonate's auditory-processing skills in the days and weeks immediately following birth also have been demonstrated by Eisenberg (1970). Her findings indicate that the newborn infant not only is capable of detecting auditory stimuli, but also can make gross discriminations between various auditory signals on the basis of frequency and intensity parameters. This process of selective listening is extended to phonemic signals within a few weeks following birth (Eimas, 1975; Eisenberg, 1976; Moffitt, 1971). The rather rapid emergence of auditory skills, as described by Northern and Downs (1994), is crucial for the development of speech and language in the infant. Without the benefit of ample auditory stimulation, however, the development of language will be seriously affected. And although the basic auditory skills necessary for the normal acquisition of language and speech are present to some degree at birth or shortly thereafter, these skills are sharpened further during the early years of an individual's life.

Perception of Nonspeech Stimuli

Although the human auditory system has sophisticated perceptual capabilities, it is limited, to some extent, in terms of the signals it can process. Optimally, the normal human ear is capable of perceiving auditory signals comprising frequencies between about 20 and 20,000 Hz. Stimuli made up entirely of frequencies below and above these limits cannot be detected. Intensity limits, as shown in Figure 3.2, vary as a function of the frequency of the auditory stimulus. The maximum range of intensity we are capable of processing occurs at 3000–4000 Hz, and varies from about 0–140 dB SPL. Signals with intensity of less than 0 dB SPL are generally not perceived; in contrast, signals in excess of 140 dB SPL produce the sensation of pain rather than of hearing.

In addition to the detection of acoustic signals, the human ear is also able to discriminate different stimuli on the basis of only minor differences in their acoustical properties. The study of our ability to discriminate differences in auditory signals has centered around three parameters of sound; namely, frequency, intensity, and duration. Results of such investigations have revealed a complex interaction among these variables. Thus, our ability to discriminate changes in the frequency, intensity, or duration of a signal is influenced by the magnitude of each of the other factors. Stevens and Davis (1938) estimated that the normal ear is capable of perceiving approximately 340,000 distinguishable tones within the audible range of hearing. This total number was based only on frequency and intensity variations of the stimuli, and it suggests that our auditory system possesses amazing discrimination powers.

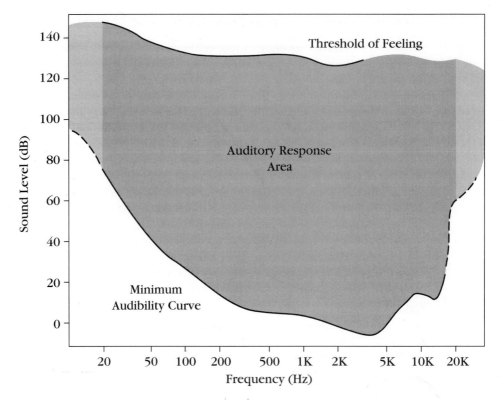

Figure 3.2 The auditory response area for persons with normal hearing.

Durrant J.D. & Lovrinic J.H. (1984), *Bases of Hearing Science* (2nd ed), Baltimore, MD: Williams & Wilkins. Reprinted by permission.

Acoustics of Speech

Knowledge about the acoustical properties of speech is important for understanding how speech is perceived. Therefore, basic information relevant to this process will be covered in the following sections.

Intensity Parameters of Speech. The human ear is capable of processing signals within an intensity range approaching 130–140 dB; however, the range of intensity normally found in speech is relatively small. Fletcher (1953) reported that the average intensity of connected speech, when measured at a distance of approximately 1 meter from the speaker, approximates 65 dB SPL. This corresponds to a value of about 45 dB HL when expressed audiometrically. The average shout will approach 85 dB SPL (65 dB HL), while faint speech occurs at about 45 dB SPL (25 dB HL). Thus, a range of about 40 dB typifies the softest to the loudest connected speech we are exposed to in common communication situations. Factors such as distance between the speaker and listener can influence the intensity levels for a given communication situation.

Considerable variability also exists in the acoustical energy normally associated with individual speech sounds. Table 3.1 lists the relative phonetic powers of the

TABLE 3.1 *Relative Phonetic Power of Speech Sounds as Produced by an Average Speaker*

ɔ	680	l	100	t	15
ɑ	600	ʃ	80	g	15
ʌ	510	ŋ	73	k	13
æ	490	m	52	v	12
ʊ	460	tʃ	42	ð	11
ɛ	350	n	36	b	7
u	310	dʒ	23	d	7
ɪ	260	ʒ	20	p	6
i	220	z	16	f	5
r	210	s	16	θ	1

Source: Speech and Hearing in Communication by H. Fletcher, 1953, Princeton: D. VanNostrand.

phonemes, as reported by Fletcher (1953). As illustrated, the most powerful phoneme, /ɔ/, possesses an average of about 68 times as much energy as the weakest phoneme, /θ/, representing an average overall difference in intensity between the two speech sounds of approximately 28 dB. Since a considerable amount of variability also exists in the intensity of individual voices, Fletcher estimated that, collectively, different speakers may produce variations in the intensity of these two phonemes as great as 56 dB. The relative power of vowels, according to Fletcher, is significantly greater than that of consonants, with the weakest vowel, /i/, having more energy than the most powerful consonant or semivowel, /ɝ/. Further, typical male speakers produce speech with an overall intensity that is about 3 dB greater than that of female speakers.

Frequency Parameters of Speech. The overall spectrum of speech, as seen in Figure 3.3, is composed of acoustical energy from approximately 50–10,000 Hz (Denes & Pinson, 1993). Closer examination of this figure also reveals that the greatest amount of energy found in speech generally occurs below 1000 Hz. Above this frequency region, the energy of speech decreases at about a 9-dB/octave rate. The concentration of energy in the lower frequencies can be largely attributed to the fundamental frequency of the adult human voice (males—130 Hz, females—260 Hz; Zemlin, 1981) and the high intensity and spectral characteristics associated with the production of vowels. It should be noted that the fundamental frequency of children is substantially higher than that of adults, around 450 Hz (McGlone, 1966). As a result, the major energy concentration for this age group occurs higher on the frequency scale than for adults.

The vowels in English are composed mainly of low- and mid-frequency energy and, as indicated earlier, contribute most of the acoustic power in speech. Specifically, the frequency spectrum of each vowel contains at least two or three areas of energy concentration that result from the resonances that occur in the vocal tract during phonation. These points of peak amplitude are referred to as *formants,* and their location on the frequency continuum varies for each vowel. Figure 3.4 illustrates the approximate location of the major formants associated with the vowels, as spoken by

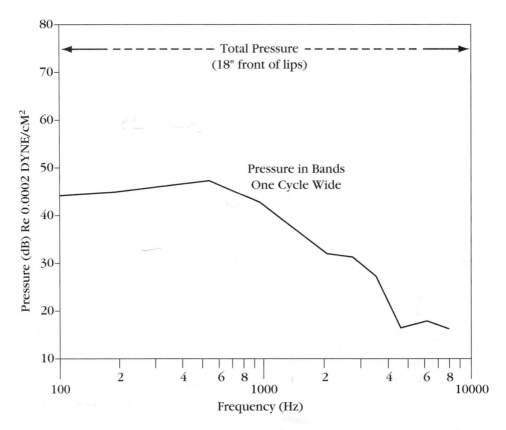

Figure 3.3 Long-interval acoustic spectrum of male voices. Measurement made with microphone 17 inches from speaker's lips.

Miller, G.A. *Language and Communication.* New York: McGraw-Hill. p. 87. (1951).

adult males. It is important to note that even though vowels generally have several formants, we need only hear the first two or three to be able to perceive accurately the vowel spoken (Peterson & Barney, 1952).

The consonants in English display a broader high-frequency spectral composition than do vowels. This is particularly true for those consonants for which voicing is not utilized and whose production involves substantial constriction of the articulators. Although they contain relatively little overall energy when compared with vowels, consonants are extremely important in determining the intelligibility of speech. Consequently, accurate perception of consonants is vital.

Figure 3.5 contains estimates of the combined intensity and frequency values associated with the individual speech sounds in English. Specifically, the vertical axis presents the intensity levels in dB HL of the major components of each sound (if a particular sound has more than one major frequency component, each is noted by the same phonetic symbol), while the horizontal axis expresses the general frequency region for each speech sound. A close inspection of this figure discloses, as indi-

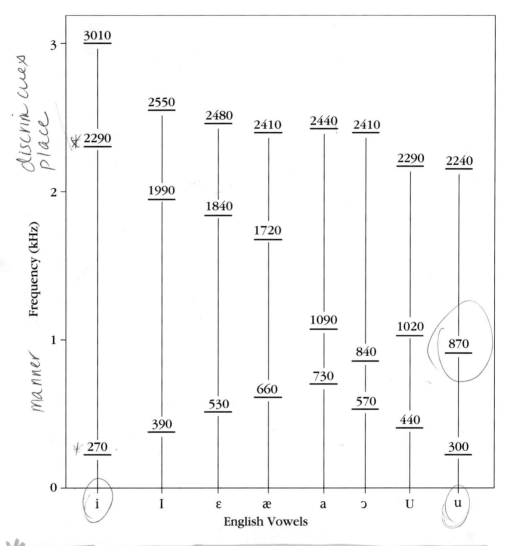

Figure 3.4 Mean values of formant frequencies of vowels of American English for adult males.

Peterson, G. E., & Barney, H. L. (1952). Control methods used in the study of the vowels. *Journal of the Acoustical Society of America, 32*, 693–703.

cated earlier, that the vowels can generally be characterized as having considerable acoustic energy, for the most part confined to the low- and mid-frequency range. On the other hand, the consonants demonstrate decidedly less intensity overall and a much more diffuse frequency distribution as a group. The voiced consonants generally possess a greater amount of low- and mid-frequency energy, while the unvoiced consonants are made up of mid- and high frequencies. All consonants appear in the upper portion of the figure, reflecting their weaker intensity values.

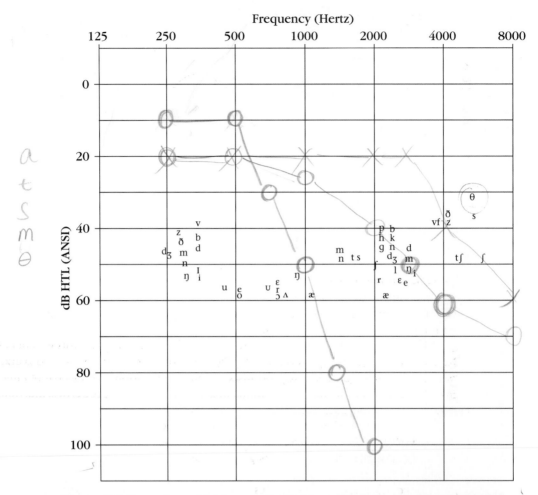

Figure 3.5 Intensity and frequency distribution of speech sounds in the English language. The values given should be considered only approximations, and are based on data reported by Fletcher (1953) and Ling & Ling (1978). Sounds with more than one major component appear in more than one location in the figure.

In addition to the spectral properties associated with each of the consonants, it is important to identify the frequency characteristics related to the distinctive features of these phonemes. Miller and Nicely's (1955) classification system includes five features: voicing, nasality, affrication, duration, and place of articulation. According to Boothroyd (1978), the voiced/voiceless distinction, as well as cues for nasality and affrication, are primarily carried by low-frequency energy. Information about place of articulation, on the other hand, is contained in the higher frequencies. Table 3.2 categorizes each consonant phoneme by its place and manner features and voicing.

Finally, as indicated by Ling (1978), the important suprasegmental aspects of speech (e.g., intonation, rhythm, pitch, stress) are conveyed primarily by the low-frequency components of speech.

TABLE 3.2 *Categorizing Consonants on the Basis of Mannner and Place of Articulation and Voicing*

Manner of Articulation	Place of Articulation						
	Bilabial	*Labiodental*	*Linguadental*	*Alveolar*	*Palatal*	*Velar*	*Glottal*
Plosives or Stops	p b			t d		k g	
Fricatives		f v	θ ð	s z	ʃ ʒ		h
Affricative					tʃ dʒ		
Nasal	m			n		ŋ	
Liquid				l,r			
Glide	w				j		

Note: Voiceless consonants are listed first, with voiced consonants underneath.

Temporal Parameters of Speech. The duration of individual speech sounds in our language covers a range from about 30–300 msec (Lehiste, 1976). A number of factors can significantly influence the duration of a given phoneme, making the direct comparison of duration among phonemes difficult. Yet the research of Crandall (1925), as cited by Fletcher (1953) and Lisker (1957), suggests that vowels generally have a longer duration than consonants. Fletcher considered vowels to have average durations of between 130 and 360 msec, while the duration of consonants ranges from 20–150 msec. In spite of variations in absolute durational properties, individual phoneme duration does contribute toward speech perception. For instance, Minifie (1973) pointed out that the duration of stop consonants (examples: /p/ and /b/) varies systematically in a vowel-consonant-vowel context, with correct perception of the speech sound depending, to a degree, on the durational property of the phoneme produced.

As we all know, speakers' rates of speech differ considerably. The research of Goldman-Eisler, as discussed by Lehiste (1970), demonstrates that the average rate of speech used during connected discourse will result in the production of about 4.4 to 5.9 syllables per second. The normal rate of speech, as expressed in phoneme output, can result in the production of as many as 15 phonemes per second (Orr, Friedman, & Williams, 1965). Thus, the articulatory process is swift and capable of producing a flood of speech sounds and words that must be processed as effectively by the receiver, or listener, as they were produced by the speaker. Both of these are challenging tasks!

Transitional Cues. The acoustic properties of a given phoneme spoken in isolation are altered significantly when the phoneme is produced in connected discourse or conversational speech. In connected discourse the dynamic movements of the articulators in the production of adjacent phonemes produce acoustical byproducts, termed *transitional cues.* These cues make up a large portion of the total speech signal and are utilized extensively in the perception of speech, since they contain valuable information related to individual phoneme perception.

For example, the second and third formants of vowels often contain transitions in frequency produced by the flowing movement of the articulators that signal the presence of particular consonants that immediately follow. These formant transitions occur as the vocal resonances shift during articulation of vowels and consonants, which are combined in speech. Likewise, the durational aspects of vowels in connected speech can be altered to convey information regarding the phoneme to follow. For example, a voiced consonant in the final position is often accompanied by increased duration of the vowel immediately before it. The prolonged vowel duration contributes to our perception of voicing in the consonant which follows. This is an example of why transitional cues are a vital part of the speech signal and are quite important for speech perception.

Speech Perception/Comprehension

Our discussion has emphasized the segmental and suprasegmental aspects that constitute speech. The organization and production of these crucial elements into a meaningful oral message by the speaker and the accurate reception of this dynamic signal by the listener represent a highly complex, sophisticated process. However, mere reception of the speech stimuli by a listener does not result in proper perception of the message. Perception of speech implies understanding and comprehension, and the reception of speech signals by the auditory mechanism is only a first step in its perception.

In its most basic form, the perception/comprehension of speech may be thought of as involving a number of components. Among these are:

Detection.   This aspect of auditory perception involves experiencing the awareness of sound. Our ability to detect speech is influenced by our hearing acuity and the intensity level of the speech signal.

Discrimination.   Speech discrimination refers to the ability to distinguish among the individual speech stimuli (phonemes, syllables, etc.) of our language. How accurately we perceive the individual elements of speech is of relevance.

Identification.   The ability to identify or label what one has heard by repeating, pointing to, or writing a word or sentence.

Attention.   A fundamental ingredient in the perception of speech relates to attending to or focusing on the speaker and the message being conveyed. The degree and quality of the listener's attention will influence how well speech is perceived.

Memory.   A key component in speech perception is the ability to retain or store verbal information for relatively brief periods or, in some instances, extended lengths of time. Memory is also fundamental to other components of speech perception and enables us to combine individual speech units for the purpose of deriving meaning from an entire verbal message, rather than from each individual unit of the message.

Closure.   The speech elements which are received, properly discriminated, and retained for further processing must be brought together into a meaningful whole. This is a difficult task at best, but when we do not adequately receive all the contents of a verbal message, as often occurs with a hearing loss, closure can still occur through a process wherein missing information is deduced by the listener on the basis of the available context.

Our task in audiologic rehabilitation should be to take into consideration what is currently known concerning speech perception as we work with individuals with hearing impairments.

Speech Perception and Hearing Loss

Our success in processing speech stimuli is closely related to our ability to receive the coded acoustical information which constitutes the signal. Hence, hearing impairment may have grave implications for proper speech perception. In the following section, we shall consider the effects of physical properties of speech, redundancy, and constraints on speech perception.

Physical Properties.   Information concerning the physical properties of speech is most relevant when considering the relationship between the perception of speech and hearing loss, for the degree of our success in processing speech stimuli appears closely related to our ability to receive the coded acoustical information which makes up the signal.

The normal ear is well equipped to receive and process speech in most situations. Since speech is normally presented at average intensity levels of around 45 dB HL, it is well within the sensitivity range of the normal human ear. Also, although we are capable of hearing auditory signals ranging in frequency from about 20–20,000 Hz, only a portion of the entire range is required for the reception of speech, since speech contains energy from roughly 50–10,000 Hz. Consequently, in most listening conditions, those with normal hearing will have no difficulty in adequately receiving the speech sounds found in oral communication.

The same does not hold true for persons with hearing impairment. No longer are the intensity and frequency ranges of the impaired ear always sufficient to provide total perception of the speech signal. One or both of these stimulus parameters may be limited such that it becomes difficult to hear specific speech sounds adequately for identification purposes. For example, a person with 50-dB thresholds from 2000–8000 Hz would have considerable difficulty perceiving the phonemes with spectral compositions that primarily involve those higher frequencies. The information in Figure 3.5 regarding the relative frequency and intensity characteristics of individual speech sounds as spoken at a typical conversation level is significant in explaining why this occurs.

While factors such as type of hearing loss and test materials can influence the outcome of investigations concerning hearing loss and the perception of phonemes, some general patterns of speech-perception difficulties have been observed for persons with hearing loss. For instance, most hearing-impaired listeners experience only minimal difficulty in vowel perception (Owens, Benedict, & Schubert, 1971).

Specifically, in their research the vowel phonemes /ɛ/ and /o/ were found to have the highest probability of error. Only when the degree of impairment is severe to profound does the perception of vowels become significantly altered (Erber, 1979). Consonant perception, however, presents a far more difficult listening task for those with hearing impairment. Owens (1978) found phonemes such as /s/, /p/, /k/, /d/, and /θ/ to be among the most frequently missed by adults with sensorineural hearing loss. He also found discrimination errors to be more frequent for phonemes in the final position of words than in the initial position. The most common errors in consonant phoneme discrimination occur with the place of articulation feature (Boothroyd, 1978; Byers, 1973; Owens, 1978), followed by manner of articulation. Errors in the perception of nasality and voice among consonants are generally far less frequent.

Owens and his colleagues conducted a series of investigations regarding the perception of consonants. In one such study Owens et al. (1972) examined the relationship between the configuration of the audiogram and the specific consonant perceptual errors made by a group of hearing-impaired individuals. The /s/, /ʃ/, /ʧ/, /ʤ/ and the /t/ and /θ/ in the initial position only, were found to be difficult for listeners with sloping configurations on the audiogram. The authors noted that these phonemes became increasingly difficult to hear accurately as the steepness of the sloping high-frequency hearing loss increased. Correct recognition of /s/ and the initial /t/ and /θ/ were found to be closely related to hearing sensitivity above 2000 Hz, while perception of /ʃ/, /ʧ/, and /ʤ/, was very dependent on sensitivity between 1000–2000 Hz. These findings point out the crucial role which hearing in this frequency region plays in the perception of several consonant phonemes. A similar study by Sher and Owens (1974) with listeners having high-frequency impairments confirmed that individuals with normal hearing to 2000 Hz and a sharp-sloping sensitivity loss for frequencies above that experience difficulty in adequately hearing a number of consonant phonemes. These authors pointed out that information concerning phoneme errors is useful in establishing audiologic rehabilitation strategies for persons with hearing losses of this type.

As can be seen, the actual overall degree of difficulty in speech perception imposed on an individual is related to the intensity and frequency features of the hearing loss found on the conventional audiogram. However, this difficulty can also be influenced by other related variables, which will be discussed elsewhere in this chapter and throughout the text. Therefore, although research by Walden and Montgomery (1975) and Bilger and Wang (1976) supports the notion that the audiogram is our most useful single predictor of a person's speech perception abilities, predictions made based only on the results of pure-tone audiometry must be done with caution as they are prone to some degree of error (Sher & Owens, 1974).

Redundancy and Noise.   The perception of speech is a highly complex process that involves more than the acoustics of speech or the hearing abilities of the listener, even though these are important variables, to be sure. Ultimately, for oral communication to be successful, sufficient information must be present in the message of interest for it to be perceived. The amount of information available for a given communication situation is closely associated with the concepts of redundancy and noise.

TABLE 3.3 *A Partial List of Factors that Can Influence the Amount of Redundancy in Speech*

Within the Speaker	• Compliance with the rules of the language • Use of appropriate articulation, intonation, stress • Size/appropriateness of the vocabulary used to convey the message
Within the Message	• Number of syllables, words, etc. • Amount of context • Frequency composition of the speech signal • Intensity of the speech signal
Within the Communication Environment	• Amount of acoustic noise • Degree of reverberation • Number of situational cues present that are related to the message
Within the Listener	• Familiarity with the rules of the language • Familiarity with the vocabulary of the message • Knowledge of the topic of conversation • Hearing abilities

Adapted from Sanders, 1971.

Conversational speech generally can be described as being highly redundant. That is, it contains information from a variety of sources which is available for a listener to use in perceiving the essence of a message, even though portions of the communication may not have been heard. The degree of redundance in oral communication varies from one expression to the next, so the extent to which a listener can predict what was said will also vary. Basically, the more redundant a message, the more readily it can be perceived by the listener, especially in difficult listening situations. A number of factors present in a given communication situation can influence the amount of redundancy present, and Table 3.3 provides a list of some of these.

Among the many factors associated with the redundancy, or predictability, found in conversational speech for the listener to use for perception are structural, semantic, and situational constraints. Structural constraints relate to the predictable manner in which linguistic units are chained together according to the rules associated with acceptable English. The selection and use of phonemes and words in an utterance are strongly influenced by these rules, making it easier for the listener to predict what is to follow after having heard only the initial portion of the sentence. Such syntactic clues can be used in conjunction with another factor related to redundancy, namely semantic constraints, which allow the listener to predict the type of vocabulary and expressions to be used based on the general semantic content of the expression. When the topic of conversation is food, for example, the listener can expect to hear a rather restricted range of vocabulary peculiar to that particular topic. Use of this small range of words will increase the redundancy in what is said. Situational constraints also create redundancy. Our conversational partner, the location of the conversation, the time of day it takes place, and other similar factors all influence what we say and how we say it, which also can make conversational speech somewhat predictable. All of these types of constraints, along with other factors listed in

TABLE 3.4 *Some Potential Sources of Noise in Oral Communication*

Within the Speaker	• Poor syntax
	• Abnormal articulation
	• Improper stress/inflection
Within the Communication Environment	• Abnormal lighting
	• Competing/distracting visual stimuli
	• Competing/distracting auditory stimuli
	• Reverberation
Within the Listener	• Lack of familiarity with the rules of the language
	• Inability to identify the topic of the message
	• Poor listening skills

Adapted from Sanders, 1971.

Table 3.3, collectively produce the redundancy that makes the perception of speech easier for us all.

Noise in oral communication refers to a host of factors that can actually reduce the amount of information present for the listener to use. In this context, "noise" refers to a variety of variables that can be counterproductive to communication, not just competing auditory noise. Table 3.4 provides a partial list of the potential sources of noise associated with oral communication with which the listener must contend. Each of these factors may reduce the amount of information in a spoken message, thus reducing the amount of redundancy, or predictability, which is available for the listener to use in perceiving speech.

Thus, the degree of information available for the listener to use in perceiving a message is influenced in a positive or negative manner by a number of related variables that are part of oral communication. For the listener, particularly one with hearing impairment, the importance of each of these variables to the process of speech perception cannot be overstated.

AUDITORY TRAINING AND PERSONS WITH HEARING IMPAIRMENT

Traditionally, auditory training has been considered a major component of the audiologic rehabilitation process. Thus, its potential in assisting those with hearing loss has been expressed in major textbooks within the field of audiology, both in the past (Davis & Silverman, 1960; Oyer, 1966; Davis & Hardick, 1981) and recently (Alpiner & McCarthy, 1993; Hull, 1992; Sanders, 1993). Yet, even though auditory training is considered to be an integral part of audiologic rehabilitation, its actual benefits for the person with hearing impairment have rarely been fully assessed (Walden & Grant, 1993). This lack of validation, in part, serves to explain why some forms of auditory training are not utilized more frequently with individuals with hearing loss.

The intent of the next major section of this chapter is to familiarize the reader with both the traditional and the current forms of auditory training and how they fit into the entire audiologic rehabilitation process.

Definition/Application of Auditory Training

Numerous attempts have been made to define auditory training in the past. Though similar in some respects, these definitions vary considerably according to the orientation of the definer and special considerations dictated by factors associated with hearing loss, such as its degree and time of onset.

Goldstein (1939), for example, worked primarily with deaf children and felt that auditory training involved a development and/or improvement in the ability to discriminate various properties of speech and nonspeech signals. These properties include loudness, pitch, rhythm, and inflection. Goldstein's approach was directed toward facilitating the perception of speech, and included the use of a variety of verbal and nonverbal stimuli during therapy.

Probably the most commonly referred-to definition of auditory training is attributed to Carhart (1960), who considered auditory training a process of teaching the child or adult with hearing impairment to take full advantage of available auditory clues. As a result, Carhart recommended an emphasis in therapy on developing an awareness of sound, gross discrimination of nonverbal stimuli, and gross and fine discrimination of speech.

More recently, in discussing the use of auditory training with children, Erber (1982) described it as

> the creation of special communication conditions in which teachers and audiologists help hearing-impaired children acquire many of the auditory perception abilities that normally hearing children acquire naturally without their intervention. (p. 1)

Erber stated further that:

> Our intent is to help the hearing-impaired child apply his or her impaired auditory sense to the fullest capacity in language communication, regardless of the degree of damage to the auditory system. Usually progress is achieved through careful application of amplification devices and through special teaching techniques. (p. 29)

When considering auditory training for adults, two general objectives are usually relevant: (a) learning to maximize the use of auditory and other related cues available for the perception of speech, and (b) adjustment and orientation to facilitate the optimum use of amplification, including cochlear implants and tactile devices. Inherent in the various views of auditory training, as well as those of other professionals in audiologic rehabilitation, is the notion that persons with hearing impairment can be trained to maximize the use of whatever amount of hearing they possess. The ultimate aim of auditory training is, therefore, to achieve maximum communication potential by developing the auditory sensory channel to its fullest. Although the primary goal of auditory training is usually to maximize receptive communication abilities, it is important to point out that achieving this basic goal can result in other important achievements, including acquisition of more proficient speech and language skills, educational and vocational advancement, and successful psychosocial adjustment. As indicated earlier, if the communication skills of persons with hearing impairment can be improved, other areas of concern, such as educational progress, will be facilitated as well.

Historical Overview

The earliest efforts in auditory training date back to the 18th century. Individuals in Europe used auditory training with the hearing impaired throughout the 1800s, with some success noted. Impressed with their accomplishments, Goldstein (1939) introduced a similar approach to auditory training in the United States in the late 1890s and early 1900s. Known as the Acoustic Method, this approach centered around systematic stimulation with individual speech sounds, syllables, words, and sentences to improve speech perception and to aid deaf persons in their own speech production. The Acoustic Method was utilized in a number of facilities throughout the country, including the Central Institute for the Deaf in St. Louis, Missouri, which Goldstein founded. Goldstein exerted a significant influence on the thinking of many professionals over the years regarding the potential of auditory training with persons with hearing impairment.

Early applications of auditory training were directed almost exclusively toward children with severe to profound hearing loss in a deaf-education setting. In recent times, however, use of auditory training has been expanded to include those with less severe impairments, as well as the inclusion of auditory-training activities in the rehabilitative management of hard-of-hearing adults and children. This has occurred, in part, as a result of significant improvements in hearing aids and the development of other electronic devices for persons with hearing impairment, such as the cochlear implant, which have made it possible for more persons to use their hearing effectively for communication. Growth in the use of auditory training can also be associated with the emergence of audiology as a profession following World War II, and the interest shown by audiologists in maximizing the use of residual hearing in persons with varying degrees of hearing loss as a part of the audiologic rehabilitation process. Thus, what was once perceived as a procedure to be used only with deaf children has become a somewhat more widely utilized aspect of audiologic rehabilitation for persons of varying ages and degrees of hearing impairment.

THE AUDITORY TRAINING PROCESS

As indicated, the definition and goals of auditory training have varied over the years, due, in part, to (a) the environment in which auditory training takes place (educational or clinical), (b) the age of the individual receiving services (child or adult), and (c) the degree of hearing loss involved (mild-moderate or severe-profound). These issues, as well as other related factors, including the need for speech/language development and adjustment to a new hearing aid or cochlear implant, have been responsible for the many diversified approaches to auditory training that have evolved. The next section, on implementation of auditory training, will include a summary of the procedures commonly utilized to evaluate the auditory abilities of persons with hearing impairment as a preliminary step to auditory training, as well as a review of the key features of selected traditional and more current approaches to auditory training therapy.

Assessment of Auditory Skills

An integral part of a comprehensive auditory-training program is the assessment of the client's performance. Before, during, and at the conclusion of auditory training the clinician should attempt to evaluate the auditory abilities of the person with hearing impairment. Information of this nature is of the utmost importance for several reasons, including:

1. Determining whether or not auditory training appears warranted.
2. Providing a basis for comparison with post-therapy performance, to assess how much improvement in auditory performance, particularly speech perception, has occurred.
3. Identifying specific areas of auditory perception to concentrate on in future auditory training.

The nature of the auditory testing that takes place will vary considerably depending upon a number of variables, such as the age of the client, his or her language skills, and the type and degree of the hearing loss. The clinician must exercise care in selecting test materials for the individual patient, particularly with regard to the language levels required for a given test. This individuation requires that a variety of tests of auditory perception, both formal and informal, be available for assessment purposes so that the particular needs of each client can be met adequately.

Evaluating Children. Both the degree and the sophistication of testing appropriate for young children are limited by their physical and cognitive development. Therefore, informal testing and observation are relied upon heavily with this age group. For the infant, the initial goal of assessment for auditory training purposes may not center on speech perception. Rather, an effort may be made to identify the extent to which auditory skills have emerged, such as gross discrimination and localization of a variety of stimuli. Once this information is known, a specific program for developing auditory skills, such as that described in Chapter 8, can be implemented in conjunction with therapy related to development of speech and language.

For older children, more formal, in-depth assessment of overall speech perception abilities generally is possible. Specifically, materials have been developed that require the child to respond in a prescribed manner to individual words or phonemes presented at a comfortable listening level. Some of the commonly used formal tests of this type which have been designed for assessing children with hearing impairment include:

1. *Word Intelligibility by Picture Identification (WIPI) by Ross and Lerman (1970).* The authors of the WIPI modified an existing test for children (Myatt &

Landes, 1963) so as to include only vocabulary appropriate for children with hearing impairment. The WIPI includes four lists that each contain 25 monosyllabic words. The child provides a picture-pointing response in a closed-set format. According to the authors, the test is suitable for use with hearing-handicapped children with limited receptive and expressive language abilities.

2. *Northwestern University Children's Perception of Speech (NU-CHIPS) by Katz and Elliott (1978).* This test consists of 50 monosyllabic nouns which have been scrambled to form four individual lists. Like the WIPI, the NU-CHIPS uses a response format that requires that the child point to the one picture from several options which best represents the test items. Because of the basic vocabulary included and the non-verbal response format, use of the NU-CHIPS with many children with hearing loss appears appropriate.

3. *Five Sound Test by Ling (1976; 1989).* Five isolated phonemes (/a/, /u/, /i/, /s/, and /ʃ/) are spoken to the child at a normal conversational level. Those with usable residual hearing up to 1000 Hz should be able to detect the vowels. Children with some residual hearing up to 2000 Hz should detect /ʃ/, and those with residual hearing up to 4000 Hz (not worse than 90 dB HL at 4000 Hz) should detect /s/. In certain instances, Ling (1989) has advocated the use of a sixth sound, /m/, to obtain more information concerning the perception of low-frequency stimuli.

Additional test batteries are designed to assess aspects of auditory perception ability. Examples include:

1. *Test of Auditory Comprehension (TAC), developed by the Audiologic Services of the Los Angeles County Schools (Tramwell & Owens, 1977).* Designed for children ages 4–12 years with moderate to profound hearing losses, the TAC is the evaluation part of a comprehensive auditory skills instructional plan. The instrument assesses several areas of auditory perception, including speech discrimination, memory sequencing, figure-ground discrimination, and story comprehension. Results of TAC subtests are used to establish baseline performance and direction for the companion auditory-training curriculum.

2. *Glendonald Auditory Screening Procedure (GASP), developed at the Glendonald Auditory School for the Deaf in Australia (Erber, 1982).* GASP is based on a model of auditory perception described in the next section of this chapter (see Figure 3.6) and consists of three subtests of speech perception: (a) phoneme detection, (b) word identification, and (c) sentence comprehension.
The GASP phoneme-detection subtest is similar in format to the Five Sound Test developed by Ling (1976). According to Erber, the results from GASP can aid in planning auditory training because the child's performance on the subtests is predictive of other, related auditory tasks.

3. *Pediatric Speech Intelligibility Test (PSI) by Jerger and colleagues (1980).* The PSI consists of 20 monosyllabic words and 20 sentences presented in quiet, and with competing sentence messages at varying message-to-competition ratios (MCRs). The child points to the one picture from five options which corresponds to the test word or sentence heard. Investigations of PSI results (Jerger, Jerger,

Speech Stimulus

	Speech Elements	Syllables	Words	Phrases	Sentences	Connected Discourse
Detection	1					
Discrimination						
Identification			2			
Comprehension					3	

Response Task

Figure 3.6 An auditory stimulus-response matrix showing the relative positions of the three GASP subtests: Phoneme Detection (1), Word Identification (2), and Sentence (Question) Comprehension (3).

From N. Erber (1982). *Auditory Training.* Washington, DC: Alexander Graham Bell Association for the Deaf. Reprinted by permission.

& Abrams, 1983) suggest that in addition to the test's utility in assessing speech perception with children having peripheral hearing impairments, it shows promise for detecting central auditory dysfunction as well.

These tests all attempt to take into account the limitations of hearing-impaired youngsters' receptive vocabulary level and their ability to respond orally. However, the variability observed in the receptive and expressive communication skills of these children makes it unwise to draw any firm generalizations about the specific age range of children for whom any of these tests are suited. Vocabulary age rather than chronological age is a key consideration in selecting the appropriate test to use.

Evaluating Adults. A number of formal tests of speech perception are available for use with adults. Any of the traditional monosyllabic word lists, such as the CID W-22s (Hirsh, et al., 1952) or the Northwestern University Auditory Test No. 6 (Tillman & Carhart, 1966), may be employed to evaluate overall word-recognition abilities.

Other tests allow for more in-depth assessment of the perception of consonants, which can be especially difficult for persons with hearing impairment to perceive accurately. One example, the Nonsense Syllable Test (Levitt & Resnick, 1978; Resnick, et al., 1976), consists of seven subtests, each having seven to nine nonsense syllables, as shown in Figure 3.7. Test items were selected in an effort to include those consonants known to present difficulty to adults with hearing impairment. Each subtest

1	2	3	4	5	6	7
af	uθ	iʃ	ab	fa	la	na
aʃ	up	if	að	ta	ba	va
at	us	it	ad	pa	da	ma
ak	uk	ik	am	ha	ga	za
as	ut	is	az	θa	ra	ɡa
ap	uf	iθ	ag	tʃa	ja	ba
aθ	uʃ	ip	an	sa	dʒa	ða
			aŋ	ʃa	wa	da
			av	ka		

Figure 3.7 Test items comprising the NST. Each column represents a subtest of the NST.

From S. Resnick, et al. (1976). *Phoneme identification on a closed-response syllable test.* Houston, TX. Reprinted by permission.

uses a closed-set response format, with the foils consisting of all the other syllables within the subtest. Edgerton and Danhauer (1979) developed a similar test made up of nonsense syllables, which appears appropriate for use with both adults and children (Danhauer, Lewis, & Edgerton, 1985).

Owens and Schubert (1977) produced a 100-item, multiple-choice consonant-perception test called the California Consonant Test (CCT). Thirty-six of the test items assess consonant perception in the initial word position, while 64 items test perception in the final position. Research by Schwartz and Surr (1979) demonstrated that, compared to the NU-6's, the CCT is more sensitive to the speech-recognition difficulties experienced by individuals with high-frequency hearing loss. Consequently, the CCT is often relied on in assessing the speech-recognition abilities of adult patients.

Tests which employ sentence-type stimuli also can be informative. Kalikow, Stevens, and Elliott (1977) developed a test called Speech Perception in Noise, or SPIN. This test is unique in that it attempts to assess a listener's utilization of both linguistic and situational cues in the perception of speech. Sentence material is presented against a background of speech babble, with the listener's task being to identify the final word in the sentence. Ten 50-item forms of SPIN have been generated, each version containing sentences with either high or low predictability relative to the final word in each sentence. Examples of each are shown in Figure 3.8. Bilger, and

Sentence	Level of Predictability
The honey bees swarmed round the *hive*.	High
The girl knows about the *swamp*.	Low
The cushion was filled with *foam*.	High
He had considered the *robe*.	Low

Figure 3.8 Examples of low- and high-predictability sentences from the SPIN Test. Kalikow, Stevens, & Elliott (1977).

colleagues (1979) have revised the forms to make them more equivalent to each other. The SPIN test can provide important information concerning how effectively a given listener makes use of contextual information in the perception of speech, in addition to providing insight regarding how the listener perceives the acoustical properties of speech.

The Central Institute for the Deaf (CID) Everyday Speech Sentences (Davis & Silverman, 1978) have been used extensively to evaluate a listener's ability to perceive connected discourse. They consist of ten 10-sentence sets that vary in length and form; the sentences possess several characteristics associated with typical conversation.

Results of these tests, as well as others, such as the Modified Rhyme Test (House, et al., 1965) and the Multiple Choice Discrimination Test (MCDT) (Schultz & Schubert, 1969), should provide the clinician with specific information concerning a client's consonant perception in a word and/or sentence context. Although not as commonly confused, vowel perception in persons with hearing impairment should also be evaluated, particularly if a severe hearing loss is present. This can be accomplished by utilizing a multiple-choice format and generating lists of monosyllabic words that systematically vary either the vowel or the diphthong while keeping the consonant environment consistent. The following list is an example of this type of material:

hat	hit	hot	hate
ball	bell	bull	bowl
nut	not	neat	night
tool	tall	tell	tale
see	sew	saw	Sue

Additional information about speech perception can be gained by introducing competing noise to the test situation and varying the degree of redundancy in the test material. Also, addition of visual cues via speechreading during administration of these tests in a bisensory condition can provide useful information regarding a person's overall integrative skills (Garstecki, 1980; see Chapters 4 and 9).

Owens and coworkers (1981) developed a comprehensive set of tests, the Minimal Auditory Capabilities (MAC) Battery, for assessing auditory and visual skills of patients with severe to profound hearing impairment. The level of difficulty of the MAC is suitable for individuals for whom conventional speech perception tests are too challenging, such as with persons having profound hearing loss. Included in the MAC battery are the following 14 subtests: Question/Statement, Accent, Noise/Voice, Spondee Same/Different, Vowels, Initial Consonants, Final Consonants, Four-Choice Spondee, Environmental Sounds, Spondee Words, CID Everyday Sentences, Words in Context, Monosyllabic Words, and Visual Enhancement (speechreading). The battery has been slightly revised (Owens, et al., 1985), and is presently being widely used in the evaluation of cases considered for a cochlear implant (see Chapter 12). Another assessment battery developed for this purpose is the Iowa Cochlear Implant Battery (Tyler, Reece, & Lowder, 1984).

Traditional Auditory Training Methods

Wedenberg. An example of an early approach to auditory training used with children with severe to profound hearing loss was described by Wedenberg (1951). It was Wedenberg's view that systematic auditory training serves to exploit whatever residual hearing a child possesses. Wedenberg's approach was eventually labeled unisensory, since he advocated that speechreading not be consciously emphasized until the child developed a proper listening attitude. The preliminary efforts in Wedenberg's auditory training program were, therefore, directed toward increasing the child's attention to sound. Both environmental and speech sounds were used in the early stages, with what Wedenberg referred to as *ad concham amplification.* This involved speaking directly into the child's ear at a close range (one to two inches) rather than having the child use a hearing aid. Training also included exercises which helped the child become aware of and attend to sound at increasing distances. All these activities were intended to make the client more auditorily oriented. Vowels and voiced consonants whose formants were thought to be within the hearing-impaired child's audible range were presented in isolation. Syllables were used in a variety of formal therapeutic activities, as well as informal settings at home. Combining individual vowels and consonants learned in isolation resulted in perception of a limited number of words. At this point, Wedenberg advocated part-time use of a hearing aid. Later, training progressed to short sentences formed by words already recognized by the child acoustically. Although not a direct focus, speechreading could be utilized by the child to supplement the information derived through the auditory channel. Wedenberg was convinced that children with a strong auditory orientation would eventually become as proficient at speechreading as those receiving intensive speechreading instruction early in life. In fact, he believed that his students' increased auditory vocabulary made them better able to utilize visual information than children with a background of multisensory training. An excellent example of the principles involved in Wedenberg's approach is contained in a summary of the work done with Staffan, a profoundly deaf son of the Wedenbergs (Wedenberg & Wedenberg, 1970).

Wedenberg's method, then, was directed toward development of auditory, speech, and language skills in children with either a congenital or prelingual hearing loss of severe to profound proportions. In these respects it was similar to other auditory-training methods proposed by Goldstein (1939), Whitehurst (1966), Watson (1961), and others. However, features such as his emphasis on unisensory management of the deaf child made Wedenberg's rehabilitative methods unique.

Until World War II, the primary focus of auditory training was its use with severely/profoundly deaf children in an effort to facilitate speech and language acquisition and increase their educational potential. However, the activities that occurred at VA audiology centers during World War II served to demonstrate on a large scale that adults with mild to severe hearing impairments could profit from auditory training as well.

Carhart. Expansion of auditory training to encompass both children and adults continued after World War II. The thinking at that time concerning auditory training was perhaps best manifested in the approach to its use with both young and older individuals, as described by Carhart (1960). Carhart made one of the first extensive attempts to describe the role of auditory training in the rehabilitation process within an audiological context, and his theories were to have a significant and enduring impact on the profession.

Carhart's auditory-training program for prelingually impaired children was based on his belief that since listening skills are normally learned early in life, the child possessing a serious hearing loss at birth or soon after will not move through the normal developmental stages important in acquiring these skills. Likewise, when a hearing loss occurs in later childhood or in adulthood, some of the person's auditory skills may become impaired even though they were intact prior to the onset of the hearing loss. In each instance, Carhart believed that auditory training was warranted.

CHILDHOOD PROCEDURES. Carhart outlined four major steps or objectives involved in auditory training for children with prelingual deafness. These are:

1. Development of awareness of sound
2. Development of gross discriminations
3. Development of broad discriminations among simple speech patterns
4. Development of finer discriminations for speech

Development of an awareness of auditory stimuli and the significance of sound involves having the child acknowledge the presence of sound and its importance in his/her world. The development of gross discrimination initially involves demonstrating with various noisemakers that sounds differ. Once the child can successfully discriminate grossly different sounds, he/she is exposed to finer types of discrimination tasks that include variation in the frequency, intensity, and durational properties of sound. When the child is able to recognize the presence of sound and can perceive gross differences with nonverbal stimuli, Carhart's approach calls for the introduction of activities directed toward learning gross discrimination for speech signals. The final

~28C?

phase consists of training the child to make fine discriminations of speech stimuli in connected discourse, and integrating an increased vocabulary to enable him/her to follow connected speech in a more rapid and accurate fashion. Carhart felt that unlike the unisensory approach, speechreading by the child should be encouraged in most auditory-training activities.

ADULT PROCEDURES. Because adults who acquire a hearing loss retain a portion of their original auditory skills, Carhart recommended that auditory training with adults focus on re-educating a skill diminished as a consequence of the hearing impairment. Initially, Carhart felt that it was important to establish "an attitude of critical listening" in the individual. This involves being attentive to the subtle differences among sounds and can involve a considerable amount of drill work on the perception of phonemes that are difficult for the adult with hearing impairment to perceive. Lists of matched syllables/words which contain the troublesome phonemes, such as she-fee, so-tho, met-let, or mash-math, are read to the individual, who repeats them back. Such training should also include phrases and sentences, with the goal of developing as rapid and precise a recognition of the phonetic elements as is possible within the limitations imposed by the person's hearing loss. Speechreading combined with a person's hearing was also encouraged by Carhart during a portion of the auditory training sessions.

Because we often communicate under less-than-ideal listening circumstances, Carhart advocated that auditory-training sessions for adults be conducted in three commonly encountered situations: (a) relatively intense background noise, (b) the presence of a competing speech signal, and (c) listening on the telephone. This emphasis on practice in speech perception under listening conditions with decreasing amounts of redundancy has been emphasized more recently by Sanders (1993) and numerous other audiologic rehabilitationists.

According to Carhart, the use of hearing aids is vital in auditory training, and he recommended that they be utilized as early as possible in the auditory-training program. These recommendations were consistent with Carhart's belief that systematic exposure to sound during auditory training was an ideal means of allowing a person to adequately adjust to hearing aids and assist in using them as optimally as possible.

Persons interested in more specific information concerning Carhart's auditory-training strategies should review his chapter in the second edition of Davis and Silverman's *Hearing and Deafness* (1960).

More Recent Approaches to Auditory Training

The basic intent of auditory training is to maximize communication potential by developing to its fullest the auditory channel of the person with hearing impairment. Several other approaches to this form of audiologic rehabilitation have emerged in recent years, representing some departure from the traditional methods just described. In this section we will identify and overview the underlying features of a selected number of these approaches for providing auditory training.

The more current approaches to auditory training vary considerably. According to Blamey and Alcantara (1994), it is possible to categorize them into one of four general categories, based on the fundamental strategy stressed in therapy:

1. *Analytic*: attempts to break speech into smaller components (phoneme, syllable, word) and incorporate these separately into auditory-training exercises.
2. *Synthetic*: emphasizes a more global approach to speech perception, stressing the use of clues derived from the syntax and context of a spoken message to derive understanding. Training synthetically involves the use of meaningful stimuli (words, phrases, sentences).
3. *Pragmatic*: involves training the listener to control communication variables, such as the level of speech, the signal-to-noise ratio, and the context/complexity of the message, in order to obtain the necessary information via audition for understanding to occur.
4. *Eclectic*: includes training that combines most or all of the strategies previously described.

While the auditory training programs to be described all have analytic, synthetic, or pragmatic tendencies, most would best be described as eclectic, since more than one general strategy for the training of the hearing channel typically is used with a given child or adult.

Erber. A flexible and widely used approach to auditory training designed primarily for use with children has been described by Erber (1982). This adaptive method is based on a careful analysis of a child's auditory perceptual abilities through the use of the GASP assessment battery (described briefly in the portion of this chapter devoted to assessment). Recall that GASP's approach to evaluating a child's auditory perceptual skills takes into account two major factors: (1) the complexity of the speech stimuli to be perceived (ranging from individual speech elements to connected discourse), and (2) the form of the response required from the child (detection, discrimination, identification, or comprehension). Several levels of stimuli and responses are involved, as shown in Figure 3.6. The GASP test battery evaluates only the three stimulus-response combinations indicated in the figure. However, Erber encourages the use of other available test materials to evaluate other stimulus-response combinations from the matrix in Figure 3.6, when appropriate.

Once the child's auditory capabilities are determined, an auditory-training program is outlined using the same stimulus-response model when establishing goals and beginning points for therapy. Erber's approach is flexible and highly adaptable to children with a wide variety of auditory abilities, since the stimulus and response combinations range from the simplest (phoneme-detection) to the most complex (sentence-comprehension) perceptual tasks.

Erber also described three general styles which the clinician may use during auditory training, depending on the communication setting. These styles differ in

TABLE 3.5 *Three General Auditory Training Methods*

Natural conversational approach	1.	The teacher eliminates visible cues and speaks to the child in as natural a way as possible, while considering the general situational context and ongoing classroom activity.
	2.	The auditory speech-perception tasks may be chosen from any cell in the stimulus-response matrix, for example, sentence comprehension.
	3.	The teacher adapts to the child's responses by presenting remedial auditory tasks in a systematic manner (modifies stimulus and/or response), derived from any cell in the matrix.
Moderately structured approach	1.	The teacher applies a closed-set auditory identification task, but follows this activity with some basic speech development procedures and a related comprehension task. Thus, the method retains a degree of flexibilty.
	2.	The teacher selects the nature and content of words and sentences on the basis of recent class activities.
	3.	A few neighboring cells in the stimulus/response matrix are involved (for example, word and sentence identification and sentence comprehension).
Practice on specific tasks	1.	The teacher selects the set of acoustic speech stimuli and also the child's range of responses, prepares relevant materials, and plans the development of the task — all according to the child's specific needs for auditory practice.
	2.	Attention is directed to a particular listening skill, usually represented by a single cell in the stimulus-response matrix (for example, phrase discrimination).

Source: Auditory Training by N. Erber, 1982, Washington, D.C.: Alexander Graham Bell Association for the Deaf. Reprinted by permission.

specificity, rigidity, and direction, and are described in Table 3.5. Adaptive procedures, where the child's responses to speech stimuli are used to determine the next activity, can be employed with any of these styles. In attempting to develop a child's auditory abilities, Erber (1982) stated:

> Auditory training need not follow a developmental plan where, for instance, you practice phoneme detection first and attempt comprehension of connected discourse last. Instead, you might use the "conversational approach" during all daily conversation, and apply the "moderately structured approach" as a follow-up to each class activity. During each activity, you will note consistent errors. Later, you might provide brief periods of specific practice with difficult material. In this way, you can incorporate auditory training into conversation and instruction, rather than treat listening as a skill to be developed independently of communication. (p. 105)

Erber's emphasis on integrating the development of auditory skills into all activities with children with hearing impairment is shared by many, including Sanders (1993) and Ling and Ling (1978), who recommend that auditory training "be viewed as a supplement to auditory experience and as an integral part of language and speech training" (p. 113).

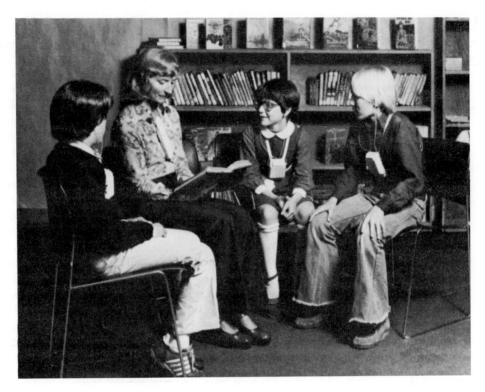

Group auditory training session.

Courtesy of H.C. Electronics.

DASL II. Stout and Windle (1986; 1992) have developed a sequential, structured auditory-training program called the Developmental Approach to Successful Listening II, or DASL II. Like Erber's (1982) approach, the DASL II consists of a hierarchy of listening skills that are worked on in relatively brief, individualized sessions.

The DASL II curriculum can be used with persons of any age, but mainly has been utilized with preschool and school-age youngsters using either hearing aids or cochlear implants. Three specific areas of auditory skill development are focused on:

1. *Sound awareness:* deals with the development of the basic skills of listening for both environmental and speech sounds. The care/use of hearing aids and cochlear implants are also included.
2. *Phonetic listening*: includes exposure to fundamental aspects of speech perception such as the duration, intensity, pitch, and rate of speech. The discrimination and identification of vowels/consonants in isolation and in words are included in this area.
3. *Auditory comprehension*: emphasizes the understanding of spoken language by the child with hearing impairment. Includes a wide range of audi-

tory processing activities from basic discrimination of common words to comprehension of complex verbal messages in unstructured situations.

The authors have developed a placement test that enables the clinician to evaluate the child's auditory skills relative to each of these three main areas. Specific subskills are tested, making it possible to determine the particular listening skills which a child has or has not acquired. As with the GASP approach, information from the DASL II placement test enables the clinician to determine the appropriate placement of the child within the auditory skills curriculum. The test's developers provided numerous activity suggestions for the clinician. These address each of the many subskills of the three main areas of listening which make up DASL II. These are organized from the simplest to the most difficult listening task. The following example is a list of subskills related to sound awareness that are included in the DASL II. Similar subskill lists and related activities are provided by the developers for all components of DASL II.

Developing Sound-Awareness Subskills

1. Responds to the presence of a loud, low-frequency gross environmental sound. (Example: loud banging on a hard surface)
2. Responds to the presence of a loud speech syllable or word.
3. Responds to the presence of a variety of different gross environmental sounds.
4. Indicates when on-going environmental sounds stop.
5. Indicates when a sustained speech syllable or word stops.
6. Indicates when teacher or parent turns both hearing aids (or processor) on or off.
7. Discriminates between presence of spoken syllable or word and silence.
8. Discriminates between a variety of familiar environmental sounds in a set of two choices.
9. Discriminates between a variety of familiar environmental sounds in a set of three choices.
10. Discriminates between a variety of environmental sounds in a set of four choices.
11. If the student is amplified binaurally, locates the direction of sound on the same plane.
12. If the student is amplified binaurally, locates the direction of sound on different planes.
13. Identifies common environmental sounds.
14. If the student is amplified binaurally, he/she can detect when one aid is on vs. both aids on in a structured situation.

A team approach is encouraged with DASL II, with the audiologist, speech-language pathologist, classroom teacher and parents working in a coordinated fashion on relevant subskills. This makes it vital that frequent communication occur among the team members.

TABLE 3.6 *The Four Phases and Eleven Skills of the SKI-HI Auditory Program*

The approximate time line indicates the estimated amount of time spent by a profoundly deaf infant in each phase. The age of the child upon entry into the program and the amount of hearing loss are among the factors which will affect the time needed to progress through the four phases.

Phases	Skills
Phase I (4-7 months)	1. *Attending:* child aware of presence of home and/or speech sounds but may not know meanings; stops, listens, etc.
	2. *Early Vocalizing:* child coos, gurgles, repeats syllables, etc.
Phase II (5-16 months)	3. *Recognizing:* child knows meaning of home and/or speech sounds but may not be able to locate; smiles when hears Daddy home, etc.
	4. *Locating:* child turns to, points to, locates sound sources.
	5. *Vocalizing with Inflection:* high/low, loud/soft, and/or, up/down
Phase III (9-14 months)	6. *Hearing at Distances and Levels:* child locates sounds far away and/or above and below
	7. *Producing Some Vowels and Consonants*
Phase IV (12-18 months)	8. *Environmental Discrimination and Comprehension:* child hears differences among and/or understands home sounds
	9. *Vocal Discrimination and Comprehension:* child hears differences (a) among vocal sounds, (b) among words, or (c) among phrases and/or understands them
	10. *Speech Sound Discrimination and Comprehension:* child hears differences among and/or understands distinct speech sounds
	11. *Speech: Use* child imitates and/or uses speech meaningfully

Source: Watkins and Clark, 1993.

SKI-HI. Clark and Watkins (1985) developed a comprehensive identification and home-intervention treatment program for infants with hearing impairment and their families, that is in wide use nationally (see Chapter 8 for more details). One of the major components of SKI-HI's treatment plan is a developmentally-based auditory stimulation/training program. It is utilized in conjunction with language/speech stimulation and consists of 4 phases and 11 general skills, which are listed in Table 3.6. Although these phases and skills are organized developmentally, infants may not always move sequentially from one phase or skill on the list to the next higher one in a completely predictable manner. SKI-HI provides an extensive description of activities which the clinician and parent/caregiver may utilize in working on subskills related to each of the specific general skills included in each phase of the auditory training program. The structure and completeness of SKI-HI's auditory training component make it "user-friendly" for parents under the guidance of clinicians. Table 3.7 provides a summary of an example of listening activities which are part of SKI-HI's comprehensive auditory stimulation program.

TABLE 3.7 *A Lesson in SKI-HI's Auditory Stimulation/Training Program*

Recognition of objects and events from sound source (Phase II, Skill 3, Subskill 6)

Parent Objective	Parent will provide repeated meaningful opportunities for their child to associate environmental and speech sounds with their source.
Child objective	Child will demonstrate recognition of environmental and speech sounds by realizing their source.
Lesson	Review with the parents the sounds/activities you have been utilizing for previous work on attending. Continue these activities, insuring that the child is aware of the source of the sound and that the sounds are relevant to the child.
Materials	Naturally-occurring environmental sounds and voice.
Activities	1. Ask everyone who comes to visit to knock several times, pause, and knock again. When someone knocks, take your child to the door and say, "listen," etc.
	2. Encourage the child to discover different sounds that toys make by providing him/her play time with several different sound toys.
	3. Stimulate the child to produce sounds by manipulating objects/toys (banging pans, squeezing toy, etc.) and stimulate vocalization by making sounds as you play with the toys.
	4. Imitate the child's actions, such as shaking a rattle, and imitate all vocalizations.
	5. Associate speech with all major movements (e.g., saying "roll" each time you roll the child over and "up" when you pick him/her up).
	6. Stimulate association of particular voices with particular people by having siblings/relatives use voice as they play with the child.

Adapted from Clark and Watkins, 1985; Watkins and Clark, 1993.

Foundations in Speech Perception (Foundations). Foundations (Brown, 1994) is a newly-introduced interactive software system designed for the evaluation/ development of listening skills in children who use hearing aids, tactile aids, or cochlear implants. Color graphics and high-quality audio are available with more than 1000 lessons, which have been developed for this purpose.

The first of the two major components of Foundations, Integrated Curriculum Plans, uses non-speech and speech stimuli to develop fundamental auditory skills. Speech stimuli are presented in series which target pattern, word, syllable, and phoneme perception, and the auditory mode can be supplemented with varying degrees of visual support (pictures, sign language) as well to facilitate performance and learning. The child interacts with the computer via keyboard, touchscreen, or mouse interfaces. Stories, the second major component of Foundations, incorporates spoken and written connected language in the form of stories. The child listens to stories with basic topics (family, animals) and is encouraged to process the information auditorily/visually and repeat back verbally individual words, phrases, and entire stories. Foundations includes the capacity to record the child's vocalizations, providing a means for the child to compare his/her own vocal productions to the recordings on the computer. This feature is especially effective in facilitating the acquisition of speech and language skills simultaneous with the development of auditory abilities.

All activities can be highly individualized so that lessons become tailored to meet the particular perceptual level of a given child. An ongoing record of each child's percent correct score and time spent on individual lessons is kept, allowing for accurate monitoring of his/her rate of progress at all levels.

The computer-based approach to auditory training, as with Foundations in Speech Perception, appears to have considerable potential in the management of individuals of all ages with hearing impairment, and it is anticipated that clinicians will use this mode of therapy at an increasing rate in the near future.

Consonant-Recognition Training. This form of auditory training relies primarily on an analytic approach to facilitate improved speech perception, and often incorporates speechreading into a combined auditory-visual training approach. Walden, Erdman, Montgomery, Schwartz, and Prosek (1981) originally described consonant-recognition training as it was utilized initially at Walter Reed Army Medical Center. Briefly, a large number of training exercises were developed and each exercise concentrates on a select number of consonants presented in a syllable context. The listener's task is to make same-different judgments between syllable pairs and to identify the nonsense syllables presented individually. The position of the consonants within the syllable is varied between exercises. The person with hearing impairment receives immediate feedback regarding the correctness of his/her response. This general procedure allows for intense drill to occur for a select number of consonants during a relatively short therapy session.

Walden and others presented data to support the efficacy of this approach to auditory training. They noted an 11.6% average improvement in consonant recognition. More impressively, a 28.2% average improvement was found in perception of sentences presented in a combined auditory-visual mode. A follow-up study (Montgomery, et al., 1984) utilized a similar training protocol for consonant recognition which combined work on speechreading and auditory training. Using sentence material to assess performance, they noted a substantial improvement in speech recognition for adults with hearing impairment.

Another investigation (Rubenstein & Boothroyd, 1987) also examined the effectiveness of consonant-recognition training as part of a larger study comparing analytic and synthetic approaches to improving speech perception. Rubenstein and Boothroyd found that consonant-recognition training did produce modest improvement in speech perception for a group of adults with hearing impairment, but the amount of improvement observed was not any greater than was achieved with a synthetic approach to auditory training.

More research needs to be focused on the relative merits of consonant-recognition training as it is used in attempting to improve auditory perception. Also needed is further clarification of the basic roles played by auditory and visual speech perception, both individually and when utilized in a combined manner, in the processing of speech by persons with hearing impairment (Walden & Grant, 1993; Gagne, 1994). In the meantime, interest in using consonant-recognition training continues, and its use has been extended in recent years to include computer-based programming as well (Tye-Murray, et al., 1990; Lansing & Bienvenue, 1994).

Communication Training/Therapy. A common form of audiologic rehabilitation, currently provided to some adults with hearing impairment, that emphasizes the role of pragmatics for successful communication, is generally referred to as communication training or therapy. Rather than routinely providing traditional forms of auditory training or speechreading that focus primarily on improving an individual's perceptual skills through focused exercises and drills, the emphasis in communication therapy is on sharing information of relevance concerning the communication process, and what persons with hearing impairment can do to assist in facilitating speech perception within a conversation context. This shift in the approach used with many adults who are hard of hearing has occurred, in part, because of persistent questions raised concerning the efficacy of rehabilitation methods that concentrate on attempting to enhance auditory (or visual) perceptual skills (Walden and Grant, 1993).

Most communication-therapy programs are offered to small groups of adults with hearing impairment in several sessions that typically are scheduled over a relatively short total period of time. Information is shared on a variety of topics, including hearing loss and speech perception, effective use of hearing aids, potential benefits of assistive listening devices, how vision can be used with hearing to facilitate speech perception, and psychosocial issues related to hearing disability (Giolas, 1982; see also Chapter 13).

Another important component of communication therapy which has received much attention in recent years is termed *communication strategies training*. Here the hearing-impaired person is provided with a number of options which he/she can exercise in conversations when communication difficulties are anticipated or actually experienced. These techniques are often referred to as *anticipatory and repair strategies*. Some of the common strategies available include the following:

1. Asking the talker to repeat a phrase, sentence, or key word.
2. Asking the talker to rephrase a sentence.
3. Requesting that a sentence be restated in a simpler form.
4. Requesting additional information.
5. Asking the talker to use a more moderate speaking rate.
6. Requesting the speaker to face the listener when talking.
7. Turning down, or off, a competing signal such as a television.

Table 3.8 (Erber, 1993) provides a list of problems routinely encountered by listeners, as well as suggested strategies for coping with each. Persons with hearing impairment are encouraged to employ these communication strategies when necessary, which does require some degree of assertiveness on their part as they communicate with others. Successful use of communication strategies also requires that they be used in a diplomatic manner as well.

DeFilippo and Scott (1978) developed a technique called *speech tracking*, which can be used in therapy to provide practice in utilizing communication repair strategies in a conversation context. As it is used in therapy centered on improving auditory-speech perception, speech tracking involves having a listener repeat a phrase or sentence presented by a clinician in an auditory-only condition. To assist in perceiv-

TABLE 3.8 *Some Communication Problems Commonly Experienced by Hearing Impaired People, and Associated (specific) Requests for Clarification*

What was the communication problem?	*How you can ask for help*
You understood only part of the message.	Repeat the part you understood; ask for the part you didn't understand. (e.g., "You flew to *Paris*?")
You couldn't see the speaker's mouth.	"Please put your hand down."
The person was speaking too fast.	"Please speak a little slower."
The person's speech was too soft.	"Please speak a little louder."
The sentence was too long.	"Shorter, please."
The person's speech was not clear.	"Speak a little more clearly, please."
The sentence was too complicated.	"Please say that in a different way."
You don't know what the problem was.	"Please say that again."

Source: Erber, 1993.

ing 100% of the message, the listener can use various repair strategies, such as requesting that the entire sentence, or portions, be repeated or rephrased, until the complete utterance is comprehended. Visual cues may be added for bisensory training as well. Performance in the speech-tracking procedure is monitored by calculating the number of words correctly repeated by the listener per minute over a set period of time. An example of the tracking method as applied in a therapy session is provided below. (The topic of the sentence is fishing).

Clinician:	Dry flies float on the surface.
Listener:	Dry . . . on the . . . ? Please repeat it.
Clinician:	Dry flies float on the surface.
Listener:	Dry flies . . . on the . . . ? Please repeat the word after "flies".
Clinician:	Float.
Listener:	Float?
Clinician:	Yes.
Listener:	Dry flies float on the water.
Clinician:	No. On the surface of the water.
Listener:	Oh. Dry flies float on the surface.
Clinician:	Yes.

In recent years, audiologists have frequently included condensed variations of communication training/therapy as an important aspect of audiologic rehabilitation for adults at the time they are fitted with new hearing aids. Many think that sharing information with the patient about the role of hearing and vision and the use of communication strategies in communicating is a timely and appropriate adjunct to the hearing-aid orientation process, and audiologists have begun to do this on a more frequent basis (Schow, et al., 1993). In a recent article, Montgomery (1994) discussed the rationale for providing a brief exposure to auditory rehabilitation at the time the patient who is hard of hearing is fitted with a hearing aid. Montgomery uses the acronym WATCH for his program, which includes the following key elements of AR: W: Watch the talker's mouth (lipreading); A: Ask specific questions (conversation-repair strategies); T: Talk about your hearing loss (admission of hearing loss); C: Change the situation (situation control); and H: Health-care knowledge (consumer education-awareness). The program, which takes about one hour to share with the new hearing-aid user, is designed to provide important tips for successful communication, as well as to "encourage or empower the hearing-impaired patient to take charge of his or her communication behavior and take responsibility for its success." Audiologists are encouraged to consider providing this brief, but valuable, form of AR more routinely as they work with adults who are hard of hearing.

SUMMARY

This chapter has presented an overview of the role of audition in the communication process, and the part auditory training plays in audiologic rehabilitation of the hearing disabled. Specifically, the complexity of speech perception was emphasized along with the ways in which a variety of auditory training techniques, both traditional and more pragmatically oriented, can be utilized to maximize the contribution of the impaired auditory channel to overall communication. Its potential for improving the communication skills of persons with hearing impairment is substantial. Application of auditory training and its importance in the total audiologic rehabilitation process will be further discussed in later chapters.

RECOMMENDED READINGS

Blamey, P., & Alcantara, J. (1994). Research in auditory training. In J.-P. Gagne and N. Tye-Murray (Eds.), Research in Audiological Rehabilitation [Monograph]. *Journal of the Academy of Rehabilitative Audiology*, 27, 161–192.

Erber, N. (1982). *Auditory training.* Washington, DC: Alexander Graham Bell Association for the Deaf.

Erber, N. (1988). *Communication therapy for hearing-impaired adults.* Abbotsford, Vic. 3067/Australia: Clavis Publishing.

Erber, N. (1993). *Communication and adult hearing loss.* Abbotsford, Vic. 3067/Australia: Clavis Publishing.

Giolas, T. (1994). Aural rehabilitation of adults with hearing impairment. In J. Katz (Ed.), *Handbook of clinical audiology* (4th ed.). Baltimore: Williams & Wilkins.

Tye-Murray, N. (1994). Communication strategies training. In J. Gagne & N. Tye-Murray (Eds.), Research in Audiological Rehabilitation [Monograph]. *Journal of the Academy of Rehabilitative Audiology*, 27, 193–208.

REFERENCES

Alpiner, J., & McCarthy, P. (Eds.). (1993). *Rehabilitative audiology: Children and adults* (3rd ed.). Baltimore: Williams and Wilkins.

Bench, R. (1968). Sound transmission to the human fetus through the maternal abdominal wall. *Journal of Genetic Psychology, 113*, 85–87.

Bilger, R., Rzcezkowski, C., Nuetzel, J., & Rabinowitz, W. (November, 1979). Evaluation of a test of speech perception in noise (SPIN). Paper presented at the convention of the American Speech-Language-Hearing Association, Atlanta, GA.

Bilger, R., & Wang, M. (1976). Consonant confusions in patients with sensorineural hearing loss. *Journal of Speech and Hearing Research, 19*, 718–748.

Blamey, P., & Alcantara, J. (1994). Research in auditory training. In J.-P. Gagne & N. Tye-Murray (Eds.), Research in Audiological Rehabilitation [Monograph]. *Journal of the Academy of Rehabilitative Audiology, 27*, 161–192.

Boothroyd, A. (1978). Speech perception and sensorineural hearing loss. In M. Ross & T. Giolas (Eds.), *Auditory management of hearing-impaired children*. Baltimore: University Park Press.

Brown, C. (1994). *Foundations in speech perception*. Iowa City, Iowa: Breakthrough, Inc.

Byers, V. (1973). Initial consonant intelligibility by hearing impaired children. *Journal of Speech and Hearing Research, 16*, 4–55.

Carhart, R. (1960). Auditory training. In H. Davis & R. Silverman (Eds.), *Hearing and deafness* (2nd ed.). New York: Holt, Rinehart & Winston.

Clark, T., & Watkins, S. (1985). *Programming for hearing impaired infants through amplification and home visits* (4th ed.). Logan, UT: Utah State University.

Crandall, I. (1925, October). Sounds of speech. *Bell System Technical Journal*, 586–626.

Danhauer, J., Lewis, A., & Edgerton, B. (1985). Normally hearing children's responses to a nonsense syllable test. *Journal of Speech and Hearing Disorders, 50*, 100–103.

Davis, J., & Hardick, E. (1981). *Rehabilitative audiology for children and adults*. New York: Wiley and Sons.

Davis, H., & Silverman, R. (1960). *Hearing and deafness* (2nd ed.). New York: Holt, Rinehart & Winston.

Davis, H., & Silverman, R. (1978). *Hearing and deafness* (4th ed.) New York: Holt, Rinehart & Winston.

DeFilippo, C., & Scott, B. (1978). A method for training and evaluating the reception of ongoing speech. J*ournal of the Acoustical Society of America, 63*, 1186–1192.

Denes, P., & Pinson, E. (1993). *The speech chain* (2nd ed.). New York: Freeman & Co.

Edgerton, B., & Danhauer, J. (1979). *Clinical implications of speech discrimination testing using nonsense stimuli*. Baltimore: University Park Press.

Eimas, P. (1975). Developmental studies in speech perception. In L. B. Cohen & P. Salapatek (Eds.), *Infant perception* (Vol. 2). New York: Academic Press, 193–231.

Eisenberg, R. (1965a). Auditory behavior in the human neonate. I. Methodologic problems and the logical design of research procedures. *Journal of Auditory Research, 5*, 159–177.

Eisenberg, R. (1965b). Auditory behavior in the human neonate. II. *Journal of International Audiology, 4*, 65–68.

Eisenberg, R. (1970). The development of hearing in man: An assessment of current status. *Asha, 12*, 110–123.

Eisenberg, R. (1976). *Auditory competence in early life*. Baltimore: University Park Press.

Erber, N. (1979). Speech perception by profoundly hearing-impaired children. *Journal of Speech and Hearing Disorders, 122*, 255–270.

Erber, N. (1982). *Auditory training*. Washington, DC: Alexander Graham Bell Association for the Deaf.

Erber, N. (1993). *Communication and adult hearing loss*. Abbotsford, Victoria: Clavis Press.

Fletcher, H. (1953). *Speech and hearing in communication*. Princeton: D. VanNostrand Co.

Gagne, J.-P. (1994). Visual and audiovisual speech perception training: Basic and applied research needs. In J.-P. Gagne & N. Tye-Murray (Eds.), Research in audiological rehabilitation [Monograph]. *Journal of the Academy of Rehabilitative Audiology, 27*, 133–160.

Garstecki, D. (1980). Alterative approaches to measuring speech discrimination efficiency. In R. Rupp & C. Stockdell (Eds.), *Speech protocols in audiology*. New York: Grune Stratton, 119–144.

Giolas, T. (1982). *Hearing-handicapped adults*. Englewood Cliffs, NJ: Prentice Hall.

Goldstein, M. (1939). *The acoustic method of the training of the deaf and hard of hearing child*. St. Louis: Laryngoscope Press.

Hirsh, I., Davis, H., Silverman, S. R., Reynolds, E., Eldert, E., Bensen, R. (1952). Development of materials for speech audiometry. *Journal of Speech and Hearing Disorders, 17*, 321–337.

House, A., Williams, C., Hacker, M., Kryter, K. (1965). Articulation-testing methods: Consonantal differentiation with a closed-response set. *Journal of the Acoustical Society of America, 37*, 158–166.

Hull, R. (Ed.). (1992). *Aural rehabilitation*. San Diego, CA: Singular Publishing.

Jerger, S., Jerger, J., & Abrams, S. (1983). Speech audiometry in the young child. *Ear and Hearing, 4*, 56–66.

Jerger, S., Lewis, S., Hawkins, J., & Jerger, J. (1980). Pediatric speech intelligibility test I. Generation of test materials. *International Journal of Pediatric Otorhinolaryngology, 2*, 217–230.

Kalikow, D., Stevens, K., & Elliott, L. (1977). Development of a test of speech intelligibility in noise using sentence materials with controlled word predictability. *Journal of the Acoustical Society of America, 61,* 1337-1351.

Katz, D., & Eliott, L. (1978, November). Development of a new children's speech discrimination test. Paper presented at the convention of the American Speech-Language-Hearing Association, Chicago.

Lansing, C., & Bienvenue, L. (1994). Intelligent computer-based systems to document the effectiveness of consonant recognition training. *Volta Review, 96,* 41-49.

Lehiste, I. (1970). *Suprasegmentals.* Cambridge: The MIT Press.

Lehiste, I. (1976). Suprasegmental features of speech. In N.J. Lass (Ed.), *Contemporary issues in experimental phonetics.* New York: Academic Press, Inc., 225-242.

Levitt, H., & Resnick, S. (1978). Speech reception by the hearing impaired. Methods of testing and the development of new tests. *Scandinavian Audiology, 6* (Suppl. 1), 107-130.

Ling, D. (1976). *Speech and the hearing-impaired child: Theory and practice.* Washington, DC: Alexander Graham Bell Association for the Deaf.

Ling, D. (1978). Auditory coding and recoding: An analysis of auditory training procedures for hearing-impaired children. In M. Ross & T. Giolas (Eds.), *Auditory management of hearing-impaired children.* Baltimore: University Park Press.

Ling, D. (1989). *Foundations of spoken language for hearing-impaired children.* Washington, DC: Alexander Graham Bell Association for the Deaf.

Ling, D., & Ling, A. (1978). *Aural rehabilitation.* Washington, DC: Alexander Graham Bell Association for the Deaf.

Lisker, L. (1957). Closure duration and the intervocalic voiced-voiceless distinction in English. *Language, 33,* 42-49.

McGlone, R. (1966). Vocal pitch characteristics of children aged one and two years. *Speech Monographs, 33,* 178-181.

Miller, G., & Nicely, P. (1955). Analysis of perceptual confusions among some English consonants. *Journal of the Acoustical Society of America, 27,* 338-352.

Minifie, F. (1973). Speech acoustics. In F. Minifie, T. Hixon, & F. Williams (Eds.), *Normal aspects of speech, hearing and language.* Englewood Cliffs, NJ: Prentice Hall.

Moffitt, A. (1971). Consonant cue perception by twenty- to twenty-four week-old infants. *Child Development, 42,* 717-732.

Montgomery, A. (1994). WATCH: A practical approach to brief auditory rehabilitation. *The Hearing Journal, 47*(10), 53-55.

Montgomery, A., Walden, B., Schwartz, D., & Prosek, R. (1984). Training auditory-visual speech recognition in adults with moderate sensorineural hearing loss. *Ear and Hearing, 5,* 30-36.

Myatt, B., & Landes, B. (1963). Assessing discrimination loss in children. *Archives of Otolaryngology, 77,* 359-362.

Northern, J., & Downs, M. (1994). *Hearing in children* (4th ed.). Baltimore: Williams & Wilkins.

Orr, D., Friedman, H., & Williams, J. (1965). Trainability of listening comprehension of speeded discourse. *Journal of Educational Psychology, 56,* 148-156.

Owens, E. (1978). Consonant errors and remediation in sensorineural hearing loss. *Journal of Speech and Hearing Disorders, 43,* 331-347.

Owens, E., Benedict, M., & Shubert, E. (1971). Further investigation of vowel items in multiple-choice discrimination testing. *Journal of Speech and Hearing Research, 14,* 814-847.

Owens, E., Benedict, M., & Shubert, E. (1972). Consonant phoneme errors associated with pure tone configurations and certain types of hearing impairment. *Journal of Speech and Hearing Research, 15,* 308-322.

Owens, E., Kessler, D., Roggio, M., & Schubert, E. (1985). Analysis and revision of the Minimal Auditory Capabilities (MAC) battery. *Ear and Hearing, 6,* 280-287.

Owens, E., Kessler, D., Telleen, C., & Shubert, E. (1981). The Minimal Auditory Capabilities (MAC) battery. *Hearing Journal, 34*(9), 32-34.

Owens, E., & Shubert, E. (1977). Development of the California Consonant Test. *Journal of Speech and Hearing Research, 20,* 463-474.

Oyer, H. (1966). *Auditory communication for the hard of hearing.* Englewood Cliffs, NJ: Prentice Hall.

Peterson, G. E., & Barney, H. L. (1952). Control methods used in the study of the vowels. *Journal of the Acoustical Society of America, 32,* 693-703.

Resnick, S., Dubno, D., Howie, G., Hoffnung, S., Freeman, L., & Slosberg, R. (November, 1976). Phoneme identification on a closed-response nonsense syllable test. Paper presented at the convention of the American Speech-Language-Hearing Association, Houston.

Ross, M., & Lerman, L. (1970). A picture identification test for hearing impaired children. *Journal of Speech and Hearing Research, 13,* 44-53.

Rubenstein, A., & Boothroyd, A. (1987). Effect of two approaches to auditory training on speech recognition by hearing-impaired adults. *Journal of Speech and Hearing Research, 30,* 153-160.

Sanders, D. (1971). *Aural rehabilitation.* Englewood Cliffs, NJ: Prentice Hall.

Sanders, D. (1993). *Management of Hearing Handicap* (3rd ed.). Englewood Cliffs, NJ: Prentice Hall.

Schow, R., Balsara, N., Smedley, T., & Whitcomb, C. (1993). Aural rehabilitation by ASHA audiologists: 1980-1990. *American Journal of Audiology, 2,* 28-37.

Schultz, M., & Schubert, E. (1969). A multiple choice discrimination test (MCDT). *Laryngoscope, 79,* 382-399.

Schwartz, D., & Surr, R. (1979). Three experiments on the California Consonant Test. *Journal of Speech and Hearing Disorders, 44,* 61-72.

Sher, A., & Owens, E. (1974). Consonant confusions associated with hearing loss above 2,000 Hz. *Journal of Speech and Hearing Research, 17,* 669-681.

Stevens, S., & Davis, H. (1938). *Hearing: Its psychology and physiology.* New York: John Wiley & Sons.

Stout, G., & Windle, J. (1992). *Developmental Approach to Successful Listening II*. Englewood, CO: Resource Point, Inc.

Tillman, T., & Carhart, R. (1966). An expanded test for speech discrimination utilizing CNC monosyllabic words. Northwestern University Auditory Test No. 6 (Technical Report No. SAM-TR55). Brooks Air Force Base, TX: USAF School of Aerospace Medicine.

Tramwell, L., & Owens, S. (November, 1977). The test of auditory comprehension (TAC). Paper presented at the annual convention of the American Speech-Language-Hearing Association, Chicago.

Tye-Murray, N., Tyler, R., Lansing, C., & Bertschy, M. (1990). Evaluating the effectiveness of auditory training stimuli using a computerized program. *Volta Review*, *92*, 25–30.

Tyler, R., Preece, J., & Lowder, M. (1983). The Iowa cochlear implant tests. Iowa City, Iowa: University of Iowa Press.

Walden, B., Erdman, l., Montgomery, A., Schwartz, D., & Prosek, R. (1981). Some effects of training on speech recognition by hearing-impaired adults. *Journal of Speech and Hearing Research*, *24*, 207–216.

Walden, B., & Grant, K. (1993). Research needs in rehabilitative audiology. In J. Alpiner & P. McCarthy (Eds.), *Rehabilitative audiology: Children and adults*. Baltimore: Williams & Wilkins.

Walden, B., & Montgomery, A. (1975). Dimensions of consonant perception in normal and hearing-impaired listeners. *Journal of Speech and Hearing Research*, *18*, 111–155.

Watkins, S., & Clark, T. (1993). SKI-HI Resource Manual: Family-Centered Home-Based Program for Infants, Toddlers & School-Aged Children with Hearing Impairment. Login, VT: Hope, Inc.

Watson, T. (1961). *The use of residual hearing in the education of deaf children*. Washington, DC: The Volta Bureau.

Wedenberg, E. (1951). Auditory training of deaf and hard of hearing children. *Acta Otolaryngologica* (Suppl. 110).

Wedenberg, E., & Wedenberg, M. (1970). The advantage of auditory training. In F. Berg & S. Fletcher (Eds.), *The hard of hearing child*. New York: Grune & Stratton, 319–330.

Whitehurst, M. (1966). *Auditory training for children*. Washington, DC: Alexander Graham Bell Association for the Deaf.

Zemlin, W. (1981). *Speech and hearing science* (2nd ed.). Englewood Cliffs, NJ: Prentice Hall.

4

Visual Stimuli in Communication

NICHOLAS M. HIPSKIND

Contents

INTRODUCTION

When engaged in conversation, we tend to rely primarily on our hearing to receive and subsequently comprehend the message being conveyed. In addition, given the opportunity, we look at the speaker in order to obtain further information related to the topic of conversation. The speaker's mouth movements, facial expressions, and hand gestures, as well as various aspects of the physical environment in which the communication takes place, are potential sources of useful information. Humans learn to use their vision for communication to some extent, even though most of us enjoy the benefits of normal hearing and find it unnecessary in most situations to depend on vision to communicate effectively.

The person with hearing impairment, on the other hand, is much more dependent on visual cues for communication. The degree to which persons with hearing impairment need visual information when conversing is proportional to the amount of information that is lost due to hearing impairment. In other words, a person with a severe hearing loss is likely to be more dependent on visual information to communicate than is an individual with a mild auditory impairment.

Visual information may be transmitted by means of a manual or an oral communication system. In oral communication, the listener uses visual cues by observing the speaker's mouth, facial expressions, and hand movements to help perceive what is being said. This process is referred to by such terms as *lipreading, visual hearing, visual communication, visual listening,* and *speechreading.* Among lay personnel the most popular of these terms is *lipreading.* The term seems to imply the use of only visual cues for purposes of identifying various articulatory gestures. However, since the use of vision for communication involves more than watching the speaker's mouth, most professionals prefer the term *speechreading.* Thus, *speechreading* is used in this chapter to refer to visual perception of oral communication. An exception to this is a highly specialized form of speechreading termed TADOMA, in which the speechreader uses tactile cues for speech perception by placing the fingers and hand on the speaker's lips, face, and neck. This method has proven successful with some individuals who are both deaf and blind (Reed, et al., 1985).

Manual communication, or "sign language," also relies on a visual system. Manual communication is transmitted via special signs and symbols made with the hands and is received visually. This complex form of communication allows for transfer of information via the visual channel when both the sender and the receiver are familiar with the same system of symbols.

This chapter discusses the advantages and limitations of vision as part of the audiologic rehabilitation process. Emphasis will be given to the factors that affect speechreading, as well as to a discussion of manual communication methods. The reader is reminded that persons with hearing impairment comprise two populations: persons who are hard of hearing, and those who are deaf. Although frequently classified under the generic term "hearing impaired," these groups have different communication needs and limitations. Therefore, it is unrealistic to expect that a single rehabilitation method can satisfy all their communication needs. Ultimately, it is the clinician's responsibility to select appropriate strategies that will enable persons who are hard of hearing and persons who are deaf to use vision to enhance their communicative skills effectively, to achieve educational and vocational success, and to mature emotionally and socially.

FACTORS RELATED TO SPEECHREADING

The variables that affect the speechreading process usually fall into one of four general areas: the speaker, the signal code, the environment, and the speechreader. While research has contributed to a better understanding of how speech is processed visually, some of the findings are equivocal and have been found to be difficult to duplicate in the clinical setting (Alpiner & McCarthy, 1993). This is not to imply that audiologic rehabilitationists should ignore available laboratory findings; rather, they must realize the significance of these findings in order to provide individualized patient programming. The following section presents selected experimental evidence regarding factors that have been reported to influence the efficacy of speechreading. Figure 4.1 provides a summary of these factors.

Speaker

Differences among speakers have a greater effect on speechreading than on listening. Over 50 years ago, a positive correlation was shown to exist between speaker-listener familiarity and the information received from speechreading (Day, Fusfeld, & Pintner, 1928). That is, speechreading performance improved when the speaker was familiar to the receiver (speechreader). Speakers who used appropriate facial expressions and common gestures and who positioned themselves face to face or within a 45-degree angle of the listener also facilitated communication for the speechreader (Berger, 1972a; Stone, 1957; Woodward & Lowell, 1964).

The rate of normal speech results in the production of as many as 15 phonemes/sec (Orr, Friedman, & Williams, 1965). Evidence suggests that the eye is capable of recording only 8 to 10 discrete movements/sec (Nitchie, 1951). Thus, a speaker's normal speaking rate may exceed the listener's visual reception capabilities. The normal rate of speech may be too fast for optimum visual processing; on the other hand, slowed and exaggerated speech production does not assure improved comprehension. Rather, investigators have reported that speakers who use a normal speech rate accompanied by precise, not exaggerated, articulation are the easiest for the speechreader to understand (O'Neill, 1951; Rios-Escerla & Davis, 1977). Recently, Montgomery (1993) has noted that the rapidity of speech may not be as limiting a factor in determining speechreading success as was once thought because each phoneme does not produce a discrete visual stimulus. The speaker also should avoid simultaneous oral activities such as chewing, smoking, and yawning when conversing with a hearing-impaired person. While the "masking effects" of these coincidental activities have not been documented, they seem likely to complicate an already trying task. With respect to the gender of speakers, Berger and DePompei (1977) found evi-

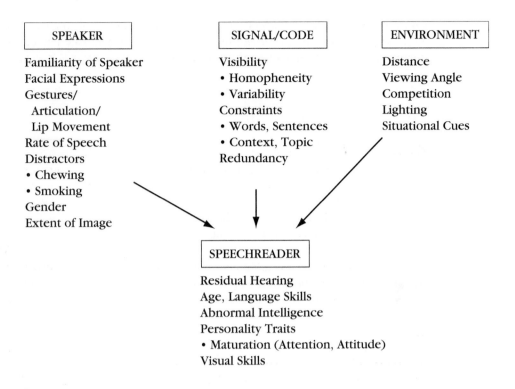

Figure 4.1 Summary of various factors related to speechreading performance. *Note:* Arrows have been drawn from the Speaker, Signal/Code, and Environmental lists to Speechreader to signify that all these factors influence the speechreader's performance, in addition to those variables that are directly related to the speechreader.

dence to suggest that male speechreaders often find female speakers to be more difficult to speechread than male speakers. However, little evidence exists which clarifies the potential influence that gender-related variables associated with the speaker, such as a moustache or the use of lipstick, may have on speechreading success.

The speaker may enhance conversational efficiency by complementing speechreading with appropriate facial expressions and gestures (Sanders, 1993). From infancy, we learn that the spoken word "no" can be accompanied by a stern facial expression and shaking of the head and/or index finger from side to side. Salutations are often made in conjunction with a smile and the extension or wave of the hand, opening of the arms and/or puckering of the lips. Similarly, shrugging of the shoulders has become a universal gesture that augments the verbal phrases, "I don't know" or "I don't care." Consequently, appropriate nonverbal communication is closely associated with the verbal message and is used simultaneously with speech to provide emphasis and redundancy. This means that situations where the speechreader can observe both the head and body of the speaker generally will be more productive for the speechreader. Nitchie (1912) was one of the first teachers of speechreading to stress that persons with hearing impairment must learn to be cognizant of nonverbal cues when attempting to understand speech that to them is acoustically and visually distorted.

Signal/Code

Speech consists of acoustic information that is efficiently received and effectively interpreted by the normal auditory mechanism. It possesses physical characteristics that are compatible with the receptive capabilities of the normal ear. The basic units of speech are consonants and vowels, classified as *phonemes*. A given phoneme has distinctive acoustic features that enable the listener to distinguish it from all other speech sounds.

Vowels embody the major concentration of acoustic energy found in speech, and are termed resonated phonemes. Vowel production is accomplished by the speaker's directing vocalizations through the oral cavity, which is altered in shape and size by different tongue and lip positions. These subtle alterations are responsible for providing each vowel with specific acoustic features.

Consonants, which are primarily responsible for the intelligibility of speech, are termed articulated phonemes, since their production involves the manipulation of the various articulators—lips, tongue, and teeth. As pointed out in Chapter 3, these phonemes possess articulatory features that permit a listener to recognize them. Miller and Nicely (1955) classified these features as voicing, nasality, affrication, duration, and place of articulation. Except for place of articulation, the identifying characteristics of consonants are perceived well on the basis of acoustic information. Although difficult to distinguish acoustically, the place of articulation may be processed to some extent visually due to the visibility of the articulators.

 Since many of the approximately 40 phonemes used in English demonstrate ambiguous or very limited visible features, an individual who relies solely on vision to understand speech faces much uncertainty. Knowledge of the visual components of speech depends, for the most part, on research using small speech units, that is, consonant-vowel combinations or monosyllabic words (e.g., Jackson, 1988; Owens & Blazek, 1985).

Visemes. The cues for distinctive visual features of vowels and consonants are reduced to the shape of the mouth for vowels and the place of articulation for consonants. Since the perception of phonemes is primarily an auditory function based on acoustic features, Fisher (1968) coined the term *viseme* to indicate the distinguishable visual characteristics of speech sounds. A viseme, therefore, is the visual correlate of a speech sound (phoneme) that has been classified by its place of articulation or by the shape of the mouth. This creates a major limitation for the observer of speech compared to the listener. Whereas combinations of auditory distinctive features are unique to each phoneme, several phonemes yield the same viseme, thus limiting the speechreader to the conclusion that one of a group of sounds was uttered.

Woodward (1957) and Woodward and Barber (1960) concluded that, since groups of consonants are produced at the same points of articulation, the phonemes within these groups cannot be differentiated visually without grammatical, phonetic, or lexical information. These visually confusable units of speech are labeled homophemes—different speech sounds that look the same. Similarly, words that look alike are referred to as homophenous words. Look in the mirror and say aloud or have a friend utter the syllables /p/, /b/, and /m/. As you watch and listen simultaneously, the syllables sound so different that you may not notice their visual similarities. However, when these same syllables are formed without voice, you will note that their visual characteristics are indistinguishable. This same type of confusion occurs often among word groups (e.g., *pet*, *bed*, and *men*; *tip*, *limb*, and *dip*; and *cough* and *golf*). However, it has been demonstrated that talkers significantly influence the number of visemes (Kricos & Lesner, 1982). That is, some talkers are easier to speechread than others because they produce more distinctively different viseme groups. It has been estimated that, regardless the number of viseme categories reported by various authors, in conversational speech nearly 50% of the words are indistinguishable visually (Berger, 1972b).

Consonant Visemes. A number of studies have been conducted to determine the number of visemes in spoken English. Woodward and Barber (1960) were the first to classify consonants into four visually contrastive groups based on their place of articulation: bilabials, rounded labials, labiodentals, and nonlabials. Fisher (1968) later tested for confusion among these same consonants when they occurred in the initial and final positions of words. In general, his results were in agreement with Woodward and Barber's (1960) classification of homophenous groupings; however, his viseme classes resulted in five clusters, rather than four, for both the initial and final positions. Erber (1974), Binnie, Montgomery, and Jackson (1974), Binnie, Jackson, and Montgomery (1976), Walden, et al. (1977), Walden, et al. (1981), Owens and Blazek (1985), and Lesner, Sandridge, and Kricos (1987) found that their viewers were able to recognize from five to nine distinct groups of consonants. Table 4.1 lists the homophenous classifications proposed by several authors. Table 4.1 also illustrates the chance for error a listener has when required to interpret phonemes visually. Except for the *independent visemes* of /h/, /r/, /w/, and /j/ reported by Binnie, et al. (1976) and Jeffers and Barley (1971), all visemes contain at least two phonemes. Consequently, on the average, the speechreader has at best a 50% chance of correctly identifying a specific isolated phoneme within any group when relying solely on vision.

Vowel Visemes. Although vowels are not considered articulated phonemes, Jeffers and Barley (1971) suggested that vowels can be visually recognized by their movements, that is, by "a recognizable visual motor pattern, usually common to two or more speech sounds" (p. 42). These authors observed seven visible movements when the vowels were produced at a slow rate accompanied by pronounced movement

TABLE 4.1 *Visemes for English Consonants Determined by Various Researchers*

Viseme Groups			
Jeffers and Barley (1971)	*Fisher (1968)*		*Binnie et al. (1976)*
	Initial*	*Final***	
1. /f, v/	1. /f, v/	1. /f, v/	1. /f, v/
2. /p, b, m, d/	2. /p, b, m, d/	2. /p, b/	2. /p, b, m/
3. /p, b, m/	3. /hw, w, r/	3. /ʃ, ʒ, dʒ, tʃ/	3. /w/
4. /θ, ð/	4. /ʃ, t, n, l, s,	4. /t, d, n, θ, ð,	4. /l, n/
5. /ʃ, ʒ, tʃ, dʒ/	z, dʒ, j, h/	s, z, r, l/	5. /ʃ, ʒ/
6. /s, z/	5. /k, g/	5. /k, g, ʒ, m/	6. /r/
7. /j/			7. /θ, ð/
8. /t, d, n, l/			8. /t, d, s, z/
9. /k, g, ŋ/			9. /k, g/

*Observed in the initial position

**Observed in the final position

The order of the visemes is based on Binnie and coworkers (1976) rank-ordering of the visual clustering of these phonemes.

and normal rhythm. When the same phonemes were produced in conversational speech, the number of different movements was reduced to four. The distinctive visible characteristics of vowels as determined by Jeffers and Barley (1971) and Jackson, et al. (1976) are shown in Table 4.2.

In general, it has been demonstrated that there are consistent visual confusions among vowels, frequently with vowels that have similar lip positions and movement (Jackson, et al., 1976; Montgomery & Jackson, 1983). Furthermore, there are vowels that are seldom recognized visually and, as might be expected, the vowels that are perceived correctly in isolation are not necessarily comprehended visually in conversational speech.

In summary, most of the individual phonemes in our language are not unique visually, resulting in considerable confusion and misperception on the part of the speechreader.

Visual Intelligibility of Connected Discourse. Researchers have enumerated the visemes that viewers can identify at the syllable and word levels, but they are less certain about what is visibly discernible when these units are portions of lengthier utterances. The visual properties of isolated speech units change when placed in sentence form, as does the acoustic waveform itself. Unless there is a visible pause between words, a speechreader presumably perceives an uninterrupted series of lip movements of varying degrees of inherent visibility. This sequence is broken only when the speaker pauses, either deliberately or for a breath. As a result, the written message, "There is a blue car in our driveway," is spoken, /ðɛrɪzəblukarɪnaʊɚdraɪvweɪ/. Connected speech contains numerous articulatory positions and movements that occur in a relatively short period of time. The major

TABLE 4.2 *Visemes for English Vowels, as Determined by Two Separate Studies*

Viseme Groups	
Jeffers and Barley (1971)	*Jackson, Montgomery, and Binnie (1976)*

Ideal Viewing Conditions

1. Lips Puckered-Narrow Opening—/u, ʊ, o, oʊ, ɝ/
2. Lips Back-Narrow Opening—/i, ɪ, eɪ, e, ʌ/
3. Lips Rounded-Moderate Opening—/ɔ/
4. Lips Relaxed-Moderate Opening to Lips Puckered-Narrow Opening—/aʊ/
5. Lips Relaxed-Moderate Opening—/ɛ, æ, a/
6. Lips Rounded-Moderate Opening to Lips Back-Narrow Opening—/ɔɪ/
7. Lips Relaxed-Moderate Opening to Lips Back-Narrow Opening—/aɪ/

Usual Viewing Conditions

1. Lips Puckered-Narrow Opening—/u, ʊ, o, oʊ, ɝ/
2. Lips Relaxed-Moderate Opening to Lips Puckered-Narrow Opening—/aʊ/
3. Lips Rounded-Narrow Opening—/ɔ, ɔɪ/
4. Lips Relaxed—Narrow Opening—/i, ɪ, eɪ, ʌ, E, æ, a, aɪ/

Dimension 1 Lip Shape—from Lips Extended to Lips Rounded—/aɪ, æ, a, eɪ, ɛ, ʌ/ vs. /u, ʊ, ɝ, aʊ, oʊ, ɔɪ/

Dimension 2 Vertical Dimension of the Lips—/i, ɪ, ɛ/vs./aɪ, æ, a/

Dimension 3 General Size of Mouth Opening—Small vs. Large—/u, ʊ, ɝ, i/ vs./æ, a, ɛ/

Dimension 4 Size of Movement from Nucleus 1 to Nucleus 2 in Diphthong Production--/aɪ/ vs./eɪ/

Dimension 5 Size of Lip Opening for Nucleus 2 in Dipthong Production—/aʊ/ vs./aɪ/

ity of phonemes in conversational speech occur in the medial position. The example just given contains an initial consonant /ð/, a final diphthong /eɪ/, with numerous sounds (positions and movements) between these phonemes. Ironically, researchers have not determined the number of visemes identifiable when phonemes occur in the medial position.

The nature of grammatical sentence structure imposes constraints on word sequences that are not present when the words exist as isolated units. These word-arrangement rules change the probabilities of word occurrence. Thus, the receiver's task is altered (theoretically easier) because of the linguistic information and redundancy provided by connected discourse. Language is structured in a way that provides more information than is absolutely necessary to convey a given meaning or thought. Even if certain fragments of the spoken code are missed, cues or information inherent in the message may assist the receiver in making an accurate prediction of the missing parts. That is, oral language is an orderly process that is governed by the rules of pragmatic, topical, semantic, syntactic, lexical, and phonological constraints that are the sources for linguistic redundancy (Boothroyd, 1988).

Briefly, the pragmatic constraints of language (context, intent) allow two or more individuals to share thoughts and information orally. Similarly, the topical constraints, which are also referred to as contextual and situational constraints, limit conversation to a specific topic, which, in turn, governs the vocabulary that is appropriate to describe the topic. We use this rule consistently, even though we frequently introduce it in a negative manner. For example, how many times have you said, "Not to change the subject," and then promptly deviated from the original topic of conversation? You are engaging the rule of contextual information, and regardless of how it is initiated, it provides your receiver with a preparatory set that allows her/him to expect a specific vocabulary concerned with a specific event. The situation/environment determines the manner in which the speaker will describe a certain event. Comedians are masters at using this rule; they alter the language of their "stories" based on the make-up of their audience. Contextual and situational constraints are closely allied and are used interchangeably by some authors. For example, during a televised sporting event when a coach disputes a decision by a referee, have you noticed how well you perceive what the coach says even though you only have limited auditory and visual cues available? Contextually you perceive an argument while the situation causes the coach to express himself by using a rather limited and "heated" vocabulary that enables you to predict the words being used. As illustrated in this instance, the situation in which the conversation occurs provides information that otherwise you may not have been able to obtain by relying solely on the articulatory features of the message.

Redundancy, the result of these constraints, contributes significantly to the information afforded by oral language. Thus, redundancy allows the receiver to predict missed information from the bits of information that have been perceived. To illustrate, "Dogs going" means the same as "The dogs are going away." The latter is grammatically correct and contains redundant information. Plurality is indicated twice (dogs, are), present tense twice (are, going), and the direction twice (going, away). Consequently, it would be possible to miss the words "are" and "away" while yet comprehending the message ("dogs going"). If we miss part of a message, linguistic redundancy can enable us to synthesize correctly what we missed. However, as will be mentioned in the discussion of perceptual closure, a minimum amount of information must be perceived before accurate predictions can be made. In the preceding example, the words *dogs* and *away* would have to be processed visually in order for the speechreader to conceptualize the message, "The dogs are going away."

While the constraints of language do not enhance the physical visibility of oral sentences, they assist the receiver in visually understanding or speechreading what has been said. Albright, Hipskind, and Schuckers (1973) demonstrated that speechreaders actually obtain more total information from the redundancy and linguistic rules of spoken language than from phoneme and word visibility. This finding has been supported by Hipskind (1977). Clouser (1976) concluded that the ratio between the number of consonants and vowels did not determine the visual intelligibility of sentences; rather, he found that short sentences were easier to speechread than longer sentences. In another study related to visual perception of speech, Berger (1972b) determined that frequently used words were identified visually more often than were words used infrequently. Additional information on redundancy is provided in Chapter 3 (see Tables 3.3 and 3.4).

Environment

Circumstances associated with the environments in which the speechreader must communicate can influence the speechreading process considerably. For example, investigators have demonstrated that such factors as distance and viewing angles between the speaker and receiver affect speechreading performance. Erber's (1971c) study regarding the influence of distance on the visual perception of speech revealed that speechreading performance was optimal when the speaker was about 5 feet from the speechreader. Although performance decreased beyond 5 feet, it did not drop significantly until the distance exceeded 20 feet. Similarly, there is evidence that simultaneous auditory and visual competition can have an adverse effect on speechreading under certain conditions (O'Neill & Oyer, 1981). Although the amount of lighting is not an important factor in speechreading, provided a reasonable amount of light is present, Erber (1974) suggested that, for optimal visual reception of speech, illumination should provide a contrast between the background and the speaker's face.

Based on independent studies, Pelson and Prather (1974) and Garstecki (1977) concluded that speechreading performance improved when the spoken message was accompanied by relevant pictorial and auditory cues. This finding was given further support by Garstecki and O'Neill (1980), whose subjects had better speechreading scores when the CID Everyday Sentences were presented with appropriate situational cues. In essence, environmental cues provide speechreaders with contextual and situational information, thereby increasing their ability to predict what is being conveyed verbally.

Speechreader

Reduction of a person's ability to hear (auditory sensitivity) auditory stimuli is only one of several parameters that contribute to the handicapping effects of hearing impairments. Other factors, such as auditory perception abilities (recognizing, identifying, and understanding), age of onset of the hearing loss, progressivity, site(s) of lesions, and the educational/therapeutic management all contribute toward making the hearing-impaired population extremely heterogeneous (Hipskind, 1978). This heterogeneity appears to extend to speechreading, since individuals with hearing impairment demonstrate considerable variation in their ability to use vision to speechread. Individual differences in speechreading abilities are large. This body of research is summarized by Dodd and Campbell (1987). Some persons possess amazing speechreading abilities, while others are able to perceive very little speech through the visual channel. Since the inception of using speechreading as an educational and clinical approach to audiologic rehabilitation, clinicians and researchers have attempted to determine what personal characteristics of the speechreader account for success/failure in speechreading, including variables such as age, intelligence, personality traits, and visual acuity (Berger, 1972a; O'Neill & Oyer, 1981). In general, it was impossible to clarify totally the characteristics associated with success in speechreading. The following is a sampling of the research that has been conducted in this area related to the speechreader.

Hearing. Unfortunately, persons with hearing impairment generally are not any better at speechreading than are those with normal hearing. Among persons with hearing impairment, however, there is a slight relationship between speechreading proficiency and the degree of hearing loss present. Those persons with significant amounts of residual hearing remaining have the potential to speechread more successfully than those with very limited hearing. This is due to the fact that speechreading is enhanced by the availability of simultaneous auditory cues contained in speech. This enhancement is especially apparent in persons beginning to use either a cochlear implant or a tactile device, where speechreading performance often improves dramatically relative to what it had been previously.

Age. There appear to be some interactions between a speechreader's age and other attributes that contribute to speechreading ability. Specifically, evidence suggests that speechreading proficiency tends to develop and improve throughout childhood and early adulthood and appears to be closely associated with the emergence of language skills (Berger, 1978; Jeffers & Barley, 1971). Even though their speechreading abilities are not fully developed, younger children, even infants, may use speechreading to some extent (Pollack, 1985).

Some older people demonstrate phonemic regression, that is, an inability to understand speech that is not consistent with their audiometric profiles (Gaeth, 1948). This same type of phenomenon may account, in part, for the finding that older individuals do less well in speechreading than their counterparts who are between the ages of 21 and 30 (Garstecki, 1983; Pelson & Prather, 1974). Shoop and Binnie (1979) suggested that the elderly perform more poorly on experimental speechreading tasks, because of the lowered ability to process abstract stimuli and unfamiliarity with the stimuli used to assess speechreading ability. Finally, the decreased visual acuity which accompanies aging may also contribute to reduced speechreading skill.

Intelligence. An abundance of research describes the relationship between speechreading and mental abilities. Generally, no demonstrable positive correlation has been found between understanding speech visually and intelligence, assuming intelligence levels in or above the "low normal" range (Lewis, 1972). However, a study conducted by Smith and his colleagues (1964) with a population of individuals with mental impairment revealed that much-reduced intelligence levels did result in significantly poorer speechreading performance.

Personality Traits. As may be expected from the preceding discussion, investigators have not been able to ferret out specific personality traits that differentiate among levels of speechreading proficiency. While motivation is tenuous to assess, most clinicians intuitively concur that highly motivated (competitive) clients tend to speechread more effectively than do unmotivated clients. Nitchie (1912, 1950) and Kinzie (1931) discussed the necessity of motivation in their methods of teaching speechreading. However, various persons have concluded that good and poor speechreaders cannot be predicted based on personality patterns (Giolas, Butterfield, & Weaver, 1974; O'Neill, 1951).

Visual Skills. Since speechreading is a visual activity, acuity of vision is critical in the decoding process. As discussed in the Visual Assessment section of this chapter, vision has received meager attention from researchers in audiologic rehabilitation.

VISUAL ACUITY. In 1970 Hardick, Oyer, and Irion determined that they could rank-order successful and unsuccessful speechreaders on the basis of visual acuity. Furthermore, these authors observed a significant relationship between eye blink rate and speechreading ability, with poorer speechreaders demonstrating higher eye blink rates. Just prior to this research, Lovering (1969) demonstrated that even slight visual acuity problems (vision of 20/40 and poorer) had an appreciable, negative effect on speechreading scores. Most recently, Johnson and Snell (1986) showed that distance has a significant effect on visual acuity. These authors report that children with visual acuity of 20/80 or better should be able to speechread at 5 feet with an adequate degree of accuracy. When the speechreader is positioned 22 feet from the talker, it is necessary that the speechreader have visual acuity no poorer than 20/30. If, however, the speechreader has one eye of 20/30 or better, he or she should be able to speechread at a level comparable to that of individuals with normal binocular vision under similar viewing conditions.

In support of the argument that good visual acuity is important for successful speechreading performance, Romano and Berlow (1974) concluded that visual acuity must be at least 20/80 before speech can be decoded visually. A line of research also has compared visually evoked responses and speechreading ability. According to the results of this research, a viewer's ability to process speech visually is, in part, a function of the rapidity (latency) with which physical visual stimuli are transduced to neural energy for interpretation at the cortical level (Samar & Sims, 1983, 1984; Shepard, 1982; Shepard, et al., 1977; Summerfield, 1992). While the clinical applicability of this research has not yet been fully realized, visually evoked responses can assist the clinician in understanding a client's ability to process visually oriented information. Potentially, visually evoked responses may provide audiologic rehabilitationists with information regarding a viewer's ability to speechread various types of oral stimuli.

VISUAL PERCEPTION. Based on Gibson's (1969) definition of perception, our eyes receive visual stimuli that are interpreted at a cortical level and provide us with visual information. This information, in turn, enables us to make a selective response to the original stimuli. Thus, when interpreting speech visually, the speechreader first "sees" the movement of the lips, which the cortex classifies as speech. The accuracy of the speechreader's response to these stimuli is partially a function of how well the peripheral-to-central visual process enables her/him to discriminate among the speaker's articulatory movements.

At present, explanations of the way in which the perceptual process develops are theoretical. However, two strategies appear predominant in connection with obtaining information from the environment. The first, figure-ground patterning, is achieved by identifying a target (meaningful) signal embedded in similar, but ambient, stimuli. Observe the following letters:

W A B R I O D R A Z

O P A I B L O H Y E

L I P R E A D I N G

L R A C R A X O L

M U A L Y O C E P L

The letters within this rectangle are of the same case (capitals) and are placed in an order that meets the criteria of structural ordering. That is, all the letter combinations are possible and probable in written English. As noted, however, there is only one string of letters that creates a meaningful word: *LIPREADING* (line 3). Thus, this sequence of printed symbols is the figure while all the other letters are merely spurious background stimuli. The development of figure-ground patterning permits persons with hearing impairment to separate meaningful visual and auditory events from ambient stimuli.

As early as 1912, Nitchie claimed that successful speechreaders are intuitive and able to synthesize limited visual input into meaningful wholes. Later, Sanders and Conscarelli (1970), Sharp (1972), and Hipskind (1977) concurred that effective speechreaders possess the ability to visually piece together fragmented pictorial and spoken stimuli into meaningful messages. This ability, termed closure, is yet another strategy used to obtain information from environmental events. Before this strategy can be used effectively, we must receive at least minimal stimulation, and, more importantly, must have had prior experience (familiarity) with the whole. Both of the following sentences require that the reader use closure to obtain accurate information:

1. Humpty _____ _____ _____ _____ wall.
2. When you ___*kill*___ time, you murder *opportunity*.

In all probability you had little difficulty supplying the four words, "Dumpty sat on a", to the first sentence. The second sentence may have been more difficult unless you are familiar with the adage, "When you kill time, you murder opportunity." The first sentence provides considerably fewer physical cues than does the second; but experience with and exposure to nursery rhymes permitted you to perceive the whole figure. Effective visual closure skills are essential for persons with hearing impairment, because, due to their disorder and the limited visual cues afforded by speech, they receive fragmented/distorted auditory and visual stimuli. In trying to understand the role of prediction or predictability it is probably very important to realize that we do not merely get some information by perception (processing the stimuli) and some from the context (prediction), and then add the two. If we did, the total information received would be equal to, or less than (because of redundancy, or correlation) the sum of what we can get from either channel alone. The fact that the total is greater than the sum of both channels (as measured above) implies a facilitating or "feedback" effect from one to the other: The audiologic information facilitates visual processing, and the visual information enhances auditory processing.

It is apparent that numerous factors have an impact on speechreading success. The successful clinician will be familiar with these and take each into account when assisting persons with hearing impairment in effectively using visual information for communication.

SPEECHREADING AND PERSONS WITH HEARING IMPAIRMENT

Assessing speechreading ability and providing effective speechreading instruction to persons with hearing impairment are two primary responsibilities of the audiologic rehabilitationist. The next section outlines some of the ways in which a person's visual communication ability can be evaluated. It also describes several traditional and current approaches to speechreading instruction.

Assessment of Speechreading Ability

Because of the complexities associated with the process, accurate evaluation of speechreading performance is difficult. Although professionals have attempted for several decades to develop a means of reliable and valid measurement, to date no universally acceptable test or battery of tests has emerged for this purpose. Nevertheless, clinicians recognize the importance of assessing speechreading ability to determine if visual communication training is warranted for a particular individual as well as to evaluate the effectiveness of speechreading training. Consequently, a number of formal and informal approaches to measuring speechreading ability are currently in use.

Formal Speechreading Tests. Since the mid-1940s, speechreading tests have been developed, published, and used. These tests, designed either specifically for adults or for children, may consist of syllables, words, sentences, stories, or a combination of these stimuli. Speechreading tests are presented either in a vision-only condition (without acoustic cues) or in a combined visual-auditory test condition in which the stimuli are both seen and heard by the speechreader. These formal tests sometimes are presented via pre-recorded video tape, but often are administered in a live, "face-to-face" situation, where the clinician presents the test stimuli. While test contents remain constant, the manner of presentation may vary considerably among clinicians when tests are administered live. These variations can make interpretation of the results less secure due to use of different speakers to present the test stimuli (Kricos & Lesner, 1982; Montgomery, et al., 1987; Spitzer, et al., 1987). Some of these tests are listed in Table 4.3 and in the appendices of this chapter.

only use as an informal tool to let you know their relative ability to speechread.

TABLE 4.3 *Chronological Listing of Speechreading Tests for Adults and Children*

Not very reliable

Date Developed	Title of Test	Author(s)	Content Format
	Adults		
1946	How Well Can You Read Lips?*	Utley	Words Sentences Stories
1957	A Film Test of Lipreading	Taaffe	Sentences
1967	Multiple-Choice Test of Lipreading	Donnelly and Marshall	Sentences
1971	Barley-CID Sentences	Barley	Sentences
1976	Lipreading Screening Test	Binnie, Jackson and Montgomery	CV-Syllables
1978	Denver Quick Test of Lipreading Ability*	Alpiner	Sentences
	Children		
1949	Cavender Test of Lipreading Ability	Cavender	Sentences
1957	Costello Test of Speechreading	Costello	Words Sentences
1959	Semi-Diagnostic Test	Hutton, Curry, and Armstrong	Words
1964	Craig Lipreading Inventory*	Craig	Words Sentences
1968	Butt Children's Speechreading Test	Butt and Chreist	Questions Commands
1970	Diagnostic Test of Speechreading	Myklebust and Neyhaus	Words Phrases Sentences

*See Appendix Four C for more information.

Informal Speechreading Tests. Informal tests are developed by the clinician, who selects stimulus materials of her/his choosing. Contents should vary as a function of the client's age and the information sought by the rehabilitationist. Clinicians use a variety of speech forms, including lists of words presented in isolation or sentences. Sentence items may include statements like "What is your name?" or "Show me a toothbrush." Informal assessment allows the tester to select stimuli that are more pertinent for a particular client than items on formal speechreading tests. However, as a result of the loose format and the intent of these tests, the obtained results do not lend themselves well to comparative analysis. Sanders (1971, 1982) presents a thorough discussion of informal speechreading assessment. The reader is encouraged to consult this source for additional information.

Whether formal or informal speechreading tests are used, it is important that the stimuli not be so difficult that they discourage the client, nor so easy that test scores reflect a ceiling effect (100% correct for each viewer). Materials should be selected so that they approximate various types of stimuli encountered by the individual in everyday situations. For children and certain adults (such as those with severe speech or writing problems) the response mode should involve pointing with a multiple-choice format; most adults are capable of responding to (writing or repeating) open-set tests. Because of the various shortcomings of existing speechreading tests, these instruments cannot be expected to provide completely valid measures of speechreading ability, but may yield data of some clinical usefulness.

The use of live, face-to-face presentation, while widespread, should be conducted carefully with optimal consideration for distance (5–10 feet), lighting (no shadows), and viewing angle (0–45 degrees). Even following these precautions, speaker variability will introduce uncertainty into the test situation. Not only will two speakers produce the same speech stimuli differently, but a single talker, producing the same stimuli twice, will not do so in precisely the same manner each time. Therefore, it is difficult to compare a person's skills from one testing to another (pre- and post-therapy) or to compare directly the performance of two individuals. Scores obtained through face-to-face test administration, while useful, need to be interpreted carefully.

Assessment of speechreading can involve the presentation of visual stimuli without any associated acoustic cues. While this method yields meaningful information regarding the basic skill of speechreading, additional testing of speechreading ability in a combined auditory/visual fashion is also advocated, since it more closely resembles ordinary person-to-person communication. Such testing provides a measure of how well a person integrates visual and auditory information (Garstecki, 1983; see also Chapter 9).

Visual Assessment and Speechreading Measurement

It is obvious that assessment of speechreading skills must be preceded by a measure of visual acuity. As discussed, there is clear evidence that even mild visual acuity problems can have adverse effects on speechreading performance. It is amazing, therefore, that audiologic rehabilitationists have given only limited attention to measuring visual abilities in connection with assessment/instruction of speechreading for persons with hearing impairment. Concern for this is further reinforced by research on visual disorders among those with hearing loss. Thus, evidence indicates that the incidence of ocular anomalies among students with hearing impairment is greater than for normally hearing children of the same age (Johnson & Caccamise, 1982). Campbell and her associates (1981) surveyed the literature and found that 38–58% of persons with hearing impairment reportedly have accompanying visual deficiencies. Even more alarming are data from the National Technical Institute for the Deaf showing that of the total number of students entering in 1978 and 1979, 65% demonstrated defective vision (Johnson, et al., 1981). (Additional information by Karp [1983] concerning visual defects among individuals with hearing loss is provided in Chapter 13 of this text.)

Riggs (1965) suggested that visual tasks of detection, recognition, resolution, and localization are fundamental when assessing a person's visual acuity. Each of these measurements uses static stimuli; that is, the viewer describes specific characteristics of stationery targets that measure a certain aspect of the viewer's visual acuity. Although research on the relationship between visual acuity and speechreading has concentrated on visual *recognition* (commonly referred to as *far visual acuity*), at least for some clients it may be prudent to determine their ability to *detect*, *resolve*, and *localize* visual test stimuli prior to initiating speechreading therapy.

Hearing Impairment and Dependence on Vision

The degree to which persons with hearing impairment depend on vision for information is related to the extent of their hearing loss. To paraphrase Ross (1982), there is a world of difference between persons who are deaf, who must communicate mainly through a visual mode (speechreading or manual communication), and persons who are hard of hearing, who communicate "primarily" (albeit imperfectly) through an auditory mode.

Persons Who Are Deaf. The deaf, who receive quite limited meaningful auditory cues, must rely more on their vision to keep in contact with their environment. Persons who are deaf, by the nature of their disorder, use their vision projectively and are visually oriented. However, as stated throughout this chapter, vision generally is less effective than audition to decode spoken language. Furthermore, for persons who are congenitally deaf, English usually is *not* the native language. ASL is their native language, as is explained later in this chapter, as well as in Chapter 6. Therefore, these individuals must learn to decode a foreign language without the benefit of auditory cues. As stated in the following chapter, English competency, which is most effectively and efficiently developed via the auditory channel, is essential to communication in our society. By definition, "speechreading is an inherently linguistic activity" (Boothroyd, 1988). Persons who are deaf therefore are further handicapped in that, before they can gain meaning from speechreading English, they must develop the linguistic rules of English, which, in turn, are most naturally acquired through aural stimulation. In summary, to benefit from speechreading, the listener/viewer must have a fairly extensive language background. Without this, he/she is unable to fill in the gaps providing information not obtained through speechreading or hearing (Bevan, 1988). Thus, persons who are deaf face the monumental challenge of having to speechread words that they may never have conceptualized.

Persons Who Are Hard of Hearing. Individuals who are hard of hearing, by definition, possess functional residual hearing, which permits them to receive and ultimately perceive more auditory stimuli within their environment than do persons who are deaf. This enhanced ability would suggest that they are less dependent on their vision than are persons who are deaf when perceiving speech. Even so, the hard of hearing, who employ their vision to supplement distorted and reduced acoustic stimuli, receive considerably more information from the spoken code (speech) than is provided solely by their auditory channel.

Various investigators have assessed the advantages that audition, vision, and a combination of these sensory modalities afford the receiver when decoding spoken stimuli (CHABA, 1991; Massaro, 1987; Qiu, 1992). Few would disagree that using these senses simultaneously produces better speech perception than using either alone. Likewise, it is clear that vision provides information to the receiver when decoding speech in the absence of auditory cues. More importantly, however, even limited auditory input allows the listener to establish a referent from which additional information can be gained visually. Thus, the contributions made by these sensory mechanisms as receptors of speech fall into a hierarchy. That is, when both residual hearing and speechreading are available, the listener with impaired hearing tends to do better on a communicative task. For example, if a person achieves a speech recognition score of 50% with hearing alone and a speechreading score of 20% using similar test material, that individual may achieve a combined auditory/visual score that could approach 90%. In other words, there is more than a simple additive effect from the combination of auditory and visual information. Consequently, speechreading used as a unisensory approach (visual only) to rehabilitate persons who are hard of hearing is normally not encouraged. A point forgotten by many clinicians is that the ultimate goal is to provide their clients with experiences that will alleviate limitations, rather than stressing a procedure that exaggerates the existing impairment. The utility of vision in decoding speech should be exploited in audiological communication training. However, this particular decoding process generally should not be emphasized at the expense of denying auditory input, except under special circumstances.

Traditional Speechreading Methods

During the early 1900s, four methods of teaching speechreading were popularized in the United States (O'Neill & Oyer, 1981). Three of these methods were nurtured by individuals who had normal hearing until adulthood, at which time they acquired significant hearing losses. Initially, they sought assistance to overcome the limitations placed on them by their sensory deprivation. Subsequently, they became interested in assisting other persons with hearing impairment to develop speechreading skills, eventually establishing methods that bear their names: the Bruhn method (1929), the Kinzie method (1931), and the Nitchie method (1912). Later, Bunger (1944) wrote a book describing the Jena method, developed by Brauckman in Jena, Germany. Although the original four speechreading methods are now seldom used as they were originally conceived, it is recommended that the interested reader refer to French-St. George and Stoker (1988) for a historical chronicle of speechreading and these early methods.

Analytic and Synthetic Approaches. Each of the above original methods for teaching speechreading, as well as the recent approaches used currently, primarily makes use of one of two general approaches (analytic or synthetic) for speechreading instruction. The analytic approach is based on the concept that before an entire word, sentence, or phrase (the whole) can be identified, it is necessary that each of its basic parts be perceived. That is, since a speaker constructs a word by placing phonemes in a given sequential order, and a sentence (thought) by correctly order-ing words, it is essential that the viewer initially visually identify phonemes in isolation before attempting to perceive words. Likewise, we must be able to identi-fy individual words before attempting to recognize strings of words (sentences/ phrases). Said differently, this approach considers the syllable to be the basic unit of speech; therefore, these units must be recognized in isolation before comprehension of the whole is probable.

Conversely, the synthetic approach emphasizes that the perception of the whole is paramount regardless of which of its parts is perceived visually. Consequently, the speechreader is encouraged to comprehend the general meaning of oral utterances rather than concentrating on accurately identifying each component within the oral message. As noted earlier, many English phonemes are not visible or distinguishable on the speaker's lips; thus, the receiver must predict and synthesize information from fragmented visual input. The synthetic approach therefore considers the sentence/ phrase to be the basic unit and backbone of visual speech perception.

Recent Trends in Speechreading Instruction

The improvements in hearing aids, assistive listening devices (ALDs), vibrotactile devices, and cochlear implants that have occurred during the past two decades have made it possible for persons with hearing impairment, especially those with moder-ate to severe losses, to more effectively use their hearing in an integrated manner with speechreading. In a sense, this increased potential to greatly improve the com-munication abilities of those with hearing loss through hearing aids has led to less emphasis on speechreading therapy in rehabilitation programs for many individuals than in the past, particularly those with mild to moderate hearing impairments. However, speechreading is still viewed as a potentially significant component of audiological rehabilitation, and therapy designed to facilitate speechreading skills is recommended for some persons with hearing impairment. The next two sections briefly discuss some of the more recent ways in which speechreading has been incor-porated into rehabilitation strategies for both children and adults.

Children. Since children with hearing impairment constitute such a heterogeneous population, there is a dearth of information concerning speechreading strategies for them (Yoshinaga-Itano, 1988). Early therapeutic approaches used for children with hearing impairment focused almost exclusively on maximizing the use of the audito-ry channel (Wedenberg, 1951; Huizing, 1952; Griffith, 1964; and Pollack, 1964, 1985). As noted in Chapter 3, this auditory-only, unisensory philosophy of management for persons with hearing impairment is sometimes referred to as the acoupedic approach. Despite the unisensory orientation of these approaches, children trained by them often emerged with effective speechreading skills. Neither Wedenberg nor Pollack generally prevented their students from speechreading, although the teaching clearly focused on processing and using auditory input. Nonetheless, speechreading appears to develop synergistically with the acquisition of auditory and language skills (Pollack, 1964).

Yoshinaga-Itano (1988) suggests using what she terms a *holistic approach* when teaching children who are hard of hearing to speechread. This method differs from the traditional approaches to speechreading, in that rather than using a single technique for all young clients, it focuses on each individual child's motivation, tolerance and sense of responsibility for communicating. Yoshinaga-Itano refers to this as *functional therapy*, while other authors classify it as a *naturalistic approach*. Consequently, the stimuli used are client oriented, and therapy is based on each client's capabilities and needs rather than on "canned" exercises. Therefore, clinical activities must address the individual needs of each child. In addition, the activities must be interesting and give the child the opportunity to experience success by correctly perceiving what is being presented. Figure 4.2 is an example of an activity that may be appropriate for *some* children who are hard of hearing. The child is given a worksheet with a picture on it and asked to speechread the key words presented by the clinician, or by other children if it is being used in a group session. Beyond providing contextual and situational information, the picture has the potential to stimulate client motivation and interest. As a reward, the clinician may ask the child to color the picture. The clinician is reminded that this is only an example, and the idea/format should be adapted to meet the needs and interests of her/his clients.

Currently, methods that incorporate both auditory and visual input are frequently favored. This bisensory stimulation is supported by such researchers and clinicians as Alpiner and McCarthy (1993) and Rodel (1985), even though the auditory input often receives the initial emphasis (Pollack, 1985). In short, the use of visual stimuli in remediation of children with hearing loss continues to be an important component in early training. However, there is a tendency mainly to allow speechreading to develop naturally in conjunction with the acquisition of auditory, speech, and linguistic skills (see Chapter 8). Thus, more emphasis is placed on improving the integration of auditory and visual cues that are available rather than exclusive work in isolation on either speechreading or auditory skills. A considerable amount of research also exists that illustrates the positive effects of using simultaneous vibrotactile or cochlear implant stimulation, along with visual information, to enhance a listener's speechreading skills (see CHABA, 1991).

Adults.   In the past, speechreading instruction was often provided to adults with hearing impairment in an intensive manner over a long period of time, which sometimes extended over several months. This older approach is still used in some instances, such as the program at the National Technical Institute for the Deaf (NTID) (Jacobs, 1982; Sims, 1985), and speechreading therapy conducted with some individuals at Walter Reed Army Hospital (Walden, et al., 1977, 1981). Interest has been growing, however, in including limited speechreading instruction as part of a general orientation to effective communication skills (Alpiner, 1982). This type of program is comparatively short-term and emphasizes a number of key components of effective communication, including the importance of speechreading in communicating, as well as providing basic information about how to enhance speechreading performance in a variety of communicative situations. (Giolas outlines such an approach in Chapter 13 of this book.) Fleming (1972) and Hardick (1977) also described similar methodologies.

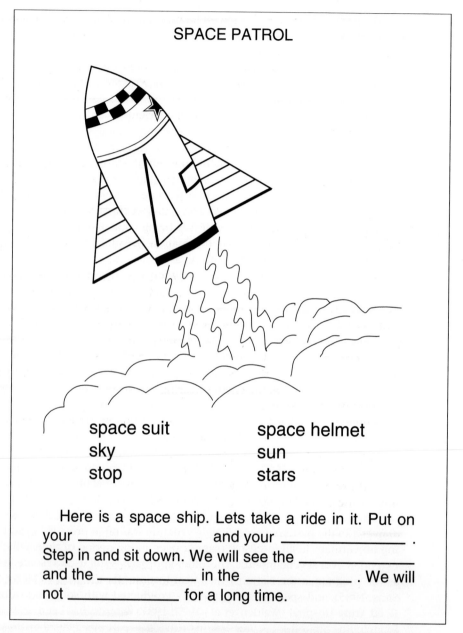

SPACE PATROL

space suit   space helmet
sky   sun
stop   stars

Here is a space ship. Lets take a ride in it. Put on your _____ and your _____ . Step in and sit down. We will see the _____ and the _____ in the _____ . We will not _____ for a long time.

Figure 4.2 An example of an exercise used in speechreading therapy with children.

Whether speechreading therapy is conducted over the short or long term, or is carried out in an analytic or synthetic manner, several researchers (Garstecki, 1983; Montgomery & Sylvester, 1984) have expressed a growing awareness of the wisdom of working with adults on integration of *auditory and visual speech perception skills*.

In emphasizing the need for integration of visual and auditory training, Sanders (1982) stated:

> Except for the person with little or no residual hearing, visual communication train-
> ing is inseparable from auditory training. To consider it as a separate aspect of com-
> munication requiring separate training sessions is to ignore the indisputable finding
> that audiovisual speech processing is superior to auditory or visual processing alone
> under degraded listening conditions. (p. 436)

Since a frequent complaint by persons who are hard of hearing is that they have difficulty understanding speech in noise or during group conversations, conducting speechreading therapy in the presence of controlled competition is a useful and practical technique in developing speechreading skills. This may be accomplished by developing one tape (auditory only) of meaningful sentences, and another tape of multi-talker speech babble. Next, a sample of meaningful sentences (targets) is presented to the client (auditorily and visually). These may be delivered live or on videotape. The target sentences and the competition (speech babble or similar signal) are introduced simultaneously at various signal/competition ratios. The competition is more effective and creates a more realistic environment when sentences of the same topic as the target sentences are used. That is, Competition: "We saw a horse at the farm"; Target: "The brown horse didn't run very far." Or Competition: "Successful students develop good study habits"; Target: "The student was successful in achieving good grades." Rehabilitationists must select appropriate signal-to-competition ratios for each client, based on the client's hearing and visual abilities (see Chapter 9 for further discussion regarding adults).

Binnie's (1976) *pseudo-dialogue format* is an effective strategy for developing listener/viewer confidence. This procedure involves selecting a specific topic such as carpentry, cooking, economics, hobbies, natural resources, and so forth, from which a number of questions and answers are developed. The client reads (out loud to him/ herself) a question prepared by the clinician, such as: "What type of leisure-time activities do you enjoy?" The client then observes the clinician who replies, without voice, "My favorite summer activity is golfing." The client then writes down what he or she thinks the clinician has said, and reads the next question, which may be, "How often do you get to play?" to which the clinician may answer, without voice, "I usually play on Saturday morning." The client's next printed question would be, "Is that all you get to play?", to which the clinician's "mouthed" response would be, "Every now and then I sneak out during the week." This give-and-take provides the listener with a preparatory set while attempting to interpret speech visually.

In describing the general strategies to use with the adult with hearing impairment in the management process, Alpiner (1982) introduced the *progressive approach*. This is a client-centered, individualized format to rehabilitation which emphasizes an interactive rather than a directive approach between the clinician and the client. Although Alpiner (1982) describes the progressive approach as a counseling-oriented methodology to improve oral communication, other authors feel that this approach specifically includes: determining each client's needs, aspirations, attitude,

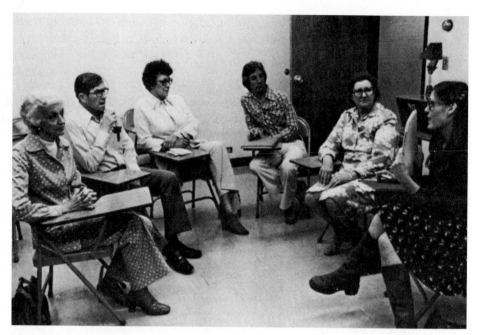

The clinician presents speech in an auditory-only condition to demonstrate the loss of information when speechreading is not possible.

and motivation; problem-solving; developing client self-responsibility; involving the client's significant others, including colleagues, employer and clergy; and designing homework activities (Cherry & Rubinstein, 1988). Consequently, the premise of the progressive approach is to assist adults who are hard of hearing to maintain and improve their oral communication skills in their everyday activities by using those same everyday activities to enhance these skills. Specifically, Alpiner (1978) states "that the goals of therapy in the progressive approach are to modify either the client's behavior and attitudes or his environment or a combination of both" (p. 98). This modification, as it pertains to speechreading, may be achieved by explaining to the adult clients with hearing impairment that speechreading is a supplement to the fragmented auditory information they receive. It will assist them to synthesize auditory and visual information to understand better what people are saying. As Nitchie (1912, 1950) pointed out, speechreading is a combined physical and mental activity that enables the listener's mind to interpret the available information in order to make a predictable judgement of what was said. Cherry and Rubinstein (1988) state that the speechreader must use two types of information: (1) the portion of the conversation that is unequivocally understood, and (2) any additional cues—the speaker's facial expressions, gestures, postures, and movements; and the situation in which the conversation occurs. This second type of information will be enhanced when the speechreader uses repair strategies that are developed by her/his knowing the topic being discussed, using her/his knowledge of language, keeping abreast of current events, and developing a level of confidence that will alleviate the fear of making a "best guess." Alpiner suggests that it is paramount to educate the client's significant others. This is accomplished by: (1) having family members accompany the client to therapy, (2) permitting the clinician to explain to the client's employer the handicapping effects of her/his hearing loss and how the work site can be adjusted to accommodate the employee, and (3) allowing the clinician to do public relations-type services within the community to inform the populace about the ramifications of hearing impairments.

The procedure, known as *Continuous Discourse Tracking* (CDT), or simply *tracking*, was developed by DeFilippo and Scott (1978). Originally, it was used for assessing and training a listener's ability to process conversational speech auditorily. This procedure is now being used in speechreading assessment and therapy. Tracking requires the listener who is hard of hearing to speechread verbatim passages presented by the clinician either without voice or in a combined auditory-visual manner. A performance score is derived by counting the number of words per minute (wpm) that the listener/viewer correctly identifies. An example of how tracking is applied in a therapy session is presented in Chapter 3. Owens and Telleen (1981), Robbins, et al. (1985) and Levitt, et al. (1986) confirmed that their subjects demonstrated significant learning effects when using the tracking procedure. However, there is some controversy about requiring the listener to respond verbatim in a communicative situation. DeFilippo (1988) defends the scoring procedure by stating that: (1) "it removes the responsibility of determining which deviations from a stimulus are acceptable" and (2) "verbatim reception can be both satisfying and instructive" (p. 234). Owens and Raggio (1987) and Tye-Murray and Tyler (1988) feel that verbatim responses are not appropriate in communicative activities. These authors state that the listener's ability to perceive the gist of the conversation rather than correctly identifying each word within the conversation is a much more realistic activity and should be the goal of rehabilitation. Although DeFilippo agrees that communication is an exchange of information and ideas, she believes that if the tracking procedure is used, then it should be scored as a verbatim words per minute task. If another scoring procedure is followed then the task should be referred to as something other than tracking. It is interesting to note that Fenn and Smith (1987) have developed a scoring procedure that includes *penalty points* when the speechreader is unable to perceive a stimulus word.

Another innovative approach to speechreading training is referred to as *computer-assisted interactive video* (CAIV) instruction. The use of computer-driven video and laser-disc units has received considerable attention and application in hearing rehabilitation during the past decade (Wynne and Richardson, 1989). Mahshie (1987) defines interactive video as a "video program that can be controlled by the person using it." However, for this methodology to be useful, it must be capable of controlling complex protocols tailored to the rehabilitative needs of individual students/clients. Therefore, CAIV must incorporate a variety of teaching strategies and client-response formats (Sims, 1988). The advantage of laser videodisc is the rapidity and accuracy in which specific stimuli can be accessed from the videodisc. According to Sims and his associates (1985), it takes approximately one second to access any one of 54,000 video frames. Fifteen years ago, the first interactive video for speechreading was developed at the National Technical Institute for the Deaf by Cronin and his colleagues (1979). This system was known as DAVID (Dynamic Audio Video Interactive Device). Since the first use of this technology, researchers and clinicians have used interactive video systems to determine the benefits of cochlear implants and vibrotactile devices on speechreading. In 1986, laser videodisc technology was introduced as a speechreading-training protocol (Kopra, et al., 1986). It is not within the scope of this chapter to discuss in detail the various CAIV programs now available. However, the following are other examples of the more current interactive video speechreading programs: Auditory-Visual Laser Videodisc Interactive System (ALVIS), developed by Kopra and associates (1987); Computer-Assisted Speech Perception Evaluation and Training (CASPER), designed by Boothroyd and his coworkers (Boothroyd, 1987); Computer-Aided Speechreading Training Program (CAST) designed by Pichora-Fuller and Benguerel (1991); and Computerized Laser Videodisc Programs for Training Speechreading and Assertive Communication Behaviors, developed at The University of Iowa Hospitals by Tye-Murray and her associates (1988). Most of these CAIV programs include both analytic and synthetic-based activities for speechreading instruction, including a tracking component. These programs show great promise, but the reader should be aware that many are still in various stages of development and may not be "user-friendly" for some time.

Other Considerations. It is not unusual for clinicians to lament the lack of carryover between successive therapy sessions, or between therapy and everyday activities. One reason for this is that little may be occurring in therapy that is appropriate for the client to carry over, or apply to the real world. Materials presented during speechreading therapy should be meaningful and useful, and applicable to the client's daily needs. If they are, the odds of successful carryover are greatly increased.

To increase further the chances of carryover, clinicians are encouraged to conduct a portion of the therapy sessions on speechreading outside the confines of the therapy cubicle. Frequently, therapy becomes unduly artificial because of where, as well as how, it is conducted. Most clients with hearing impairment communicate adequately, if not normally, during individual therapy sessions. Yet many of these same clients experience considerable difficulty conversing in everyday situations. Clinicians may learn a great deal by taking their clients to auditoriums, playgrounds, coffee shops, shopping malls, and other community locations.

MANUAL COMMUNICATION

Physical gestures and facial expressions have always been used by humans to express emotions and to share information. Historically, the transmission of thoughts in this manner undoubtedly preceded verbal communication. As stated earlier in this chapter, manual communication comprises specific gestural codes. That is, a message is transmitted by the fingers, hands, arms, and bodily postures using specific signs and/or fingerspelling.

In general, manualism is used by a high percentage of persons who are deaf and profoundly hard of hearing to communicate among themselves and others with these skills. The various forms of manual communication are used in isolation or in combination with speech.

Types of Manual Communication

Numerous forms of manual communication have evolved. The major types, along with spoken English, are briefly described and compared in Table 4.4 (Smith, 1984). Smith pointed out that the only two pure languages represented in this group are English and American Sign Language.

American Sign Language, also referred to as *ASL* or *Ameslan*, was the first form of manual communication established, independent of existing oral languages, by persons who are deaf. Consequently, the original sign language was indeed a unique "natural" language. Approximately one-half million deaf and hearing individuals use this language (Baker & Cokely, 1980). Interestingly, most individuals learn ASL via their peers and associates who are deaf rather than from their parents. Padden (1980) reports that it is probably the only language that is not learned from parents. Nonetheless, most adults who are deaf are proud that they communicate via ASL and are annoyed by teachers and others who are averse to its use (Vernon & Andrews, 1990).

The signs associated with ASL possess four identifying physical characteristics: hand configuration, movement, location, and orientation. In fact, Stokoe (1978) claims that there are 19 basic symbols for handshapes, 12 basic symbols for locations, and 24 basic symbols for movement. While these parameters, referred to as *cheremes* by Stokoe and associates (1965), are different from spoken lexical items, they may be viewed as analogous to the distinctive features of speech. These features are illustrated in Figure 4.3. The prosodic features of ASL are provided by facial expressions, head tilts, body movement, and eye gazes (Vernon & Andrews, 1990).

Since ASL is a language, it consists of words. However, there is not a corresponding sign to represent each English word, just as there is no unique relationship between the words used in English and any other language, such as French, Portuguese, Cantonese, or Japanese.

Historically, all languages were developed using a common code for exchange of information. Also, the structure of each language is as unique as is its vocabulary (code). Thus, "Ni qui guo zhong-guo mei-you?" probably looks and sounds "peculiar" and unintelligible to English-speakers, but the sentence is logical and meaningful to someone in Taiwan. Similarly, ASL is not a form of English, but rather a language produced manually that requires just as unique a translation of English as does any other foreign language.

Some of the over 6000 signs that are part of ASL can be decoded intuitively. These signs are classified as iconic, meaning that they are visual images of English words. The signs in Figure 4.4 will be familiar to most readers, even those who have never been exposed to manual communication—specifically ASL.

TABLE 4.4 Forms of Manual and Spoken Communication

American Sign Language (ASL)	Pidgin Sign Language (PSE)	Signed English	Linguistics of Visual English (LOVE)	Signing Exact English (SEE 2)	Seeing Essential English (SEE 1)	Finger Spelling	Cued Speech	English
Independent language; visual manual mode; own grammar; own syntax; signs are meaning based; has dialects, regionalisms, slang, puns; can be written; wide range of vocabulary covering minute differences in meaning; may borrow from other languages; is verbal, but also makes use of nonverbal elements.	A combination of elements from ASL and the sign systems, ranging from the more ASL-like (occasionally called Ameslish) to the more English-like (sometimes called CASE—Conceptually Accurate Signed English). Usually contains few if any sign markers (see Signed English), yet makes frequent use of finger-spelled English words. Used in conjunction with speech in interpreting and college teaching. Signs are meaning based.	Signed in accordance with English grammar, but signs are meaning based; specially invented sign markers for important affixes in English; invented by Bornstein; used widely in education.	Essentially the same as SEE 2, but has a method of writing each sign; used in education; invented by Wampler; usage is diminishing.	Signs are word based; special signs for all affixes in English; signed in strict accordance with English; invented by Zawolkow, Pfetzing and Gustason; widely used in education; very influential.	Signs are based on word roots (morphemes) (trans/port/a/tion); an extreme form of word-based signs; invented by Anthony; not popular in U.S., but still common in Iowa and Colorado schools for the deaf; signs for all affixes.	Manual representation of the written language; one hand shape for each letter of alphabet; used to borrow English words in ASL; when used with speech and speechreading, it is called the Rochester Method.	Employs 8 hand shapes in 4 positions on the face, and used in conjunction with lip movements to enable a deaf person to lipread more easily; based on sound with the syllable as the basic unit; devised by Orin Cornett at Gallaudet College.	Independent language; aural-oral mode; own grammar; own syntax; words are meaning based; contains dialects, regionalisms, slang, puns; can be written; wide range of vocabulary covering minute differences in meaning; may borrow from other languages; is verbal, but also makes use of nonverbal elements.

Artificial pedagogical systems, invented for educational purposes

Nonverbal communication: natural gestures, facial expression, body movements, body language, pantomime

Source: From W. H. Smith, personal communication, 1984.

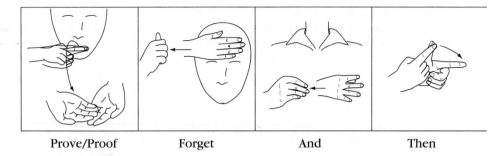

| Prove/Proof | Forget | And | Then |

Figure 4.3 Four signs used in ASL representing the features of handshape (DEZ), movement/signation (SIG), tabulation where sign is produced (TAB), and palmar direction of the hands.

From L. Riekehof (1978). *The Joy of Signing*. Springfield, MO: Gospel Publishing House.

Signed English Systems. There is evidence that only adults who are deaf are truly proficient at using ASL. When most English-speaking individuals with normal hearing attempt to communicate manually using ASL with persons who are deaf, they tend to use the signs of ASL in a manner that more closely resembles English structure. This counterpart to ASL is commonly referred to as *Pidgin Sign Language*. In other words, Pidgin Sign Language involves combining ASL with English to some extent. If the signer makes considerable English-related modifications, then the result is Pidgin Signed English.

Other attempts have been made to seriously alter ASL so that it closely resembles English. The results are referred to as sign systems. Sign systems, which have been developed mainly by educators for use in educating persons who are deaf, are contrived and have not evolved naturally, so they are not considered languages.

Signed English, for example, is a system where the English words that appear in a message are signed in the same order as in spoken English. To indicate tense, person, plurality, and possession, a sign-marker is used as a suffix to the signed word.

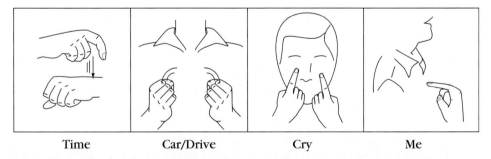

| Time | Car/Drive | Cry | Me |

Figure 4.4 Four iconic signs. The signs are visual images of the English words they represent.

From L. Riekehof (1978). *The Joy of Signing*. Springfield, MO: Gospel Publishing House.

Seeing Essential English (SEE I) was developed by David Anthony, an individual who was deaf, as a means of presenting English visually to persons who are deaf in the same way as it is presented auditorily to children with normal hearing. Anthony suggested that the word order of the message parallel that used in English. *Signing Exact English (SEE II)* is an outgrowth of SEE I. The purpose of this system is to maintain the syntactic structure of SEE I without making the system unintelligible for those using ASL.

Linguistics of Visual English (L.O.V.E.) was established at approximately the same time that SEE II was initiated. Again, this was an attempt to refine another sign system aimed at approximating English. L.O.V.E.'s vocabulary is more limited than that of SEE I and SEE II. It attempts to mirror spoken English by making signed movements that correspond to the number of syllables uttered in a spoken word. Yet, L.O.V.E. is primarily a manual system, similar to SEE II. The reader is urged to read the works of Scheetz (1993) and Vernon and Andrews (1990) for a historical and more detailed discussion of these systems.

Fingerspelling. Another method of communicating manually is to have senders spell the words with their fingers. That is, instead of using pencil and paper, persons spell their message in the air by using various handshapes to represent the letters in the English alphabet. This mode of communication, fingerspelling, represents the 26 letters of the English alphabet by 25 handshapes and two hand movements (see Figure 4.5). Collectively, these are also referred to as the *manual alphabet.* The letters *i* and *j* are produced by the same handshape, with the *j* being produced by moving the hand in a hook- or *j*-like motion. The letter *z* is made by moving a unique handshape in the form of a *z*. Although fingerspelling is an exact and effective means of communication, it is the least efficient form of manual communication, since each letter of each word must be individually produced. This makes it a relatively laborious means of communicating. Since no additional characters are included in the alphabet, nor digits in the numeric system, a person can learn to transmit a message via fingerspelling in a relatively short time. However, because of the rapidity in which one learns to "spell" a message and because of the similarity in the production of *e, o, m,* and *n,* and of *a* and *s,* the reception of fingerspelling requires considerable practice and concentration. As mentioned in the discussion of speechreading, the similarity among letters and sounds becomes more confounding during discourse than in isolation. But, as in every other form of communication, predictability mitigates this problem. Today, fingerspelling is used to supplement all forms of manual communication by expressing proper names, technical terms, and events that cannot be conveyed by signs. One application of fingerspelling is the Rochester Method, in which the teachers and students simultaneously "spell" what they are expressing orally.

Cued speech. Some professionals have promoted the use of cued speech as an ancillary tool in speechreading instruction (Cornett, 1967, 1972; Ling & Ling, 1978). The intent of Cornett's (1967) cued speech system (some would prefer to classify it as a manual system) is to use hand cues to reduce the confusion produced by speechreading homophenous phonemes, making speechreading more accurate and

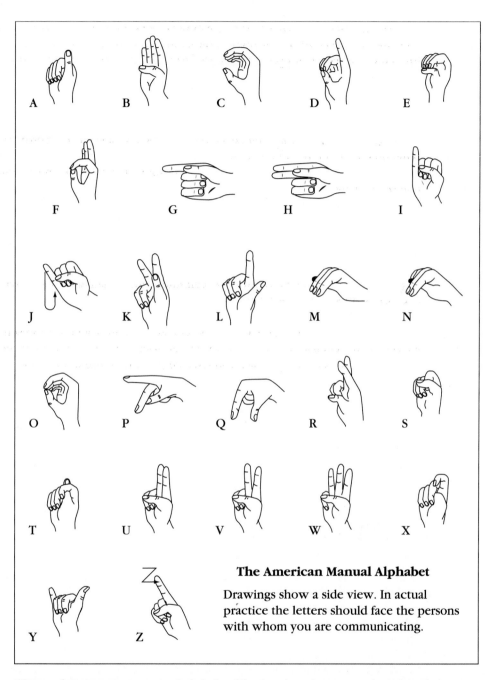

The American Manual Alphabet

Drawings show a side view. In actual practice the letters should face the persons with whom you are communicating.

Figure 4.5 American manual alphabet. The hand positions are shown as they appear to the person reading them.

Courtesy of Gallaudet College, Washington, DC.

Chart I
Cues for English Vowels

	Group I (Base Position)		Group II (Larynx)		Group III (Chin)		Group IV (Mouth)	
Open	[a:]	(fäther) (gŏt)	[a]	(thăt)	[o:]	(fôr) (ought)		
Flattened-Relaxed	[ʌ] [ə]	(but) (the)	[i]	(is)	[e]	(gĕt)	[i:]	(feet) (meat)
Rounded	[ou]	(note) (boat)	[u]	(gŏŏd) (put)	[u:]	(blue) (food)	[ə]	(ûrn) (hĕr)

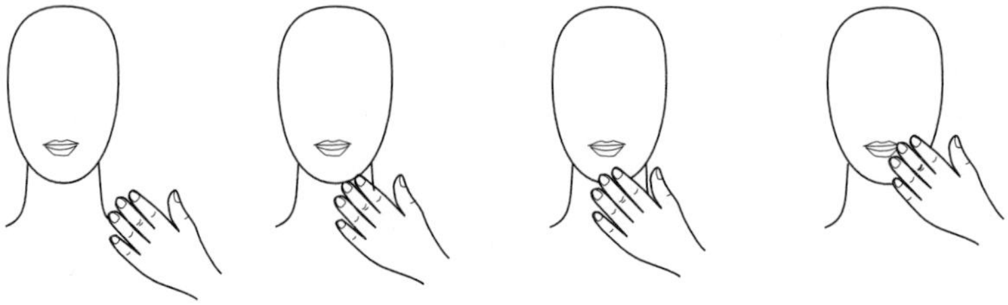

Chart III
Cues for English Consonants

T Group*	H Group	D Group	ng Group	L Group	K Group	N Group	G Group
t	h	d	(ng)	l	k	n	g
m	s	p	y (you)	sh	v	b	j
f	r	zh	ch	w	th (the)	hw**	th (thin)
					z		

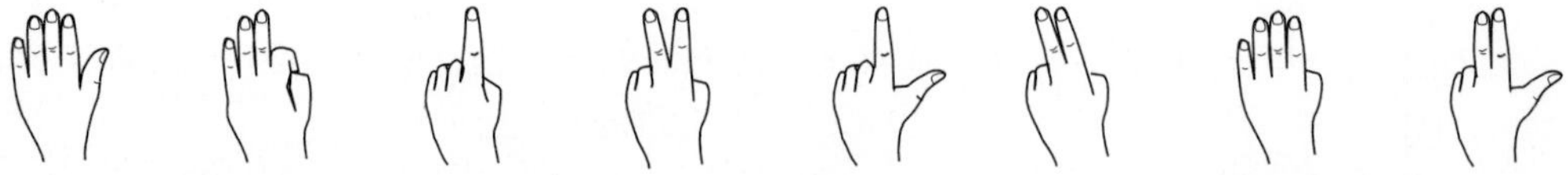

*Note: The T group cue is also used with an isolated vowel — that is, an initial vowel not run with a final consonant from the preceding syllable.

Figure 4.6 An illustration of the hand positions and handshapes used in cued speech.

From R. Cornett (1967). Cued speech. *American Annals of the Deaf, 112,* 3–13.

effective. Cornett selected four hand positions and eight handshapes near the mouth to accompany spoken vowels and consonants respectively (see Figure 4.6). These cues are used in combination and presented simultaneously with speech as a supplement to the visual information already present for the speechreader. Kipila and Williams-Scott (1988) state,

> A basic rule of cueing is to cue what you say, the way you say it, when you say it. Cued speech is based on spoken language, including dialects, accents and colloquialisms. Anything uttered within the accepted phoneme system of a spoken language can be cued.

Vernon and Andrews (1990) cite several disadvantages of this system. Among these are: (1) the information provided by the cues is totally dependent on the listener's ability to speechread; (2) it eliminates group communication since the speechreader must face the talker; (3) difficulty occurs when the speaker attempts to synchronize hand movements with production of homophenous speech sounds; and (4) the speechreader must have command of English. As was stated earlier, a prerequisite to speechreading is familiarity with the linguistic rules of the oral language being speechread. These authors conclude that cued speech may provide benefits when articulation is being taught or during speechreading training; however, they emphasize that it is not a viable aid to manual communication or to speech in a program that uses signs and speech.

SUMMARY

This chapter has reviewed information related to the various ways in which vision can be utilized effectively by persons with hearing impairment. Philosophies differ considerably concerning the role of vision and the way it is utilized in audiologic rehabilitation. Yet, most would urge the use of the visual channel in some fashion to facilitate communication in the overall rehabilitation of hearing loss.

RECOMMENDED READINGS

Alpiner, J., & McCarthy, P. (Eds.). (1993). *Rehabilitative audiology: Children and adults* (3rd ed.). Baltimore: Williams and Wilkins.

DeFilippo, C., & Sims, D. (1988). New reflections on speechreading. *Volta Review*, *90*(5), 3–313.

Gagne, J.-P., & Tye-Murray, N. (Eds.). (1994). Research in audiological rehabilitation: Current trends and future directions [Monograph]. *Journal of the Academy of Rehabilitative Audiology*, *27*.

Hipskind, N. (1978). Aural rehabilitation for adults. *Otolaryngologic Clinics of North America*, *11*, 823–834.

Jeffers, J., & Barley, M. (1971). *Speechreading*. Springfield, IL: Charles C. Thomas.

Vernon, M., & Andrews, J. (1990). *The psychology of deafness*. New York: Longman.

Vernon, M. (1987). Controversy within sign language. *The Deaf American*, *28*(1), 22–25.

REFERENCES

Albright, P., Hipskind, N., & Schuckers, G. (1973). A comparison of visibility and speechreading performance on English and Slurvian. *Journal of Communication Disorders, 6*, 44–52.

Alpiner, J. G. (1978). *Handbook of adult rehabilitative audiology*. Baltimore: Williams & Wilkins.

Alpiner, J. G. (1982). *Handbook of adult rehabilitative audiology* (2nd ed.). Baltimore: Williams & Wilkins.

Alpiner, J. G., & McCarthy, P. (Eds.). (1987). *Rehabilitative audiology: Children and adults*. Baltimore: Williams & Wilkins.

Alpiner, J. G., & McCarthy, P. (Eds.). (1993). *Rehabilitative audiology: Children and adults* (2nd ed.). Baltimore: Williams & Wilkins.

Baker, C., & Cokely, D. (1980). *American sign language: A teacher's resource test on grammar and culture*. Silver Spring, MD: T. J. Publishers.

Berger, K. (1972a). *Speechreading: Principles and methods*. Baltimore: National Educational Press.

Berger, K. (1972b). Visemes and homophenous words. *Teacher of the Deaf, 70*, 396–399.

Berger, K., DePompei, R. A., & Droder, J. L. (1970). The effect of distance on speechreading performance. *Ohio Journal of Speech and Hearing, 5*, 115–122.

Bevan, R. C. (1988). *Hearing-impaired children: A guide for parents and concerned professionals*. Springfield, IL: Charles C. Thomas Publishers.

Binnie, C. A. (1976). Relevant aural rehabilitation. In J. L. Northern (Ed.), *Hearing disorders* (pp. 213-227). Boston: Little, Brown & Co.

Binnie, C. A., Jackson, P., Montgomery, A. (1976). Visual intelligibility of consonants: A lipreading screening test with implications for aural rehabilitation. *Journal of Speech and Hearing Disorders, 41*, 530–539.

Boothroyd, A. (1987). CASPER, computer-assisted speech perception evaluation and training. In *Proceedings of the 10th Annual Conference of the Rehabilitation Society of North America*, Washington, DC: Association for Advancement of Rehabilitation Technology.

Boothroyd, A. (1988). Linguistic factors in speechreading [Monograph]. In C. L. DeFilippo & D. G. Sims (Eds.). *New Reflections on Speechreading. The Volta Review, 90*(5), 77-87.

Bruhn, M.E. (1929). *The Mueller-Walle method of lip reading for the deaf*. Lynn, MS: Nicholas Press.

Bunger, A.M. (1944). *Speechreading—Jena method*. Danville, IL: The Interstate Co.

CHABA, Working Group on Communication Aids for the Hearing-Impaired. (1991). Speech-perception aids for hearing impaired people: Current status and needed research. *Journal of the Acoustical Society of America, 90*, 637-685.

Cherry, R., & Rubinstein, A. (1988). Speechreading instructions for adults: Issues and approaches [Monograph]. In C. L. DeFilippo & D. G. Sims (Eds.). *New Reflections on Speechreading. The Volta Review, 90*(5), 289–306.

Clouser, R.A. (1976).The effects of vowel-consonant ratio and sentence length on lipreading ability. *American Annals of the Deaf, 121*, 513–518.

Cornett, R. O. (1967). Cued speech. *American Annals of the Deaf, 112*, 3–13.

Cornett, R. O. (1972). *Cued speech parent training and follow-up program.* Washington, DC: Bureau of Education for the Handicapped, DHEW.

Cronin, B. (1979).The DAVID system:The development of an interactive video system at the National Institute for the Deaf. *American Annals of the Deaf, 124*, 615–618.

Day, H., Fusfeld, I., & Pintner, R. (1928). *A survey of American schools for the deaf 1924-25.* Washington, DC: National Research Council.

DeFilippo, C. L. (1988).Tracking for speechreading training [Monograph]. In C. L. DeFilippo & D. G. Sims (Eds.). *New Reflections on Speechreading. The Volta Review, 90*(5), 215–236.

DeFilippo, C. L., & Scott, B. (1978).A method for training and evaluating the reception of ongoing speech. *Journal of the Acoustical Society of America, 63*(4), 1186–1192.

Dodd, B., & Campbell, R. (1987). *Hearing by eye: The psychology of lip-reading.* London: Erlbaum.

Erber, N. P. (1971). Effects of distance on the visual reception of speech. *Journal of Speech and Hearing Research, 14*, 848–857.

Erber, N. P. (1974). Effects of angle, distance and illumination on visual reception of speech by profoundly deaf children. *Journal of Speech and Hearing Research, 17*, 99–112.

Erber, N. P. (1979).Auditory-visual perception of speech with reduced optical clarity. *Journal of Speech and Hearing Research, 22*, 212–223.

Fenn, G., & Smith, B. Z. D. (1987).The assessment of lipreading ability: Some practical considerations in the use of the tracking procedure. *British Journal of Audiology, 21*, 253–258.

Fisher, C. G. (1968). Confusions among visually perceived consonants. *Journal of Speech and Hearing Research, 12*, 79600.

Fleming, M. (1972).A total approach to communication therapy. *Journal of the Academy of Rehabilitative Audiology, 5*, 28–31.

Gaeth, I. H. (1948). A study of phonemic regression in relation to hearing loss (Unpublished doctoral dissertation, Northwestern University).

Garstecki, D. (1977). Identification of communication competence in the geriatric population. *Journal of the Academy of Rehabilitative Audiology, 10*, 36–45.

Garstecki, D. (1983). Auditory, visual and combined auditory-visual speech perception in young and elderly adults. *Journal of the Academy of Rehabilitative Audiology, 16*, 221–233.

Garstecki, D., & O'Neill, J. J. (1980). Situational cues and strategy influence on speechreading. *Scandinavian Audiology, 9*, 1–5.

Gibson, E. J. (1969). *Principles of perceptual learning and development*. New York: Appleton-Century-Crofts.

Giolas, T., Butterfield, E. C., & Weaver, S. J. (1974). Some motivational correlates of lipreading. *Journal of Speech and Hearing Research, 17*, 18–24.

Griffith, C. (1964). The auditory approach for pre-school deaf children. *The Volta Review, 66*, 387.

Hardick, E. J. (1977). Aural rehabilitational programs for the aged can be successful. *Journal of the Academy of Rehabilitative Audiology, 10*, 51–66.

Hardick, E. J., Oyer, H. J., & Irion, P.E. (1970). Lipreading performance is related to measurements of vision. *Journal of Speech and Hearing Research, 13*, 92.

Hipskind, N. M. (1977, November). The relationship of linguistic redundancy to speechreading. Paper presented at the Speech-Language-Hearing Association National Convention, Chicago.

Hipskind, N. M., Nerbonne, G. P., & Gravel, J. S. (1973). The intelligibility of C.I.D. Auditory Test W-1 words as speechreading stimuli. *Journal of Communication Disorders, 6*, 1–10.

Jackson, P. L. (1988). The theoretical minimal unit for visual speech perception: Visemes and coarticulation. *The Volta Review, 90*, 99–115.

Jackson, P. L., Montgomery, A. A., & Binnie, C. A. (1976). Perceptual dimensions underlying vowel lipreading performance. *Journal of Speech and Hearing Research, 19*, 796–812.

Jacobs, M. (1982). Visual communication for the severely and profoundly hearing-impaired young adult. In D. Sims, G. Walter, & R. Whitehead (Eds.). *Deafness and communication: Assessment and training*. Baltimore: Williams & Wilkins.

Jeffers, J., & Barley, M. (1971). *Speechreading*. Springfield, IL: Charles C. Thomas Publisher.

Johnson, D., & Caccamise, F. (1982). *Visual assessment of hearing-impaired persons: Options and implications for the future*. Chicago: John C. Winston.

Johnson, D., Caccamise, F., Rothblum, A., Hamilton, L., & Howard, M. (1981). Identification and follow-up of visual impairments in hearing-impaired populations. *American Annals of the Deaf, 126*, 321–360.

Johnson, D., & Snell, K. B. (1986). Effects of distance & visual acuity problems on the speechreading performance of hearing-impaired adults. *Journal of the Academy of Rehabilitative Audiology, 19*, 42–55.

Karp, A. (1983). Aural rehabilitation strategies for the visually and hearing impaired patient. *Journal of the Academy of Rehabilitative Audiology, 16*, 23–32.

Kipila E., & Williams-Scott, B. (1988). Cued speech and speechreading [Monograph]. In C. L. DeFilippo & D. G. Sims (Eds.). *New reflections on speechreading. The Volta Review, 90*(5), 179–189.

Kinzie, C. E., & Kinzie, R. (1931). *Lipreading for the deafened adult*. Chicago: John C. Winston.

Kopra, L., Kopra, M., Abrahamson, J., & Dunlop, R. (1986). Development of sentences graded in difficulty for lipreading practice. *Journal of the Academy of Rehabilitative Audiology, 19*, 71–86.

Kopra, L., Kopra, M., Abrahamson, J., & Dunlop, R. (1987). Lipreading drill and practice software for an auditory-visual videodisc interactive system (ALVIS). *Journal for Computer Users in Speech and Hearing, 3*, 58-68.

Kricos, P. B., & Lesner, S. A. (1982). Differences in visual intelligibility across talkers. *The Volta Review, 84*, 219-225.

Lesner, S., Sandridge, S., & Kricos, P. (1987). Training influences on visual consonant and sentence recognition. *Ear and Hearing, 8*, 283-287.

Levitt, H., Waltzman, S. B., Shapiro, W., & Cohen, N. L. (1986). Evaluation of a cochlear prosthesis using connected discourse tracking. *Journal of Rehabilitation Research, 23*(1), 147-154.

Lewis, D. N. (1972). Lipreading skills of hearing impaired children in regular schools. *Volta Review, 74*, 303-311.

Ling, D., & Ling, A. (1978). *Aural rehabilitation: The foundations of verbal learning in hearing-impaired children.* Washington, DC: Alexander Graham Bell Association for the Deaf.

Lovering, L. (1969). Lipreading performance as a function of visual acuity (Unpublished doctoral dissertation, Michigan State University).

Mahshie, J. J. (1987). A primer on interactive video. *Journal for Computer Users in Speech and Hearing, 3*, 39-57.

Massaro, D. M. (1987). *Speech perception by ear and eye: A paradigm for psychology inquiry.* Hillsdale, NJ: Lawrence Erlbaum Associates.

Miller, G. A., & Nicely, P. E. (1955). An analysis of the perceptual confusions among some English consonants. *Journal of the Acoustical Society of America, 27*, 338-352.

Montgomery, A. (1993). Management of the hearing-impaired adult. In J. Alpiner & P. McCarthy, (Eds.). *Rehabilitative audiology: Children and adults* (2nd ed.). Baltimore: Williams & Wilkins.

Montgomery, A. A., & Jackson, P. L. (1983). Physical characteristics of the lips underlying vowel lipreading performance. *Journal of the Acoustical Society of America, 73*, 2134-2144.

Montgomery, A. A., Walden, B. E., Schwartz, D. M., & Prosek, R. A. (1984). Training auditory-visual speech reception in adults with moderate sensorineural hearing loss. *Ear and Hearing, 5*, 30-36.

Montgomery, A., & Sylvester, S. (1984). Streamlining the aural rehabilitation process. *Hearing Instruments, 35*, 46-50.

Nitchie, E. B. (1912). *Lip reading: Principles and practice.* New York: Frederick A. Stokes Co.

Nitchie, E. B. (1950). *New lessons in lip reading.* Philadelphia: J.B. Lippincott.

O'Neill, J. J. (1951). An exploratory investigation of lipreading ability among normal-hearing students. *Speech Monographs, 18*, 309-311.

O'Neill, J. J., & Oyer, H. J. (1981). *Visual communication for the hard of hearing* (2nd ed.). Englewood Cliffs, NJ: Prentice Hall.

Orr, D., Friedman, H., & Williams, J. (1965). Trainability of listening comprehension of speeded discourse. *Journal of Educational Psychology, 56*, 148-156.

Owens, E., & Blazek, B. (1985). Visemes observed by hearing-impaired and normal hearing adult viewers. *Journal of Speech and Hearing Research, 28*, 381–393.

Owens, E., & Raggio, M. (1987). The UCSF tracking procedure for evaluation and training of speech reception by hearing impaired adults. *Journal of Speech and Hearing Disorders, 52*, 120–128.

Owens, E., & Telleen, C. (1981). Tracking as an aural rehabilitation process. *Journal of the Academy of Rehabilitative Audiology, 34*(11), 9.

Padden, C. (1980). The deaf community and the culture of deaf people. In C. Baker & R. Battison (Eds.), *Sign language and the deaf community: Essays in honor of William Stokoe*. Silver Spring, MD: National Association of the Deaf.

Pelson, R. O., & Prather, W. (1974). Effects of visual message-related cues, age and hearing impairment on speechreading performance. *Journal of Speech and Hearing Research, 17*, 518–525.

Pichora-Fuller, M. K., & Benguerel, A-P. (1991). The design of CAST (computer-aided speechreading training). *Journal of Speech and Hearing Research, 34*, 202–212.

Pollack, D. (1964). Acoupedics. *The Volta Review, 66*, 400.

Pollack, D. (1985). *Educational audiology for the limited hearing infant and preschooler*. (2nd ed.). Springfield, IL: Charles C. Thomas.

Qiu, W. W. (1992). Relationships between auditory-alone and visual-alone speech perception and cognitive abilities (Unpublished master's thesis, Indiana University, Bloomington).

Reed, C. M., Rabinowitz, N. I., Braida, L. D., Conway-Fithian, S., & Schultz, M. C. (1985). Research on the Tadoma method of speech communication. *Journal of the Acoustical Society of America, 77*(1), 247–257.

Riggs, L. (1965). Visual acuity. In C. Graham (Ed.), *Vision and visual perception* (pp. 321–349). New York: John Wiley & Sons.

Rios-Escalera, A., & Davis, J. (1977). An investigation of lipreading performance as a function of speaking rate. In K. Berger (Ed.), *Research studies in speechreading* (pp. 60–70). Kent, OH: Herald Publishing House.

Robbins, A., Osberger, J. J., Miyamoto, R., Kienle, M., & Myers, W. (1985). Speech-tracking performance in single-channel cochlear implant subjects. *Journal of Speech and Hearing Research, 28*(4), 565–578.

Rodel, M. (1985). Children with hearing impairment. In J. Katz (Ed.), *Handbook of clinical audiology* (3rd ed., pp. 1004-1016). Baltimore: Williams & Wilkins.

Romano, P., & Berlow, W. (1974). Vision requirements for lipreading. *American Annals of the Deaf, 119*, 393–386.

Ross, M. (1982). *Hard of hearing children in regular schools*. Englewood Cliffs, NJ: Prentice-Hall.

Samar, V. J., & Sims, D. G. (1983). Visual evoked response correlates of speechreading performance in normal-hearing adults: A replication and factor analytic extension. *Journal of Speech and Hearing Research, 26*, 2–9.

Samar, V. J., & Sims, D. G. (1984). Visual evoked response components related to speechreading and spatial skills in hearing and hearing impaired adults. *Journal of Speech and Hearing Research, 27*, 23–26.

Sanders, D. A. (1971). *Aural rehabilitation.* Englewood Cliffs, NJ: Prentice Hall.

Sanders, D. A. (1982). *Aural rehabilitation* (2nd ed.). Englewood Cliffs, NJ: Prentice Hall.

Sanders, D. A., & Conscarelli, J. E. (1970). The relationship of visual synthesis skill to lipreading. *American Annals of the Deaf, 115*, 23–26.

Scheetz, N. A. (1993). *Orientation to deafness.* Boston, MA: Lenstok Press.

Sharp, E. Y. (1972). The relationship of visual closure to speechreading. *Exceptional Children, 38*, 729-734.

Shepherd, D. C. (1982). Visual-neural correlate of speechreading ability in normal-hearing adults: Reliability. *Journal of Speech and Hearing Research, 25*, 521-527.

Shepherd, D. C., DeLavergne, R. W., Fruek, F. X., & Clobridge, C. (1977). Visual-neural correlate of speechreading ability in normal-hearing adults. *Journal of Speech and Hearing Research, 20*, 752-765.

Shoop, C., & Binnie, C. A. (1979). The effects of age upon the visual perception of speech. *Scandinavian Audiology, 8*, 3-8.

Sims, D. G., Kopra, L. L., Dunlop, R. J. & Kopra, M. A. (1985). A survey of microcomputer applications in aural rehabilitation. *Journal of the Academy of Rehabilitative Audiology, 18*, 9-26.

Smith, R. (1964). An investigation of the relationships between lipreading ability and the intelligence of the mentally retarded (Unpublished master's thesis, Michigan State University).

Spitzer, J. B., Leder, S. B., Milner, P., Flevaris-Phillips, C., & Giolas, T. G. (1987). Standardization of four videotaped tests of speechreading ranging in task difficulty. *Ear and Hearing, 8*, 227-231.

Stokoe, W. C. (Ed.). (1978). *Sign and culture, a reader for students of American sign language.* Silver Spring, MD: Lenstok Press.

Stokoe, W. C., Casterline, D., & Croneberg, C. (1965). *A dictionary of American sign language on linguistic principles.* Washington, DC: Gallaudet College Press.

Stone, L. (1957). *Facial clues of context in lipreading.* Los Angeles, CA: John Tracy Clinic Research Papers, V.

Summerfield, Q. (1992). *Lipreading and audio-visual perception.* Philosophical Transactions of the Royal Society of London, January 29, 71-78. Royal Society of London.

Tye-Murray, N., & Tyler, R. S. (1988). A critique of continuous discourse tracking as a test procedure. *Journal of Speech and Hearing Disorders, 53*, 226-231.

Tye-Murray, N., Tyler, R. S., Bong, B., & Nares, T. (1988). Computerized laser videodisc programs for training speechreading and assertive communication behaviors. *Journal of the Academy of Rehabilitative Audiology, 21*, 143-152.

Vernon, M., & Andrews, J. F. (1990). *The psychology of deafness: Understanding deaf and hard-of-hearing people*. NY: Longman.

Walden, B., Erdman, S., Montgomery, A., Schwartz, D., & Prosek, R. (1981). Some effects of training on speech perception by hearing-impaired adults. *Journal of Speech and Hearing Research, 24*, 207–216.

Walden, B., Prosek, R., Montgomery, A., Scharr, C., & Jones, C. (1977). Effects of training on the visual recognition of consonants. *Journal of Speech and Hearing Research, 20*, 130–145.

Wedenberg, E. (1951). Auditory training of deaf and hard of hearing children. *Acta Otolaryngology* (Suppl. 94), *39*, 1–139.

Woodward, M.F. (1957). *Linguistic methodology in lip reading research*. Los Angeles, CA: John Tracy Clinic Research Papers, IV.

Woodward, M. F., & Barber, C. G. (1960). Phoneme perception in lipreading. *Journal of Speech and Hearing Research, 3*, 212–222.

Woodward, M. F., & Lowell, E. (1964). *A linguistic approach to the education of aurally-handicapped children*. Washington, DC: DHEW (Project i 907).

Wynne, M. K., & Richardson, S. (1989). Five-year summary of the journal for computer users in speech and hearing. *Journal for Computer Users in Speech and Hearing, 5*, 8–21.

Yoshinaga-Itano, C. (1988). Speechreading instruction for children [Monograph]. In C. L. DeFilippo & D. G. Sims (Eds.). New reflections on speechreading. *The Volta Review, 90*(5), 241–254.

Appendix Four A

Utley—How Well Can You Read Lips?

This text, commonly referred to as the *Utley Test*, consists of three subtests: Sentences (Forms A and B), Words (Forms A and B), and Stories accompanied by questions that relate to each of the stories. Utley (1946) demonstrated that the Word and Story subtests are positively correlated with the Sentence portion of the test. Therefore, these are the stimuli most often used and associated with the *Utley Test*.

Utley evaluated her viewers' responses by giving one point for each word correctly identified in each sentence. A total of 125 words are contained in the 31 sentences on each form (Form A and B). Consequently, a respondent's score may range from 0 to 125 points. Utley suggested that homophenous words not be accepted when scoring the sentence subtest.

Utley administered the sentence subtest to 761 hearing-impaired children and adults, and the following descriptive statistics summarize her findings:

	Form A	Form B
Range	0–84	0–89
Mean	33.63	33.80
SD	16.36	17.53

Practice Sentence

1. Good morning.
2. Thank you.
3. Hello.
4. How are you?
5. Goodbye.

Utley Sentence Test—Form A

1. All right.
2. Where have you been?
3. I have forgotten.
4. I have nothing.
5. That is right.
6. Look out.
7. How have you been?
8. I don't know if I can.
9. How tall are you?
10. It is awfully cold.
11. My folks are home.
12. How much was it?
13. Good night.
14. Where are you going?
15. Excuse me.
16. Did you have a good time?
17. What did you want?
18. How much do you weigh?
19. I cannot stand him.
20. She was home last week.
21. Keep your eye on the ball.
22. I cannot remember.
23. Of course.
24. I flew to Washington.
25. You look well.
26. The train runs every hour.
27. You had better go slow.
28. It says that in the book.
29. We got home at six o'clock.
30. We drove to the country.
31. How much rain fell?

From "A Test of Lipreading Ability" by J. Utley, 1946, *Journal of Speech and Hearing Disorders, 11*, pp.109–116. Reprinted by permission.

Appendix Four B

The Denver Quick Test of Lipreading Ability

The *Denver Quick Test* is designed to measure adult ability to speechread 20 common everyday sentences. Sentences are presented "live" or taped by the tester and are scored on the basis of meaning recognition. No normative data are available to which individual scores may be compared; however, when the Quick Test was given without acoustic cues to 40 hearing-impaired adults, their scores were highly correlated (0.90) with their results on the *Utley Sentence Test* (Alpiner, 1982).

The Denver Quick Test of Lipreading Ability

1. Good morning
2. How old are you?
3. I live in (state of residence).
4. I only have one dollar.
5. There is somebody at the door.
6. May I help you?
7. I feel fine.
8. It is time for dinner.
9. Turn right at the corner.
10. Are you ready to order?

11. May I help you?
12. I feel fine.
13. It is time for dinner.
14. Turn right at the corner.
15. Are you ready to order?

6. Is that all?
7. Where are you going?
8. Let's have a coffee break.
9. Park your car in the lot.
10. What is your address?

16. Is this charge or cash?
17. What time is it?
18. I have a headache.
19. How about going out tonight?
20. Please lend me 50 cents.

From "Evaluation of Communication Function" by J. Alpiner. In *Handbook of Adult Rehabilitative Audiology* (pp.18–79) by J. Alpiner (Ed.), 1982, Baltimore: Williams & Wilkins. Reprinted by permission.

Appendix Four C

Craig Lipreading Inventory

The Craig Lipreading Inventory consists of two forms of 33 isolated words and 24 sentences. The vocabulary for these stimuli was selected from words used by children enrolled in kindergarten and first grade. A filmed version of the test is available. The test is usually presented "live," but may be videotaped by a clinician.

The viewer should be positioned 8 feet from the speaker. Each of the isolated words is preceded by a contextually meaningless carrier phrase, "show me." The respondent is provided with answer sheets that contain four choices for each stimulus. A single point is awarded for each of the words and sentences identified correctly. Consequently, maximum scores are 33 and 24 for the word test and sentence test, respectively.

Individual performances may be compared to the following mean scores obtained by Craig with deaf children:

	Preschool	Nonpreschool
Words	62.5%–68%	68%–69%
Sentences	52.5%–62%	61.5%–63%

Craig Lipreading Inventory
Word Recognition—Form A

1. white	12. woman	23. ear
2. corn	13. fly	24. ice
3. zoo	14. frog	25. goat
4. thumb	15. grapes	26. dog
5. chair	16. goose	27. cat
6. jello	17. sled	28. nut
7. doll	18. star	29. milk
8. pig	19. sing	30. cake
9. toy	20. three	31. eight
10. finger	21. duck	32. pencil
11. six	22. spoon	33. desk

Sentence Recognition—Form A

1. A coat is on a chair.
2. A sock and shoe are on the floor.
3. A boy is flying a kite.
4. A girl is jumping.
5. A boy stuck his thumb in the pie.
6. A cow and a pig are near the gate.
7. A man is throwing a ball to the dog.
8. A bird has white wings.
9. A light is over the door.
10. A horse is standing by a new car.
11. A boy is putting a nail in the sled.
12. A big fan is on a desk.
13. An owl is looking at the moon.
14. Three stars are in the sky.
15. A whistle and a spoon are on the table.
16. A frog is hopping away from a boat.
17. Bread, meat and grapes are in the dish.
18. The woman has long hair and a short dress.
19. The boys are swinging behind the school.
20. A cat is playing with a nut.
21. A man has his foot on a truck.
22. A woman is carrying a chair.
23. A woman is eating an apple.
24. A girl is cutting a feather.x

Craig Lipreading Inventory

Word Recognition   Name: _____

Age: _____   Date: _____   School: _____

Ex.	fish	table	baby	ball
1.	kite	fire	white	light
2.	corn	fork	horse	purse
3.	two	zoo	spoon	shoe
4.	cup	jump	thumb	drum
5.	hair	bear	pear	chair

Word Recognition			Page 2
6.	yoyo	hello	jello	window
7.	doll	ten	nail	suit
8.	pig	pie	book	pear
9.	two	toe	tie	toy
10.	flower	finger	fire	feather
11.	six	sing	sit	kiss

164   Chapter 4

Word Recognition				**Page 3**
12.	table	apple	woman	rabbit
13.	fire	tie	fly	five
14.	four	frog	fork	flag
15.	grapes	airplane	tables	cups
16.	goose	tooth	shoe	school
17.	desk	sled	leg	nest

Word Recognition   Page 4

18.	dog	sock	star	car
19.	wing	sing	ring	swing
20.	three	teeth	key	knee
21.	duck	rug	truck	gun
22.	moon	school	spoon	boot
23.	ear	hair	eye	egg

Word Recognition   Page 5

24.	horse	house	ice	orange
25.	goat	gate	kite	girl
26.	dish	duck	desk	dog
27.	cat	cake	gun	coat
28.	nail	nut	nest	ten
29.	man	bat	milk	bird

Word Recognition   Page 6

30.	egg	cake	key	car
31.	eight	egg	cake	gate
32.	pencil	picture	mitten	pitcher
33.	wet	dress	nest	desk

5

Language and Speech of the Deaf and Hard of Hearing

Deborah N. Seyfried
Patricia B. Kricos

Contents

INTRODUCTION

All of us possess personal attitudes toward language and modes of communication. These feelings form a basis for the way we choose to view the language abilities of persons with hearing loss. For example, a father of a child with profound hearing loss and a cochlear implant states, "I won't respond to my daughter unless she uses spoken words." In contrast, a family with a young daughter with severe hearing impairment realizes that she is not responding well to amplified spoken language. Mom, Dad, and the two siblings go to the library, borrow all the sign language books, and start signing. An adolescent who is deaf begins a course of study at Gallaudet University and chooses not to use spoken language because it is not accepted by the Deaf community. All of these examples reflect "family" attitudes and choices toward language.

Professionals may respond to such family attitudes and choices toward language use in various ways. For many years, professionals established language programs based on their own principles and beliefs. Only then did they enlist families' participation in these programs. With the passage of PL 99-457, however, our profession is moving in a new direction toward family-centered language programs (Crais, 1991). In family-centered programs, families are to be equal partners in language assessment, intervention, and decision-making. In order to move toward family-centered practice, professionals may find it helpful to first evaluate their own definitions of, and views toward, language and communication.

LANGUAGE AND COMMUNICATION

Communication has been defined as any behavior or set of behaviors that allows messages or ideas to be shared with others (Owens, 1990). Obviously, this definition encompasses many possible communication behaviors. Humans can communicate using language, but language is not the only means for communicating. Attitude and emotion can also be expressed by using specific intonation and stress. For example, a mother's "aaaaah" when she sees that baby has spilled juice all over a new playsuit will differ from her "aaaaah" when she sees baby peacefully sleeping. Gestures, body posture, facial expression, eye contact, head and body movement, and physical distance also allow for communication (Owens, 1990). For example, the young child raising her arms up to Dad conveys the message that she wants to be picked up. It is apparent that communication begins in infancy. Thus, professionals working with children who have hearing loss must be aware of the prelinguistic and early communication behaviors of the infant or toddler with hearing loss. These behaviors are believed to be the precursors to the development of language.

Language has been defined as a set of symbols and rules established by a community to express meaning and facilitate communication (Kretschmer & Kretschmer, 1990). For most of us in the United States, "language" is English. However, children with hearing loss may come from families that have other language backgrounds, e.g.,

Spanish, Chinese, American Sign Language, or spoken English + Manually Coded English Sign Systems. In the past, professionals often assessed only the English-language abilities of children with hearing loss. The challenge of family-centered intervention is to assess and develop the language or languages used and/or chosen by the family.

Traditionally, language has been viewed as the product of five underlying rule systems: syntax (rules for combining words into sentences), morphology (rules for combining morphemes), phonology (rules for combining speech sounds), semantics (the meaning of words and word combinations), and pragmatics (conversational rules; Owens, 1990). According to Hasenstab and Tobey (1991), pragmatics includes strategies or knowledge concerning use of appropriate eye contact, how to initiate and terminate conversations, how to repair communication breakdowns, and how to shift topics and take turns in conversations. While all five rule-systems are considered to be important and interrelated, researchers and professionals have historically focused on the assessment and treatment of only one or a few of these rule systems at a time. Changing views of what language is, how it functions, and the interaction and interrelation of these rule systems have prompted re-evaluation of such clinical practices.

Kretschmer and Kretschmer (1990) discuss how concepts about language have changed and influenced intervention with children with hearing impairment. Prior to the 1970s, the focus was on the child's knowledge and use of syntax and word types (e.g., nouns, verbs, adjectives). Consequently, clinicians providing therapy to children with hearing impairment focused on expanding vocabulary and developing the use of different sentence types. Depending on the clinician, language targets might be developed through structured drill and imitation or through natural language activities. In the 1970s and 1980s, there was a shift in focus. Greater importance was assigned to meaning (semantics) and to conversational abilities (pragmatics). However, many programs for children with hearing loss still do not reflect the trend toward holistic, pragmatic, and meaning-based treatment. Instead, they continue to focus on vocabulary and syntax drill rather than on developing conversational skills and overall communication effectiveness (Kretschmer & Kretschmer, 1989, 1990). Models do exist, however, for developing meaning and conversational abilities in children with hearing loss (Moeller & Carney, 1993; Stone, 1988). Additionally, there are models that include families in programming (Moeller, Coufal, & Hixson, 1990).

Language intervention practices used with children with impaired hearing have also been re-evaluated in view of changing theories about how language is naturally learned. The whole-language philosophy views language learning as a process that occurs in natural contexts where the young child is exposed to all rule systems simultaneously rather than through the use of vocabulary or grammar drills (Schirmer, 1994). For example, the child is not simply taught the words "eggs," "cereal," "milk," "juice," and "toast" while the clinician holds up the items or picture cards depicting the items. Instead, the child would learn about and talk about breakfast foods and the characteristics of breakfast foods while making a breakfast. The conversation might also lead to a discussion of what foods are not eaten for breakfast, such as candy bars and pizza. In this way, the child learns about all aspects of language use, not just isolated words.

The whole-language philosophy also stresses the close developmental ties between spoken language and written language (i.e., literacy development; Goodman, 1986). Contrary to popular belief, written language is not learned after spoken language. Actually, children with normal hearing begin learning about written language long before they speak their first words or are "taught to read" in school. Using a whole-language approach, a clinician would include printed materials in language activities. For example, in the breakfast routine one could show and read the labels on the breakfast foods (e.g., "egg" on the egg carton, "juice" on the juice box). The clinician and child could also read a book about eating breakfast.

Literacy development also includes learning writing skills. Consequently, activities involving prewriting and writing skills would be included when possible. Literacy activities for children with hearing impairment have been presented and advocated by several researchers (Truax, 1985; Staton, 1985).

Factors Affecting Language Acquisition

In addition to considering language and language intervention perspectives, it is also essential to consider how hearing loss affects the acquisition of spoken language. The deteriorated speech signal resulting from hearing loss robs the child with hearing impairment of information regarding the form (phonology, syntax, morphology), content (semantics), and use (pragmatics) of language. Not surprisingly, language delay is a primary consequence of this information loss.

It must be stressed that, despite their language-learning difficulties, children with hearing loss are not a homogeneous group when it comes to language acquisition. The three most obvious factors that might account for differences in language acquisition among children with hearing impairment are the degree of loss, age of onset, and whether other disabilities are present. Moeller, Coufal, and Hixson (1990), for example, noted a 30% incidence of educationally significant secondary disabilities in their population of children with hearing impairment.

In general, the greater the hearing loss, the greater the expected language delay (Norlin & Van Tasell, 1980). However, language abilities cannot be predicted solely on the basis of severity of hearing loss. Often, a range of language abilities can be observed in children with similar unaided audiograms. Surprisingly, some children with severe hearing impairment have age-appropriate language skills, while others have language difficulties that far exceed what would be expected for a given level of hearing loss. For the child with profound hearing impairment, the lack of sufficient speech information may preclude the acquisition of spoken language through audition. Even children who, at an early age, have mild fluctuating hearing losses secondary to otitis media may evidence significant delays in language development (Silva, Chalmers, & Stewart, 1986; Wallace, Gravel, McCarton, & Ruben, 1988).

Nonverbal intelligence appears to be a major factor in language development of children with severe hearing impairment (Moeller, et al., 1986; Osberger, et al., 1986; Watson, et al., 1982). The purpose of a study by Clarke and Rogers (1981) was to examine the variables that may affect knowledge of English syntax in children ages 8–19 years, whose hearing losses ranged from moderate to profound. The results of their study indicated that the syntactic abilities of children with hearing impairment are a consequence of an assortment of variables. Severity of hearing loss, additional educational handicaps, and age were found to be significantly related to syntax proficiency. Educational setting and primary mode of communication were found to be secondary in significance, adding to the effects of the previously mentioned variables.

Differences in family communication and intervention programs may also produce differing language difficulties. Moeller and Luetke-Stahlman (1990) cite a number of studies which suggest that parents' signing skills can influence a child's language learning. Their own study of the syntactic, semantic, and pragmatic features of parental signed input revealed individual patterns of strengths and weaknesses among the parents. The parents generally signed grammatically simple, short utterances to their children, and rarely used fingerspelling to introduce new words. Moeller and Luetke-Stahlman (1990) offer a number of suggestions for improving parent sign-language training programs in order to augment the language learning environment of the child who is deaf.

The following sections will discuss language characteristics and assessment issues for children with hearing impairment in two general age ranges: preschool (birth to age five), and school age (age five through adolescence). Issues related to language management for all children are presented next. While speech is the oral means for expressing language, its separate presentation in latter sections is intended to simplify the discussion.

Language Characteristics of Preschool Children with Hearing Impairment

Preverbal/Early Verbal Communication. During the first three to four months of life, infants gesture, move, cry, and produce other vocalizations that are interpreted as communication by their caregivers. These early infant behaviors represent nonverbal behaviors, whereas the later use of words or signs represent verbal behaviors. Snow (1977) found that mothers respond to infants' nonverbal behaviors (e.g., vocalizations, smiles) and verbal behaviors as if they were conversational turns in an ongoing dialogue. Infants learn to share joint attention, and to take turns in "dialogues" with their caregivers. These "dialogues" take place during everyday caregiving and play.

During the second half of the first year of life, children begin to show evidence of intentional communication. They use gesture and vocalization to achieve a goal. And they may repeat the same gesture and/or vocalization until they accomplish their goal (McAnally, Rose, & Quigley, 1987).

During the prelinguistic and one-word stage, a child with normal hearing is likely to use gestures in the vast majority of communicative acts. The use of gestures then decreases by the multiword stage. At this point, words become the predominant communication means, and gestures serve to augment the words (Wetherby, Cain, Yonclas, & Walker, 1988). In contrast, children who are hard of hearing or deaf may show an increase in the use of nonverbal communications from 6–36 months (Yoshinaga-Itano & Stredler-Brown, 1992). These investigators indicated that nonverbal communications appear to stabilize or decrease when the child with impaired hearing begins to acquire and use words and/or signs.

Parental Interaction with Preschool Children. In addition to interpreting infant behaviors as communication, caregivers also modify their communication style when talking with infants and young children. That is, parents use utterances that are short, syntactically and semantically simple, grammatical, fluent, repetitive, and relevant to the child's immediate environment (Bloom & Lahey, 1978; de Villiers & de Villiers, 1978). While these adjustments have been termed "motherese," both mothers and fathers adjust their spoken language to the language level of their children.

With children with hearing impairment, investigators have sought to explore how and if hearing loss and related communication difficulties affect parent-child interaction. If the parent and child are both deaf and use American Sign Language, then one would not expect communication to be impeded. However, the majority of children who are deaf have hearing parents (Altshuler, 1974). If the parents with normal hearing choose to use only spoken language with their children, then the child's hearing loss will reduce and/or distort the language heard. If the parents choose to use manual communication, then the parent's level of competence in using sign language will affect the language received by the child. In fact, the true benefits of simultaneous communication are difficult to ascertain because parents may have limited signing skills that in turn limit the language they use with their children (Moeller & Luetke-Stahlman, 1990).

Some investigators have compared parent-child interactions using dyads (matched pairs) with children having normal hearing and children with hearing impairment of similar ages. However, parents appear to adjust their language primarily to the child's language level rather than to chronological age, making interpretation difficult. When studies match children by language level, however, parents of children with hearing impairment have interactions generally comparable to parents of children with normal hearing. Researchers have found similarities in number of utterances addressed, mean length of utterance, and percentage of expansion or extension of utterances (Hughes & Howarth, 1980; Hughes, 1983), and communication functions expressed (Tanksley, 1993). Mothers of children with hearing impairment also appear to adjust their language to changes in their children's language. Tucker (1981) studied changes in mother-child interaction for 24 months after diagnosis of hearing loss. Mothers of children showing rapid language growth showed increased use of more complex language.

The nature of parental communication style with children with hearing impairment appears to be related to both the communication mode and competence of the parent-child dyads. Meadow, Greenberg, Erting, and Carmichael (1981) found that parent-child dyads in which both interactants had normal hearing or both were deaf exhibited similar communication interactions. These parent-child dyads had significantly longer and more complex interactions than parent with normal hearing/child with hearing impairment dyads. These results were noted regardless of communication mode (i.e., either simultaneous communication or spoken language only).

Less similarity has been found in parent-child interactions, however, when degree of participation was considered. There is evidence that normal-hearing mothers of children with hearing impairment tend to dominate interactions in two different ways: (a) by producing a high number of utterances, and/or (b) by failing to respond to their children's communication behaviors. Spencer and Gutfreund (1990) found that mothers of children with hearing impairment produced significantly more utterances than did mothers of children with normal hearing, and their children initiated fewer topics than the children with normal hearing. The investigators' impression was that the mothers of children with hearing impairment dominated the "dialogues," leaving few quiet moments during which their children could present their own topics of interest. This impression was supported by follow-up interviews in which mothers expressed the need to be "full-time teachers" to provide their infants with a continual stream of language input to compensate for what they were missing due to hearing loss.

In a similar vein, Pratt (1991) found indications of maternal dominance in non-verbal communications during play between mothers with normal hearing and their infants with hearing impairment. She found that mothers of children with hearing impairment produced significantly fewer elaborations of their children's behaviors and significantly greater elaborations of the mothers' own play behaviors. These mothers tended to sustain their own focus of interest more often than they responded to their children's focus of interest.

Further evidence of differences in parent speech to the child with impaired hearing comes from Kentworthy (1984). He reported that the vast majority of utterances used by mothers in mother with normal hearing/child with hearing impairment dyads were noncontingent. That is, mothers of children with hearing impairment often produced comments unrelated to their child's comments or apparent focus of attention. The example in Table 5.1 (presented by Kentworthy) illustrates two examples of interactions: one in which the mother's comments are noncontingent (example one) and the second, in which the mother's comments are contingent (example two). The first mother tried to establish her own conversational topic rather than talking about her child's focus of attention at the window. In contrast, the second mother focused on her child's topic at the window, resulting in an effective communicative exchange.

Blennerhassett (1984) presented a case study that indicates possible differences between maternal and paternal communication styles with an infant with hearing impairment. Prior research had suggested that both mothers and fathers used shorter utterances with young children but that mothers spoke more, were more responsive to their children's communication attempts, and used simpler words than fathers (Clarke-Stewart, 1978; Golinkoff & Ames, 1979; Kreidberg, 1975; Stein, 1973). In her study, Blennerhassett found that both parents were similar in the number and duration of topic exchanges shared with their daughter with hearing impairment, the number of turns within topics, and their proportion of topic initiations. The parents differed, however, with respect to the types of topic shifts they used while communicating with their daughter. The mother used equal numbers of focus shifts (i.e.,

TABLE 5.1 *Examples of Typical Mother-Child Interaction Sequences in Two Normal-Hearing Mother/Hearing-Impaired Child Dyads*

Example 1	Example 2
C: Bah (*points to window*).	*C:* Abah.
M: This is a nice truck (*holds up toy*).	*M:* What?
C: Bah (*repeats without pointing*).	*C:* Abah (*points to window*).
C: (*walks to window*)	*M:* You want it open?
M: Jerry. (*pause*) Jerry, Come here,	*C:* Ah (*nods head "yes"*).
(*pause*) look at this nice farm.	*M:* What do you want?
C: (*points to toy*)	*C:* Obeh.
	M: Okay. You do it. (*child looks up to window*)

    C = Child   *M* = Mother

Source: Kentworthy, 1986.

shifts to a new feature of the topic) and new-topic shifts. The father used a much greater proportion of new-topic shifts. The parents also differed in responding to their daughter's topic shifts. The father responded to 20.7% of his daughter's topic shifts while the mother responded to 47% of her daughter's topic shifts. When their daughter repeated an ignored topic, the mother responded to that topic 91% of the time whereas the father responded to that topic only 53% of the time. While this study is limited to one family, it does indicate the need to be aware of differences in parental communication style. Differing styles can undoubtedly have an impact on language acquisition and treatment programming.

Communication and Interaction with Preschool Children. Infants with hearing loss appear to follow a normal developmental pattern in learning to use vocal and non-vocal behaviors for communication (Tait & Wood, 1987; Wood, Wood, Griffiths, & Howarth, 1986). The nature of their vocal and nonvocal behaviors differs in some ways, however, from those of children with normal hearing. Data are limited because until recently, prelingual hearing loss generally has not been identified until the age of approximately two years (Elsmann, Matkin, & Sabo, 1987). Spencer (1993) studied the gestural/tactile and vocal/verbal communication behaviors of 36 mother-infant dyads. Mothers all had normal hearing while infants in half the dyads had hearing loss in the moderate to profound range. Unlike many children with hearing impairment, the children in this study were identified and provided with language programming and amplification prior to the age of 12 months. Interactive play sessions between mother-infant dyads were videorecorded when the children were 12 and 18 months of age.

The two groups of infants did not differ significantly with respect to the overall number of intentional communication behaviors (i.e., combined vocal and gestural behaviors), the frequency of use of gestures, or the total number of communicative vocalizations. The groups did differ, however, with respect to the nature of their vocal and verbal productions. Children with normal hearing produced significantly greater

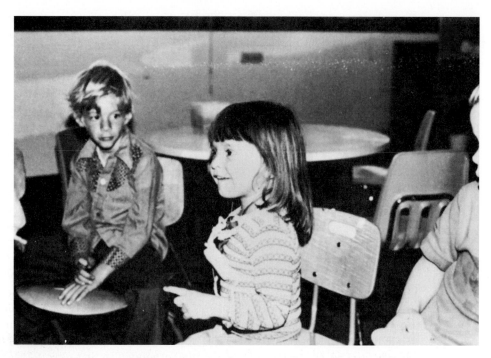

Children work on communication skills in a pre-school classroom for the hearing impaired.

numbers of canonical syllables (i.e., a consonant-like sound paired with a vowel), conventional vocalizations (imitations of animal sounds, vehicle noises, and nonrepresentational vocalizations like "uh-oh"), and single-element or multi-element spoken or sign utterances. Correspondingly, Yoshinaga-Itano and Stredler-Brown (1992) also reported an overall low number of verbal communications (words and signs) for children with hearing impairment through the age of 18 months.

Because preschoolers with impaired hearing often have limited verbal abilities (words and/or signs), investigators have looked at the range of meanings (semantic functions) and communicative intentions (pragmatic functions) that these children can express through both verbal means and nonverbal means. Verbal means can include speech and/or sign, and nonverbal means include gestures, facial expressions, and vocalizations. Children with normal hearing predominately use gesture and vocalization to communicate prior to word development (prelinguistic) and during the one-word stage. They then shift to the predominant use of words when they reach the multiword stage (Wetherby, Cain, Yonclas, & Walker, 1988). In addition, children with normal hearing typically use multiword utterances (i.e., exhibit mean length of utterances [MLUs] of 2.0 or more) between the ages of two and two-and-a-half (Miller, 1981). Because children with hearing impairment may reach the multiword or multi-sign stage at a later age, the shift from the predominant use of nonverbal communication to words/signs may occur at a later age also.

Knowledge of Schema in Preschool Children. It has been suggested that early child language development is established through the use of daily routines in the child's life (Schirmer, 1994). The child, for example, experiences typical sequences of events and communication at dinner time, bath time, and bed time. Over time, the child stores and remembers a body of knowledge (called "schema") about these events and forms (Yoshinaga-Itano & Downey, 1986). Children with impaired hearing often have limited schemata for two main reasons. First, they have limited access to the language used by parents and siblings during daily routines. Children with hearing impairment who receive spoken language often will receive incomplete and distorted messages, while those receiving primarily signed or signed and spoken language will often receive incomplete and distorted messages because of the limited signing skills of family members. Second, children with hearing loss miss out on incidental learning opportunities. The child with normal hearing can overhear mom and dad talking about cleaning up the dinner dishes. The child with hearing loss may hear little of conversations unless they are directed toward him/her. In addition, parents using simultaneous communication may not sign communications if they are not directed toward their child (Yoshinaga-Itano & Downey, 1986). Thus, children with hearing impairment have reduced language input and the language they miss leads them to miss out on knowledge about their world.

Semantic and Pragmatic Functions in Preschool Children. Several investigators have reported that preschool children with hearing impairment exhibit a full range of pragmatic functions but limited semantic functions using nonverbal and verbal communication behaviors (Skarakis & Prutting, 1977; Curtiss, Prutting, & Lowell, 1979). These investigations involved observation of children with hearing impairment during play and preschool activities in oral-training programs. Analysis of communication acts was based on Greenfield and Smith's (1976) semantic function categories (e.g., agent action, object, performative) and Dore's (1974) pragmatic function categories (e.g., labeling, response, request/demand). Most of the children expressed their meanings and intentions primarily through the use of gestures. In fact, children with hearing impairment were able to communicate a full range of communicative intents by the age of two. In contrast, their limited verbal abilities (average MLU of 1.8–1.85 for children from 1.8–5 years) appeared to limit their ability to code different semantic meanings. Such meanings are more difficult to express nonverbally (Curtiss, Prutting, & Lowell, 1979). Thus, children with hearing impairment between the ages of two and four years were expressing the same semantic and pragmatic functions as children with normal hearing in the pre-linguistic and one-word stage (i.e., children with normal hearing typically younger than two years of age; Skarakis & Prutting, 1977).

Use of communicative intentions has also been studied in children with profound hearing impairment learning Manually Coded English (Day, 1986; McKirdy & Blank, 1982). Both studies involved analysis of play sequences. However, children in the Day (1986) study were videotaped while playing with their mothers. The children in the McKirdy and Blank (1982) study were videotaped while playing with peers with hearing impairment. (McKirdy and Blank reasoned that peers with hearing impairment often have more proficient signing skills than parents, and that more extensive communication might be viewed with peer-peer interactions.) Another difference between these studies is the systems used for categorizing communication acts: Day used an elaboration of Dore's (1977) pragmatic categories, and McKirdy and Blank used Blank and Franklin's (1980) speaker-initiator and speaker-responder categories. Day found that use of pragmatic functions by the children with hearing impairment was generally comparable to that of children with normal hearing. However, the children with impaired hearing used more conversational devices (e.g., looking at the communication partner or at the focus of the partner's comment, or imitating part of the partner's comment to maintain the conversation), and fewer "wh" questions (e.g. who, what, where, why, etc.). He postulated that children with hearing impairment may have a greater need for ensuring that communication is maintained by directing the parent's attention, checking the parent's attention, and imitating the parent's response to take a conversational turn. The less frequent use of "wh"-questions has been attributed to the reduced number of "wh"-questions produced by mothers of children with hearing impairment (Hyde, Elias, & Power, 1980). McKirdy and Blank found that when compared to peers with normal hearing, children who were deaf were less likely to respond to comments made by their conversational partners. In addition, they used touching rather than comment to initiate conversational turns. Comments of children who were deaf were limited to objects and events in the "here and now." Many of the children who were deaf used self-generated rather than conventional signs, which would make it difficult to discuss events out of the "here and now." McKirdy and Blank urged that communication assessment of children who are deaf look beyond labeling language forms used, and look at the children's ability to participate in dialogue.

Yoshinaga-Itano and Stredler-Brown (1992) provided data concerning the frequency of use of different nonverbal and verbal communicative intentions (e.g., comment on object/action, request object/action/information, answer, acknowledgment, and protest) for children with hearing impairment during parent-child play sessions. Data were provided for the following age ranges in months: 6–12, 13–18, 19–24, 25–30, and 31–36. All 82 children in this cross-sectional sample were hard of hearing (better ear pure-tone averages less than 70 dB HL, 44%) or deaf (better ear pure-tone averages greater than 70 dB HL, 56%) and were enrolled in the Colorado Department of Health Home Intervention Program. Results showed that the overall number of nonverbal communicative intentions across categories increased with age. Children who were hard of hearing or deaf used a similar number of nonverbal communications. Verbal communication behaviors began to appear at 19 months of age, stabilized through 30 months, and then showed significant growth between 30 and 36 months. The children who were hard of hearing, however, showed significantly more verbal communications than the children who were deaf. Based on their findings, Yoshinaga-Itano and Stredler-Brown proposed the overall stages of development of communication intent in children with hearing impairment shown in Table 5.2.

Early Vocabulary in Preschool Children. Few studies have investigated the early vocabulary of children with hearing loss. Profound hearing loss appears to limit

✶TABLE 5.2 *Proposed Stages of Development of Communicative Intent in a Hearing-Impaired Population*   *What should we know.*

Stage One	• 6 through 12 months
	• Acquisition of pragmatic categories
	• Comments and request for action or object
	• Answering/Acknowledgment/Protest
	• Pointing/Showing/Giving
Stage Two	• 12 to 24 months
	• Complete differentiation of non-verbal
	• Increases in quantity in all nonverbal categories
	• Acquisition of non-verbal requests for information
	• Emergence of symbolic (often non-communicative) gestures: symbolic representations of objects or actions, such as stirring, drinking, hammering, sleeping (may be used in sequence)
Stage Three	• 18 to 30 months
	• Onset of verbal communicative intention
	• Category differentiation
	• Stabilization of non-verbal communicative intention categories
	• Critical transition from nonverbal to verbal communication
Stage Four	• 24 to 36 months
	• Completed differentiation of verbal categories
	• Increased quantity in all verbal categories

Source: Yoshinaga-Itano and Stredler-Brown, 1992

greatly the size of spoken vocabulary in young children. Schafer and Lynch (1980) studied four deaf children between the ages of 15 and 34 months. Two of the children were enrolled in oral programs, and two were enrolled in total communication programs. At 18 months of age, the children were using from 0 to 9 words. In contrast, normal hearing children have between 20 and 50 words at that age (Lenneberg, 1966; Nelson, 1973). At 22 months, the children in the total communication program had approximately 60 signed or spoken words, and the children in the oral program used approximately 10 spoken words. The types of words/signs learned first were similar to those learned first by children with normal hearing.

Griswold and Cummings (1974) noted that four-year–old deaf children had an expressive vocabulary of approximately 158 spoken words. In contrast, children of kindergarten age with normal hearing may have a vocabulary of 2,000 words (Dale, 1976).

Howell (1984) examined parent reports (Maryland School for the Deaf preschool vocabulary list) of sign vocabulary for 4 four-year–old deaf children. All four children participated in a total communication program and had parents using sign language at home. Two of the children had parents who were deaf and who had signed with them since birth. The other two children had parents who had begun signing with them at one and three years of age, respectively. The children with parents who were deaf and had early exposure to sign had sign vocabularies of 1301 and 1269 signs, while the children with hearing parents and later exposure to sign had sign vocabularies of 750 and 945 signs. All four children showed the greatest use of nominals, verbals, and modifiers with limited or no use of temporals, spatials, negations, questions, connectives, and pronouns. While children had productive vocabularies differing in size, their proportionate use of different types of vocabulary items was similar.

Syntax in Preschool Children. Studies of syntactic abilities in children with hearing impairment have been conducted with school-age children rather than children in the 0–5 age range. The syntactic abilities of the school-age child with impaired hearing is discussed in a later section.

Pre-Literacy and Literacy Issues. Another issue in language development for the child with impaired hearing is the development of literacy (reading and writing) skills. Low reading- and writing-proficiency skills for children with hearing impairment have been related to limited oral language skills that serve as a base for literacy. Children with hearing loss also may not be exposed to the range and amount of pre-reading and reading activities as children with normal hearing (Limbrick, McNaughton, & Clay, 1992). Unfortunately, little attention has been directed toward establishing the precursors to reading and writing in this population.

Children with normal hearing learn about printed materials when they are very young. Infants and toddlers see and are shown letters and words on pictures, toys, and television, and in books. Parents read story books, traffic signs, and television ads (van Kleeck & Schuele, 1987). In contrast, children with hearing impairment may not have the same amount of exposure to these literacy experiences. This may be due to an unintentional overemphasis on spoken-language development in the early years with the expectation that reading and writing will be taught later in the elementary-school setting. Literacy development and literacy facilitation activities are discussed by van Kleeck and Schuele (1987) and Schuele and van Kleeck (1987). Ewoldt (1985) has described a school-based literacy program for children with hearing impairment that included story telling, story creation, and free time for drawing and writing. Such activities may be crucial because reading is a critical skill for the child with hearing impairment. It provides for vocabulary expansion throughout life (Schirmer, 1994). Reading skills also allow the child who is deaf access to captioned television and the teletype device for the deaf (TDD).

Language Characteristics of School-Age Children with Hearing Impairment

The literature pertaining to the acquisition and use of language by school-age children who have hearing impairment is extensive and establishes a number of important concerns. Three major aspects of language have been evaluated in this population: (a) lexical/semantic skills, (b) syntactic/morphologic skills, and (c) pragmatic, or functional communication skills. Each of these will be briefly discussed.

Lexical/Semantic Skills of School-Age Children. The acquisition of the semantic component of language by children with hearing impairment may be mildly to profoundly delayed. Reduced vocabulary is common among individuals with hearing loss. Moeller, Osberger, and Eccarius (1986) and Osberger, Moeller, Eccarius, Robbins, and Johnson (1986) administered a large battery of expressive- and receptive-language tests to children and young adults ranging in age from 4.5–20 years. Severe delays in the acquisition of lexical/semantic skills were observed across all age groups. On the average, the children's performance on the various measures of word knowledge was similar to that of a six- to eight-year-old child with normal hearing. Marked difficulties with the semantic/lexical aspects of language have been documented by other investigators (Brenza, Kricos, & Lasky, 1981; Conway, 1990; Davis, 1974; Nunnally & Blanton, 1966; Templin, 1966). Conway (1990), for example, examined the semantic relationships expressed in the word-meanings of children with hearing impairment. Children with profound hearing impairment, ranging in age from 6 to 11 years, provided definitions for 10 common nouns. Although significantly more semantic relationships were produced by the older children, the younger and older children did not differ in the types nor the complexity of relationships expressed, and their definitional abilities remained relatively immature.

In a sample of 40 children with mild to moderate hearing impairments, scores on the Peabody Picture Vocabulary Test (PPVT) (Dunn, 1959) were also found to indicate delays in vocabulary development (Davis, Elfenbein, Schum, & Bentler, 1986). Vocabulary delays ranged from a delay of approximately one year for older children with moderate hearing losses to greater than three years for older children with severe hearing impairment.

Syntactic/Morphologic Skills of School-Age Children. The difficulties in acquisition of English syntactic/morphologic skills by children who have hearing impairment have been extensively documented, and are even more pronounced than this population's difficulties with the semantic/lexical aspects of language. Descriptive studies of the syntactic abilities in this population have shown evidence of the following:

1. Restricted knowledge of word classes as evidenced by overuse of nouns and verbs and omission of function words.
2. Restricted knowledge of syntax as evidenced by overuse of the subject-verb-object sentence structure.
3. Syntactic delay with subsequent plateau in regard to syntactic abilities.
4. Deviant syntax in children with profound hearing impairment, e.g., misuse of morphological markers, omission of major sentence constituents, and asequential word order.

In their study of 145 children and young adults, ages 4.5–20 years, Moeller, et al. (1986) found that few students evidenced language ages greater than 5–7 years in receptive syntax. Children with severe to profound hearing losses seem to grasp the simpler aspects of English syntax, such as the concept of sentences consisting of subject-verb-object. However, it has been repeatedly documented that they have substantial difficulties with the more complex, subtle aspects of syntax (Kretschmer & Kretschmer, 1978; Moeller, et al., 1986; Osberger, et al., 1986; Quigley & King, 1981; Quigley, Power, & Steinkamp, 1977; Wilbur, Goodhart, & Fuller, 1989). Given the seeming inconsistencies in English syntax, it is not surprising that such difficulties are experienced by individuals with severe hearing impairment. Consider, for example, the following sentences: "I am going home." — "I am going to school." — "I am going to the store." It is no wonder that individuals with impaired hearing have difficulty sorting through the irregularities of the English language, ultimately generating sentences such as "I am going school" or "I am going to home."

Pragmatic Skills of School-Age Children. The abilities of school-age children with impaired hearing to control the pragmatic aspects of language have, until fairly recently, received less attention from researchers. The limited research that has been conducted with older children, however, has delineated a number of concerns with the pragmatic aspects of language. Duchan (1988) reviews these studies, which show that many school-age children with hearing loss have difficulties with conversational turn-taking and topic initiations and maintenance. Studies of the pragmatic abilities of children who have been educated in a Total Communication program were reviewed by Johnson (1988). Although difficulties in turn-taking, topic identification, and communication repair were noted in these studies, there is at least some evidence that there is a steady progression of conversational skills in children with hearing impairment as they become older. Prinz and Prinz (1985) found that children's communication competence increased from ages 3–11 years (the ages of their subjects) as a result of their improved American Sign Language discourse strategies.

Plateau in Language Acquisition for School-Age Children. More disturbing than the delays in the development of language skills in children with hearing impairment is the apparent plateau in development of these skills, which has been documented in numerous studies (Boothe, Lasky, & Kricos, 1982; Clarke & Rogers, 1981; Davis, 1974; Moeller, Osberger, McKonkey, & Eccarius, 1981; Watson, Sullivan, Moeller, & Jensen, 1982). For example, Clarke and Rogers (1981) administered the Test of Syntactic Abilities, a test specifically designed to assess the syntactic abilities of children with hearing impairment, to 382 students between the ages of 8 and 19 years. With the effect of degree of hearing loss controlled, no increase in score was exhibited for the children beyond 11 years of age. Similarly, Moeller, et al. (1986) found little growth in semantic and syntactic skills of children with severe hearing losses after 12–13 years. Plateaus have even been noted in children with less severe hearing losses. Davis (1974) evaluated the performance of children, ages six to nine years, who were hard of hearing, on a test of basic concepts. Not only was their knowledge of basic concepts extremely poor, there was also no difference in performance between the younger and older children.

Although there is strong evidence to support the existence of a plateau in the acquisition of language skills by children with hearing impairment, Boothe, et al.

(1982) discovered that language abilities may improve in young adults with hearing impairment once they leave the formal education environment. Boothe, et al. (1982) compared the comprehension and production of syntactic structures in three age groups of individuals with severe to profound hearing loss: 8–11 years, 17–19 years, and 22–30 years. The two younger age groups performed similarly on the syntactic tasks, but the 22–30 year group performed significantly better on all measures. The results of this study showed that although there was a plateau in the development of syntactic skills in the school-age subjects, there was improvement in these skills in young adults who had been away from formal education for at least two years.

General Issues in Language Assessment

Measures used for assessing the language of children with hearing impairment can be categorized as follows: (a) communication checklists, (b) formal language tests, and (c) communication/language sample analyses. Many of the assessments most commonly used with young children with hearing impairment are those developed and standardized for use with children with normal hearing (Abraham & Stoker, 1988). Use of these assessments allows one to consider the language skills of children with hearing loss with reference to their normal-hearing peers. One could determine, for example, that Johnny, age seven, who has hearing impairment, has a vocabulary score typical of a 4.5-year-old child with normal hearing. Standard assessments typically indicate that spoken-language proficiency is usually delayed in children with impaired hearing. Assessments standardized on children with hearing impairment do exist. These assessments are likely to be most available to clinicians working in settings with a steady caseload of children with hearing impairment.

Because relatively few measures of language are specifically designed for children with hearing impairment, the clinician often needs to consider use of language-evaluation measures that were devised for and standardized with children with normal hearing. Language measures such as the Peabody Picture Vocabulary Test (PPVT; Dunn, 1981), the Expressive One-Word Picture Vocabulary Test-Revised (EOWPVT-R; Gardner, 1990), and the Test of Language Development (TOLD; Newcomer & Hammill, 1977) can be administered to children with impaired hearing. However, caution in the administration, scoring, and interpretation of test results is warranted when these tests are administered to children who have impaired hearing. For example, one should not compute or use mental ages or I.Q. scores for the child with impaired hearing, because low scores usually reflect only the child's language delay.

A few language assessments have been developed for and normed on children with hearing impairment. Most of these tests have been developed for school-age children with hearing loss. Some language specialists question the importance of comparing the performance of a child with impaired hearing to the heterogeneous population of children with hearing loss (Waldron, 1994). The question arises as to whether we want to view the child's language function in relation to that of peers with normal hearing or of other children with hearing loss and probable language delays. For example, is it more important to know that seven-year-old Johnny's vocabulary score is typical for children of his age with hearing impairment, or to know that

Johnny's vocabulary score on a standard assessment indicates that his vocabulary is more limited than that of his classmates with normal hearing?

Limitations/Cautions in Using Formal Language Measures. Receptive language tests typically involve oral presentation of a word or sentence and require a picture-pointing response by the child. If a child with impaired hearing responds incorrectly, it is difficult to determine whether a language or a perceptual problem is responsible. Using printed stimulus items puts too much reliance on the child's reading abilities, making it difficult to ascertain whether a language or a reading problem is responsible for the child's errors. Even signing of the stimulus items is not without difficulties. Moeller, et al. (1986) point out that the iconic nature of some signs may help the child to match the sign with the pictured response; thus, a true measure of the child's linguistic skills is not accomplished.

The speech intelligibility of the child being tested is frequently a problem when using expressive language measures. The story-retell procedure described by Osberger, et al. (1986) can be useful in helping the examiner to decipher the child's linguistic sample, because the examiner has a better idea of its content than with open-ended conversation or narrative.

Osberger (1986) stressed that most formal measures of language involve assessment of the comprehension and production of words and sentences in isolation, with little contextual information available. Thus, they may not provide a true measure of a child's linguistic skills in everyday conversations, in which the child has access to situational and linguistic cues to help decipher what is being said. Osberger (1986) also points out that the pragmatic aspects of language, such as repair strategies and discourse skills, are rarely tapped by formal language measures. The need to combine formal and informal strategies for language assessment of children with hearing impairment is delineated in an excellent article by Moeller (1988). De Villiers (1988), Duchan (1988), and Kretschmer and Kretschmer (1990) provide numerous suggestions for evaluation of the pragmatic aspects of language.

Essential Conditions for Evaluating the Language Abilities. Several factors must be kept in mind when evaluating the language of a child with hearing impairment. First, sensory devices such as hearing aids or cochlear implants should be checked for proper function. Second, the test environment should be optimized by reducing noise and other environmental distractions. Third, when spoken language is used during testing, the clinician should make a conscious effort to allow the child full access to speechreading cues. This might necessitate allowing the child time to look down at a picture and then look back at the tester's face prior to presentation of the test item.

An extremely important factor in language evaluation is that persons administering language tests be proficient users of the child's primary communication mode and language, whether that be spoken language only, spoken language + Cued Speech, spoken language + Signed English, or American Sign Language. Otherwise, test results will be invalid, reflecting misunderstanding of test instructions and desired responses rather than language ability. Luetke-Stahlman and Luckner (1991) have emphasized the concept of "first-language" assessment. That is, children with severe hearing impairment may not necessarily develop English as their first or native language. If their parents are manually-communicating adults who are deaf, the child's first language may be American Sign Language (ASL). Even if their parents have normal hearing, which is true in the majority of cases, the children may not necessarily have acquired English skills, but rather, developed their own manner of communication including gesture, invented and formal sign language, and/or oral words (Luetke-Stahlman & Luckner, 1991). The assessment procedures that have been outlined in this chapter apply mainly to English-language acquisition, and may not be appropriate for a child who has developed another form of communication. Ideally, either the examiner will have signing skills, including ASL and manually-coded English, or someone with these skills will be available to assist in the language evaluation, when necessary. "Normal" language development may not be revealed in children whose primary language is non-English when they are tested with measures based on standard English acquisition. This dilemma presents a challenge to the examiner, but must be recognized if one is to obtain an accurate profile of the child's language abilities. This is not to suggest that children with hearing loss should not be expected to develop functional English skills. Rather, an effort should be made to determine the child's present status in both his/her "native" language *and* the target language, which is frequently English.

Other Considerations in Language Assessment. In addition to language measures, other considerations and observations are critical for assessing the language skills of children with impaired hearing. It is essential to obtain as much information as possible about factors that may have affected a child's language development and that may affect the child's potential for further growth in linguistic skills. Luetke-Stahlman and Luckner (1991) advise that the examiner function as a sort of private investigator, gathering as much information as possible from a variety of sources so that the most appropriate educational program can be developed for the child. Some of the factors to be considered are:

1. review of past audiological records to determine the nature of the hearing loss and the child's functional auditory skills;
2. speechreading abilities;
3. family support;
4. visual processing skills such as visual-motor integration and visual memory;
5. review of past records to determine the child's patterns of language learning;
6. nonverbal intellectual abilities;
7. presence of additional language-learning disabilities, such as attentional deficits, impulsivity, and difficulty making transitions;
8. presence of behavior problems;
9. social skills and experience;
10. speech intelligibility; and
11. reading abilities.

Language Assessment for Preschool Children With Hearing Impairment

Communication Checklists. Communication checklists typically are provided to allow parents and/or teachers the opportunity to observe and identify communication behaviors the child uses in real-world settings such as home and school. Information from checklists can be related to results from formal language tests and/or language samples. Abraham and Stoker (1988) found that the Receptive-Expressive Emergent Language Scale (REEL; Bzoch & League, 1970), and Scales of Early Communication Skills for Hearing-Impaired Children (SECS-HI; Moog & Geers, 1975) are commonly used to assess the young child with impaired hearing. The SECS-HI was developed for use by a child's teacher. It provides normative data for children with hearing impairment between ages 2.0 and 8.11 years. Another checklist, The Teacher Assessment of Grammatical Structures Pre-Sentence Level (Moog & Kozak, 1983), was developed to indicate the understanding and use by the child with impaired hearing of single words, two-word combinations, three-word combinations, "wh"-questions, pronouns, and tense markers.

Several newer checklists, the McArthur Communicative Development Inventory: Words and Gestures (Developmental Psychology Lab San Diego State University, 1992), the Macarthur Communicative Development Inventory: Words and Sentence (Developmental Psychology Lab San Diego State University, 1992), and the Eco Interview (MacDonald & Gillette, 1989) can also provide useful information on infant/toddler communication. The McArthur Communicative Development Inventories are intended for use by parents/caretakers. Both of these inventories assess the child's use of actions, gestures, and words. The Eco Interview includes two checklists: one serving to indicate the child's social and communicative behaviors (Infant Social and Communicative Survey) and the other serving to indicate the caregiver's communication interaction with the child (Eco Adult Communication Evaluation). Checklists based on parent report (REEL, McArthur, and Eco Interview) are particularly appealing since treatment includes emphasizing strong family involvement in assessment and management.

Formal Language Tests for Preschool Children. According to Abraham and Stoker (1988), "formal" language performance tests commonly used with infants (birth to two years) with hearing impairment include the Preschool Language Scale (Zimmerman, Steiner, & Pond, 1979), Bankson Language Screening Test (Bankson, 1977), Peabody Picture Vocabulary Test (Dunn & Dunn, 1981), and the Assessment of Children's Language Comprehension (Foster, Giddan, & Stark, 1973). For preschool children, the following formal language tests were most commonly employed (Abraham & Stoker, 1988): Preschool Language Scale, Peabody Picture Vocabulary Test, Assessment of Children's Language Comprehension, and Test for Auditory Comprehension of Language (Carrow, 1973). None of these tests has norms for children with hearing impairment, but all can be used to indicate baseline language abilities. The Grammatical Analysis of Elicited Language-Pre Sentence Level (GAEL-P; Moog, Kozak, & Geers, 1983) is one of the few language tests developed specifically for young children with severe to profound hearing loss. Age ranges for this test are 3–6 years. Understanding and use of single words and short sentences are assessed.

Language Sample Analysis for Preschool Children. The most common form of language assessment used for children with hearing impairment between birth and five years of age is language sample analysis (Abraham & Stoker, 1988). While various language sample analyses are available, one would want to choose an analysis procedure that would allow for consideration of both nonverbal and verbal communication behaviors. As previously discussed, young children with hearing impairment may extensively use gestures, facial expressions, actions, and vocalizations rather than words to communicate. The two communication sample analyses presented in the following discussion focus on the analysis of both the child's and parent's communication behaviors. Some investigators (Prinz & Prinz, 1985; McKirdy & Blank, 1982) have suggested the need for also assessing child-peer interactions. The majority of children who are deaf with parents who have normal hearing, for example, may exhibit greater communication abilities with peers who are deaf, who have more extensive signing skills than the child's parents.

One useful analysis system designed for use with young children with hearing impairment is a videotape analysis procedure developed by Cole and St. Clair-Stokes (1984). The procedure calls for videotaping the child playing with a caregiver in the home or other very familiar setting for approximately 15 minutes. Cole and St. Clair-Stokes recommend that clinicians review the entire videotape to evaluate turn-taking, motherese alterations, and strategies for maximizing communication. However, they indicate that only a two-to-three minute sample of the videotape needs to be transcribed for in-depth analysis. Substantially more information is gained, however, if a larger portion of the play session is transcribed. Transcription includes making note of all vocal and nonvocal behaviors exhibited by the child and the caregiver. Cole and St. Clair-Stokes provide guidelines for assessing gaze behaviors, contingency of communication behaviors, attention-getting behaviors, and the functional nature of comments. Table 5.3 shows the outcome of this analysis for Tina and Scott, two preschoolers with hearing impairment who are similar in age and degree of hearing loss, but dissimilar with respect to child-parent communication (Seyfried & Waldron, 1993.)

A second communication sample analysis useful with the young child with impaired hearing is the ECOScales Assessment (MacDonald & Gillette, 1989). The benefit of using the ECOScales Assessment is twofold. First, it can be used in conjunction with the Eco Interview. Second, specific communication-intervention goals for the child and intervention strategies for the parent are provided. Table 5.4 shows the analysis outcome and intervention strategies suggested by the ECOScales Assessment for Tina and Scott (Seyfried & Waldron, 1993).

TABLE 5.3 *Example of Cole and St. Clair-Stokes Analysis*

General Observations

Scott	Tina
Mom talked within appropriate communicative distance.	Both parents talked within appropriate communicative distance.
Mom used normally pitched unexaggerated voice	Both parents used normally pitched unexaggerated voice.
Mom used some gestures.	
Mom let Scott direct his own play.	Mom used many gestures.
Mom interpreted Scott's cry, but not gestures, eye gaze, or some vocalizations.	Both parents provided pauses for Tina to take turns.
	Parents let Tina direct her own play.
	Both responded readily to Tina's eye gaze, gestures, and vocalizations.

Caregiver Attention-Getting Behaviors (AGBs)

Scott	Tina
10/17 of Mom's AGBs were vocal and unsuccessful.	27/41 of Mom's AGBs were vocal.
1/17 of Mom's AGBs were tactile and successful.	9/17 of Dad's AGBs were vocal.
5/17 of Mom's AGBs combined tactile/vocal were successful.	14/58 of Mom's and Dad's tactile and vocal AGBs were successful.

Child's Attention-Getting Behaviors (AGBs)

Scott	Tina
4/6 of Scott's AGBs were vocal and most were successful.	18/35 of Tina's AGBs with Mom were vocal.
	24/42 of Tina's AGBs with Dad were visual.
	Almost all AGBs were successful.
	Facial expression was very successful.

Child's Communicative Intentions

Scott	Tina
Nonverbal – Vocalizing	Nonverbal – Facial
Requesting action	Expression and gesture
Responding	Requesting action, information
Attention seeking to objects	Responding
Protesting	Protesting
	Informing
No Verbal Communication	**Verbal Communication**
Used no words.	Used greeting (bye-bye), naming (doll) and repeating (hot).
Did not call, greet, request information, inform, or comment.	Did not call, comment or request answer.
Speech	**Speech**
Short productions .5 to 1.5 seconds mostly vowels, a few consonants	Short productions .5 to 1.5 seconds
	Short CV forms, C:/b, n, m, g, d/

TABLE 5.4 *Example of ECOScales Assessment*

Interactive Problems

Children and Adults

Scott	Tina
Lack of playfulness	Task-oriented activities
Lack of active togetherness	Poor conversations

Adult

Scott	Tina
Not interpreting child behaviors	Directive, controlling style
Lack of sensitive responding	Take majority of turns
	Little waiting for child communication

Child

Scott	Tina
Low interactive participation	Low verbal skills
Playful but not social: plays on own activity	Uses single words more than phrases or sentences
Lack of give and take with actions	Speech hard to understand
Failure to keep attending to shared activity	Narrow range of vocabulary
Brief contacts during activity	
Low communicative participation	
Communication too instrumental: focuses primarily on getting needs met	

Communicative Intervention Strategies

Child Goals

Scott	Tina
Stay with others in play	Begin to communicate verbally
Imitate others	Use a range of meanings with words
Show a turntaking play style	Send clear understandable messages
Intentionally communicate with others	Make self understood
Communicate nonverbally	
Begin to communicate verbally: signing	
Make self understood	

Adult Strategies

Scott	Tina
Play in childlike ways	Play in childlike ways
Communicate in ways close to the child	Communicate in ways close to the child
Communicate about immediate experiences	Communicate about immediate experiences
Maintain and balance turntaking	Comment more than question or command
Match the child's behavior	Match the child's behavior
Wait, signal, expect	Wait, signal, expect
	Match child communication progressively (use models to code intentions child already communicates)

Language Assessment for School-Age Children With Hearing Impairment

Despite the well-documented language-learning difficulties of children who are hearing impaired, relatively few language assessment tools are specifically designed for and normed with this population. The Test of Syntactic Ability (TSA; Quigley, Steinkamp, Power, & Jones, 1976) was specifically designed to be used with school-aged children with hearing loss, and has norms for children with hearing loss and for children with normal hearing. The TSA has two screening versions and 20 subtests that assess the student's knowledge of the major syntactic structures in English. It consists of a series of multiple-choice paper and pencil tasks (thus requiring some reading ability), such as judging grammaticality of sentences and construction of sentences (e.g., forming one sentence from two). The screening version requires approximately one hour to complete, and can be followed with any of the subtests for more in-depth probing of a particular syntactic area.

Another test specifically designed for and normed with children who are hearing impaired is the Grammatical Analysis of Elicited Language (GAEL; Moog & Geers, 1979, 1981). The GAEL for school-aged children is available in two versions: the simple sentence level, and the complex sentence level (a preschool version is also available). Each version consists of target sentences which the examiner attempts to elicit through use of props, a modelled script, and imitation. By analyzing the child's production of the various morphological and syntactic structures within the target sentences, problem areas can be noted and teaching goals formulated. The GAEL tests were standardized using children who communicate orally as well as children who use total communication.

Several authors have proposed models for assessment of the language production of children with hearing loss. Moog and Kozak (1983) developed a series of checklists called the Teacher Assessment of Grammatical Structures (TAGS), which cover the pre-sentence, simple-sentence, and complex-sentence levels. The TAGS checklists are based on the development of syntax and morphology in children with normal hearing, and help the teacher to rate the child's use of grammatical structures in classroom activities. The TAGS checklists are appropriate for spoken and/or signed English, and are useful for planning the sequence of teaching of grammatical structures.

A blueprint for the assessment of the spontaneous language of children with hearing impairment is provided by Kretschmer and Kretschmer's (1978) Spontaneous Language Analysis Procedure (SLAP). The SLAP involves obtaining a spontaneous language sample, preferably through conversational interactions. The SLAP protocol is then used to describe precisely the language output and competence of the child who is hearing impaired. Both expressive and receptive language are analyzed in the six sections of the SLAP: preverbal categories (when appropriate), single- and two-word combinations, single propositions, complex sentences, communication competence, and restricted forms. The SLAP provides for description of the syntactic devices, semantic content, and pragmatic skills used by the child. Although time-consuming, the SLAP yields valuable information for description of the child's current language competency and for the formulation of teaching goals.

Although language sampling and analysis can be useful in the evaluation of children with hearing loss, the procedure is not without drawbacks. Chief among these are the difficulties in analyzing the language sample of children whose speech is nearly unintelligible, and the limited number and complexity of productions that may appear in the spontaneous sample. To combat these problems, a story retell procedure was developed by Malinda Eccarius at the Boys Town National Institute (Osberger, et al., 1986). The procedure entails the use of five cartoon picture plates and an accompanying narrative outline. The story is modelled by the examiner and the child is asked to retell the story, first frame-by-frame, and then in its entirety. Thus, prompts are given to elicit more complex language from the child, and knowledge of the story helps the examiner to decipher the child's speech. The child with severe speech intelligibility problems can be asked to retell the story in written form.

Communication/Language Management for Preschool and School-Age Children with Hearing Impairment

In addition to considering the general format of language intervention appropriate for children with hearing impairment, it is essential to establish a family-centered approach to management. Whenever possible, family members should be involved in reviewing assessment information; planning communication, language, and speech goals; and in monitoring and changing goals. Such involvement is necessary regardless of specific remediation techniques.

Two traditional intervention formats have predominated in language intervention with children with hearing impairment: One emphasizes syntactic mastery and stresses the need for drill and practice, and the other emphasizes the need for a more natural or experiential approach to language learning (Kretschmer & Kretschmer, 1990). While language drills may be employed in the elementary and upper school years, they are of little meaning or interest to the young child with hearing impairment. In addition, heavy use of highly structured drills does not allow children time for social interaction and conversation (Moeller, Osberger, & Morford, 1987).

Children with normal hearing have a wide range of conversational skills that children with hearing impairment may not have. Drilling on vocabulary labels or simple sentence forms does not allow a child with hearing loss to discover how to hold and maintain a conversation. Consequently, exposure to communication functions/forms/structures in everyday contexts should be the primary goal of early communication-development programs. As noted previously, children with hearing impairment may miss out on a great deal of incidental learning (e.g., others' conversations). Thus, an important part of language facilitation with the young child with impaired hearing is creating experiences that allow the child to discover and learn about a wide range of everyday events and reasons to communicate about them. Language-facilitation strategies are applicable to all children with hearing impairment regardless of whether they are developing spoken and/or signed language.

It is important for parents, teachers, and clinicians to facilitate rather than directly teach language targets/forms (Norris & Damico, 1990). Rather than drill or dictate what the child says, adults can learn to facilitate the child's use of conversational skills. True conversation is characterized by contingent and relevant responses, shared topics, and a mutual frame of reference (Garvey & Berninger, 1981). For example, instead of requiring the child to label all the fruit in the fruit bowl, mom can show the child the bowl of fruit and follow the child's conversational lead.

Adults may need to learn to be responsive and contingent. Parents who talk, talk, talk may believe that they are teaching lots of language. In the meantime, where is the child's opportunity to talk or communicate? The parents can miss out on the child's special interest and focus, or on the child's attempt to enter the conversation. If the child does use words and/or gestures, then the adult needs to acknowledge the communication. For example, if the child reaches for the apple in the fruit bowl the parent could respond, "Oh, you want the red apple" rather than ignoring the child and continuing to instruct "Now, this is a red apple, and this a green pear, and this is a yellow banana."

Even with knowledgeable language modelers and an abundance of contextually-rich communication exchanges, some structure and practice will be necessary for language to develop in children who are hearing impaired, especially those with more severe losses. However, syntactic and semantic principles must be presented under appropriate pragmatic conditions. Wilbur, et al. (1989) attribute many of the difficulties children with impaired hearing have with linguistic structures to the practice of teaching them language using sets of unrelated sentences, with each sentence presented in isolation, devoid of any pragmatic or semantic context. A focus on isolated sentences may ultimately teach the child syntactic word order for certain syntactical devices, such as determiners, indefinite pronouns, and modals, but fails to teach the child under what pragmatic situation it would be appropriate and useful to employ the device. Conway (1990) argues similarly that the traditional use of definitions of lists of words should be replaced with the children's learning the words in semantically rich contexts.

The signing abilities of parents, instructors, and clinicians is critical to language development for children using a total communication approach. Moeller and Luetke-Stahlman (1990) studied parental use of simultaneous communication with their preschoolers who were deaf. All parents had sign language MLUs that were lower than their own child's MLU. Parents rarely signed or spoke syntactically or semantically complex utterances. And, unlike parents who were deaf, these parents with normal hearing rarely used fingerspelling to introduce new words. This writer remembers the comment of one father of a deaf child who said, "I don't need to know much sign language because my son only knows five signs." Clinicians and educators need to find ways to help parents gain, and understand the importance of, sign-language proficiency. For example, videotape sign series are now available to help families learn sign language (e.g., *Sign With Me: A Family Sign Language Curriculum*; Moeller & Schick, 1993). Challenging as it may be, the instructor(s), parents, and siblings must be proficient in sign language in order for the child to develop language at a normal rate. If those communicating with the child are proficient in signing, every conversation can serve to aid language proficiency in the child with hearing impairment.

Strategies for Developing Conversational Skills. Schirmer (1994) discusses several different conversational approaches that facilitate language development. These approaches encourage the child's practice as a conversation partner learning how and when to initiate, take turns, and end conversations. The strategies employ real and role-played conversations. As such, they help the child become more communicatively proficient with all language aspects, not just syntax or morphology.

One technique discussed by Schirmer was "recasting." Adults communicating with the child target syntactic-semantic structures for development. If and when the child uses incomplete or inappropriate forms during conversation, the adult recasts the utterance maintaining the child's meaning but providing the appropriate form. For example, if the child says, "Daddy eated cookie" the parent responds, "Yes, daddy ate the cookie." The parent does not require the child to correct his/her original utterance. This technique has been found to facilitate language development in children with hearing impairment (Prinz & Masin, 1985).

Another conversational strategy is the use of minimal conversational encouragers by the adult. The adult, for example, could say, "Oh, that's interesting," nod her head, or repeat the child's comment. Use of this strategy has been found to result in greater conversational participation, and greater asking of questions by children who are deaf (Wood & Wood, 1984).

Children with hearing impairment often have under-developed schema or limited knowledge concerning everyday events like what happens during a trip to the doctor's office (Yoshinaga-Itano & Downey, 1986). Schema can be developed by purposefully planning experiential learning events. For example, Dad could read a book about a trip to the doctor for a check-up, Dad and child could talk about visiting the doctor for a check-up, prepare for the trip to the doctor (e.g., take a bath and leave at the appointed time), visit the doctor and talk about the office and check-up, and later remember and tell Mom about the visit to the doctor's office.

When real-life schema-building experiences cannot be arranged, adults can set up conversational scenarios or imaginary play scenes. The child and adult can pretend a "going-to-the-doctor scene" including what happens prior to and during the visit. The role-played scene still allows the child to learn about language and conversation in that setting. Use of role-playing scenarios is discussed further by Stone (1988).

Practical suggestions for teaching language use, content, and form are also provided by Luetke-Stahlman and Luckner (1991). They point out that much of the success in teaching the pragmatic aspects of language will depend on the teacher's and caretaker's ability to create an abundance of meaningful language opportunities for the child to communicate in routine situations. Several saboteur strategies are suggested to provide the child with opportunities to use language that has been mastered. One type of activity, for example, is to violate a routine event. At the dinner table, set the table by placing the plates and silverware on the chairs, or forget to put the child's favorite, mashed potatoes, on the table. These sabotaging activities provide opportunities for the child to protest, request, comment, and tease, and ensure that the child has ample opportunity to use language in a meaningful context.

The same requirement to create real needs in the context of natural settings is stressed by Luetke-Stahlman and Luckner (1991) for the semantic and syntactic aspects of language. Suggestions for helping children expand their English vocabularies are provided. One technique is the use of semantic mapping, in which a new word, such as *satisfactory*, is explained in graphic form using words the child already knows, such as *excellent* and *terrible*. Communication games, such as barrier games, can provide opportunities for children to use their emerging syntactic skills in a fun, meaningful way.

Pre-Literacy and Literacy Activities. In addition to facilitating conversational skills, parents and clinicians will also want to provide early pre-literacy and literacy activities for the young child with hearing impairment. Words on labels and traffic signs can be pointed out to the child, and story reading and retelling can be used to develop early awareness of reading and print. Children should also be allowed the opportunity to draw pictures and trace letters, and watch their stories be written down by their parents. Literacy activities for children with hearing impairment have been presented by Truax (1985) and Staton (1985), and general early literacy activities are presented by Gibson (1989).

Bilingual Education for Children Who are Deaf. The history of education of children who are deaf has been marked by continual controversy regarding communication approach. For years, the argument was centered mainly on whether oral or manual communication was more appropriate for children with severe and profound hearing losses. In recent years, educators have increasingly embraced a bilingual-bicultural approach to communication with education of these children. Interest in the bilingual approach was sparked by Johnson, Liddell, and Erting (1990), who suggested that the academic curriculum would be more accessible to children who are deaf if it was presented in American Sign Language (ASL), which they felt should be the child's primary language. Under the model proposed by Johnson, et al. (1990), ASL would be used for academic instruction and interpersonal communication in the classroom. English skills would be taught through written language, with explanations given using ASL. Johnson, et al. (1990) argue that it is time to stop pathologizing deafness, and that acceptance of ASL as the primary language of children who are deaf will yield better academic success *and* ultimately greater English language competency than presenting instruction solely in English. An excellent discussion of rehabilitative issues in the bilingual education of children who are deaf is presented by Lieberth (1990). She poses a number of unanswered questions regarding the bilingual education model, including whether competency in English can be developed through writing, how parents with normal hearing will acquire competency in sign language, and how the relationship between children who are deaf and their parents with normal hearing will be affected by the child's bilingualism. Stewart (1993) emphasizes that bilingual-bicultural programs should not have exclusive use of ASL as the ultimate goal, but rather should provide for consistent and complete linguistic input in the target language as well. Thus, ASL and English-based signing could serve as complementary communication tools. Like Lieberth (1990), Stewart (1993) raises a number of questions regarding the current move in deaf education toward a bilingual education model. It is only through the gathering of data from controlled investigations that we will be able to answer these questions and to document the efficacy of a bilingual model of education for children who are deaf.

SPEECH CHARACTERISTICS, ASSESSMENT, AND MANAGEMENT

Many clinicians and parents advocate the development of oral communication skills to whatever extent possible. The focus of this chapter section reflects that attitude. However, this perspective is not meant to deny that other means of communication, such as sign language, are beneficial and essential. Indeed, not all children with hearing impairment will be able to become oral communicators. Thus, this section will not apply to remediation for all children with hearing impairment. Within that cautionary framework, the following discussion will address early vocalizations of the child with hearing impairment, speech intelligibility, speech characteristics of those with mild–moderate and severe–profound hearing impairment, speech behaviors, and assessment and management concerns.

Early Vocalizations of the Child. In order to consider early vocalizations of the child with impaired hearing, it is essential to review briefly the typical vocalizations produced by infants with normal hearing. Babies with normal hearing develop vocalizations in an ordered sequence from birth to their first words (Stoel-Gammon & Otomo, 1986). They move through the following sequence of sound productions: crying and vegetative sounds (burps, coughs, sneezes), cooing and laughing, reduplicated babbling (same CV [consonant-vowel] syllable produced in a repetitive string, and variegated babbling (CV-syllable change within a string) with sentence-like intonation (Oller, 1980; Stark, 1983). Between 11 and 14 months, children produce some speech sound combinations called "vocables" to consistently represent meaning (Owens, 1990). For example, the child may call her blanket "bee" on a consistent basis. Some time around the first birthday the child will begin producing his or her first words.

Children with hearing impairment vocalize also, but the nature of their early vocalizations is not clearly understood (Stoel-Gammon & Otomo, 1986). The study of early vocal development in infants with hearing impairment is further confounded by the fact that childhood hearing loss is often not identified until 18 months of age or older (Elsmann, Matkin, & Sabo, 1987). A review of studies suggests that there are similarities and dissimilarities in the vocal development of infants with normal hearing and those with hearing impairment. Similarities noted include the finding that both babies with normal hearing and babies with impaired hearing coo, squeal, growl, and babble (Lenneberg, 1966; Rebelsky & Nichols, 1965; Oller, et al., 1985; Stoel-Gammon & Otomo, 1986), produce similar vowel positions and greater proportion of velar/back consonants at 12–15 months (Smith, 1982), and show similar development of place of articulation of consonants and in the frequency of reduplicated babbling (Smith, 1982). However, studies have also found differences in vocal production for the two groups, including restricted range of speech-like sounds (Stark, 1983; Oller, Eilers, Bull, & Carney, 1985; Stoel-Gammon & Otomo, 1986).

In contrast to infants with normal hearing, infants with hearing impairment produce fewer consonant-like sounds from 6–10 months of age (Stoel-Gammon & Otomo, 1986; Oller & Eilers, 1988; Kent, Osberger, Netsell, & Hustedde, 1987). Oller and Eilers, for example, reported that while babies with normal hearing started canonical babbling (i.e., using reduplicated consonant-like sounds with vowels) between 6 and 10 months of age, babies with hearing impairment showed onsets between 11 and 25 months and showed fewer instances of canonical babbling than babies with normal hearing. Kent and his associates (1987) reported on the babbling samples of identical twins, one with normal hearing and the other with a profound hearing loss that was aided when he was three months of age. Babbling samples were video- and audio recorded when the twins were 8, 12, and 15 months of age. The first and second formants of vowel productions for both twins changed over time from 8 months to 15 months. For the twin with normal hearing, the most notable change was in the lowered range of first formants used at 15 months. In contrast, the vowels of the twin with impaired hearing were characterized by a lowering of both the first and second formants by the 15th month. At 8 months, the twin with normal hearing produced a number of CV syllables while the productions of the twin with impaired hearing were almost all in the vowel or diphthong category. This overwhelming majority of vowel or diphthong productions persisted for the twin with hearing impairment until 20 months of age, when increased use of consonant-vowel syllables was noted. Frequency of occurrence for place of articulation was compared for the boys at 24 months. Alveolar consonants were predominant in the productions of the twin with hearing impairment, accounting for 77% of all productions, with bilabials next, accounting for 15%. In contrast, the twin with normal hearing produced a more uniform frequency of occurrence for different places of articulation at this age.

Speech Intelligibility. Speech intelligibility refers to the proportion of speech that can be understood by a listener (Kelly, Dancer, & Bradley, 1986). Although the intelligibility of speech of a child with hearing impairment may not be predicted solely on the basis of the child's hearing levels, research supports a cautious general distinction between the speech of children with mild to moderate hearing impairment (25–70 dB HL) and that of children with severe to profound hearing impairment (≥70 dB HL). Nober (1967), for example, reported substantially poorer performance on the Templin-Darley Test of Articulation (Templin & Darley, 1969) for children with hearing levels greater than 80 dB HL versus children with lesser degrees of hearing impairment. Similarly, as seen in Table 5.5, a nationwide survey by Jensema, et al. (1978) indicated considerably poorer speech-intelligibility ratings for children with hearing levels exceeding 70 dB HL. Further, inspection of Table 5.5 reveals that a majority of children with hearing levels of 70 dB HL or better demonstrated intelligible or "very intelligible" speech. Intelligibility ratings, however, can be more variable in the population of children with hearing levels exceeding 70 dB HL (Jensema, et al., 1978; Monsen, 1983). In fact, children with severe to profound hearing losses may span the whole range from *very intelligible* to *very unintelligible* (Monsen, 1983).

While the hearing thresholds mentioned previously indicate unaided hearing, aided audiometric thresholds should provide a better indicator/predictor of a child's speech intelligibility. Plotting of the aided audiogram on the Familiar Sounds Audiogram (see Figure 5.1), for example, can allow one to predict what speech sounds might be available auditorily to serve as a basis for speech development. In addition to aided thresholds, onset of hearing loss, intervention strategies, and family attitudes can also influence speech intelligibility. The following discussion will address the speech characteristics, assessment, and management concerns for two categories of children with hearing impairment: those with mild to moderate hearing loss (i.e., unaided pure tone losses ≤ 70 dB HL), and those with severe to profound hearing loss (unaided losses > 70 dB HL).

Children with Mild to Moderate Loss

Characteristic Speech Errors of Children with Mild-Moderate Loss While published data are relatively sparse, children with mild to moderate hearing loss generally appear to have intelligible speech (Jensema, et al., 1978; Elfenbein, Hardin-Jones, & Davis, 1994; Markides, 1970). The primary speech errors of this population are related to the misarticulation of single consonants (Markides, 1970; Elfenbein, Hardin-Jones, & Davis, 1994) and consonant blends (Cozad, 1974). Vowel-production errors are rare (Markides, 1970), and voice quality and suprasegmental features are generally either normal or mildly deviant (Elfenbein, Hardin-Jones, & Davis, 1994; Weiss, et al., 1985).

Knowledge of speech acoustics and the typical sloping audiometric configuration would suggest that errors might be made most commonly with sounds characterized by low intensity, high frequency, and/or short duration. Complexity of formation, visibility, and developmental order of acquisition are also considerations in the speech errors of this population. Sounds most commonly in error are the affricates, fricatives, and blends (Markides, 1970; Elfenbein, Hardin-Jones, & Davis, 1994). Markides (1970) reported that the greatest number of errors were related to final-consonant omissions and the distortion of fricatives and affricates. Elfenbein, et al. (1994) also found that fricatives and affricates were most often in error, but that the most common error types were substitutions (57%), followed by distortions (29%), and omissions (14%). Stop-plosives, nasals, and glides are less mistaken (McGarr, 1987; Elfenbein, et al., 1994). In fact, the speech errors made by children with mild to moderate hearing impairment are similar to errors made by younger children with normal hearing (McDermott & Jones, 1984).

Phonologic assessments have been made of children with hearing impairment to indicate rule-governed speech error patterns (Abraham, Stoker, & Allen, 1988). Two sets of researchers have reported phonologic analyses of children with mild to

TABLE 5.5 Speech Intelligibility Ratings as a Function of Age

Age in Years[a]	Very Intelligible		Intelligible		Barely Intelligible		Not Intelligible		Would Not Speak		Total	
	N	%	N	%	N	%	N	%	N	%	N	%
≤7	18	9.7	66	35.5	34	18.3	36	19.4	32	17.2	186	100.0
8–11	67	17.8	100	26.6	83	22.1	88	23.4	38	10.1	376	100.0
12–15	37	15.1	69	28.2	58	23.7	49	20.0	32	13.1	245	100.0
≥16	28	16.6	52	30.8	39	23.1	27	16.0	23	13.6	169	100.0
All Categories	150	15.4	287	29.4	214	21.9	200	20.5	125	12.8	976	100.0

$x^2 + 19.146, df = 12, p > .05$ (nonsignificant)

[a]The age of two students was not available.

Source: *The Rated Speech Intelligibility of Hearing-Impaired Children: Basic Relationships* by C. J. Jensema, M. A. Karchmer, and R. J. Trybus, 1978, Washington, DC: Gallaudet College of Demographic Studies.

FAMILIAR SOUNDS AUDIOGRAM ©

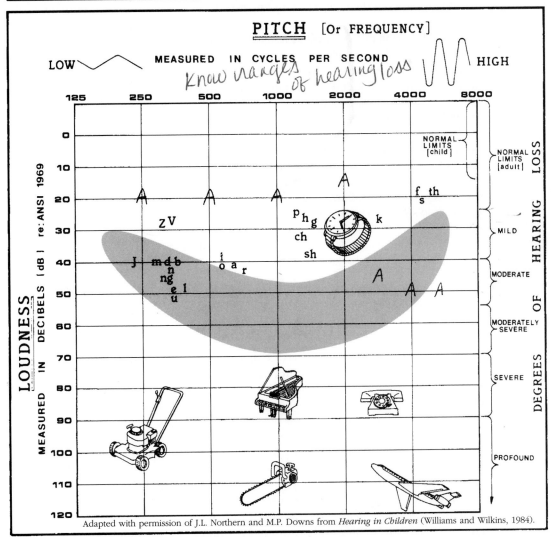

NAME	DATE

PITCH [Or FREQUENCY]

LOW — MEASURED IN CYCLES PER SECOND — HIGH

Know ranges of hearing loss

LOUDNESS MEASURED IN DECIBELS [dB] re: ANSI 1969

DEGREES OF HEARING LOSS

Adapted with permission of J.L. Northern and M.P. Downs from *Hearing in Children* (Williams and Wilkins, 1984).

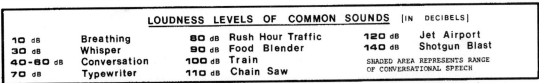

LOUDNESS LEVELS OF COMMON SOUNDS [IN DECIBELS]

10 dB	Breathing	80 dB	Rush Hour Traffic	120 dB	Jet Airport
30 dB	Whisper	90 dB	Food Blender	140 dB	Shotgun Blast
40-60 dB	Conversation	100 dB	Train	SHADED AREA REPRESENTS RANGE OF CONVERSATIONAL SPEECH	
70 dB	Typewriter	110 dB	Chain Saw		

LDOS Familiar Sounds Audiogram Form-2, 6/84   B.A. Chaudoin, S.S., CCC-A
To reorder, call or write: Louisville Deaf Oral School, 414 W. Ormsby, KY, 40203, 1-502-636-2084

Figure 5.1 Aided thresholds (A) plotted on the Familiar Sounds Audiogram.

moderate hearing loss (Oller & Kelly, 1974; West & Weber, 1974). These investigators compared the phonological processes of a child with impaired hearing to those of a child with normal hearing. Both children reportedly produced accurate vowels. The consonant errors of the children with impaired hearing were similar to phonological processes used by younger children with normal hearing, (e.g., voicing avoidance, fronting of consonants). Oller and Kelly tentatively proposed that children who are hard of hearing develop and use speech sounds in the same order as children with normal hearing. These findings have implications for the assessment and remediation of speech errors in the child with mild to moderate hearing impairment.

Speech Assessment of Children with Mild to Moderate Loss. The child with mild to moderate hearing impairment and the articulation-delayed or phonologically-delayed child with normal hearing apparently share common speech errors. Therefore, the practice of using standard articulation tests and phonologic analyses appears justified. One caution for the tester is to consider the vocabulary level of the stimulus words or items used, and the need for replacing words/items not within the child's vocabulary. Assessment of vowel production, voice quality, and suprasegmental features would depend on the needs of the individual child. (These latter types of assessments are described in the assessment section for children with severe to profound hearing impairment.)

Speech Management of Children with Mild to Moderate Loss. With early and appropriate amplification, many children with mild to moderate hearing losses can be expected to have highly intelligible speech. Children whose losses remain undetected and/or not amplified may be expected to manifest more extensive speech errors. In many cases, the clinician's major efforts may often be directed toward improving intelligibility by focusing on articulation or phonological treatment. Standard articulation and/or phonological treatment techniques are generally appropriate with some special considerations/modifications to programming.

Several considerations should be kept in mind while undertaking such treatment. First, children with normal hearing who have articulation or phonologic disorders are capable of using auditory feedback cues. Children with hearing loss may need visual, tactile, and kinesthetic cues to compensate for their inability to hear certain speech sound distinctions. Second, the clinician must be familiar with the child's aided thresholds in order to identify which speech sounds are not likely to be within the child's hearing range. This information can be gained by plotting the child's aided-hearing threshold levels on the Familiar Sounds Audiogram (see Figure 5.1). For sounds not within the child's aided-hearing range, nearly total reliance on other cues for speech sound production may be necessary. Third, the clinician should be familiar with the impact of co-articulation, since speech sounds change when paired with different speech sounds. Consequently, training on isolated speech-sound production should be limited and instead should move quickly to the production of sounds in meaningful words and phrases. For children with hearing impairment in the birth-to-three-year age range, Cole (1992) advocates use of the following guidelines (p. 74):

1. Selecting and sequencing the child's speech targets based on normal developmental information;
2. Maximizing and ensuring optimal residual hearing;
3. Having parents and clinicians target spoken-language goals during normal everyday activities.

Children with Severe to Profound Loss

Speech Characteristics of Children with Severe to Profound Loss. Studies have indicated that the average intelligibility of children with severe to profound hearing loss is approximately 20%, although ratings for individual children vary from 0–100% (Carney, 1986). These children may exhibit difficulties with consonant production, vowel and diphthong production, and voice quality (Hudgins & Numbers, 1942; Markides, 1970). For purposes of discussion, speech characteristics in this population will be discussed under the categories of respiration, resonance, phonation, and articulation. While this categorization simplifies the discussion, one must remain aware that respiratory, resonatory, phonatory, and articulatory behaviors are interactive and co-occur during on-going speech. Smith (1982) cautions that the speech of children who are deaf actually represents "stacks of errors which are complex and interrelated" (p. 27). Children with severe to profound hearing loss also exhibit faulty suprasegmental features. The discussion of suprasegmental errors in this population will be followed by assessment and management considerations.

RESPIRATION. Clinicians and investigators have noted that individuals with severe to profound hearing loss may speak only a few syllables on a single exhalation of air (Forner & Hixon, 1977). Few studies, however, have explored the underlying physiologic adjustments for speech breathing in this population. Cavallo, Baken, Metz, and Whitehead (1991) studied chest-wall movements before phonation (i.e., vowel production) in seven adult males with severe to profound hearing loss. Ribcage and abdominal movements were recorded, and lung volume was estimated based on measures from a mercury strain gauge. Before phonation, the speakers with hearing impairment demonstrated expansion of the ribcage and contraction of the diaphragm comparable to that seen in speakers with normal hearing. However, measures showed that speakers with hearing impairment lost significantly more air during the short adjustment period immediately prior to phonation. Cavallo, et al. proposed that this loss might be due to a delay in the adduction of vocal folds prior to phonation that would normally limit loss of air. They further indicated that this air loss might explain why some speakers with hearing impairment initiate speech at or below functional residual capacity for the lungs (a finding reported by Forner and Hixon, 1977).

Forner and Hixon (1977) studied abdomen and ribcage movement in 10 young adult males with severe to profound hearing losses. Unlike speakers with normal hearing, subjects with impaired hearing who had poor speech intelligibility initiated speech at low lung volumes, uttered only a few syllables at a time with air wastage during the pauses between segments, and continued to speak with lung volumes well below functional residual capacity. The air wastage during pauses was related to the lack of appropriate laryngeal valving (i.e., vocal fold adduction) prior to speaking. Hutchinson and Smith (1976) noted high air-flow rates during production of some consonantal segments, suggesting lack of sufficient vocal fold adduction in some speakers with hearing impairment. In summary, studies of respiration have indicated that some speakers with hearing impairment initiate speech on low volumes of air, waste air during pauses and during spoken segments, and continue to speak on very low lung volumes. Interestingly, the air wastage appears to be related to lack of sufficient vocal fold adduction rather than faulty respiratory moves.

RESONANCE. Both hyponasality and hypernasality have been noted in the speech of speakers with hearing impairment (Smith, 1975). The presence of resonance problems is interesting, given that acoustic information on nasality is found in the lower frequencies, where speakers with hearing impairment may have more residual hearing (Borden, Harris, & Raphael, 1994). In these cases, individuals might be trained to make use of auditory cues to nasality resulting in improved resonance.

PHONATION. Studies of respiration led investigators to link air wastage prior to and during the production of speech with insufficient vocal fold adduction rather than to respiratory difficulties. Inadequate vocal fold adduction has been directly observed in speakers with hearing impairment when producing vowels (Metz, Whitehead, & Whitehead, 1984). This incomplete closure can result in the overall perception of breathy voice quality, and in the perception of voiceless sounds being substituted for voiced sounds (McGarr & Whitehead, 1992).

Control of fundamental frequency of the voice is also primarily a function of laryngeal events (Shipp, 1975; Shipp & McGlone, 1971). While speaking, persons who are deaf may use higher fundamental frequency than their counterparts with normal hearing. Angelocci, Kopp, and Holbrook (1964) measured fundamental frequency in two groups of 18 male subjects (some with normal hearing, some with hearing impairment) ranging in age from 11–14 years. Their results confirmed that this group of boys who were deaf had fundamental frequencies that were noticeably higher than those of the boys with normal hearing. In contrast, others have reported normal overall fundamental frequency for some groups of speakers with hearing impairment (Boone, 1966; Monsen, 1979).

Another observation is that the range of fundamental frequencies produced during speech is reduced in the speech of the deaf. In fact, Hood and Dixon (1969) found reduced variability as evidenced by the comparison of fundamental frequency change across an utterance as spoken by speakers with both normal and impaired hearing (see Figure 5.2).

Speech intensity, another aspect of phonation, is also primarily a function of laryngeal activity (Isshiki, 1964; Hirano, Ohala, & Vennard, 1969). Unfortunately, data on voice intensity for speakers with hearing impairment are limited. Reduced intensity, excessive intensity, and reduced intensity variation across utterances have all been observed in this population. Calvert and Silverman (1975) suggested that over-

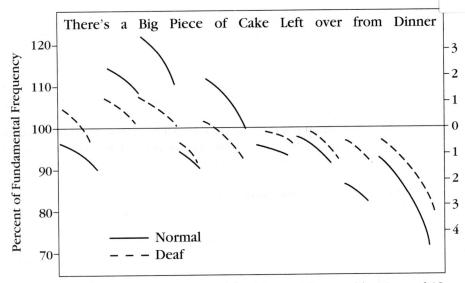

Figure 5.2 Mean intonation patterns of 6 subjects with normal hearing and 12 subjects with hearing impairment during production of the sentence, "There's a big piece of cake left over from dinner."

From R. B. Hood & R. F. Dixon (1969). Physical characteristics of speech rhythm of deaf and normal-hearing speakers. *Journal of Communication Disorders, 2,* 224.

all intensity is generally reduced in persons who are deaf. The presence of pervasive breathiness and low lung volume during speech could be related to reduced voice intensity. In contrast, Penn (1955) found excessive voice intensity to be a common speech characteristic in his study of 1086 subjects with hearing impairment. Excessive intensity might be related to excessive glottal resistance. Hood and Dixon (1969) reported reduced variability in intensity for subjects who are deaf when speaking sentences. Lack of auditory feedback may be one reason for this decreased variability. Individuals with hearing impairment who speak on low lung volumes may also be unable to produce appropriate stress.

ARTICULATION. Variability seems to be one of the hallmarks of speech production among those with severe to profound hearing loss. This is certainly true of articulation. Despite the variability, however, some difficulties may be expected in most children with severe to profound hearing loss. First, patterns of both consonant and vowel errors can be identified in this population. Second, consonant misarticulation is much more common than vowel or diphthong misarticulation.

The following categorizations of vowel error patterns, offered originally by Hudgins and Numbers (1942), have been substantiated in more recent research (Markides, 1970, 1983; Smith, 1975):

1. vowel substitution and neutralization (i.e., the tendency for all vowels to resemble the neutral schwa /ə/);

2.   dipthongalization (e.g., /aI/ for /a/);
3.   diphthong distortion (e.g., /a/ for /aI/);
4.   nasalization of vowels.

The perception of vowel neutralization has been verified by acoustic and physiologic studies. Perceptually, the first two formant frequencies of vowels are critical to the identification of different vowels (Borden, Harris, & Raphael, 1994). Hearing sensitivity in individuals with hearing loss is typically poorest above 1000 Hz, reducing the ability to perceive second formant frequencies. Because the second formant frequency is primarily a result of tongue height, a feature not easily seen during on-going speech, talkers with hearing impairment tend to use a centralized tongue position (Dagenais & Fletcher, 1989). Monsen (1976) reported that second formant frequencies for adolescents with hearing impairment clustered around 1800 Hz for all vowel productions. Tye-Murray (1991), using cinefluorography and x-ray microbeam, found that speakers who were deaf moved their tongues when shifting from consonants to vowels in CVC syllables, but that tongue-movement patterns were similar for different vowels. Dagenais (1992) also noted tongue positions located in the middle of the oral cavity for different vowels produced by a group of children with profound hearing impairment.

Children with hearing impairment produce consonants less accurately than vowels on both spontaneous and imitative tasks (Geffner & Freeman, 1980). Hudgins and Numbers (1942) categorized the most common consonant errors of children who are deaf in the following manner:

1.   voicing errors (e.g., substitution of /b/ for /p/);
2.   omission and distortion of consonants (e.g., omission of velars and final consonants);
3.   omission of consonants in blends; (e.g., /tʌk/ for /trʌk/);
4.   nasalization of consonants.

Although the majority of investigators report a greater proportion of voiced/voiceless errors (Gold, 1980), the voiceless/voiced error may also be observed in the speech of children who are deaf. Voicing errors noted include voiced/voiceless confusions, devoicing of final consonants, and omission of final voiced consonants (Hutchinson, et al., 1978; Hutchinson & Smith, 1979; Stark, 1979; Oller, Jensen, & Lafayette, 1978; McGarr & Osberger, 1978; Nober, 1967).

Studies of tongue placement during consonant production have been conducted, using a technique called "palatometry." Palatometry involves the placement of a thin custom-fit pseudo-palate over the child's hard palate and maxillary teeth. The pseudo-palate has a set of 96 electrodes which, when contacted by the tongue, show as contact points on a display screen. Results of these studies have indicated that children with profound hearing impairment have idiosyncratic tongue-to-palate contacts as compared to speakers with normal hearing (Dagenais & Critz-Crosby, 1991; Fletcher, Dagenais, & Critz-Crosby, 1991a).

In addition to individual phoneme errors, speech of persons who are deaf is sometimes characterized by reduced coarticulatory movements (Whitehead & Jones, 1978; Tye-Murray, 1987). The production of a speech sound in an utterance can be influenced by both preceding sounds (perseveratory coarticulation) and subsequent sounds (anticipatory coarticulation). Recent data indicate that children with profound hearing impairment produce both types of coarticulatory effects, but that coarticulation effects are much smaller than those produced by children with normal hearing (Baum & Waldstein, 1991; Waldstein & Baum, 1991). Reduced coarticulation has been related to two possibilities: (a) the tendency of some individuals with hearing impairment to speak on a word-by-word basis, and (b) poor coordination of articulators (Baum & Waldstein, 1991).

SUPRASEGMENTAL ASPECTS. Suprasegmental errors (i.e., errors in the relative variation of duration, intensity, and fundamental frequency across an utterance) may contribute substantially to the poor intelligibility of the child who is deaf (Gold, 1980; Hudgins & Numbers, 1942; Smith, 1975). Suprasegmentals can communicate an individual's emotional intent or the urgency of a message, or encode linguistic stress (Lehiste, 1976). According to Allen (1975), linguistic stress allows a listener to "organize the incoming acoustic elements into coherent packages which allow for the perceptual separation of words and phrases" (p. 84). Consequently, suprasegmental errors of the child who is deaf may be expected to reduce speech intelligibility.

Individuals who are deaf speak at an overall rate 1.5–2 times slower than that of speakers with normal hearing (Tye-Murray, 1992). Slow speaking rate has been related to the prolongation of individual phonemes and the presence of lengthy pauses within utterances (Markides, 1983; Voelker, 1935). Tye-Murray (1992) cited several studies that indicated that speakers who are deaf do not produce longer open posture steady-states for vowels than speakers with normal hearing. It is interesting to note that some investigators have reported improved intelligibility for slower speaking rates (Osberger & Levitt, 1979). Thus, overall slow speaking rate may, in part, serve as an appropriate compensatory adjustment. On the other hand, excessively slow rates can interrupt the perceived cohesiveness of speech, thus reducing intelligibility. Markides (1983) noted that "a considerable number of children with hearing impairment's oral reading was so slow that the listeners had difficulty in organizing the speech of the children into meaningful wholes" (p. 188).

Speakers with hearing impairment have been found to use more and longer pauses in addition to within-phrase pauses during utterances (John & Howarth, 1965; Miller, 1980). Speakers with normal hearing, in contrast, tend to avoid the use of within-phrase pauses (Osberger & Levitt, 1979). Although speakers who are deaf often exhibit abnormal pause behaviors, Osberger and Levitt found little effect of abnormal pauses on speech intelligibility.

Differences in intonation of deaf speakers have been consistently associated with reduced speech intelligibility (Formby & Monsen, 1982; Monsen, Engbretson, & Vemulla, 1979; Wingfield, Buttett, & Sandoval, 1979). Both excessive pitch variation and less than normal pitch variation have been observed (Boone, 1966; Formby &

Monsen, 1982; Green, 1956; Miller, 1980; Monsen, 1979; Voelker, 1935). When required to produce sentences with either falling intonation (e.g., declarative sentence) or rising intonation (e.g., question), children with hearing impairment are better able to produce sentences with falling intonation (Rubin-Spitz & McGarr, 1990; Most & Frank, 1991). The rising intonation pattern necessitates vocal fold tensing rather than the relaxation of the vocal folds at the end of an utterance (Most & Frank, 1991).

In summary, speakers who are deaf may have difficulty adjusting duration, intensity, and intonational cues within an utterance. These suprasegmental difficulties may result in faulty linguistic stress and reduce speech intelligibility. Atypical intonation, in particular, has been associated with lower overall speech intelligibility (Formby & Monsen, 1982).

Speech Assessment of Children with Severe to Profound Loss. Comprehensive speech evaluation of those with severe to profound hearing loss should include perceptual measures of intelligibility, articulation and phonology, suprasegmental features, and voice characteristics. The additional use of acoustic and/or physiologic measures typically depends on the availability of the appropriate equipment. In this section, then, four general areas of evaluation will be considered. First, attention will be directed toward procedures for assessing the physiological and acoustic dimensions of speech production. Second, measures of speech intelligibility will be considered. Third, strategies for assessing articulation and phonology will be reviewed. Fourth, several methods of perceptual assessment of the voice will be offered.

ACOUSTIC AND PHYSIOLOGIC MEASURES. It is beyond the scope of this chapter to discuss fully the instrumentation and procedures used to measure the acoustic and physiologic aspects of speech. Realistically, these measures often are not taken because budgetary constraints prevent clinicians from obtaining the necessary equipment for making the assessments. Nevertheless, a brief overview will be presented.

Instrumentation providing displays of acoustic characteristics of speech are generally more likely to be available to clinicians than physiologic instrumentation. Commonly used equipment that displays acoustic features includes the Visi-Pitch (Kay Elemetrics, Inc.), which can indicate fundamental frequency and intensity, and the IBM SpeechViewer (see Figure 5.3), which can indicate the mean frequency and standard deviation of frequency across an utterance, mean intensity (in % saturation) and standard deviation of intensity across an utterance, and percentage of utterance voiced. Physiologic instrumentation, when available, can be used to assess respiratory function, nasality, and tongue-to-palate contacts. A spirometer can be used to assess speech initiatory lung volumes and other patterns of respiratory adjustment used by a hearing-impaired speaker. A nasometer can be used to determine the presence of hyponasality or hypernasality. And a palatometer can be used to indicate whether an individual is making appropriate tongue-to-palate contacts.

MEASURES OF SPEECH INTELLIGIBILITY. Assessment and improvement of speech intelligibility would appear to be important program goals for speakers with hearing

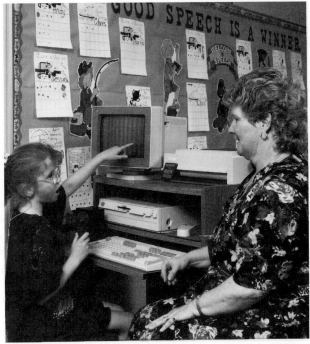

Figure 5.3 An example of an acoustic display device, the IBM SpeechViewer, and a physiologic display device, the Palatometer.

impairment. Surprisingly, it is often not assessed in audiologic rehabilitation programs (Monsen, 1981). When speech intelligibility is assessed, "percent intelligible word" scores and intelligibility rating scales are the most widely used procedures (Kelly, Dancer, & Bradley, 1986). Difficulties arise with each of these assessment procedures.

With the percent intelligible word scores, a listener/judge or set of listeners/judges identifies words produced by a speaker with hearing impairment. The score is then established by computing the overall percent of words correctly identified. The main complication with this procedure is that a large set of factors can influence the percent intelligibility score. The score can vary depending upon whether (a) simple sentences, sentences with consonant clusters, polysyllabic words, or complex syntax are used, (b) judges are experienced or inexperienced in listening to speech of speakers with hearing impairment, (c) sentences are in or out of context, and (d) sentences are presented auditorily only or with visual cues (Monsen, 1983). Thus, one score will typically represent the intelligibility for that speaking/listening context only. Markides (1978) cautioned that speech intelligibility scores can also be poor when children with hearing impairment are asked to read a passage or set of sentences. In fact, the effects of reading difficulties and change in normal speech rhythm that occurs when children shift to a "reading aloud" register may suppress intelligibility scores for some children. Other options include assessment of intelligibility based on a conversational sample or a picture description.

TABLE 5.6 *Sets of Words Used in the SPINE Test*

1. feel	fail	fill	fell
2. pain	pan	pen	pine
3. net	Nat	nut	not
4. look	lack	luck	lock
5. ride	right	wide	white
6. pull	pole	pool	Paul
7. bed	bad	bet	bat
8. bid	bead	bit	beat
9. bit	bid	but	bud
10. ten	ton	den	done

Another type of assessment tool, the rating scale, has been presented by the National Technical Institute for the Deaf (NTID) as a rapid and efficient means for assessing intelligibility (Subtelny, 1975). This procedure requires a set of listeners/judges who first must be trained in the use of a five-point rating scale. The scale ranges from 1 (speech cannot be understood) to 5 (speech is completely intelligible). NTID provides a set of training audiotapes to allow listeners to anchor their rating judgments with various levels of speech intelligibility. Obviously, the need for a group of trained judges limits the use of this technique.

A third option for measuring speech intelligibility involves use of a forced-choice procedure (Carney, 1986). The CID Picture SPINE: Speech Intelligibility Evaluation (Monsen, 1981) provides a rapid and easy forced-choice assessment of speech intelligibility for children as young as six years of age (see Table 5.6 for a listing of the words depicted on the CID Picture SPINE). The examiner shuffles a set of picture cards and deals each card to the child in such a way that the examiner cannot see the word depicted on the card. The child says the word depicted on the card and the examiner writes the word s/he believes was spoken. Once all of the picture cards are dealt, the examiner takes the pile of cards and writes the target words next to the words recorded. The examiner then computes the percentage of words correctly produced and this represents the overall percent intelligibility for that child.

Assessment of intelligibility for picture-description tasks or conversational samples can indicate how the child's knowledge of spoken language (e.g., syntax, suprasegmental features) affects speech intelligibility. One can use these samples to calculate the number of totally intelligible utterances, number of totally unintelligible utterances, and numbers of intelligible and unintelligible words.

MEASURES OF ARTICULATION/PHONOLOGY. Standard articulation tests have been used in the assessment of children with hearing impairment. A survey by Abraham, Stoker, and Allen (1988) indicated that the following tests were most commonly used with children with hearing impairment: Goldman Fristoe Test of Articulation (Goldman & Fristoe, 1969), Fisher-Logemann Test of Articulation Competence (Fisher & Logemann, 1971), Photo Articulation Test (Pendergast, Dickey, Selmar, & Soder, 1969), Arizona Articulation Proficiency Scale (Fudula, 1970), Templin-Darley Tests of Articulation (Templin & Darley, 1969), and the Deep Test of Articulation (McDonald, 1964). None of these tests has normative data for children with hearing impairment. Use of such tests can, however, indicate phonemes produced accurately, phonemes produced inaccurately, and the types of speech sound errors (substitution, distortion, omission, or addition). One major concern with respect to use of these tests with children with hearing impairment is the vocabulary level of the assessments. Geffner and Freeman (1980) recommended restricting test stimuli to words known to be in the vocabulary of young children who are deaf. Speech production in children with hearing impairment may also be rule-governed rather than reflecting simple phoneme confusions. Phonological process analysis allows clinicians to identify patterns such as final consonant deletion, cluster reduction, and stopping. These processes occur naturally in the speech of young children, and have also been noted in the speech of children with hearing impairment. Analysis of processes can guide therapy decisions. Phonological process assessments such as the Assessment of Phonological Processes (Hodson, 1980) and the Phonological Process Analysis (Weiner, 1979) have been used to assess children with hearing impairment from ages 3–18 years (Abraham, et al., 1988).

Ling (1976) developed the Phonetic Level Evaluation and Phonologic Level Evaluation specifically for use with children who have severe to profound hearing loss. The Phonetic Level Evaluation requires the child to imitate meaningless syllables presented orally by the tester. Test stimuli include consonants and consonant blends in the initial and final positions of syllables, and vowels and diphthongs. This assessment is lengthy; consequently Ling generally begins with a speech-production task that the clinician knows the child can perform (Ling, 1981) and ends when the clinician has identified a set of immediate speech treatment objectives (Tye-Murray & Kirk, 1993).

Ling's Phonologic Level Evaluation requires that a spontaneous language sample of 50 utterances be obtained. The clinician determines whether vowels, diphthongs, consonants, and consonant blends are produced with accuracy on a consistent or inconsistent basis during the sample. Phonologic processes, however, are not identified. According to the survey by Abraham, et al. (1988), the Phonetic Level and Phonologic Level Evaluations and the Goldman-Fristoe Test of Articulation are the most commonly used speech assessments with children with hearing impairment. Unfortunately, the Phonetic Level Evaluation has been found to have unacceptable interobserver reliability (i.e., different clinicians give different scores; Shaw & Coggins, 1991), and the scoring/coding system may need to be modified.

PERCEPTUAL ASSESSMENT OF SUPRASEGMENTALS AND VOICE CHARACTERISTICS. Speech and voice characteristics are most often assessed by clinicians who rate characteristics of a spoken passage or spontaneous speech sample produced by the individual with hearing impairment. Both Ling evaluations include a general rating of the acceptability of various suprasegmental features. Some clinicians may even use the voice-rating system developed by Wilson (1977). In this system, clinicians rate clients with regard to laryngeal valving ("laryngeal air wastage" to "extreme tension"), pitch, nasality, intensity variability, and pitch variability. In addition, Wilson urges the clinician to check for the presence of voice deviations such as diplophonia, audible inhalation, pitch breaks, and phrasing irregularities.

An alternative approach is to use a formal test procedure. The Prosodic Feature Production Test (Stark & Levitt, 1974), for example, allows one to evaluate the child's ability to produce simple prosodic contrasts. Four short sentences are marked in relation to the presence of the following: (a) statement, (b) question with a final rising pitch, (c) specified pauses, and (d) different stress patterns.

Speech Management.   Nearly all investigators who have studied speech production in persons who are deaf are struck by the extreme variability in error patterns between subjects (Miller, 1980; Miller & Hutchinson, 1982). Such variability highlights the importance of individualizing speech management procedures. A second critical concern is that speech training be as meaningful as possible. Speech is used to express meaning. Speech sounds that cannot be heard and developed through the use of optimal amplification may require additional visual and/or tactile cues. However, training should not focus on lengthy motor drills of sounds in meaningless syllables. Speech-sound training should move quickly to use in meaningful words. In accord with a whole-language philosophy, speech targets should appear in words that a child would learn about in natural contexts. A child, for example, would not simply learn the label "duck" when working on production of the /d/ and produce it each time the clinician showed a toy duck or picture of a duck. The child would read about ducks, play with ducks, go see ducks at the duckpond, and talk about birds that are ducks and birds that are not ducks. In addition, the development of sounds in different phonetic contexts is also important to ensure the development of coarticulation.

Four major approaches may enhance speech-sound training in persons with hearing impairment: (a) optimal use of residual hearing, (b) anatomic and pictorial monitoring, (c) visual stimulation, and (d) use of complex feedback aids. These strategies are not mutually exclusive, and their combined use may be warranted.

Most individuals with hearing impairment possess some residual hearing, and its use should be maximized. An important question to ask is, "Does the client's hearing aid/FM system/cochlear implant/vibrotactile system provide him or her with as many speech sounds as possible?" It would be ideal if clinicians could assume that clients are receiving the most speech sounds possible with the assistance of their sensory devices. But the fitting of devices, particularly in children, can be a tricky bit of educated guesswork. Feedback from parents and clinicians is essential to establish effectiveness of these devices. According to Ling (1989), many children require adjustments of hearing aids in order to provide hearing for a greater range of speech sounds. The responsibility for providing optimal speech reception lies in the hands of the audiologist. However, the responsibility for audiologic consultation/referral when sensory systems do not appear to be optimal lies in the hands of the clinician (i.e., usually a speech-language pathologist). The clinician might plot the child's aided thresholds on the Familiar Sounds Audiogram and notice that few speech sounds are audible, or notice that the child is not responding to sounds in his environment. Observations like these signal the need to consult with the child's audiologist.

Anatomic and pictorial modeling have also been used to help establish speech sound productions. Anatomic charts, sagittal sections of the head with a mobile tongue, and pictures of tongue shape may be useful in some cases. Some of these

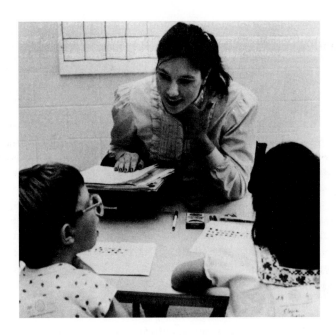

Speech therapy emphasizing voicing with a hearing-impaired child.

models are available commercially, but they can also be made without undue expense. The problem with these aids is that they provide a static picture whereas the production of a speech sound is not static. It may be wise to use these types of models only in the initial stages of sound production, and only as a last resort.

Another approach to improving speech production is visual stimulation by the clinician and/or visual monitoring with the use of a mirror. Some information concerning speech production is available visually; however, excessive attention to visual feedback may be hazardous. The visual characteristics of sounds change dramatically as a function of context. For example, /ʃ/ looks considerably different in the words "shoe" and "she."

Complex feedback aids or devices have also been used to assist in training speech production in the hearing impaired. Most devices allow for visual monitoring of acoustic or physiologic features of speech production. The VisiPitch and IBM SpeechViewer are two devices that provide feedback on the acoustic characteristics of speech. The VisiPitch, for example, allows for display of fundamental frequency of the voice and intensity variation across an utterance. The child may try to match her fundamental frequency tracing to the clinician's. The IBM SpeechViewer allows for child-friendly displays with loudness indicated by the changing size of a balloon, pitch indicated as changes on a thermometer, and vowel accuracy indicated by a monkey dropping a coconut from a tree. Although vowel-treatment effects have been documented with the use of the IBM SpeechViewer (Pratt, Heintzelman, & Deming, 1993;

Ryalls, Michallet, & Le Dorze, 1994), there is no proof that the system is more effective than traditional therapy approaches. In addition, children appear to lose interest in the monkey and coconut dropping over multiple sessions (Pratt, et al., 1993). Also, there is no evidence that speech behaviors practiced in treatment carry over to everyday life. Consequently, these types of devices may be of most benefit as a supplementary treatment tool.

Acoustic displays do not show individuals how to articulate speech sounds properly. Fletcher and Hasegawa (1983) suggested that physiologic feedback devices can provide more direct information on speech movements to persons with impaired hearing. Glossometry and palatometry represent two types of physiologic feedback systems (Dagenais, 1992). Both systems require the speaker to wear a pseudopalate, a custom-fit thin plate fit over the speaker's hard palate and maxillary teeth. The palatometry pseudopalate contains 96 contact electrodes which can indicate tongue-to-palate contact points during consonant production (for a description of the glossometry pseudopalate, see p. 204). When electrodes are contacted, the contacted points are subsequently indicated on the video display monitor. Reports of glossometry and palatometry training with children who are deaf have been promising, but the system is not widely available for use (Fletcher, Dagenais, & Critz-Crosby, 1991a, 1991b; Dagenais, 1992). Dagenais suggested that speech training might begin with use of these systems to establish correct articulatory placements of sounds in nonsense syllables and single-syllable words, and then move to more traditional speech exercises that emphasize words and utterances varying in complexity.

Speech in the Adventitiously Hearing Impaired. Descriptions of speech abilities in individuals with acquired hearing loss have not been well documented in the literature but generally consist of anecdotal reports instead. Adventitious deafness in those with well-developed speech appears to produce a gradual, rather than immediate deterioration of speech in a small percentage of cases. Zimmerman and Rettaliata (1981) suggested that "while auditory information may not be necessary on a gesture-to-gesture basis, it plays a critical role in the long-term monitoring and maintenance of speech coordination" (p. 177). The apparently wide variation in speech production may be attributed to the degree of hearing loss, age at onset of hearing loss, hearing-aid history, and other factors (Cowie, Douglas-Cowie, & Kerr, 1982; Jackson, 1982). According to Calvert and Silverman (1975), typical speech errors in this population affect production of sibilants, final consonants, voice quality, loudness, and speech rhythm. Some deafened adults may show little deterioration of speech sound production (Goehl & Kaufman, 1984).

Cowie and Douglas-Cowie (1983) reported data from their assessment of the speech of 13 adults with severe or profound adventitious hearing losses. Speech intelligibility was assessed by first having the speakers with hearing impairment read a series of short passages. Judges with normal hearing then listened to a passage and immediately repeated what they heard. The percent of words correctly identified was averaged for 10 listener judges. Intelligibility scores ranged from below 10% to above 90%. Age at onset was related to the rank ordering of speakers by intelligibility, with those deafened before 18 years of age generally less intelligible than those deafened later. Cowie and Douglas-Cowie noted that both reduced intelligibility and negative reactions to voice quality/slurring were associated with the speech of these adventitiously deafened adults.

SUMMARY

Who should be responsible for speech and language intervention with hearing-impaired individuals? Is there one professional who should be solely responsible for speech and language intervention? The audiologist, speech-language pathologist, teacher of the hearing-impaired, and family members may all be involved in the management of the child with hearing loss. All have complementary and sometimes overlapping contributions toward language facilitation. The audiologist may have the greatest expertise in monitoring the child's hearing loss, establishing and ensuring that sensory devices are providing the maximum amount of speech acoustic cues, and communicating to others about the aspects of spoken language that may be audible to the child. The speech-language pathologist will often have the strongest background and training in current language-intervention practices, including ways to establish more family-centered intervention. The teacher of the hearing-impaired may have the greatest expertise in enhancing language abilities essential in the school setting, and may be the most proficient of the professionals with respect to knowledge and use of sign language. The family is the constant in the child's life (Crais, 1991), and as such the family's needs and choices are critical to the success and carryover of language intervention. The true challenge of family-centered intervention is working out the collaboration and consultation between the family and professionals involved in the management of the child with hearing loss.

RECOMMENDED READINGS

Bernstein, L. E., Goldstein, M. H., & Mahshie, J. J. (1988). Speech training aids for hearing-impaired individuals: I. Overview and aims. *Journal of Rehabilitation Research and Development, 25*, 4, 53–62.

Bunch, G. O. (1987). *The curriculum and the hearing-impaired student: Theoretical and practical considerations.* Austin, TX: Pro-Ed.

Damico, J. S. (1992). *Whole language for special needs children.* Buffalo, NY: Educom Associates, Inc.

King, C. M., & Quigley, S. P. (1985). *Reading and deafness.* Austin, TX: Pro-Ed.

McAnally, P. L., Rose, S., & Quigley, S. P. (1987). *Language learning practices with deaf children.* Austin, TX: Pro-Ed.

Osberger, M. J., Moeller, M. P., Eccarius, M., Robbins, A. M., & Johnson, D. (1986). Expressive language skills. In M. J. Osberger (Ed.), *Language and learning skills of hearing-impaired students* (pp. 54–65). *ASHA Monographs*, 23. Washington, DC: ASHA.

Osberger, M. J., Robbins, A. M., Lybolt, J., Kent, R. D., & Peters, J. (1986). Speech evaluation [Monograph 23]. In M. J. Osberger (Ed.), *Language and learning skills of hearing-impaired students* (pp. 24-31). ASHA Monographs. Washington, DC: ASHA.

Quigley, S. P., & Paul, P. V. (1984). *Language and deafness.* San Diego: College-Hill Press.

Thompson, M., Biro, P., Vethivelu, S., Pious, C., & Hatfield, N. (1987). *Language assessment of hearing impaired school age children.* Seattle: University of Washington Press.

REFERENCES

Abraham, S., & Stoker, R. (1988). Language assessment of hearing-impaired children and youth: Patterns of test use. *Language, Speech, and Hearing Services in the Schools, 19,* 160-173.

Abraham, S., Stoker, R., & Allen, W. (1988). Speech assessment of hearing-impaired children and youth: Patterns of test use. *Language, Speech, and Hearing Services in the Schools, 19,* 17-27.

Allen, G. D. (1975). Speech rhythm: Its relation to performance universals and articulatory timing. *Journal of Phonetics, 3,* 75-86.

Altshuler, K. (1974). The social and psychological development of the deaf child: Problems, their treatment, and prevention. *American Annals of the Deaf, 119,* 365-376.

Ammons, R. B., & Ammons, H. S. (1948). *Full-Range Picture Vocabulary Test.* Missoula, MT: Psychological Test Specialists.

Angelocci, A. A., Kopp, G. A., & Holbrook, A. (1964). The vowel formants of deaf and normal-hearing eleven-to-fourteen year old boys. *Journal of Speech and Hearing Disorders, 29,* 156-170.

Bankson, N. (1977). *Bankson Language Screening Test.* Baltimore: University Park Press.

Bargstadt, G. H., Hutchinson, J. J., & Nerbonne, M. A. (1978). Learning visual correlates of fricative production by normal-hearing subjects: A preliminary evaluation of the video articulator. *Journal of Speech and Hearing Disorders, 43,* 200-207.

Baum, S. R., & Waldstein, R. S. (1991). Perseveratory coarticulation in the speech of profoundly hearing-impaired and normally hearing children. *Journal of Speech and Hearing Research, 34,* 1286-1292.

Bernstein, L. E., Goldstein, M. H., & Mahshie, J. J. (1988). Speech training aids for hearing-impaired individuals: I. Overview and aims. *Journal of Rehabilitation Research and Development, 25*(4), 53-62.

Blank, M., & Franklin, E. (1980). Dialogue with preschoolers: A cognitively-based system of assessment. *Applied Psycholinguistics, 1,* 127-150.

Blanton, R. L., & Nunnaly, J. C. (1964). Evaluational language processes in the deaf. *Psychological Reports, 15,* 891-894.

Blennerhassett, L. (1984). Communicative styles of a 13-month-old hearing-impaired child and her parents. *Volta Review, 5*, 217–227.

Bloom, L., & Lahey, M. (1978). *Language development and language disorders*. New York: John Wiley and Sons.

Boehm, A. E. (1971). *Boehm Test of Basic Concepts*. New York: The Psychological Corporation.

Boone, D. R. (1966). Modification of the voices of deaf children. *Volta Review, 68*, 686–692.

Boothe, L., Lasky, E., Kricos, P. (1982). Comparison of the language abilities of deaf children and young deaf adults. *Journal of Rehabilitation of the Deaf, 15*, 10–15.

Borden, G. J., Harris, K. S., & Raphael, L. J. (1994). *Speech Science Primer: Physiology, acoustics, and perception of speech* (3rd ed.). Baltimore: Williams and Wilkins.

Brannon, J. B. (1968). Linguistic word classes in spoken language of normal, hard-of-hearing and deaf children. *Journal of Speech and Hearing Research, 11*, 279-287.

Brannon, J. B., & Murray, T. (1966). The spoken syntax of normal, hard of hearing and deaf children. *Journal of Speech and Hearing Research, 9*, 604-610.

Brenza, B. A., Kricos, P. B., & Lasky, E. Z. (1981). Comprehension and production of basic semantic concepts by older hearing-impaired children. *Journal of Speech and Hearing Research, 24*, 414–419.

Brown, R. (1973). *A first language: The early stages*. Cambridge, MA: Harvard University Press.

Bzoch, K., & League, R. (1970). *Receptive-Expressive Emergent Language Scale*. Gainesville, FL: Computer Management Corp.

Calvert, D. R., & Silverman, S. R. (1975). *Speech and deafness*. Washington, DC: Alexander Graham Bell Association for the Deaf.

Campbell, M., Boothroyd, A., McGarr, N. S., & Haris, K. S. (1992). Articulatory compensation in hearing-impaired speakers. *Journal of the Acoustical Society of America*, (A).

Caniglia, J., Cole, N. J., Howard, W., Krohn, E., & Rice, M. (1972). *Apple tree: A patterned program of linguistic expanse through reinforced experiences and evaluations*. Beaverton, OR: Dormac, Inc.

Carney, A. E. (1986). Understanding speech intelligibility in the hearing impaired. *Topics in Language Development, 6*(3), 47–59.

Carrow, E. (1973). *Test of Auditory Comprehension of Language*. Austin, TX: Learning Concepts.

Cavallo, S. A., Baken, R. J., Metz, D. E., & Whitehead, R. L. (1991). Chest wall preparation for phonation in congenitally profoundly hearing-impaired persons. *Volta Review, 12*, 287–299.

Charrow, V. R. (1977). A psycholinguistic analysis of "deaf English". *Sign Language Studies, 7*, 139–150.

Clarke, B. R., & Rogers, W. T. (1981). Correlates of syntactic abilities in hearing-impaired students. *Journal of Speech and Hearing Research, 24*, 48–54.

Clarke-Stewart, K.A. (1978). And daddy makes three: The father's impact on mother and young child. *Child Development, 49*, 466–478.

Cole, E. B. (1992). Promoting emerging speech in birth to three year-old hearing-impaired children. *Volta Review, 94*, 63–77.

Cole, E. B., & St. Clair-Stokes, J. (1984). Caregiver-child interactive behaviors: A videotape analysis procedure. *Volta Review, 86*, 200–216.

Conway, D. F. (1990). Semantic relationships in the word meanings of hearing-impaired children. *Volta Review, 92*, 339–349.

Cooper, R. (1967). The ability of deaf and hearing children to apply morphological rules. *Journal of Speech and Hearing Research, 10*, 77–86.

Cooper, W. E., & Sorensen, J. M. (1977). Fundamental frequency contours at syntactic boundaries. *Journal of the Acoustical Society of America, 62*, 783–792.

Cowie, R. I. D., & Douglas-Cowie, E. (1983). Speech production in profound postlingual deafness. In M. E. Lutman & M. P. Haggard (Eds.), *Hearing science and hearing disorders*. New York: Academic Press.

Cowie, R. I. D., Douglas-Cowie, E., & Kerr, A. G. (1982). A study of speech deterioration in post-lingually deafened adults. *Journal of Laryngology and Otology, 96*, 101–112.

Cozad, R. L. (1974). *The speech clinician and the hearing-impaired child*. Springfield, IL: Charles C. Thomas.

Crais, E. R. (1990). World knowledge to word knowledge. *Topics in Language Disorders, 10*, 3, 45–62.

Crais, E. R. (1991). Moving from "parent involvement" to family-centered services. *American Journal of Speech-Language Pathology, 9*, 5–8.

Curtiss, S., Prutting, C. A., & Lowell, E. L. (1979). Pragmatic and semantic development in young children with impaired hearing. *Journal of Speech and Hearing Research, 22*, 534–552.

Dagenais, P.A. (1992). Speech training with glossometry and palatometry for profoundly hearing-impaired children. *Volta Review, 94*, 261–282.

Dagenais, P. A., & Critz-Crosby, P. (1991). Consonant lingual-palatal contacts produced by normal-hearing and hearing-impaired children. *Journal of Speech and Hearing Research, 34*, 1423–1435.

Damico, J. S. (1992). *Whole language for special needs children*. Buffalo, NY: Educom Associates, Inc.

Davis, J. (1974). Performance of young hearing-impaired children on a test of basic concepts. *Journal of Speech and Hearing Research, 17*, 342–352.

Davis, J., & Blasdell, R. (1975). Perceptual strategies employed by normal-hearing and hearing-impaired children in the comprehension of sentences containing relative clauses. *Journal of Speech and Hearing Research, 17*, 281–295.

Davis, J. M., Elfenbein, J., Schum, R., & Bentler, R. A. (1986). Effects of mild and moderate hearing impairments on language, educational and psychosocial behavior of children. *Journal of Speech and Hearing Disorders, 51*(1), 53–62.

Day, P. S. (1986). Deaf children's expression of communicative intentions. *Journal of Communication Disorders, 19*, 367–386.

de Villiers, P. A. (1988). Assessing English syntax in hearing-impaired children: Eliciting production in pragmatically-motivated situations. In R. R. Kretschmer & L. W. Kretschmer (Eds.), Communication assessment of hearing-impaired children: From conversation to classroom [Monograph]. *Journal of the Academy of Rehabilitative Audiology, 21*(Suppl.), 41–73.

de Villiers, J. G., & de Villiers, P.A. (1978). *Language acquisition*. Cambridge, MA: Harvard University Press.

Dore, J. (1974). A pragmatic description of early language development. *Journal of Psycholinguistic Research, 3*, 343–350.

Duchan, J. F. (1988). Assessing communication of hearing-impaired children: Influences from pragmatics. In R. R. Kretschmer & L. W. Kretschmer (Eds.), Communication assessment of hearing-impaired children: From conversation to classroom [Monograph]. *Journal of the Academy of Rehabilitative Audiology, 21*(Suppl.), 19–41.

Dunn, C., & Newton, L. (1986). A comprehensive model for speech development in hearing-impaired children. *Topics in Language Development, 6*(3), 25–46.

Dunn, L., & Dunn, L. (1981). *Peabody Picture Vocabulary Test* (Revised). Circle Pines, MN: American Guidance Service.

Elfenbein, J. L., Hardin-Jones, M.A., & Davis, J. M. (1994). Oral communication skills of children who are hard of hearing. *Journal of Speech and Hearing Research, 37*, 216–226.

Elsmann, S. R., Matkin, N. D., & Sabo, M. P. (1987). Early identification of congenital sensorineural hearing impairment. *Hearing Journal, 40*, 13–17.

Ewoldt, C. (1985). A descriptive study of the developing literacy of young hearing-impaired children. *Volta Review, 87*(5), 109–125.

Fisher, H., & Logemann, J. (1971). *Fisher-Logemann Test of Articulation Competence*. Boston, MA: Houghton-Mifflin.

Fletcher, S. G. (1989). Visual articulatory training through dynamic orometry. *Volta Review, 91*, 47–64.

Fletcher, S. G., Dagenais, P.A., & Critz-Crosby, P. (1991a). Teaching consonants to profoundly hearing-impaired speakers using palatometry. *Journal of Speech and Hearing Research, 34*, 929–942.

Fletcher, S. G., Dagenais, P.A., & Critz-Crosby, P. (1991b). Teaching vowels to hearing-impaired speakers using glossometry. *Journal of Speech and Hearing Research, 34*, 942–956.

Fletcher, S. G., & Hasegawa, A. (1983). Speech modification by a deaf child through dynamic orometric modeling and feedback. *Journal of Speech and Hearing Disorders, 48*, 178–185.

Formby, C., & Monsen, R. B. (1982). Long-term average speech spectra for normal and hearing-impaired adolescents. *Journal of the Acoustical Society of America, 71*, 196–202.

Forner, L. L., & Hixon, T. J. (1977). Respiratory kinematics in profoundly hearing-impaired speakers. *Journal of Speech and Hearing Research, 20*, 373–407.

Foster, R., Giddan, J., & Stark, J. (1972). *Assessment of Children's Language Comprehension*. Palo Alto, CA: Consulting Psychologists Press.

Fudula, J. (1970). *Arizona Articulation Proficiency Scale*. Los Angeles: Western Psychological Services.

Gardner, M. F. (1990). *Expressive One-Word Picture Vocabulary Test-Revised*. Novato, CA: Academic Therapy Publications.

Geers, A. E., Miller, J. D., & Gustus, C. (November, 1983). Vibrotactile stimulation—Case study with a profoundly deaf child. Paper presented at the American Speech-Language-Hearing Association, Cincinnati.

Geers, A. E., & Moog, J. S. (1992). Speech perception and production skills of students with impaired hearing from oral and total communication education settings. *Journal of Speech and Hearing Research*, *35*, 1384–1393.

Geffner, D. S., & Freeman, L. R. (1980). Assessment of language comprehension of six-year-old deaf children. *Journal of Communication Disorders*, *13*, 455–470.

Gillette, Y. (1989). *Ecological programs for communication partnerships: Models and cases*. San Antonio, TX: Special Press, Inc.

Goehl, H., & Kaufman, D. K. (1984). Do the effects of adventitious deafness include disordered speech? *Journal of Speech and Hearing Disorders*, *49*, 58–64.

Gold, T. (1980). Speech production in hearing-impaired children. *Journal of Communication Disorders*, *13*, 397–418.

Goldman, R., & Fristoe, M. (1969). *The Goldman-Fristoe Test of Articulation*. Circle Pines, MN: American Guidance Service.

Golinkoff, R. M., & Ames, G. J. (1979). A comparison of fathers' and mothers' speech with their young children. *Child Development*, *50*, 28–32.

Goodman, K. (1986). *What's whole in whole language?* Portsmouth, NH: Heinemann.

Goodman, M., Davis, J., &, Raffin, M. (1980). Use of common morphemes by hearing-impaired children exposed to a system of manual English. *Journal of Auditory Research*, *20*, 57–69.

Goss, R. (1970). Language used by mothers of deaf children and mothers of hearing children. *American Annals of the Deaf*, *115*, 93-96.

Green, D. S. (1956). Fundamental frequency characteristics of the speech of profoundly deaf individuals. Unpublished doctoral dissertation, Purdue University.

Greenberg, M. T. (1980). Social interaction between deaf preschoolers and their mothers: The effects of communication method and communication competence. *Developmental Psychology*, *5*, 465–474.

Greenfield, P., & Smith, H. (1976). *The structure of communication in early language development*. New York: Academic Press.

Griswold, E., & Cummings, J. (1974). The expressive vocabulary of preschool deaf children. *American Annals of the Deaf*, *119*, 16–28.

Hasenstab, M. S., & Tobey, E. A. (1991). Language development in children receiving nucleus multichannel cochlear implants. *Ear and Hearing*, *12*(Suppl.), 55S-65S.

Hirano, M., Ohala, J., & Vennard, W. (1969). The function of laryngeal muscles in regulating fundamental frequency and intensity of phonation. *Journal of Speech and Hearing Research, 12,* 616-628.

Hochberg, I., Levitt, H., & Osberger, M. J. (Eds.), (1983). *Speech of the hearing impaired: Research, training, and personal preparation.* Baltimore: University Park Press.

Hodson, B. (1980). *The assessment of phonological processes.* Danville, IL: Interstate.

Hood, R. B., & Dixon, R. F. (1969). Physical characteristics of speech rhythm of deaf and normal-hearing speakers. *Journal of Communication Disorders, 2,* 20-28.

Howell, R. F. (1984). Maternal reports of vocabulary development in four-year-old deaf children. *American Annals of the Deaf, 12,* 459-465.

Hudgins, C. V., & Numbers, F. C. (1942). An investigation of the intelligibility of speech of the deaf. *Genetic Psychology Monographs, 25,* 289-392.

Hughes, M. E. (1983). Verbal interactions between mothers and their hearing-impaired children. Unpublished master's thesis. University of Manchester.

Hughes, M. E., & Howarth, J. N. (1980). Verbal interaction between mothers and their young hearing-impaired children, *Proceedings of the International Congress on Education of the Deaf,* Hamburg, *2,* 527-532.

Hutchinson, J. M., & Smith, L. L. (1976). Aerodynamic functioning during consonant production by hearing-impaired adults. *Audiology and Hearing Education, 2,* 16-24.

Hutchinson, J. M., Smith, L. L., Kornhauser, R. L., Beasley, D. S., & Beasley, D. C. (1978). Aerodynamic functioning in consonant production in hearing-impaired children. *Audiology and Hearing Education, 4,* 23-31.

Hyde, M., Elias, G., & Power, D. (1980). *The use of verbal and nonverbal control techniques by mothers of hearing-impaired infants.* Mt. Gavatt, Australia: Mt. Gavatt College of Advanced Education, Center for Human Development.

Isshiki, N. (1964). Regulatory mechanism of voice intensity variation. *Journal of Speech and Hearing Research, 7,* 17-29.

Jackson, P. L. (1982). Techniques for speech conservation. In R. Hull (Ed.), *Rehabilitative audiology* (pp. 129-152). New York: Grune and Stratton.

Jensema, C. J., Karchmer, M. A., & Trybus, R. J. (1978). *The rated speech intelligibility of hearing-impaired children: Basic relationships.* Washington, DC: Gallaudet College Office of Demographic Studies.

John, J. E., & Howarth, J. N. (1965). The effect of time distortion on the intelligibility of deaf children's speech. *Language and Speech, 8,* 127-134.

Johnson, D. D. (1985). Communication characteristics of NTID students. *Journal of the Academy of Rehabilitative Audiology, 8*(1), 17-32.

Johnson, H. A. (1988). A sociolinguistic assessment scheme for the total communication student. In R. R. Kretschmer & L. W. Kretschmer (Eds.), Communication assessment of hearing-impaired children: From conversation to classroom [Monograph]. *Journal of the Academy of Rehabilitative Audiology, 21*(Suppl.), 101-129.

Johnson, R. E., Liddell, S. K., & Erting, C. J. (1990). *Unlocking the curriculum: Principles for achieving access in deaf education*. Gallaudet Research Institute Working Paper 89-3. Washington, DC: Gallaudet University.

Kelly, C., Dancer, J., & Bradley, R. (1986). Correlation of SPINE test scores to judges' ratings of speech intelligibility in hearing-impaired children. *Volta Review*, 145–150.

Kent, R. D., Osberger, M. J., Netsell, R., & Hustedde, C. G. (1987). Phonetic development in identical twins differing in auditory function. *Journal of Speech and Hearing Disorders*, *52*(1), 64–75.

Kentworthy, O. T. (1986). Caregiver-child interaction and language acquisition of hearing-impaired children. *Topics in Language Disorders*, *6*(3), 1–11.

Koplin, J. H., Odom, P. B., Blanton, R. L., & Nunnally, J. C. (1967). Word association test performance of deaf subjects. *Journal of Speech and Hearing Research*, *10*, 126–132.

Kretschmer, R. R., & Kretschmer, L. W. (1978). *Language development and intervention with the hearing impaired*. Baltimore: University Park Press.

Kretschmer, R., & Kretschmer, L. W. (1989). Communication competence: Impact of the pragmatics revolution on education of hearing-impaired individuals. *Topics in Language Disorders*, *9*(4), 1–16.

Kretschmer, R. R., & Kretschmer, L. W. (1990). Language. In S. R. Silverman & P. B. Kricos (Eds.), The Alexander Graham Bell Association for the Deaf: A Centennial Review [Monograph]. *The Volta Review*, *92*(4), 56–71.

Kricos, P., & Aungst, H. (1984). Cognitive and communication development in hearing impaired preschool children. *Sign Language Studies*, *43*, 121–140.

Lach, R., Ling, D., Ling, A., & Ship, N. (1970). Early speech development in deaf infants. *American Annals of the Deaf*, *115*, 522–526.

Lehiste, I. (1976). Suprasegmental features in speech. In N. J. Lass (Ed.), *Contemporary issues in experimental phonetics* (pp. 225–239). New York: Academic Press.

Lenneberg, E. H. (1967). *Biological foundations of language*. New York: Wiley Press.

Lenneberg, E. H., Rebelsky, G. F., & Nichols, I. A. (1965). The vocalizations of infants born to deaf and hearing parents. *Human Development*, *8*, 23–37.

Lieberth, A. K. (1990). Rehabilitative issues in the bilingual education of deaf children. *Journal of the Academy of Rehabilitative Audiology*, *23*, 53–61.

Limbrick, E. A., McNaughton, S., & Clay, M. M. (1992). Time engaged in reading: A critical factor in reading achievement. *American Annals of the Deaf*, *137*(4), 309–314.

Ling, D. (1974). Discussant comment. In R. E. Stark (Ed.), *Sensory capabilities of hearing-impaired children* (pp. 185–217). Baltimore: University Park Press.

Ling, D. (1976). *Speech and the hearing-impaired child: Theory and practice*. Washington, DC: Alexander Graham Bell Association for the Deaf.

Ling, D. (1981). Early speech development. In G. T. Mencher & S. E. Gerber (Eds.), *Early management of hearing loss*. New York: Grune and Stratton.

Ling, D. (1989). *Foundations of spoken language for hearing-impaired children*. Washington, DC: Alexander Graham Bell Association for the Deaf.

Ling, D., & Milne, M. M. (1980). The development of speech in hearing-impaired children. In F. Bess (Ed.), *Amplification in education*. Washington, DC: Alexander Graham Bell Association for the Deaf.

Luetke-Stahlman, B. (1988). Documenting syntactically and semantically bimodal input to hearing-impaired subjects. *American Annals of the Deaf*, 230–234.

Luetke-Stahlman, B., & Luckner, J. (1991). *Effectively educating students with hearing impairments*. New York: Longman.

Lund, N. J., & Duchan, J. F. (1983). *Assessing Children's Language in Naturalistic Contexts*. Englewood Cliffs, NJ: Prentice-Hall.

MacDonald, J. D., Gillette, Y., & Hutchinson, T. A. (1989). *ECOScales Manual*. San Antonio, TX: Special Press, Inc.

MacGuintie, W. (1964). Ability of deaf children to use different word classes. *Journal of Speech and Hearing Research*, 141–150.

Markides, A. (1967). The speech of deaf and partially-hearing children with special reference to factors affecting intelligibility. Unpublished master's thesis, University of Manchester.

Markides, A. (1970). The speech of deaf and partially hearing children with special reference to factors affecting intelligibility. *British Journal of Disorders of Communication*, *5*, 126–140.

Markides, A. (1978). Assessing the speech intelligibility of hearing-impaired children. Oral reading vs. picture description. *Journal of the British Association of Teachers of the Deaf*, *2*, 185–189.

Markides, A. (1983). *The speech of hearing-impaired children*. Oxford: Manchester University Press.

McAnally, P. L., Rose, S., & Quigley, S. P. (1987). *Language learning practices with deaf children*. Boston: College-Hill Press.

McCarr, D. (1973). *I can write*. Beaverton, OR: Dormac, Inc.

McDermott, R. P., & Jones, T. A. (1984). Articulation characteristics and listener's judgement of the speech of children with severe hearing loss. *Language, Speech and Hearing Services in Schools*, *15*, 110–126.

McDonald, E. (1964). *Articulation testing and treatment: A sensory-motor approach*. Pittsburgh, PA: Stanwix House.

McGarr, N. S., & Osberger, M. J. (1978). Pitch deviancy and intelligibility of deaf speech. *Journal of Communication Disorders*, *11*, 237–248.

McGarr, N. S. (1987). Communication skills of hearing-impaired children in schools for the deaf [Monograph 26]. In H. Levitt, N. McGarr, & D. Geffner (Eds.), *Development of language and communication skills in hearing-impaired children* (Asha Monographs, pp. 91–107). Washington, DC: American Speech-Language-Hearing-Association.

McGarr, N. S., & Whitehead, R. (1992). Contemporary issues in phoneme production by hearing-impaired persons: Physiologic and acoustic aspects. *Volta Review*, *94*, 33–45.

McKirdy, L. S., & Blank, M. (1982). Dialogue in deaf and hearing preschoolers. *Journal of Speech and Hearing Research*, *25*, 487–499.

Meadow, K. P., Greenberg, M. T., Erting, C., & Carmichael, H. (1981). Interactions of deaf mothers and deaf preschool children: Comparisons with three other groups of deaf and hearing dyads. *American Annals of the Deaf*, *126*, 454–468.

Menyuk, P. (1977). Effects of hearing loss on language acquisition in the babbling stage. In B. Jaffe (Ed.), *Hearing loss in children* (pp. 621–629). Baltimore: University Park Press.

Metz, D., Whitehead, R., & Whitehead, B. (1984). Mechanics of vocal fold vibration and laryngeal articulatory gestures produced by hearing-impaired speakers. *Journal of Speech and Hearing Research*, *27*, 62–69.

Miller, J. F. (1981). *Assessing language production in children experimental procedures*. Baltimore: University Park Press.

Miller, M. L. (1980). Deviant vocal parameters in the speech of hearing-impaired children and adolescents. Unpublished master's thesis, Idaho State University.

Moeller, M. P. (1988). Combining formal and informal strategies for language assessment of hearing-impaired children. Communication assessment of hearing-impaired children: From conversation to classroom. In R. R. Kretschmer & L. W. Kretschmer (Eds.), Communication assessment of hearing-impaired children: From conversation to classroom [Monograph]. Supplement, *Journal of the Academy of Rehabilitative Audiology*, *21*, 73–101.

Moeller, M. P., Coufal, K. L., & Hixson, P. K. (1990). The efficacy of speech-language pathology intervention: Hearing-impaired children. *Seminars in Speech and Language*, *11*, 4, 227–240.

Moeller, M. P., & Luetke-Stahlman, B. (1990). Parents' use of signing exact english: A descriptive analysis. *Journal of Speech and Hearing Disorders*, *55*, 327–338.

Moeller, M. P., Osberger, M. J., & Eccarius, M. (1986). Receptive language skills [Monograph 23]. *Language and learning skills of hearing-impaired students*, *Asha Monographs*, 41–54.

Moeller, M. P., Osberger, M. J., McConkey, A., & Eccarius, M. (1981). Some language skills of the students in a residential school for the deaf. *Journal of the Academy of Rehabilitative Audiology*, *14*, 84–111.

Moeller, M. P., Osberger, M. J., & Morford, J. A. (1993). Speech-language assessment and intervention in preschool hearing-impaired children. In J. Alpiner & P. McCarthy (Eds.), *Rehabilitative Audiology: Children and Adults* (pp. 163–187). Baltimore: Williams and Wilkins.

Moeller, M. P., & Schick, B. (1993). *Sign with me parent workbook*. Omaha, NE: Center for Hearing Loss in Children.

Monsen, R. B. (1974). Durational aspects of vowel production in the speech of deaf children. *Journal of Speech and Hearing Research*, *17*, 386–398.

Monsen, R. B. (1976). Normal and reduced phonological space: The production of English vowels by deaf adolescents. *Journal of Phonetics*, *4*, 189–198.

Monsen, R. B. (1978). Toward measuring how well deaf children speak. *Journal of Speech and Hearing Research, 21*, 197-219.

Monsen, R. B. (1979). Acoustic qualities of phonation in young hearing-impaired children. *Journal of Speech and Hearing Research, 22*, 270-288.

Monsen, R. B. (1981). A usable test for the speech intelligibility of deaf talkers. *American Annals of the Deaf, 126*, 845-852.

Monsen, R. B. (1982). A usable test for the speech intelligibility of deaf talkers. *American Annals of the Deaf, 71*, 845-852.

Monsen, R. B. (1983). The oral speech intelligibility of hearing-impaired talkers. *Journal of Speech and Hearing Research, 48*, 286-296.

Monsen, R. B., Engbretson, A. M., & Vemulla, N. R. (1979). The effects of deafness on the generation of voice. *Journal of the Acoustical Society of America, 66*, 1680-1690.

Moog, J. S., & Geers, A. E. (1975). *Scales of early communication skills for hearing impaired children*. St. Louis: Central Institute for the Deaf.

Moog, J. S., & Geers, A. E. (1979). *Grammatical analysis of elicited language—Simple sentence level*. St. Louis, MO: Central Institute for the Deaf.

Moog, J. S., & Geers, A. E. (1981). *Grammatical analysis of elicited language—Simple sentence level*. St. Louis: Central Institute for the Deaf.

Moog, J.S. & Geers, A. E. (1983) *Grammatical analysis of elicited language—presentence level*. St. Louis, MO: Central Institute for the Deaf.

Moog, J. S., & Kozak, V. J. (1983). *Teacher assessment of grammatical structures*. St. Louis: Central Institute for the Deaf.

Most, T., & Frank, Y. (1991). The relationship between the perception and the production of intonation by hearing-impaired children. *Volta Review, 12*, 301-309.

Nelson, K. (1973). Structures and strategies in learning to talk. *Monographs of the Society for Research in Child Development. 38*, 149.

Newcomer, P., & Hammill, D. (1977). *Test of Language Development*. Los Angeles: Western Psychological Services.

Newton, L. (1985). Linguistic environment of the deaf child: A focus on teacher's use of nonliteral language. *Journal of Speech and Hearing Research, 28*(3), 336-344.

Nober, E. H. (1967). Articulation of the deaf. *Exceptional Child, 33*, 611-621.

Norlin, P. F., & Van Tasell, D. J. (1980). Linguistic skills of hearing-impaired children. *Monographs in Contemporary Audiology, 1*, 1-32.

Nunnally, J. C., & Blanton, R. L. (1966). Patterns of word associations in the deaf. *Psychological Reports, 18*, 87-92.

Oller, D. K. (1980). The emergence of speech sounds in infancy. In G. Yeni-Komishan, J. Kavanaugh, & C. A. Ferguson (Eds.), *Child Phonology: Vol. 1. Production* (pp. 93-112). New York: Grune and Stratton.

Oller, D., & Eilers, R. E. (1988). The role of audition in infant babbling. *Child Development, 59*, 441-449.

Oller, D. K., Eilers, R. E., Gull, D. H., & Carney, A. E. (1985). Prespeech vocalizations of a deaf infant. A comparison with normal meta-phonological development. *Journal of Speech and Hearing Research, 28*, 47-63.

Oller, D., Jensen, H., & Lafayette, R. (1978). The relatedness of phonological processes of a hearing impaired child. *Journal of Communication Disorders, 11,* 97-105.

Oller, D., & Kelly, C. A. (1974). Phonological substitution processes of a hard-of-hearing child. *Journal of Speech and Hearing Disorders, 39,* 65-74.

Osberger, M. J., Johnstone, A., Swarts, E., & Levitt, H. (1978). The evaluation of a model speech training program for deaf children. *Journal of Communication Disorders, 11,* 293-313.

Osberger, M. J., & Levitt, H. (1979). The effect of timing errors on the intelligibility of deaf children's speech. *Journal of the Acoustical Society of America, 66,* 1316-1324.

Osberger, M. J., Moeller, M. P., Eccarius, M., Robbins, A. M., & Johnson, D. (1986). Expressive language skills [Monograph 23]. In M. J. Osberger (Ed.), *Language and learning skills of hearing-impaired students* (pp. 54-65). Asha Monographs, Washington, DC: Asha.

Osberger, M. J., Robbins, A. M., Lybolt, J., Kent, R. D., & Peters, J. (1986). Speech evaluation [Monograph 23]. In M. J. Osberger (Ed.), *Language and learning skills of hearing-impaired students* (pp. 24-31). Asha Monographs, Washington, DC: Asha.

Owens, R. E. (1990). Development of communication, language, and speech. In G. H. Shames & E. H. Wiig (Eds.), *Human Communication Disorders* (pp. 30-73). Columbus, OH: Merrill Publishing Company.

Pendergast, K., Dickey, S., Selmar, J., & Soder, A. (1969). *Photo articulation test.* Danville, IL: Interstate.

Penn, J. P. (1955). Voice and speech patterns of the hard-of-hearing. *Acta Otolaryngologica* (Suppl. 124).

Pollack, D. (1970). *Educational audiology for the limited hearing infant.* Springfield, IL: Charles C. Thomas.

Pratt, S. R. (1991). Nonverbal play interaction between hearing mothers and young deaf children. *Ear and Hearing, 12* (5), 328-336.

Pratt, S. R., Heintzelmann, A. T., & Deming, S. E. (1993). The efficacy of using the IBM SpeechViewer Vowel Accuracy Module to treat young children with hearing impairment. *Journal of Speech and Hearing Research, 36,* 1063-1074.

Prinz, P. M., & Masin, L. (1985). Lending a helping hand: Linguistic input and sign language acquisition in deaf children. *Applied Psycholinguistics, 6,* 357-370.

Prinz, P. M., & Prinz, E. A. (1985). If only you could hear what I see: Discourse development in sign language. *Discourse Processes, 8,* 1-19.

Quigley, S. P., & King, C. (1981). Syntactic performance of hearing-impaired and normal-hearing individuals. *Applied Psycholinguistics, 1,* 329-356.

Quigley, S. P., Monranelli, D. S., & Wilbur, R. B. (1976). Some aspects of the verb system in the language of deaf students. *Journal of Speech and Hearing Research, 19,* 536-550.

Quigley, S. P., Power, D., & Steinkamp, M. W. (1977). The language structures of deaf children. *Volta Review, 79,* 73-84.

Quigley, S. P., Steinkamp, M. W., Power, D., & Jones, B. (1976). *Test of Syntactic Abilities*. Beaverton, OR: Dormac.

Quigley, S. P., Steinkamp, M. W., & Jones, B. W. (1978). The assessment and development of language in hearing-impaired individuals. *Journal of the Academy of Rehabilitative Audiology, 11,* 24–41.

Ryalls, J., Michallet, B., & Le Dorze, G. (1994). A preliminary evaluation of the clinical effectiveness of vowel training for hearing-impaired children on IBM's SpeechViewer. *Volta Review, 96,* 19–30.

Schirmer, B. R. (1994). *Language and literacy development in children who are deaf*. New York: Maxwell Macmillan International.

Schuele, M. A., & van Kleeck, A. (1987). Precursors to literacy: Assessment and intervention. *Topics in Language Disorders,* 7(2), 32–44.

Schum, R. L. (1987). Communication and social growth: A development model of deaf social behavior. Paper presented at the Mayo Clinic Audiology Symposium, Rochester, MN.

Schum, R. L. (1991). Communication and social growth: A developmental model of social behavior in deaf children. *Ear and Hearing,* 12 (5), 320-327.

Seyfried, D. N., & Waldron, C. (1993). Pediatric aural rehabilitation: Combining the expertise of speech-language pathologists and audiologists. Short Course offered at Speech-Language-Hearing Association of Virginia, Reston, Virginia.

Shaw, S., & Coggins, T. E. (1991). Interobserver reliability using the Phonetic Level Evaluation with severely and profoundly hearing-impaired children. *Journal of Speech and Hearing Research, 34,* 669–702.

Shipp, T. (1975). Vertical laryngeal position during continuous and discrete vocal frequency change. *Journal of Speech and Hearing Research, 18,* 707–718.

Shipp, T., & McGlone, R. (1971). Laryngeal dynamics associated with voice frequency change. *Journal of Speech and Hearing Research, 14,* 761–768.

Shriberg, L. D., & Kwiatkowski, J. (1980). *Natural process analysis*. New York: John Wiley and Sons.

Silva, P. A., Chalmers, D., & Stewart, I. (1986). Some audiological, psychological, educational and behavioral characteristics of children with bilateral otitis media with effusion: A longitudinal study. *Journal of Learning Disabilities, 19,* 165–69.

Sitler, R. W., & Schiavetti, N., & Metz, D. E. (1983). Contextual effects in the measurement of hearing-impaired speakers' intelligibility. *Journal of Speech and Hearing Research, 26,* 30-34.

Skarakis, E. A., & Prutting, C. A. (1977). Early communication: Semantic functions and communication intentions in the communication of the preschool child with impaired hearing. *American Annals of the Deaf,   122,* 392–394.

Smith, B. L. (1982). Some observations concerning pre-meaningful vocalization of hearing-impaired infants. *Journal of Speech and Hearing Disorders, 47,* 439–441.

Smith, C. R. (1975). Residual hearing and speech production in deaf children. *Journal of Speech and Hearing Research, 18,* 795–811.

Smith, C. R. (1980). Speech assessment at the elementary level: Interpretation relative to speech training. In J. D. Subtelny (Ed.), *Speech assessment and speech improvement for the hearing impaired* (pp. 18-29). Washington, DC: The Alexander Graham Bell Association for the Deaf.

Snow, C. (1977). The development of conversation between mothers and babies. *Journal of Child Language, 4,* 1-22.

Spencer, P. E. (1993). Communication behaviors of infants with hearing loss and their hearing mothers. *Journal of Speech and Hearing Research, 36,* 311-321.

Spencer, P. E., & Gutfreund, M. (1990). Characteristics of "dialogues" between mothers and prelinguistic hearing-impaired and normally-hearing infants. *Volta Review, 92,* 351-360.

Stark, R. E. (1979). Speech of the hearing-impaired child. In L. J. Bradford & W. G. Hardy (Eds.), *Hearing and hearing impairment* (pp. 209-233). New York: Grune and Stratton.

Stark, R. E. (1983). Phonatory development in young normally hearing and hearing-impaired children. In I. Hochberg, H. Levitt, & M. J. Osberger (Eds.), *Speech of the hearing impaired: Research, training, and personnel preparation* (pp. 251-266). Baltimore: University Park Press.

Stark, R. E., & Levitt, H. (1974). Prosodic feature reception and production in deaf children. *Journal of the Acoustical Society of America, 55,* 563.

Staton, J. (1985). Using dialogue journals for developing thinking, reading, and writing with hearing-impaired students. *Volta Review, 87*(5), 127-153.

Stewart, D. A. (1993). Bi-bi to MCE? *American Annals of the Deaf, 138,* 331-337.

Stoel-Gammon, C., & Otomo, K. (1986). Babbling development of hearing-impaired and normally hearing subjects. *Journal of Speech and Hearing Disorders, 51,* 33-41.

Stone, P. (1988). *Blueprint for developing conversational competence: A planning/instruction model with detailed scenarios.* Washington, DC: Alexander Graham Bell Association for the Deaf.

Subtelny, J. D. (1977). Assessment of speech with implications for training. In F. Bess (Ed.), *Childhood deafness: Causation, assessment, and management* (pp. 183-194). New York: Grune & Stratton.

Tait, D. M., & Wood, D. J. From communication to speech in deaf children. *Child Language Teaching and Therapy, 31,* 1-16.

Tanksley, C. K. (1993). Interactions between mothers and normal-hearing or hearing-impaired children. *Volta Review, 95,* 33-47.

Templin, M. O. (1966). Vocabulary problems of the deaf child. *International Audiology, 5,* 349-354.

Templin, M. O., & Darley, F. L. (1969). *The Templin-Darley Tests of Articulation.* University of Iowa, Iowa City: Bureau of Education, Research and Service.

Thompson, M., Biro, P., Vethivelu, S., Pious, C., & Hatfield, N. (1987). *Language assessment of hearing impaired school age children.* Seattle: University of Washington Press.

Tomblin, J. B. (1977). Effects of syntactic order on serial-recall performance of hearing-impaired and normal-hearing subjects. *Journal of Speech and Hearing Research, 20,* 421–429.

Truax, R. (1985). Linking research to teaching to facilitate reading-writing-communication connections. *Volta Review, 87*(5), 155–169.

Tucker, I. G. (1981). The implications for parent guidance of recent research into parent-child interaction. Proceedings of the Conference of Heads of Schools and Services for Hearing-Impaired Children, University of Manchester, Manchester.

Tye-Murray, N. (1987). Effects of vowel context on the articulatory closure postures of deaf speakers. *Journal of Speech and Hearing Research, 30,* 99-104.

Tye-Murray, N. (1991). The establishment of open articulatory postures by deaf and hearing talkers. *Journal of Speech and Hearing Research, 34,* 453–459.

Tye-Murray, N. (1992). Articulatory organizational strategies and the roles of auditory information. *Volta Review, 94,* 243–260.

Tye-Murray, N., & Kirk, K. I. (1993). Vowel and diphthong production by young users of cochlear implants and the relationship between the Phonetic Level Evaluation and spontaneous speech. *Journal of Speech and Hearing Research, 36,* 488–502.

van Kleeck, A., & Schuele, C. M. (1987). Precursors to literacy: Normal development. *Topics in Language Disorders, 7*(2), 13–31.

Voelker, C. H. (1935). A preliminary phostroboscopic study of the speech of the deaf. *American Annals of the Deaf, 80,* 243–259.

Waldron, C. (1994). Personal correspondence.

Waldstein, R. & Baum, S. (1991). Anticipatory coarticulation in the speech of profoundly hearing-impaired and normally hearing children. *Journal of Speech and Hearing Research. 34,* 1276-1285.

Wallace, I. F., Gravel, J. S., McCarton, C. M., & Ruben, R. J. (1988). Otitis media and language development at 1 year of age. *Journal of Speech and Hearing Disorders, 54,* 245–251.

Watson, B. U., Sullivan, P., Moeller, M. P., & Jensen, J. (1982). Nonverbal intelligence and English language ability in deaf children. *Journal of Speech and Hearing Disorders, 47,* 199–203.

Weiner, R. (1979). *Phonological Process Analysis.* Baltimore: University Park Press.

Weiss, A. L., Carrey, A. E., & Leonard, L. B. (1985). Perceived contrastive stress production in hearing-impaired and normal-hearing children. *Journal of Speech and Hearing Research, 28*(1), 26–35.

West, J. J., & Weber, J. L. (1974). A phonological analysis of the spontaneous language of a four-year-old hard-of-hearing child. *Journal of Speech and Hearing Disorders, 38,* 25-35.

Wetherby, A. M., Cain, D. H., Yonclas, D. G., & Walker, V. G. (1988). Analysis of intentional communication of normal children from the prelinguistic to the multiword stage. *Journal of Speech and Hearing Research, 31,* 240–252.

Whitehead, R. L. (1983). Some respiratory and aerodynamic patterns in the speech of the hearing impaired. In I. Hochberg, H. Levitt, & M. J. Osberger (Eds.), *Speech of the hearing impaired* (pp. 97-116). Baltimore: University Park Press.

Whitehead, R. L., & Jones, K. O. (1978). The effect of vowel environment on duration of consonants produced by normal-hearing, hearing-impaired and deaf adult speakers. *Journal of Phonetics, 6,* 77-81.

Wilbur, R., Goodhart, W., & Fuller, D. (1989). Comprehension of English modals by hearing-impaired students. *Volta Review, 91,* 5-18.

Wilcox, J., & Tobin, H. (1974). Linguistic performance of hard-of-hearing and normal-hearing children. *Journal of Speech and Hearing Research, 17,* 286-293.

Wilson, F. B. (1977). *Voice disorders.* Austin, TX: Learning Concepts.

Wingfield, A. (1975). Acoustic redundancy and the perception of time-compressed speech. *Journal of Speech and Hearing Research, 18,* 96-104.

Wingfield, A., Buttett, J., & Sandoval, A. W. (1979). Intonation and intelligibility of time-compressed speech: Supplementary report. *Journal of Speech and Hearing Research, 22,* 708-716.

Wood, H. A., & Wood, D. J. (1984). An experimental evaluation of the effects of five styles of teacher conversation on the language of hearing-impaired children. *Journal of Child Psychology, Psychiatry, and Allied Disciplines, 25,* 45-62.

Wood, D., Wood, H., Griffiths, A., & Howarth, I. (1986). *Teaching and talking with deaf children.* Chichester, UK: Wiley.

Young, C., & McConnell, F. (1957). Retardation of vocabulary development in hard-of-hearing children. *Exceptional Children, 33,* 268-270.

Yoshinaga-Itano, C., & Downey, D. M. (1986). A hearing-impaired child's acquisition of schemata: Something's missing. *Topics in Language Disorders, 7* (1), 45-57.

Yoshinaga-Itano, C., & Stredler-Brown, A. (1992). Learning to communicate: Babies with hearing impairments make their needs known. *Volta Review, 94,* 107-129.

Yoshinaga-Itano, C., Stredler-Brown, A., & Jancosek, E. (1992). From phone to phoneme: What can we understand from babble. *Volta Review, 94,* 283-314.

Young, C., & McConnell, F. (1957). Retardation of vocabulary development in hard of hearing children. *Exceptional Child, 23,* 368-370.

Zimmerman, G., & Rettaliata, P. (1981). Articulatory patterns of an adventitiously deaf speaker: Implications for the role of auditory information in speech production. *Journal of Speech and Hearing Research, 24,* 169-178.

6

Psychosocial Aspects of Hearing Impairment

McCay Vernon

Contents

INTRODUCTION

No professional groups have been more instrumental in establishing the attitudes that determine the psychological and social adjustments of persons with hearing loss than those representing audiology, speech-language pathology, and education of the hearing-impaired. These persons are often important in the key decision-making times of the life of a person with hearing impairment. Therefore, it is vital that those who have professional powers influence the eventual psychological and social fate of persons who are deaf or hard of hearing possess a thorough understanding of deafness and the hearing-impaired population, as well as the assessment processes that guide them at these decision points. The information presented in this chapter addresses a number of relevant psychologic and sociologic aspects of deafness, including the dynamics surrounding diagnosis and a brief review of assessment procedures and instruments.

THE HEARING-IMPAIRED POPULATION

Hearing impairment is the single most prevalent chronic physical disability in the United States. Current estimates indicate that at least 25 million people in this country have hearing impairment (see Chapter 1).

This population represents a wide variety of hearing losses, with the two key factors affecting an individual's abilities and disabilities being age at onset of the loss (pre- or postlingual) and degree of impairment, ranging from persons for whom the loss is a mild inconvenience to those who are unable to understand conversational speech in most situations. Of this latter group, those who incurred their deafness prelingually are defined as educationally and socially deaf for the purposes of this chapter.

The Deaf Population

Intelligence and Education. Extensive research has been conducted on the intelligence of persons who are deaf; results indicate that the deaf and hearing populations have essentially the same distribution of intelligence (Vernon, 1968). Thus, no causal relationship exists between hearing loss and IQ, nor do the difficulties with speech and with written language experienced by persons with hearing impairment reflect an absence of cognitive potential.

A common fallacy related to persons with hearing impairment is that they demonstrate lower capacities for abstract thought. However, research on the relationship of language and thought, as manifested in persons who are deaf or hard of hearing, demonstrates that the potential for abstract thought is as prevalent among persons who are deaf as among people with normal hearing (Furth, 1966; Lenneberg, 1967; Vernon, 1967, 1985). What is often lacking is the linguistic proficiency needed to receive and express many abstract concepts.

In some cases the disease or condition causing a hearing loss may leave residual brain damage that affects intelligence and thought patterns; for example, meningitis, complications of Rh factor, premature birth, maternal rubella, and certain genetic syndromes (Mindel & Vernon, 1987). Also, a lower overall IQ may be expected in the minority of children who are deaf and affected by chronic brain syndromes.

In sharp contrast to these facts regarding their intelligence, the educational achievement level of persons who are deaf and many who are hard of hearing has been, on the average, shockingly low. Although some have attained advanced academic degrees, most are grossly undereducated. While this is an acknowledgment, to an extent, of the tremendous challenge hearing loss and its effects on language development present to academic learning, in larger measure it is an indictment of the educational system for failing to develop the intellectual capacity of students who are deaf.

Many surveys of the educational achievement of persons who are deaf provide data indicating that children who are deaf are failing educationally (Trybus & Karchmer, 1977; Akamatsu & Fischer, 1991; Erting, 1992). Large numbers never progress beyond the elementary grade levels; until recently, an appallingly small percentage attended college.

Thus, despite having potential, too many young people with hearing impairment still do not receive adequate and appropriate opportunities to learn. The crippling psychologic and sociologic implications of this educational deprivation are self-evident; the equally dismal vocational ramifications are discussed below.

Family Patterns. The majority (roughly 90%) of children who are deaf are born to parents with normal hearing (Schein & Delk, 1974; Mallory, Zingle, & Schein, 1993). As adults, about 95% of persons who are deaf marry deaf spouses, the most frequent exceptions being those who are hard of hearing or adventitiously deafened. Marriage between two individuals who are deaf is a realistic adjustment to deafness. In turn, the majority (roughly 88%) of offspring of couples who are both deaf have normal hearing. These figures have important ramifications for the communication patterns that develop within families, and, as a corollary, the psychological health of the family unit, as discussed later.

Deaf Culture. Increasingly, people who are deaf are seeing themselves more as members of a cultural minority than as disabled individuals (Bienvenu, 1991). This view was probably crystallized in 1988 when the "Deaf President Now" movement resulted in the appointment of Dr. I. King Jordan, a man who is deaf, as President of Gallaudet University. His appointment was akin to a "revolution" in that students and faculty who were deaf took over the University and demanded a deaf president and a Board of Trustees with a predominance of deaf members (Gannon, 1989).

From around the time of the "Deaf President Now" movement, up through the present, a series of authors and deaf leaders (including Bienvenu, 1991; Holcomb, 1993; Lane, 1990 & 1993; Rosen, 1992; & Schein, 1991) have argued that there is a "deaf culture." They and others feel that this culture consists of many of the variables that comprise other cultures, e.g., its own language (American Sign Language). Some suggest that deaf culture should be studied historically, linguistically, sociologically, etc., and the resulting data taught to people who are deaf, especially in school.

"Deaf culture" is a complex and, to a certain extent, controversial topic, some dimensions of which will be briefly described later in this chapter.

Organizations of Adults Who Are Deaf. Most adults who are deaf make conscientious efforts not to leave responsibility for their welfare in the hands of others. They have formed strong organizations to meet social, psychological, and legislative needs. These people play an integral part in the lives of persons who are deaf.

The National Association for the Deaf, consisting of over 10,000 members, is the most prominent. There are chapters in every state and a permanent office in Washington, D.C., and national meetings are held regularly. This organization does much constructive work for people who are deaf. For example, it actively protects and represents bona fide interests of the deaf and organizes cultural, athletic, and social events.

The National Fraternal Society, whose membership also exceeds 10,000, is an insurance company established and managed by people who are deaf. It provides life insurance at reasonable rates for its members who are deaf and conducts social and fraternal functions.

Every state has an association of the deaf; large cities have clubs; there is a deaf Olympics; and there are deaf theatrical groups and many other similar organizations. These are formed by persons who are deaf for themselves. Another organization, the Oral Deaf Adult Section, consists of about 250 members. It is a subgroup of the Alexander Graham Bell Association for the Deaf. This group promotes the teaching of speech and speechreading. The Gallaudet University Alumni Association is a worldwide organization of former students of Gallaudet.

One of the paradoxes of adult organizations for the deaf is the presence of "oral" clubs and "speechreaders'" clubs. The basic philosophy of oralism is that it will enable people who are deaf to integrate with those with normal hearing. Hence, the need and existence of clubs exclusively for so-called "oral" adults who are deaf is ironic. At these club meetings, members who are deaf emphasize talking and speechreading in communication with each other rather than using sign language.

These organizations, large and small, national and local, play a truly important role in the lives of persons who are deaf. Their leaders and members know more about the practical implication of deafness than anyone. Yet, until recently, audiologic rehabilitationists who have so much to say about the education and status in society of the person who is deaf have rarely consulted adults who are deaf or had the exposure to them that is required to grasp the problems of deafness. An analogous situation existed with blind leaders of organizations for the blind who fought for over a hundred years for a language they could read manually so that they might read. People with normal vision opposed the idea, ignoring the views of the blind people themselves and claiming that people who were blind must read raised printed letters that were copies of the letters that people with normal vision read. Finally, a man who was blind himself, Louis Braille, found influential people who would listen to him, and the system known as Braille was developed. Thus, persons who were blind were able to read, and now they do well educationally. A breakthrough wherein hearing professionals attend to the ideas that people who are deaf have for their own welfare is only now beginning to be achieved. People who are deaf are still forced into educational patterns that are the equivalent of "reading raised printed symbols." Certainly if more professionals in deafness had extensive experience with adults who are deaf, these problems would not continue, regardless of the age of the persons who are deaf with whom they work.

The Hearing World vs. the Deaf World. Without doubt, the most common misconception among professionals in deafness is that a person who is deaf lives in either a "hearing" world or a "deaf" world. Actually there is no either/or dichotomy. Most people who are deaf work with people with normal hearing. Their work is usually task oriented and, in the case of the person who is deaf, does not require much oral communication. Many of the deaf, in fact, communicate by writing on the job to avoid confusion. Socially, most deaf people prefer others who are deaf, as indicated by the fact that 95% of their marriages are to persons who are deaf. Although most close social contacts are with other individuals who are deaf, the adult with deafness usually has some close friends with normal hearing at work and among her neighbors at home.

The issue is that people who are deaf should not be forced into a choice of a "deaf" versus a "hearing" world any more than the Rotary Club member is forced to choose between a Rotarian or non-Rotarian world, than the American of Greek descent is forced into a "Greek" world if he decides to learn the Greek language, than a Jewish youngster who wants to learn Hebrew is forced into a "Jewish" world. Granted, many ethnic, social, and professional groups prefer primary social interactions with their own. Why should persons who are deaf not have similar desires and be permitted to exercise them without mystical suggestions on our part that they are leaving the "hearing world"? People who are deaf simply may prefer the company of others who are deaf.

Vocational Trends. Despite having the same intelligence as people with normal hearing, persons who are deaf usually engage in unskilled or semi-skilled labor because of the prevailing lack of opportunity for higher-level employment. Thus, a disproportionately high percentage of the deaf are engaged in some form of manual labor, paralleled by a disproportionately small number holding white-collar jobs. Underemployment—working at jobs below one's educational level and other levels of capabilities—is a serious and chronic problem for workers who are deaf (Schein & Delk, 1974).

In planning for the vocational future of clients who are deaf, the following employment trends must be kept in mind (Vernon, 1987):

1.   There is in the overall population a general shift to increasing numbers of white-collar jobs and decreasing numbers of manual, unskilled, and semi-skilled jobs. Thus, the area where the majority of people who are deaf find employment is one of decreasing opportunity, whereas the areas of increasing opportunity are those where

persons who are deaf experience the greatest difficulty finding and maintaining employment.

2.   The urban shift imposes hardships on some individuals who are deaf. However, in general it has resulted in making a higher level of professional services more accessible.

3.   The rapid advances in technology within the world of work have important implications for persons who are deaf. The increasing need for retraining is a potential problem for workers who are deaf because of their communication problems (this may be overcome with some flexibility on the part of the employer).

4.   A growing increase in the educational requirements for employment is evident throughout the job market. This presents difficulties for persons who are deaf in view of their generally lower levels of educational achievement.

5.   Finally, employment opportunities in the service sector (education, health and medical care, hotels) are rapidly increasing. The majority of jobs in these areas are white-collar jobs, a classification where people who are deaf are not well represented. In addition, many require civil-service examinations, the language levels of which are difficult for many of the deaf.

The resolution of this vocational crisis lies in using the potential of the deaf, which is currently largely untapped. Specifically, improvement of educational techniques, of communication opportunities through manual communication and other methods, and of counseling services can do much to alleviate what otherwise seems to be a dim vocational future for many persons who are deaf.

Communication. Any analysis of the psychological and social functioning of persons with severe hearing impairment must carefully examine the issue of communication and its implications for persons with a hearing loss. Among the basic aspects of communication that must be considered, in addition to hearing, are speech, speechreading, written English, and fingerspelling and sign language.

SPEECH. Learning speech when one has significant hearing impairment is extremely difficult. A rough parallel can be drawn by imagining the problems persons with normal hearing would encounter trying to learn to speak a foreign language without being able to hear it and without being able to monitor their own voice, or with only partial and imperfect input and feedback. Because of such difficulties, many persons with prelingual deafness are unable to develop speech that can be understood in most social situations. This is not to imply that speech training should be ignored, but the reality of the extreme difficulty of this task must not be forgotten by professionals or parents.

SPEECHREADING. Although helpful, skill in speechreading has been demonstrated to be of only limited value for most persons with hearing impairment (Erber, 1979). Since 40% to 60% of English speech sounds are homophenous (i.e., they look the same on the lips), persons without a sound language base (for example, a child who is deaf) are less able to fill in the gaps, therefore understanding very little through the visual mode alone (Mindel & Vernon, 1987). This places heavy demands on individuals with hearing impairment and on those with whom they try to communicate. Again, we are not implying that the ability to speechread has no value or that opportunities to develop it should not be provided. Rather, this communication tool must be approached realistically and with a sense of balance regarding its role in the communication functioning of persons with profound hearing impairments.

WRITTEN ENGLISH. Communication by reading and writing is a severely limited outlet for many persons who are deaf, as discussed in the section on education. The reason for this is that their exposure to English is minimal, as compared to that of the person with normal hearing. Instead of hearing English continually during their entire waking day from parents, friends, or teachers, as well as on television and radio, the child (and adult) who is deaf hears almost no English. He or she sees it pronounced for fleeting moments but, lacking English competence, understands few, if any, of those lip movements. At school the child will be shown pictures matched with the appropriate words to describe them (e.g., the picture of a ball beside the printed word "ball") and receive other similar instruction. However, the actual exposure of the child who is deaf to comprehensible, syntactically correct English averages less than 30 minutes a day. Furthermore, for many children who are deaf, English instruction does not begin until after or late in the critical period for language development. Obviously this results at best in meager reading and writing skills (Commission of Education for the Deaf, 1988; Vernon & Andrews, 1990).

FINGERSPELLING AND SIGN LANGUAGE. Most people who are deaf prefer these methods of communication; those knowing the language of signs and fingerspelling do not encounter the problems of ambiguity and frustration inherent in speech and speechreading. In addition to the social and psychological benefits of a fluent and viable communication system, there is mounting evidence of educational benefits, as discussed previously.

The psychological significance of the available data on communication is crucial. Specifically, many people with normal hearing do not communicate fluently and comfortably with family members with severe hearing impairment. Very few learn sign language or other effective communication methods. Such a lack of communication is devastating educationally, psychologically, and sociologically. In addition, many school programs for the deaf turn out a high percentage of students who do not possess adequate means of communication and social interaction. As a result, too many adults who are deaf are isolated, ignorant about much of the world in which they live. (See Chapter 7 for recent trends in educational programming.)

Personality Traits and Mental Health Concerns in People Who Are Deaf. The psychological laws of learning, including how these operate in human psychodynamics, are the same for persons who are deaf and those with normal hearing. For example, if an individual, whether deaf or with normal hearing, is reinforced for a behavior, that behavior is more likely to re-occur. Similarly, frustration tends to cause anger regardless of the hearing status of the one who is frustrated. However, in

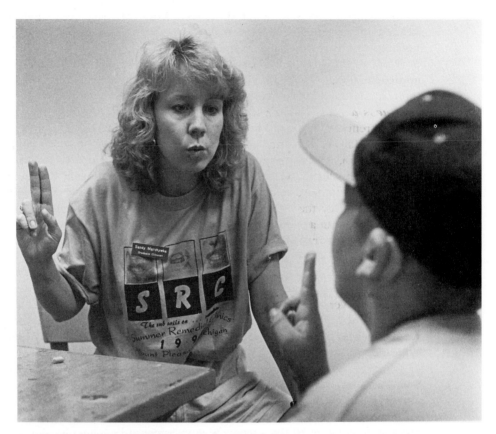

A school-age youngster practices the manual alphabet.

the human being who is deaf, the perceived environment is altered in significant ways by the lack of hearing. For example, communication is altered and reduced, the cues used in memory are in some respects different, parent and peer relationships are altered, etc.

Thus, certain behaviors appear more in the deaf than in the hearing population (Vernon & Andrews, 1990). We will examine a few of these in the next section.

Implications of Communication Limitations. Psychologically and sociologically, the significance of data presented on communication is crucial. It means that most parents do not communicate cognitively with their children who are deaf except at the most superficial level unless they learn manual communication. Relatively few do this. Hence, children who are deaf often do not receive from their parents information on ethics, on how to get along in the world, on the importance of education, on career planning, and—ad infinitum —that information which parents should provide their children. This lack of parent/child communication is devastating psychologically and sociologically.

School programs throughout the United States are turning out a high percentage of students who are deaf, who at ages 16 and up have no means of adequate communication and who have been denied peer, parent, and teacher interactions and the resultant knowledge and human interaction that occurs in most young people with normal hearing.

Deafness and Schizophrenia. If current psychological theories on the causes of schizophrenia are examined in terms of the effects of early-onset deafness (i.e., isolation, breakdown in communication with parents and others, lack of cognitive development, etc.), the obvious conclusion would be that schizophrenia should be rampant in the deaf population (Vernon & Andrews, 1990; Vernon & Rothstein, 1967). However, it is no more common among people who are deaf than those with normal hearing. Not only that, but auditory hallucinations, a frequent symptom of schizophrenia, are about as prevalent among schizophrenics who are deaf as among schizophrenics with normal hearing.

Primitive Personality. Although schizophrenia is no more common among people who are deaf than among those who hear, the condition called *primitive personality* is (Vernon & Andrews, 1990). This disorder involves a combination of extreme educational deprivation (usually functional illiteracy), minuscule social input and knowledge, including awareness of appropriate social behavior, immaturity, and a generally psychologically barren early life. While not psychotic, individuals with primitive personalities are not able to cope with life in our complex modern society. When the communication handicap of deafness is not dealt with, educationally and psychologically, primitive personality is a frequent result.

Treatment is extremely difficult. In contrast to many mental disorders where the therapist's goal is to return a mentally ill individual to a higher level of functioning, with the primitive personality it is necessary to bring the patient up to a higher level than had ever been achieved by the individual before. To do this with an illiterate patient lacking full communication skills is an awesome therapeutic challenge.

Paranoid Disorders. Research indicates that classic paranoid schizophrenia and paranoid psychoses are no more common among people who are deaf than among people with normal hearing (Vernon & Andrews, 1990). One of the myths of deafness has been that people who are deaf are paranoid.

If we go from psychotic forms of paranoid disorders to milder forms of paranoid thinking (i.e., tendencies to be suspicious), we find more of the latter behavior among people who are deaf (Grinker, 1967). However, this suspiciousness is often reality-based. Consider the life history of persons who are deaf: In most families, parents communicate very little with a child who is deaf, but rather talk about the child in front of her, knowing she does not understand. Plans such as taking her to the dentist, placing her in a residential school, and other major decisions about her life are discussed and made right in front of her but concealed from her. Siblings and peers who can hear take similar advantages. The process continues in business when co-workers are often exploitive, merchants have her sign documents she cannot understand, and so on.

Thus, most people who are deaf have experienced a history of being taken advantage of by people with normal hearing and are suspicious of them. Recognizing this pattern is important in counseling, especially where the therapist is concerned.

Depression. Classic depressive psychosis seems less prevalent among people who are deaf than among those with normal hearing (Grinker, 1967). Many think that depression is a disease caused by an overactive superego which turns anger inward; i.e., instead of getting angry at others, the depressive person directs his anger at himself. It is possible that society is unable to force upon people who are deaf the superego (childhood irrational conscience) which, in some individuals with normal hearing, leads to internalization of anger, and finally depression and suicide.

Impulse Disorders. When psychiatric hospital admissions, criminal offenses, and school dismissals of people who are deaf are studied, they yield a disproportionate number of impulsive behaviors as the precipitating incident (Vernon & Andrews, 1990). This is understandable when considered in terms of the aforementioned immaturity. Part of it can be accounted for because, quite often, the person who is deaf is unable to channel his anger through words. Whereas the person with normal hearing can "talk it out" to a whole range of people from the bartender to the psychotherapist, the options of a person who is deaf are fewer and his frustrations in putting his feelings into words greater. Thus, feelings tend to build up until they explode in some impulsive act.

Organic Factors. The leading causes of deafness are also leading causes of brain damage and other pathologies which can lead to mental illness (Vernon & Andrews, 1990). Meningitis, genetic disorders, rubella, complications of the Rh factor, and premature birth are the five major etiologies of childhood deafness. Each is associated with a high prevalence of brain lesions. For example, neurological damage is found in some genetic syndromes involving hearing loss. Of children deafened by complications of the Rh factor, 50–85% have cerebral palsy. Damage this severe has inevitable behavioral correlates. Most large state mental hospitals have one or two deaf patients who are psychotic due to chronic brain syndromes secondary to meningitis (Vernon & Andrews, 1990). There also is a proven correlation between prenatal rubella and autism.

Premature birth is associated with an increased prevalence of schizophrenia in both hearing and deaf populations (Vernon & Andrews, 1990). As children who are deaf are four times more likely to have been born prematurely than children with normal hearing, the implications for schizophrenia in the prematurely born subgroup of the deaf population are obvious.

The Hard-of-Hearing Population

The term "hard of hearing" covers a broad degree of impairments, but is generally used to refer to persons who are able, with or without amplification, to use residual hearing for purposes of communication. In addition, they may need speechreading techniques to supplement aural methods. The extent to which this definition is applicable depends on a variety of factors, including the degree and type of loss and the efficiency of amplification. Generally, persons who are hard of hearing are classified in terms of the severity of their loss, ranging from slight to mild (26–40 dB HL), mild to moderate (41–70 dB HL), and severe (71–90 dB HL). Persons with hearing losses above 90 dB demonstrate profound losses and are generally considered audiologically deaf. Regardless of degree of loss, persons may psychologically identify or consider themselves either deaf or hard of hearing; this perception, in turn, will impact preferred modes of communication and functioning.

Children who are hard of hearing face tremendous educational challenges. Unlike children who are deaf, who are more likely to receive appropriate educational placement in a school for the deaf or in a mainstreamed environment, children who are hard of hearing, depending on their individual abilities and needs, may encounter few educational or communication options. They are expected to perform as do children with normal hearing, in a mainstreamed classroom using aural and oral communication. These settings are sufficient for learning and participation only in the ideal. Often, amplification appropriate to the room size and ambient noise is not provided. In addition, the child may not be positioned close to and with a clear view of the teacher and other members of the class, and the child may miss critical educational and social learning.

The result is often boredom, and pressure from teacher and parents to perform better, leading many youngsters who are hard of hearing to counter their feelings of inadequacy with asocial behavior. Since behavior problems are common in children who are hard of hearing, audiologists should advise parents, teachers and school counselors of available means for management, including exploring classroom amplification, pursuing logistical support, and obtaining tutoring for these children. Socialization is another important part of the educational process; the child's relationship with peers and adults may also benefit from use of appropriate intervention strategies.

Adults with mild to moderate hearing losses experience persistent communication difficulties which vary in degree depending upon a number of variables. Such communication deficiencies can, in turn, lead to problems related to psychosocial adjustment. For example, the adult who is hard of hearing may experience strong feelings of frustration and inadequacy stemming from the inability to hear as effectively as before. Withdrawal from situations in which hearing difficulties often occur, such as meetings, church, and social events, therefore, is commonplace. Because the person with hearing impairment may restrict his/her activity, a sense of isolation and loneliness can result, which may eventually lead to depression. Professionals must be alert to the potential for adults who are hard of hearing to experience a variety of difficulties in adjusting to their impairment. While most will adjust reasonably well, some individuals will require counseling to resolve psychosocial problems resulting from their hearing loss.

Patterns of reaction and adjustment in adults trying to cope with hearing loss will vary. However, some patterns are commonly (though not universally) seen in initial reactions, including denial of the disability, procrastination in seeking diagnosis and treatment, and feelings of anxiety regarding the medical and personal implications of the hearing loss. Such feelings are not surprising; in fact, the same patterns may also be seen in persons experiencing other disabilities and illnesses.

Especially if hearing impairment is significant, it imposes on clients the need to adjust various aspects of their lives. As clients learn to deal with the day-to-day reality of impaired hearing, their adjustment pattern and coping strategies remain individual. This is to be expected since they bring to the experience of hearing loss the same gamut of individual variation one would encounter in the general population. A few of the myriad of factors involved in adjustment to hearing loss include such auditory factors as the degree, type, etiology, permanence, and rate of onset of the loss; in addition, personal factors such as age, sex, education, general health, socioeconomic status, and the personal and professional support systems available to the client must also be considered (Wylde, 1987).

The diversity within the hearing-impaired population should serve as a reminder that we cannot develop and impose on clients a set of stereotyped expectations regarding what people with impaired hearing are like, how they behave, and what they need. Sometimes it is easy to judge and label clients according to their behaviors, especially if they are not in keeping with our expectations. For example, the client who experiences a sudden significant hearing loss may drop certain social activities that have become stressful and unrewarding due to the hearing impairment, and adopt others that are enjoyable. Such changes may be labeled by one professional as "pathological withdrawal" or "giving in to the disability," yet another may consider the same reaction a healthy and realistic adjustment to a significant change in the client's life circumstance.

A client with hearing impairment may attempt to compensate for loss of background environmental sounds and increased difficulty in understanding speech by raising attentiveness to visual stimuli and cues, and by frequently asking what other people are saying. Such coping mechanisms have been labeled "suspiciousness" or "paranoia" by some clinicians. Such judgmental attitudes should be resisted, however; they may ultimately cause clients to feel defensive and become less able to seek and accept necessary support services.

In spite of resistance from some clients to accepting suggestions, clinicians should strive to consistently maintain client involvement in decisions regarding the direction and pace of the rehabilitation program. If such resistance exists, whatever its source, those feelings are real and cannot be overcome by "railroading" the client. It is beneficial in such situations to attend to the information only clients themselves can offer regarding the demands of their life styles and what resources are available to them (both intrapersonal and those in the environment). As they continually adjust to new ways of managing the tasks of daily living, the ability of persons with hearing impairment to turn to others for both informational and emotional support can be a key variable.

A special consideration in working with certain clients who have moderate to severe hearing loss is that they may find themselves unable to find a "niche" in which they are comfortable. Thus, many persons who are hard of hearing feel that they are "neither fish nor fowl;" they are not truly deaf and find it psychologically threatening or otherwise difficult to identify with and be accepted by the deaf community. (In fact, many members of this population have no exposure to and awareness of the deaf community.) At the same time, they discover that, because of the limitation imposed by their hearing loss, interaction with persons with normal hearing means (a) constant struggle to comprehend, (b) frequent misunderstandings, and (c) much emotional stress. Often they are encouraged by well-meaning family and professionals to push themselves to be as nearly "hearing" as possible—not to allow themselves to "be deaf."

Yet, it is not uncommon for some who are hard of hearing (more so those with a significant loss) to identify with those who are deaf. Although they may make maximal use of their residual hearing and speech skills in situations where this is appropriate, some individuals who are hard of hearing find, once they have had the opportunity to experience sign language, a sense of relief or respite in the ease and confidence of communication that is available to them only through use of manual communication systems. This need for comfortable and viable communication should not be overlooked. Although it is essential to aid each client in achieving the best possible audiologic/oral functioning, the difficulty and emotional demands that may be imposed by a hearing loss must be acknowledged and the client's feelings and wishes be considered.

COUNSELING THE CLIENT WITH HEARING IMPAIRMENT

Until recently, only limited counseling or therapeutic services were available for those who had hearing impairment, particularly for persons who were deaf. For example, patients with hearing impairment admitted to mental hospitals often faced a prolonged stay, which was more custodial than therapeutic. There still exists an acute shortage of persons who are trained in both mental health and deafness and who possess the necessary communication skills to interact and relate effectively with the deaf. However, the picture is improving as a result of new training programs, additional research on deafness, and increasing attention to deafness from psychologists as well as professionals in other disciplines.

Since the client perspective has already been examined, three other aspects of the counseling process with clients who are deaf will be examined here: the counselor, interprofessional coordination, and the counseling process.

The Counselor

Under the rubric of "counselor" may fall such diverse specialties as mental-health, vocational, and audiologic rehabilitation. In general, however, counselors share certain skills and focal areas.

First, the qualifications of counselors are rising. Thus, increasing numbers have developed familiarity with the implications of hearing impairment and sensitivity to the communication needs of their clients with hearing impairment—including learning sign language themselves. This is vital, because there can be no true counseling relationship without true communication. In addition to being willing to learn to sign (Sullivan & Vernon, 1979), counselors of the deaf also need to learn to understand and deal with the practical, everyday realities of hearing impairment, as well as to master its theoretical concepts. Overall, it is important that counselors not stereotype clients who are deaf, their abilities, or disabilities.

One of the best ways to accomplish these goals is to maintain frequent and direct contact with persons having a hearing loss.

Interprofessional Coordination in Counseling

The best provision of services often results from the combined efforts of a variety of professionals. This is true also in the provision of mental-health services for clients with hearing impairment.

Professionals with a background in audiology, speech-language pathology, and audiologic rehabilitation have valuable services to offer persons confronted with hearing impairment. Because of their involvement at crucial points in these individuals' lives, professionals from such disciplines must acquire basic grounding in the psychodynamics surrounding hearing loss and its diagnosis. At the same time, it is helpful to have as a resource a psychologist experienced in the various facets of hearing impairment. Unfortunately, such backup is rare.

One of the most frequent needs of clients with hearing impairment is psychological assessment and follow-up counseling. Another relates to parent/family therapy, either individual or group. For children, such services often fall within the realm of the school psychologist. For adults, a psychologist may be consulted in mental health centers, through vocational rehabilitation, or state agencies. Throughout, however, clients and their families are provided a disservice if these functions are carried out by mental-health professionals unfamiliar with hearing impairments. The same holds true when such services are performed by professionals experienced in hearing impairment but not in psychology. Often, state schools for the deaf are important resources, and most of them will have staff who possess the appropriate background or can provide referral information. Also, psychologists in public school programs that serve hearing-impaired children may be experienced with the population. In the absence of individuals with qualifications in both mental-health and hearing impairment, clinicians may be well served to invest time and effort on orienting relevant professionals about deafness (in return, they may gain valuable skills in the field of mental health). Such an approach offers the possible advantage of developing a pool of personnel that share professional growth and are able to work together as a team.

The Counseling Process

Assuming that the counselor possesses the basic skills necessary to be effective, what are the special considerations involved in counseling a hearing-impaired client?

Communication Modality. As noted, clients with hearing impairment present a broad range of skills, preferences, and comfort levels in communication strategies. Therefore, the counselor must initially determine the client's preferred mode of communication, assess its adequacy, and be prepared to use it. Among clients who sign, the level and type of signing used will vary greatly, and the counselor may need considerable skill to meet this challenge. If needed, an interpreter may be called in. It is rare to find a client with significant hearing impairment with whom written communication can be used effectively in the counseling relationship. Finally, the counselor must also be prepared to deal with clients who have been limited to "oral-only" communication, but have experienced limited success. In such situations, clients (and counselor) are left with severely restricted communication.

Concrete vs. Abstract. Some clients with hearing impairment may have difficulty dealing with concepts that have no immediate or specific referent. This may result from language or educational deficiencies, isolation, lack of general information, or other factors. For such clients counseling must be related directly to their concrete environment.

General Information. For some individuals with hearing impairment, hearing loss may result in the loss of a great deal of "incidental" knowledge. Therefore, professionals should be prepared for what may seem to be extreme naivete on the part of some clients, and not mistake it for a lack of intelligence.

Familiarity with Specialized Services. It is helpful for persons working with clients with hearing loss, in whatever capacity, to become familiar with area agencies and facilities that serve, or may be adapted to serve, clients with hearing impairment, as well as with regional and national resources.

PSYCHOLOGICAL ASPECTS OF DIAGNOSING HEARING LOSS IN THE CHILD

An understanding of the psychodynamics surrounding the diagnosis of a child's hearing loss is essential for all professionals who work with people with hearing loss. However, this is particularly true for those professionals who make the actual diagnosis and inform the parents of their findings.

The way in which the diagnosis of deafness, and the trauma that surrounds it, is handled has long-term consequences for both child and family. Thus, conveying such sensitive and psychologically threatening information is often very stressful for both parents and professionals. Use of a constructive approach, based on knowledge of all relevant psychodynamics and the way they develop, may help avoid irreversible psychological damage and counterproductive reactions. The discussion that follows traces the factors relevant to these parental dynamics, beginning with pregnancy.

Pregnancy

Many pregnancies are not planned, and may not be wanted. Even couples who plan and desire pregnancy sometimes feel ambivalent. High hopes, excitement, and feelings of bonding and closeness between the parents may be dampened by fearfulness and hostility toward the added responsibilities, demands, and discomfort of pending parenthood. Often, unplanned pregnancies result in one partner's blaming the other for the carelessness that led to the conception.

Such mixed feelings usually find some form of expression, ranging from simple disgruntlement over the physical discomforts of pregnancy or necessary changes in established routines to wishful fantasies that the pregnancy will somehow end prematurely. Indeed, there may be deliberate violations of the obvious canons of prenatal care, and, in some cases, more direct attempts to abort.

The point to be made here is that variations of these feelings are normal. However, they can have tremendous implications in terms of guilt and denial for parents if their child is later diagnosed as having hearing impairment.

Factors Influencing Acceptance of Hearing Loss

Diagnosis of deafness is usually made one to three years after birth. Usually, actual diagnosis is preceded by a period of gradually unfolding knowledge about the child and building suspicions that something is wrong. This process is influenced by a number of factors relevant to parental personalities and backgrounds. (For a more complete treatment of this topic, see Mindel and Feldman, 1987.)

The first relevant factor in parents' personalities is their adaptive capacities. How able are they to cope with unusual or unanticipated events, specifically, having a hearing-impaired child? The coping mechanisms of the mother and father in rearing young children may differ significantly. This results, at least partially, from the psychological processes experienced by the mother during gestation (when strong emotions, positive or negative, may be projected onto the fetus) and following the child's birth (when the newborn and parents, especially the mother, enter into a relationship that is both demanding and rewarding). The manner in which the parent deals with events in this period provides significant clues about his or her ability to cope with unanticipated events, such as those that will be encountered in having a disabled child.

Although parents' individual personalities are significant, so too are their collective personality factors, as they are influenced by the marriage relationship. The relationship of both spouses to their own mothers and fathers will also have considerable bearing on the nature of the marriage and how they handle the discovery of deafness and their child's disability.

Finally, the ordinal position of the child with hearing impairment in the family and the family's cultural background are significant. First-time parents may not know how a child should react to sound, and therefore not suspect the hearing loss as early as experienced parents. Additionally, in families where the child's language development is highly valued (especially among parents with higher levels of education), detection of hearing loss is more apt to occur earlier, because of increased attention to articulation and grammatical correctness.

The Early Years

As stated previously, actual diagnosis of hearing loss is usually preceded by a period during which parents begin to suspect a problem. They may not consider the possibility of hearing impairment, partly because many infants having significant losses demonstrate enough residual hearing to respond to gross sounds. This may mask their inability to understand speech sounds, which will have a profound impact on development. During this period, parents' anxiety will mount along with their suspicions. It is not uncommon for both parents to suspect, separately, that something is wrong, but not discuss this with one another.

When these concerns are presented to the physician, they may be interpreted as common manifestations of the anxieties experienced by many parents of normal babies. Thus, the doctor may minimize parental concerns with such comments as, "It's just a phase—she'll outgrow it"; or "Everything is fine—you're just a worrier." Although such remarks may be well intended, they serve only to increase frustration, anxiety, and confusion in the family. In addition, they also have the serious consequence of delaying diagnosis and habilitation during what is believed by many to be a crucial point in the child's psychological, linguistic, and educational development.

The high rate of misdiagnosis of hearing loss further complicates the diagnosis crisis. Some of these misdiagnoses arise out of the complex problems surrounding the differential diagnosis between brain damage, aphasia, delayed speech, autism, childhood schizophrenia, mental retardation, and deafness (Vernon & Andrews, 1990). This is especially true for the child with hearing impairment who also has additional handicaps. However, some misdiagnoses also must be attributed to errors on the part of physicians and psychologists employing inappropriate assessment techniques (Vernon & Andrews, 1990). Finally, the delay in obtaining an accurate diagnosis may result from the unconscious denial of deafness on the part of some parents who do not acknowledge the child's symptoms or associate them with hearing loss.

The Diagnosis

As stated previously, the child may be two or three years old before hearing loss is conclusively diagnosed. For some parents, the diagnosis results in a sense of relief initially, especially if the child's problem was previously believed to be retardation, autism, or some other condition perceived as being worse than deafness. For most parents, however, being confronted with the child's deafness is a traumatic disappointment, the full depth of which is rarely sensed by the professional who delivers the diagnosis.

When confronted with the realization that their child has hearing impairment, many parents experience what they often describe as "shock." Parents commonly will relate, "I don't remember a thing the doctor said after I was told my child was deaf." This reaction is a mixture of disbelief, grief, and helplessness, followed by feelings of anger and guilt. In this condition parents feel suddenly alone, set apart from the rest of society.

These feelings are an extension of the earlier period of doubts felt about the child and his condition. Thus, parents may ask themselves, "Why did this happen to me?" Consciously or unconsciously they may regard the child's hearing impairment as punishment for some supposed transgression. Specifically, the parent may recall any ambivalent feelings toward the child during pregnancy and early infancy and interpret them as somehow being the cause of the child's disability, resulting in intense feelings of guilt. Parents may torture themselves with guilt for having produced a disabled child, and seek out some reason, some cause—real or imagined.

Feelings of disappointment and frustration are common to parents having to deal with the reality of their child's disability. They experience helplessness, confusion, and either real or potential loss of some of the gratifications of parenthood. Anger is the natural consequence of this frustration. Like all emotions, anger seeks an object. While they may consciously recognize that their child is not responsible for the disability, parents will nevertheless find themselves inexplicably harboring negative feelings toward the child, which stimulates further guilt. Clearly, families in the midst of the crisis surrounding diagnosis associated with a child who is seriously and irreversibly disabled have a great deal to cope with. Extensive research by Luterman (1979), Moses (1985), and Vernon and Andrews (1990) provides some crucial general principles for helping parents and families cope better with their realization of hearing impairment.

According to the first of these principles, the patient and family can begin to cope effectively only after they are fully aware of the reality of the condition, its implications, and its irreversibility. If false hopes for a cure, or indications that the ramifications of the disability can be eliminated are extended, patients and families do not begin to develop the kind of constructive adaptations that are based on the reality of the disability. Thus, the potential for successful rehabilitation may rest, in large part, with the person who informs parents of their child's hearing impairment, and how the professional handles this delicate situation.

A second principle derived from research on reaction to disability is that certain coping mechanisms or defenses are almost universal. The most important of these is the denial of the defect or its implications. Denial is a normal coping mechanism through which we initially protect ourselves at a time of trauma. It is when denial becomes chronic that it takes on a pathological and counterproductive nature.

Parents often go through a long period of denying indications that their child has a problem, and when the deafness is finally diagnosed, it is typically initially denied. This denial syndrome is often compounded by the professional community. Frequently, in the diagnostic conference with parents, the full implications of the hearing disability are not explained (Mindel & Vernon, 1987). Perhaps almost nothing is said about what the disability will mean in the lives of the family and child. Sometimes the presentation of life with a "handicapped" child is so bleak that it becomes even more difficult for parents to confront this reality. In an effort to help parents through this difficult time, the professional often creates false impressions and hopes, glossing over the real ramifications of severe/profound hearing impairment. Consequently, parents may be led to believe that amplification and oral skills training will enable their child to function as if there were little or no hearing loss. Although subtle and usually unintentional, this leading of parents into unrealistic beliefs about the potential benefits of amplification, speech, and speechreading fosters denial and may lead to feelings of anger and frustration as parent and child eventually confront inevitable communication difficulties.

Another aspect related to diagnosis is an inevitable sense of mourning over loss of hearing. This feeling is rarely experienced as an intense grief, which is worked through psychologically (Vernon & Andrews, 1990). Thus, misdirected kindness of professionals often encourages parents to deny the loss because when the diagnosis is made parents are not given the opportunity to talk through the very intense feelings that are experienced at this time and for some time thereafter. Thus, the mourning that should be experienced is repressed, and chronic denial is substituted for constructive coping.

Constructive Coping

Debate over appropriate communication methods to be used with children who are deaf is often a hotly contested issue among professionals. Thus, parents are often given conflicting advice and forced to make decisions on how to communicate with their child without adequate objective guidance.

The professional community can do a great deal to foster a true understanding and acceptance of the hearing loss. Primary among them is presenting a realistic picture of the limitations imposed by hearing impairment, balanced by the possibility of a happy and rewarding relationship with the child if appropriate measures are taken. Counseling services that provide an accepting atmosphere and help parents understand their own emotional turmoil are of great value, as, too, are information about numerous facets of hearing disabilities and contact with both adults with hearing impairment and other parents of children with hearing loss. Centers offering a comprehensive, multidisciplinary approach can be of great help. Such programs, however, presuppose that professionals first become knowledgeable about and comfortable with persons who are deaf, and with deafness in all its aspects.

Unfortunately, it is unusual for professionals to share with parents the difficulties they and their child who is deaf will face in attempting to establish viable oral communication, often because the professionals themselves are not well informed of these facts. To present this information is painful; yet it is a reality. Until this reality is faced, denial is prolonged and constructive coping cannot begin. The consequences are a communication breakdown and a great discrepancy between parents' expectations and their child's actual achievement. This circumstance may have many sequelae: frustration, avoidance of parent-child interaction, lowered levels of academic achievement, and emotional isolation of the individual who is deaf from the family.

Two potential resolutions of the communication problems faced by many individuals with severe to profound deafness are Total Communication (TC) and Bilingual-Biculturalism. Both of these methods avoid the ambiguity inherent in deaf speech and having to depend on lipreading. They accomplish this by using manual communication. Total Communication involves signing what is said, usually in a Pidgin Sign Language, while speaking the words and providing an opportunity for speechreading, and using gestures. The Bilingual-Bicultural method involves first teaching American Sign Language (ASL) to the child who is deaf, then using ASL to teach English as a second language. The bicultural dimension of this approach consists of teaching children who are deaf about deaf history, deaf heroes, deaf mores, art produced by artists who are deaf, etc.

PSYCHOLOGICAL ASPECTS OF DIAGNOSING HEARING LOSS IN ADULTS

A majority of persons with significant hearing loss become impaired post-educationally, that is, after the age of 17. For those who had normal hearing during their formative educational and social years, a sudden loss of hearing in adult life can be a psychologically traumatic event. Unlike adults who had hearing impairments as children and for whom the disability has become part of their identity, those who face onset of hearing loss as adults identify with those who have normal hearing, even though they can no longer function as such. In addition to having an impact on personal image and identity, hearing loss in adulthood may impact significantly on social and family relationships, career, and living styles—all of which are patterned and established in the formative years for those becoming hearing impaired as youths.

For adults who lose their hearing, the term "hearing loss" has true significance, because the longer they have had normal hearing, the more they perceive its absence as a true "loss." The major loss for adults who are either deaf or hard of hearing is in communication, where easy conversation and the appreciation of music, religious liturgies, the sounds of nature, and so forth is affected. New modes of communication can be learned but, especially for those with severe hearing losses, the joy of music and the sounds of nature may be permanently lost. For those who are totally deafened, the signals that once kept them in touch with their environments—the sounds of airplanes, of sirens, of doorbells, and telephones—will be missed. So will the sounds of their own bodies, like breathing, that once, although perhaps not noticed, reassured them or alerted them to ill health.

Common reactions to hearing loss among adults may include denial, anger, guilt, and depression. They may deny their hearing impairments, insisting that communication difficulties are caused by others who do not speak clearly or loudly enough. They may be angry at physicians who cannot restore their hearing or at audiologists for not providing complete rehabilitative relief. They may turn their anger inward, feeling guilt that perhaps if they had done something differently, they could have saved their hearing. After experiencing a spectrum of emotions, and realizing that nothing can be done to restore their hearing, depression may ensue; prolonged, such depression can lead to feelings of isolation.

Adults with hearing impairment face problems related to adjustment, change, and relearning. Their success in making this adjustment depends on a combination of factors—the degree and type of hearing loss; general physical and mental health; interest in life and motivation to adapt; and support of family, friends, employers, and co-workers. These factors interact to affect the success of most rehabilitative efforts, including the fitting of hearing aids and use of other amplification devices, audiologic rehabilitation, speechreading training, fingerspelling, and/or sign language instruction.

Generally, the younger one is at the onset of hearing impairment, the easier it is to adapt. But age is a state of mind—one can be old at 45 and young at 80—and no prognosis should be assumed based solely on the client's age. The elderly, however, may face special problems adapting to hearing loss. For example, they may be more isolated by their families or by care providers in institutions. The tendency to treat elderly persons like children, using conversation only to give commands or to inquire about their basic needs, makes acceptance of a hearing loss that further isolates them even more difficult. Family members may also deny the existence of a hearing loss, even after differential diagnosis has been made by physicians and audiologists, instead attributing the elderly's behavior to senility, brain damage, or stubbornness. In addition to the mental-health and environmental-support factors affecting the elderly with hearing impairment, general physical health also affects acceptance and motivation to adapt. Thus, hearing impairment may be only one of the disabilities faced by the elderly person, and it may not be the most debilitating.

Efforts to fit elderly clients with hearing aids may be welcomed with a sense of relief—or with rebellion. Clients may complain about the earmolds or the noises the aid emits. The audiologist must take into consideration the difficulty of finding an appropriate aid for presbycusic clients (see Chapter 10), and also pay attention to the psychological components of rejecting the aid. The success of audiologic rehabilitation efforts for those who have residual hearing will depend on motivation as well as the effectiveness of amplification. Elderly clients who have not yet accepted their hearing loss are not likely to be motivated to learn compensatory methods. Similarly, speechreading efforts for clients who are deaf or hard of hearing may be thwarted by lack of client motivation and, especially with elderly clients, success may be affected by reduced visual acuity and attention span.

Regardless of the age of the person with hearing loss, many means of support are available whereby adults who are deaf or hard of hearing can improve the quality of their daily lives. For example, although the family can provide emotional and practical support, counseling is required to explain the difficulties experienced by the client as well as the family's role in providing emotional and communication support. The family or care provider should be involved in rehabilitative approaches to foster communication effectiveness outside the therapy environment. The person with hearing impairment is only one member of the communication process; to be successful, it requires willing and knowledgeable participation of family members with normal hearing. Often, the necessary participation of persons with normal hearing in the relearning process increases the guilt feelings of the person with hearing impairment upon realizing his or her dependency.

Self-help groups of adults with hearing impairment, some limited to elderly persons, are springing up across the country (see Chapter 9), providing another means of emotional support through problem sharing. These groups are most effective when they are led by a professional—a social worker or psychologist—specializing in the psychosocial aspects of hearing impairment.

Although human support is most critical to the adaptive process, many practical devices can enhance the daily lives of persons with hearing loss (see Chapter 2). Specifically, in addition to hearing aids, persons who are hard of hearing may benefit from a variety of amplification devices in various settings. The auditory loop, for example, once used only for amplification in theaters and lecture halls, has now been adapted for use on a smaller scale in meetings or even in one-to-one communication. Examples of auxiliary aids specifically mentioned in the American Disabilities Act of 1992 include: qualified interpreters, note-takers, written materials, amplifying devices, and telecommunication devices for the deaf (TTY/TDD). Today many states have relay systems which enable the deaf person to communicate by phone with others who do not have TTY/TDD phones. To do this, they call a relay operator on the TDD; this operator then dials the regular telephone of the party being called by the person who is deaf. The operator then voices the deaf person's TDD message to the caller with normal hearing. The operator also types the responses of the person with normal hearing into the TDD of the caller who is deaf. In this way, a person with a TDD can call or be called by any person with normal hearing who has a regular phone.

Communication methodology, however, is only one of the many issues parents will confront. For the vast majority, the process of revising their concept of their infant's future to one that includes realistic acknowledgment of the deafness is long and at times difficult.

PSYCHOLOGICAL ASSESSMENT OF PERSONS WHO ARE DEAF OR HARD OF HEARING

As schools, speech and hearing clinics, rehabilitation agencies, and mental health centers strive to offer coordinated, comprehensive services to persons with hearing impairment, it is vital that the professionals involved become familiar with the basic components of psychological and educational assessment: available instruments, how they should be administered with persons who are deaf and hard of hearing, what to request and expect in a psychological assessment report, and how to interpret such reports. It is the purpose of this section to provide a practical guide in these areas.

General Considerations in Assessment

A number of elements are fundamental to all types of assessment with clients who are deaf, regardless of age (Sullivan & Vernon, 1979; Vernon, 1976). Many of these testing principles also apply (although sometimes to lesser degrees) to persons who have been deafened or who are hard of hearing, who will demonstrate varying

TABLE 6.1 *Components of a Complete Psychological Assessment*

For a comprehensive psychological evaluation of a deaf person, the following data and procedures are recommended when possible.

1. Complete case history data (e.g., type of hearing loss, onset, etiology, family situation, education)
2. Comprehensive medical and audiological records
3. An assessment of intelligence
4. Evaluation of personality pyschodiagnostically and/or with behavior data and assessments and clinical observation
5. A standardized measure of educational achievement, when available
6. Communication assessment (e.g., speech intelligibility, lipreading, signing, reading, writing, etc.)
7. A neuropsychological evaluation should be given to see if neurological impairment is present, if there is reason to suspect brain damage and/or learning disability
8. Aptitude and interest measures, especially in vocational evaluations
9. The identification of additional disabilities (e.g., learning disorders, visual impairment, etc.)
10. When possible, multidisciplinary team staffings and parent-teacher conferences

degrees of hearing loss and language and communication competencies. The principles include:

1. Psychological tests involving use of oral or written language are not generally valid with clients with hearing impairment. Use of such tests will produce a score that measures the language deficiencies imposed by the client's hearing loss; therefore, it does not validly measure intelligence, emotional stability, or other aptitudes which are being assessed.

2. Tests administered by professionals who are not experienced with hearing impairment are subject to appreciably greater error than are those administered by somebody familiar with this condition.

3. Group testing with individuals who are deaf or hard of hearing is not recommended, but should be regarded as a screening technique at best.

4. Clients who are congenitally hard of hearing are often more like individuals who are congenitally deaf in terms of psychodiagnosis than their speech and response to sound seem to suggest. Therefore, these clients should be administered tests that are appropriate for both persons with profound hearing impairment and those with normal hearing. If discrepancy in the results indicates that a client performed better on the non-language measure, results of this instrument should be judged as the more valid.

Types of Testing and Their Use

Various types of information may be sought in a psychological assessment. The major types of testing and general assessment guidelines are reviewed in Table 6.1, with recommended testing batteries listed at the end of this section. A helpful reference in this area is Ziezula (1982).

Intelligence testing. Three primary guidelines apply to intelligence testing with hearing-impaired adults and children:

1.   The importance of avoiding verbal, language-based tests in evaluating the IQs of individuals with impaired hearing must be reemphasized. To be valid as measures of intelligence (rather than of language impairment), nonverbal performance-type tests must be used. With the use of such performance scales (provided they are administered correctly), it is possible to obtain valid intelligence test scores for the hearing impaired. However, "nonverbal" tests still require verbal directions (Sullivan & Vernon, 1979). Results obtained from testing a client who may be unable to understand the task are questionable, and use of such inappropriate instruments and methods has resulted in tragic misdiagnoses (Vernon, 1976). Thus, the use of American Sign Language to explain the directions of performance in IQ tests is recommended with deaf and hard-of-hearing persons who know sign language.

2.   Evaluation of clients who are hard of hearing should begin with a performance measure, followed by verbal instruments, if desired. Such procedures often result in an appreciably higher score on the former; in all probability, these instruments are more valid than the language-dependent test.

3.   The use of only the nonverbal portion of an IQ test reduces by roughly half (or more) the items used; therefore, at least two performance scales should be given to improve validity.

Special considerations in intelligence testing with children. Testing and test results obtained with children present several considerations beyond those listed previously:

1.   Test scores of preschool and early elementary-age children with hearing impairment tend to be unreliable. Therefore, these scores should be viewed as questionable, especially if low, and if no other data support them. Many factors may negatively affect a child's performance in the testing situation, leading to artificially low scores (Sullivan & Vernon, 1979).

2.   Tests that have time limits or in other ways emphasize the time factor are not as valid as those that do not. Children may respond to being timed by working very hastily, or by ignoring the time factor. Untimed tests are, therefore, preferable.

3.   The questionable validity of tests administered by those unfamiliar with deafness is even more true when working with children. These children's atypical attentive set to testing, which has been frequently cited in the literature, is felt to be one of the reasons for this (Sullivan & Vernon, 1979; Zierzula, 1982).

Several formal measures of intelligence are currently in use. A listing is provided in Table 6.2, along with comments concerning each test's utility with the hearing impaired.

Personality Assessment. Personality assessment, even with clients with normal hearing, is much more demanding and complex than assessment of intelligence.

TABLE 6.2 *Intelligence Tests Most Commonly Used with Deaf or Hard-of-Hearing Adults and Children*

Test	Age Range Covered by the Test	Evaluation of the Test
Wechsler Intelligence Scale for Adults— Revised— Performance Scale (Wechsler, 1981)	16 to Adult	This Performance Scale continues to be the single best IQ test for deaf or hard-of-hearing adults. Scores are considered to be relatively accurate. Again, Total Communication should be used if possible.
Progressive Matrices (Raven, 1948)	5 to Adult	This test is best used as a second measure of intelligence to corroborate the results of a more comprehensive test. It can be given untimed, is easy to administer, and simple to score. If the testee responds impulsively to items, the IQ will be invalid.
Test of Nonverbal Intelligence—2 (TONI-2) (Brown, Sherbenou, and Johnson, 1990)	5 to Adult	The test of Nonverbal Intelligence—2 (TONI-2) provides an estimate of nonverbal intelligence. It is best used in conjunction with a more comprehensive measure. It is one of the few nonverbal tests that require no more motor involvement than pointing and thus are useful with deaf cerebral palsied children. When testing learning disabled or impulsive children, be watchful for perseveration of response and/or impulsive responding. Because of the effect of these responses, the TONI-2 may be most appropriate for older children and adults.
The Revised Beta (Levine, 1960)	Adults	The Revised Beta is a non-language test involving mazes, spatial relations, matching, and similar performance type items. It provides an adequate measure of the intelligence of adults who are deaf.
Wechsler Intelligence Scale for Children— Third Edition Performance Scale (Wechsler, 1991)	6 to 16 years	This test has good general appeal. It can be used to evaluate relatively disturbed hard-of-hearing children who could not otherwise be tested. This test is expensive and somewhat lacking in validation. In general, however, it is an excellent test for young, hard-of-hearing children. Timing is a minor factor.
Leiter International Peformance Scale (1948 Revision) Leiter, R.D., 1979	4 to 12 years (also suitable for older mentally retarded, deaf subjects)	This test has good interest appeal. It can be used to evaluate relatively disturbed hard-of-hearing children who could not otherwise be tested. This test is expensive and lacking somewhat in validation. In general, however, it is an excellent test for young, hard-of-hearing children. Timing is a minor factor. One disadvantage is in the interpretation of the IQ scores because the mean of the test is 95 and the standard deviation is 20. This means that the absolute normal score on this test is 95 instead of 100 as on other intelligence tests. Scores of 60, for example, therefore do not indicate mental deficiency but

TABLE 6.2 *continued*

Test	Age Range Covered by the Test	Evaluation of the Test
		correspond more to about a 70 on a test such as the Wechsler or Binet. Great care must be taken in interpreting Leiter IQ scores for these reasons.
Battelle Developmental Inventory (Stock, Wnek, Guidubaldi, Svinicki, 1984)	Birth to 8 years	This is an assessment battery of developmental skills and functional abilities in young handicapped and non-handicapped children. Data collected through interviews with teachers and caregivers, and/or through direct observation of the child in his/her setting. Several items in the Cognitive Domain are language based and should be treated in the final scoring according to the procedure used in the Merrill-Palmer. Also, as items are arranged developmentally, language items should be credited up to the performance item basal. The Battelle Developmental Inventory is helpful to use with deaf and hard-of-hearing multi-handicapped children because it is possible to measure and graph progress over time. It also provides information about strengths and weaknesses which is important in developing programming.
Kaufman Assessment Battery for Children (Alan and Nadeen Kaufman, 1983)	4 years to 12 years and 5 months	An excellent test for use with preschool and elementary aged hearing impaired children. It is an individually administered measure of intelligence standardized on a large sample of normal and exceptional children aged 2 $\frac{1}{2}$ through 12 $\frac{1}{2}$ years. Validity studies with hearing impaired children are provided in the manual. There is a special Nonverbal Scale with separate norms. One major strength of the test is that, in addition to the sample item, the first two items of each subtest are teaching items in which the examiner can use any means necessary to teach the child the task. This enables the examiner to be reasonably clear about whether the child really cannot perform the task as opposed to just not understanding what is required. Another strength is that, while there are time allowances for some subtests, they are generous, and the speed of performance does not affect one's score. One caution is that, for children under the age of five, only three subtests are included in the Nonverbal Scale; thus, the nonverbal subtests from the Simultaneous Scale should be used also.

Therefore, additional information from case history data and personal experience with the client should be taken into consideration when interpreting test results in this area—especially results obtained by an examiner unfamiliar with deafness.

One of the complicating factors is that the communication problems of a person with hearing impairment make personality tests more difficult to administer (Sullivan & Vernon, 1979). In addition, many of these tests require a relatively high level of reading skills or extensive verbal exchange, in addition to assuming a level of confidence and rapport that is often difficult to achieve if the subject is unable to fully understand what is being said or written. If projective tests (such as the Rorschach) are used, it is often necessary for the examiner to be fluent in manual communication.

In an attempt to deal with the communication problems posed by clients with hearing impairment, psychologists unfamiliar with deafness sometimes use an interpreter to translate their conversations into fingerspelling and sign language. However, use of an interpreter in psychological assessments may result in conclusions of questionable validity.

Whether or not the norms established for personality structure in the general population may be appropriately applied to persons who are deaf or hard of hearing must be considered when interpreting the personality assessments of those with a hearing loss (Vernon, 1976). Although this issue remains unresolved, it is conceivable that deafness alters the environment in ways that result in a different personality organization. Consequently, the "normality" of clients with hearing impairment would differ from that of persons with normal hearing (Vernon, 1976). Current data coming from studies of deaf culture lends support to this viewpoint (Montoya, 1994).

Clinicians not familiar with the language difficulties of persons with hearing impairment may draw inappropriate conclusions based on writing samples from clients who are deaf, especially those having low levels of verbal skills. Although such samples often seem to reflect confusion and disassociation, this effect is usually the result of language difficulties, not an indication of disordered or deranged thought processes.

As a result of these factors, few personality tests have gained wide acceptance for use with persons with hearing impairment. Table 6.3 provides a review of some of the more commonly used tests of this type.

Screening for Brain Injury. Many of the major etiologies of deafness may cause other types of damage to the central nervous system (Vernon, 1987). Psychological assessments should, therefore, include testing for brain damage, supplemented with information from such sources as neurologic and audiologic diagnostic techniques.

Case History Data. Because past behavior is the best single predictor of future behavior, case history data is of critical value in a psychological assessment. This is especially true of difficult-to-test clients and those whose previous testing was done by a psychologist not experienced in deafness. Good psychological or psychiatric assessment is usually based 75% on case history.

Factors in case history that are helpful include any record of previous mental health problems, difficulties or assets habitually demonstrated in the school history, work background, and specific educational and vocational skills mastered.

TABLE 6.3 *Personality Tests and Adaptive Scales to Use with Deaf and Hard-of-Hearing Adults and/or Children*

Test	Appropriate Range Covered by the Test	Evaluation of the Test
Draw a Person	9 years to adult	A good screening device for detecting severe emotional problems. It is relatively nonverbal and probably the most practical projective personality test to use with deaf subjects. Its interpretation is highly subjective, and in the hands of a poor psychologist, it can result in rather extreme diagnostic statements about deaf clients.
Thematic Apperception Test (TAT) or Children's Apperception Test (CAT) Stein, 1955	School age to adult: can either communicate well manually or communicate skillfully in written-language	This is a test of geat potential, provided the psychologist giving it and the deaf subject taking it have fluency in manual communication. Otherwise, it is of very limited value unless the deaf subject has an exceptional command of the language. The test could be given through an interpreter by an exceptionally perceptive psychologist, although it is more desirable that the psychologist do his or her own communicating.
Rorschach Ink Blot Test (Rorschach, 1942)	Deaf subjects who communicate fluently manually or communicate with exceptional oral skill.	In order for the Rorschach to be used, it is imperative that the psychologist giving it and the deaf subject taking it be fluent in manual communication. Even under these circumstances it is debatable whether it has great value unless the subject is of above-average intelligence. It would be possible to give Rorschach through writing to a very bright deaf subject with remarkable proficiency in English, but this would be a dubious procedure.
The House Tree Test (H-T-P) (Buck, 1949)	School age to adult	This is a procedure similar to the Draw-A-Person Test. It requires little verbal communication and affords the competent clinician some valuable insight into basic personality dynamics of the subject.
Bender-Gestalt (Bender, 1938)	12 years to adult	A useful projective screening test for personality and for the detection of brain damage. Because of the rather high prevalence of brain damage among people who are deaf, it is often valuable to administer a Bender-Gestalt to clients who have severe learning problems or who give evidence of bizarre behavior.
School Behavior Check List (Miller, 1974)	Children grades 1–6	This is the best available instrument for use with deaf school-age children. It has been used in national studies (Goulder and Trybus, 1977), by knowledgeable psychologists who choose it out of all available scales.
AAMD Adaptive Behavior Scale (Nihira, Foster, Shelhaas, and Leland)	6 to 69 years	This is an excellent scale to use for deaf and hard-of-hearing children. Standarization norms include mentally-retarded, and non-retarded public-school students, and students in special education classes. It measures adaptive behavior in several areas (economic, domestic, socialization, etc.) and it includes a scale to assess maladaptive behavior.

Most state residential and large day schools for children who are deaf have excellent data on their students. Thus, these facilities are good sources of data, especially on young children. Integrated or mainstream programs that have professionals competent to teach and evaluate children who are deaf can also provide valuable data. Many of these programs, however, have psychologists, social workers, teachers, speech therapists, etc. who are experienced with youth with normal hearing but not those who are deaf. Information from such sources is often misleading.

In addition to the usual information, a child's case history should include information relevant to the disability, such as the parents' description of the nature of the problem; its etiology and onset; history of diagnosis, including past and present professional services; and communication at home. Parental interviews often offer an insight into the parents' and child's attitudes and coping behaviors toward the hearing loss.

Adult case histories should include not only routine information but also such factors as job history, family circumstances, and educational and vocational skills.

Communication Skills. Since hearing loss manifests itself most clearly in communication skills, the assessment process should include a thorough work-up in this area. Although the primary responsibility for this assessment may lie with the speech-language pathologist and audiologist, input from the psychologist, parents, and others may also be valuable.

Specifically, both receptive and expressive skills should be appraised in the following areas (in addition to an audiologic workup):

1. Ability with written language may be evaluated through use of school records, educational and language tests, or sentence completion. The verbal subtests of the Wechsler may be used by the psychologist to yield some information.

2. Speech and speechreading have considerable relevance for both the child in school and the adult at work. Thus, psychologists, counselors, and others may be involved in practical "lay" assessment in this area. Their conclusions may be questionable, however, if they are not aware of the extreme difficulty of attaining these skills. It is crucial that difficulty in communication (oral and written) not be confused with lack of intelligence. Professionals trained in these areas, especially those experienced with individuals having hearing loss, are better prepared to assess these skills and interpret the results (see Chapter 5).

3. Finally, an assessment of the client's manual communication skills is helpful in those cases where manual communication is being utilized. Manual communication is the means most often employed by adults who are deaf to communicate among themselves, and has gained increasingly wide use in school settings as part of the total communication approach. Such an assessment requires that the evaluator possess sufficient expertise to draw legitimate conclusions.

Educational Achievement. A complete assessment should also include an assessment of educational level. School records should be consulted for younger clients. In addition, numerous tests cover a wide range of content and skill areas. The most appropriate is the Stanford Achievement Test. It has norms and a special version for both hearing and deaf subjects and the Office of Demographic Studies at Gallaudet University (Washington, DC) has recently revised the test for use with students who are deaf. The Stanford is the most widely used achievement test in schools for the deaf and is easy to administer. In fact, special instructions and adaptations are provided by Gallaudet. Care must be taken that the subject understands and successfully completes the sample items in each subtest. It is also crucial that the battery chosen is at the appropriate level for the person being tested to avoid invalid results. Scores on these achievement tests, taken by subjects with hearing impairment, should be interpreted in light of the data on educational achievement presented previously in this chapter.

Aptitude and Interest Testing. Aptitude and interest are basic areas of assessment for older teens and adults because these tests assess any particular abilities and interests the client may have. Hundreds of relevant tests are available. For a more complete discussion, consult Zierzula (1982). In general, assessment for individuals with prelingual/profound hearing impairment should not be based on aptitude tests that depend on language; instead, they should measure such general areas as manual dexterity, mechanical aptitudes, and spatial relations, because these types of aptitudes are directly related to the kind of work and activity carried out by most of these individuals.

For college-bound or professional-level people who are deaf, non-verbal aptitude measures for potential in engineering, drafting, etc., exist, but the use of verbal tests for professionally related aptitudes has to be decided carefully on an individual basis.

Interest tests present a special challenge, since they are almost without exception highly verbal. One of these, the General Aptitude Test Battery (GATB), yields much misinformation when administered in its language-dependent form to persons with hearing impairment. A recent adaptation specifically for the deaf is available through the Rehabilitation Services Administration, Washington, DC.

Recommended Tests and Testing Batteries

The following test batteries are recommended for the age groups specified.

Preschool. Measurement of intelligence should be based on at least two of the following IQ tests: the Leiter International Performance Scale, the Merrill-Palmer Scale of Mental Tests, or the Randalls Island Performance Tests.

No suitable personality tests or tests for brain injury are available for preschool children who are deaf. Hence, clinical judgment and medical, audiologic, and case history data must be depended on exclusively for assessment in these areas.

Beginning School Age through Age Nine. IQ tests should include at least two of the following: the Leiter International Performance Scale, the Wechsler Intelligence

Scale for Children-Third Edition Performance Scale (WISC III), the Hiskey-Nebraska Test of Learning Aptitude, the Goodenough-Harris Drawing Test, or Raven's Progressive Matrices. Human-figure drawing interpretation and Bender-Gestalt responses should be used to screen for personality deviations and organic brain damage.

Ages 9 through 15. The most appropriate measure of intelligence for this age range is the WISC III Performance Scale (WISC III). It can best be supplemented with Raven's Progressive Matrices or the Leiter International Performance Scale. Human-figure drawings and the Bender-Gestalt become increasingly valid measures in this age range and are the best screening techniques for personality disturbance and brain damage.

Ages 16 through High-School Graduation. The Wechsler Adult Intelligence Scale-Revised (WAIS-R) stands out as the superior measure of intelligence for this age range. The second most valid measure for intelligence is Raven's Progressive Matrices. In addition, the Memory-for-Designs Test can be added to or substituted for the Bender-Gestalt and Draw-A-Person Test, and can be used as a screening measure for organic brain damage. Vocational tests should also be included at this time. Their selection is a highly individual matter that depends on the subject as well as available vocational educational facilities.

Adults. The WAIS-R, Raven's Progressive Matrices, or Revised Beta may be used as IQ tests. The Bender-Gestalt is useful for detection of brain damage and may be an effective projective test for personality, along with the Draw-A-Person and House-Tree-Person Test. The latter two require skilled interpretation. Finally, the Thematic Apperception Test may be used for personality assessment if the psychologist and the subject can communicate fluently with each other.

SUMMARY

This chapter has attempted to present some basic and practical information concerning a number of psychosocial aspects of hearing loss for both children and adults. As practitioners, our ability to work successfully with those with hearing impairment will depend a great deal on our knowledge and sensitivity concerning these issues and their impact on the persons whom we serve.

RECOMMENDED READINGS

Clark, J., & Martin, F. (Eds.). (1994). *Effective Counseling in Audiology*. Englewood Cliffs, NJ: Prentice Hall.

Erdman, S. (1993). Counseling hearing-impaired adults. In J. Alpiner & P. McCarthy (Eds.), *Rehabilitation audiology: Children and adults*. Baltimore: Williams & Wilkins.

Lane, H. (1992). *The mask of benevolence: Disabling the deaf community*. New York: Vintage Books.

Marschark, M., & Clark, M. D. (1993). *Psychological perspectives on deafness*. Hillside, NJ: L. Erlbaum Associates, Publishers.

Meadow, K. P. (1980). *Deafness and child development*. Berkeley, CA: University of California Press.

Mindel, E., & Vernon, M. (1987). *They grow in silence: Understanding deaf children and adults* (2nd ed.). San Diego: College-Hill Press.

Moores, D. F. (1996). *Educating the deaf: Psychology, principles and practices* (4th ed.). Boston: Houghton Mifflin.

Orlans, H. (Ed.). (1985). *Adjustment to adult hearing loss*. San Diego: College-Hill Press.

Padden, C., & Humphries, T. (1988). *Deaf in America: Voices from a culture*. Cambridge, MA: Harvard University Press.

Vernon, M., & Andrews, J. F. (1990). *The psychology of deafness: Understanding deaf and hard of hearing people*. New York: Longman.

REFERENCES

Akamasu, C. T., & Fischer, S. D. (1991). Using immediate recall to assess language proficiency in deaf students. *American Annals of the Deaf, 136*(5), 428–434.

Bienvenu, M. J. (1991). Can deaf people survive deafness? In M. D. Garretson (Ed.). *Perspectives on deafness: A deaf American monograph*, Silver Spring, MD: National Association of the Deaf, *41*(1, 2), 21–28.

Bender, L. (1938). *A visual motor Gestalt test and its clinical use*. New York: The American Orthopsychiatric Association.

Brown, A. L., Sherbenou, R. J., Johnsen, S. K. (1990). *Test of nonverbal intelligence-2*. Austin, TX: Pro-Ed.

Buck, J. (1949). The H.T.P. technique, a qualitative and quantitative scoring manual, *Journal of Clinical Psychology, 4, 5*.

Chess, S. (1977). Follow-up report on autism in congenital rubella. *Journal of Autism and Childhood Schizophrenia, 7*, 69–81.

Commission on Education of the Deaf. (1988). *Toward equality: Education of the Deaf*. A report to the President and the Congress of the United States. Washington, DC: U.S. Government Printing Office.

Erber, N. (1979). Auditory-visual perception of speech with reduced optical clarity. *Journal of Speech and Hearing Research, 22*, 212–223.

Erting, C. J. ((1992). Deafness and literacy: Why can't Sam read? *Sign Language Studies, 75*, 97–112.

Furth, H. G. (1966). *Thinking without language*. New York: The Free Press.

Gannon, J. R. (1989). *The week the world heard Gallaudet*. Washington, DC: Gallaudet University Press.

Gessell, A. (1956). The psychological development of normal and deaf children during the preschool years. *Volta Review*, *58*, 117-120.

Goldstein, D. (1984). Hearing impairment, hearing aids, and audiology. *Asha*, *26*, 24-35.

Grinker, R, R., Sr. (Ed.). (1969) *Psychiatric Diagnosis, Therapy, and Research on the Psychotic Deaf*. Final Report, Grant no. RD 2407 S, Social and Rehabilitation Service, Department of Health, Education and Welfare. Chicago, IL: Michael Reese Hospital.

Holcomb, T. K. (1993). The construction of a deaf identity. In M. D. Garretson (Ed.). *Deafness: A deaf American monograph*, *43*, 41-45; Silver Spring, MD: National Association of the Deaf.

Kaufman, A., & Kaufman, N. (1983). *Kaufman Assessment Battery for Children*. Circle Pines, MN: American Guidance Service.

Lane, H. (1990). Bilingual education for ASL-using children. In M. D. Garretson (Ed.). *Communication issues in deaf children: A deaf American monograph*, *40*(1, 2, 3, 4), 78-86. Silver Spring, MD: National Association of the Deaf.

Lane, H. (1993). Constructions of Deafness. In M. D. Garretson (Ed.). *Communication issues in deaf children: A deaf American monograph*, *43*, 73-81. Silver Spring, MD: National Association of the Deaf.

Lenneberg, E. H. (1967). *Biological foundations of knowledge*. New York: John Wiley & Sons.

Leiter, R. G. (1979). *Leiter International Performance Scale*. Chicago: Stoelting Company.

Levine, E. S. (1960). *The psychology of deafness*. New York: Columbia University Press.

Luterman, D. (1979). *Counseling parents of hearing-impaired children*. Boston: Little, Brown & Co.

Machover, K. (1949) *personality projection in the drawing of the human figure*. Springfield: Charles C. Thomas.

Mallory, B. L., Zingle, H. W., & Schein, J. D. (1993). Intergenerational communication modes in deaf-parented families. *Sign Language Studies*, *78*, 73-92.

Maurer, J. F. (1982). The psychosocial aspects of presbycusis. In R. H. Hull (Ed.), *Rehabilitative audiology* (pp. 221-232). New York: Grune and Stratton.

Miller, L. C. (1974). *School behavior checklist manual*. Louisville, KY: University of Louisville Press.

Mindel, E., & Feldman, V. (1987). The impact of deaf children on their families. In E. Mindel & M. Vernon (Eds.), *They grow in silence: Understanding deaf children and adults* (2nd ed.), (pp. 1-30). San Diego: College-Hill Press.

Mindel, E., & Vernon, M. (1987). *They grow in silence: Understanding deaf children and adults* (2nd ed.). San Diego: College-Hill Press.

Montoya, L. A. (1994). *Effective communication with prelingually deaf adults*. Unpublished master's thesis. New Mexico State University.

Moses, K. (1985). Dynamic intervention with families. In E. Cherow (Ed.), *Hearing-impaired children and youth with developmental disabilities* (pp. 82–98). Washington, DC: Gallaudet College Press.

Nihira, K., Foster, R., Shelhaas, M., & Leland, H. (1974). *AAMD Adaptive Behavior Scale*. Washington, DC: American Association of Mental Deficiency.

Rainer, J. D., Altschuler, K. Z., Kallmann, F. J., & Deming, W. E. (Eds.). (1963). *Family and mental health problems in a deaf population*. New York: New York State Psychology Institute.

Raven, J. (1948). *Progressive Matrices*. New York: Psychological Corporation.

Rorschach, H. (1942). *Psychodiagnostics*. Berne, Switzerland: Hans Huber.

Rosen, R. (1992). Politics of deafness: The role of and agenda for advocacy groups. In M. D. Garretson (Ed.). *Viewpoints on deafness: A deaf American monograph, 42*, 119–123. Silver Spring, MD: National Association of the Deaf.

Schein, J. D. (1991) The deaf community in the twenty-first century. In M. D. Garretson (Ed.). *Viewpoints on deafness: A deaf American monograph, 41*(1, 2), 131–134.

Schein, J. D., & Delk, M. (1974). *The deaf population of the United States*. Silver Spring, MD: National Association of the Deaf.

Siller, J. (1969). Psychological situation of the disabled with spinal cord injuries. *Rehabilitation Literature, 30*, 290–296.

Stein, M. I. (1955). *The Thematic Apperception Test*. Cambridge: Addison-Wesley Publishing Company.

Stock, W., & Guidubaldi, S. (1984). *The Battelle Developmental Inventory Manual*. Chicago: Riverside Publishing Company.

Sullivan, P., & Vernon, M. (1979). Psychological assessment of hearing impaired children. *School Psychology Digest, 8*, 271–290.

Trybus, R. J., & Karchmer, M. A. (1977). School achievement scores of hearing impaired children: National data on achievement status and growth patterns. *American Annals of the Deaf, 122*, 62–69.

Vernon, M. (1967). Prematurity and deafness: The magnitude and nature of the problem among deaf children. *Exceptional Children, 38*, 5–12.

Vernon, M. (1968). Fifty years of research on the intelligence of the deaf and hard-of-hearing. A survey of literature and discussion of implications. *Journal of Rehabilitation of the Deaf, 1*, 1–11.

Vernon, M. (1973). Psychological aspects of the diagnosis of deafness in a child. *Eye, Ear, Nose, Throat Monthly, 52*, 60–66.

Vernon, M. (1976). Psychologic evaluation of hearing-impaired children. In L. Lloyd (Ed.), *Communication assessment and intervention strategies* (pp. 195–224). Baltimore: University Park Press.

Vernon, M. (1979). Parental reactions to birth defective children. *Postgraduate Medicine, 65*, 183–189.

Vernon, M. (1985). The relationship of language and thought, bilingualism, and critical stage theory to reading. In M. Douglass (Ed.), *Proceedings of*

Claremont reading conference (pp. 21–30). Claremont, CA: Claremont Graduate School.

Vernon, M. (1987). Outcomes: Deaf people at work. In E. Mindel & M. Vernon (Eds.), *They grow in silence* (pp. 187–196). San Diego: College-Hill Press.

Vernon, M., & Andrews, J. F. (1990). *Psychology of deafness: Understanding deaf and hard of hearing people.* New York: Longman Press.

Vernon, M., & Rothstein, D. A. (1967). Prelingual deafness: An experiment of nature. *Archives of General Psychiatry, 16,* 325–333.

Wechsler, D. (1981) *Wechsler Intelligence Scale for Adults–Revised.* New York: Psychological Corporation.

Wechsler, D. (1991). *Wechsler Intelligence Scale for Children* (3rd. ed.). New York: Psychological Corporation.

Wylde, M. (1987). Psychological and counseling aspects of the adult remediation process. In J. Alpiner & P. McCarthy (Eds.), *Rehabilitative audiology: Children and adults* (3rd ed.). Baltimore: Williams & Wilkins.

Ziezula, F. R. (Ed.). (1982). *Assessment of hearing-impaired people.* Washington, DC: Gallaudet College Press.

7

Educational Options for the Deaf and Hard of Hearing

DONALD F. MOORES

Contents

INTRODUCTION

The education of persons who are deaf or hard of hearing has a long and fascinating history, longer than any other area of special education. The first documented systematic instruction of exceptional children took place in a Spanish monastery in the 1500s where a number of recessively deaf children of the Spanish aristocracy resided (Chaves & Solar, 1974). Techniques and methods related to the facilitation of speech, speechreading, language, and cognitive development were perfected in the following two centuries and were then introduced to France by the Spanish/Portuguese educator of the deaf, Pereira (Seguin, 1866). The contributions of the Spanish pioneers provided the basis for the work of the original French educators of individuals with deafness and mental retardation (Rosen, Clark, & Kivitz, 1976), which in turn provided the major guidelines for the first programs for the disabled in the United States. Specifically, the French educator Laurent Clerc, who was deaf, was the major influence on the development of educational programs in America in the early 1800s (Moores, 1996).

Throughout history, three major issues have faced educators concerned with the instruction of children and adults with hearing losses. These concern educational placement, curriculum, and modes of communication. Moores (1991) has phrased the issues in the form of three questions, as follows:

1. Where should we teach deaf and hard of hearing children?
2. What should we teach them?
3. How should we teach them?

These three questions are completely interrelated and assume increasing importance with more severe and profound hearing losses. Severe and profound hearing losses are relatively rare conditions, occurring in less than one child in a thousand in the United States. At the same time, the greater the hearing loss, the greater the probability that the child will need special instruction and training in areas such as English grammar, speech and English-language training, and utilization of residual hearing. The question then arises as to how much of the instruction should be devoted to the standard curriculum and how much should be devoted to special needs. Implicit in this is the understanding that any time devoted to special training will reduce time spent in general areas such as math, history, and science. The third question—how should children who are deaf be taught?—deals with the age-old controversy over oral and manual communication. In reality, at present, there are several schools of thought in this controversy.

It should be pointed out that most of the work with persons with hearing impairment has concentrated on individuals with severe and profound hearing losses, those who would traditionally be characterized as deaf. It is relatively easy to document trends in research, educational practices, and school placement for this population due to the enormous bodies of literature in each of these areas. Although mild and moderate hearing losses are far more frequent, much less information is available on the population traditionally classified as hard of hearing in regard to difficulties in the development of phonologic, grammatic, semantic, academic, and linguistic skills (see Chapters 5, 8, and 11). At present, a large majority of children with severe and profound hearing losses receive special services, whereas a majority of those with mild and moderate losses are underserved or not served at all.

Before addressing issues of instruction, some definition of terms is necessary as they relate to educational issues and procedures. The literature is replete with such descriptors as *deaf, hard of hearing, hearing impaired, acoustically challenged, hearing handicapped*, etc. Unfortunately, these terms mean different things to different people and there is no consistency in their use. For purposes of this chapter, we use the terms *deaf* and *hard of hearing* to accommodate the complete range of hearing loss from mild to profound. The cut-off point between *hard of hearing* and *deaf* has sometimes been placed as low as 70 dB across the speech range (Moores, 1996; Ross, 1990). Roughly, then, children with mild and moderate losses were considered *hard of hearing* and those with severe and profound losses generally were considered *deaf*. Functionally, of course, we cannot rely completely on a measure of hearing loss. Two children with identical losses may function quite differently due to a variety of factors such as age of onset of a loss, age of identification and provision of services, and presence of additional disabling conditions. Ross (1990) has argued, and the present author agrees, that the distinction between *deaf* and *hard of hearing* should be set around 90–95 dB, as noted in Chapter 6. However, some of the educational literature continues to set it around 70 dB.

In a study of procedures used in the 50 states and the District of Columbia, Bienenstock and Vernon (1994) found a bewildering lack of consistency in classification, which causes major difficulties in the provision of services throughout the country. Bienenstock and Vernon reported that Public Law 94-142 mandates the reporting by each state of the disability and educational placement of each child receiving special educational services. According to Bienenstock and Vernon, federal regulations do not use a specific measurable degree of hearing loss to establish eligibility, but rather provide the following definitions:

> Deaf—means a hearing impairment that is so severe that the child is impaired in processing linguistic information through hearing, with or without amplification, which adversely affects educational performance.

> Hard of hearing—means a hearing impairment, whether permanent or fluctuating, which adversely affects a child's educational performance, but is not included under the definition of "deaf" in this section. (p. 129)

Some states use *auditorily handicapped*, others *hearing impaired*, and yet others *hearing handicapped*. Some states use two categories—*deaf* and *hearing impaired*—while others use two other categories—*deaf* and *hard of hearing*. Massachusetts uses no category, because it does not categorize children in need of special services (p. 130). For those states that distinguish the deaf from the hard of hearing, the cutoff may be as low as 65 dB (Georgia) and as high as 92 dB (Nevada). This means that a child with a 75-dB loss is considered, for educational purposes, deaf in Georgia and hard of hearing in Nevada. Additionally, a child with a 40-dB loss may be eligible for services in one state and not in another. Finally, some states classify children with unilateral losses as eligible and others do not. Bienenstock and Vernon conclude that the inconsistencies they found across states result in meaningless, often erroneous, and inconsistent statistics, which can lead to invalid research, wasted money, and poor program planning.

DISABILITY, IMPAIRMENT, AND HANDICAP DEFINED

Part of the difficulty of securing proper services lies in the process of identification. Many children, especially those with mild losses, are misdiagnosed as mildly retarded or learning disabled. Even when correctly diagnosed, children with mild losses have not received top priority for services because they are not perceived as suffering from as great a disability as a child with more severe deafness, blindness, or highly restricted mobility. Additional difficulties arise over the confusion among the terms *impairment*, *disability*, and *handicap*. A child may have an *impairment* of the auditory mechanism. The *disability* and/or *handicap* relates to communication problems and other consequences of the loss. These two terms are used in slightly different ways, as explained in more detail in Chapter 1.

Over the past generation, there has been a movement in special education in the United States away from the use of the term *handicap* to a growing reliance on the term *disability*. An example of this change can be seen in federal legislation. In 1975, Public Law 94-142, the Education of All Handicapped Children Act, was passed. Over the years it has undergone numerous modifications, and is now referred to as the Individuals with Disabilities Education Act. Similarly, Congress has passed the Americans with Disabilities Act, guaranteeing equal access to services for disabled Americans.

The complexity of the situation concerning hearing loss was noted in Chapter 1. As suggested, two individuals may have identical audiograms while differing greatly in development of speech, use of residual hearing, academic achievement, and language. Contributing factors include age at onset of hearing loss, age at identification of loss and provision of services, appropriateness and adequacy of services, and presence of other potentially disabling conditions. Approximately 30% of children in programs for the hearing impaired in the United States suffer from additional impairments (Schildroth & Hotto, 1993). A child with hearing impairment who has additional difficulties, such as visual perception dysfunction, mental retardation, cerebral palsy, or neurologic impairment, is unlikely to respond as effectively to aural management as a child suffering from hearing impairment alone.

ESTIMATES OF INCIDENCE

Hearing loss is relatively common in the general population and most individuals experience a lessening of hearing acuity with age. Only a portion of these persons are presently in the educational system. Since the majority of hearing losses are acquired in adulthood, they are not of concern in the present chapter. Prevalence figures for the hearing-impaired school-age population are discussed in detail in Chapters 1 and 8. In terms of numbers of children actually receiving services, Schildroth and Hotto (1993) reported that from the 1991–92 Annual Survey of Hearing Impaired Children and Youth, 47,822 children who were deaf or hard of hearing were identified as receiving educational services. This represents approximately one child per thousand in the American school-age population. The degree of hearing loss for the children was as follows (p. 167):

Degree of Loss	Percentage of Total
Within Normal Limits	9%
Mild	10%
Moderate	12%
Moderately Severe	12%
Severe	18%
Profound	38%

It is interesting to note that the total number of children in programs for the deaf and hard-of-hearing declined 5% from 1985 to 1992, probably due in large part to the fact that children affected by the rubella epidemic of the mid-1960s were out of the education system by 1992. Schildroth and Hotto reported that in this period, the number of children with severe or profound losses actually decreased by 15%, while those with less than severe losses—hearing thresholds of 70 dB or lower-actually *increased* by 13%. Related to this was an increase—from 35% in 1985 to 41% in 1992—in the percentage of children taught through oral-only means. As might be expected, use of some form of manual communication is related to degree of hearing loss. In 1992, 84% of children who were deaf (severe to profound losses) were being taught by some sign-language system (Schildroth & Hotto, 1993).

It must be stressed that the numbers of children who are deaf or hard of hearing who receive special education services is lower than the actual number of these children in the school-age population. Moores (1996) has estimated that 90–95% of children who are deaf have been identified and are receiving special services, but that the situation for children who are hard of hearing is worse. Davis (1990) refers to children who are hard of hearing as "our forgotten children" and blames the problem to a great extent on financial limitations and lack of trained personnel. Ross (1990) argues that the problem is not so much that the children are forgotten, but that they are overlooked. In many cases the problems are masked because a child may communicate quite well in a face-to-face situation but not in the classroom or other group settings. Ross reports that the incidence of hearing loss from 26–70 dB in the American school age population is 16–30 per 1000. This may be extrapolated to suggest that almost 2 million children in school are hard of hearing (the total number of children with hearing loss is higher, of course, when preschool children are added; see Chapter 8). Only a very small percentage receive special educational services. At this time, we cannot state with confidence how many *should* be receiving special services, but it is clear that large numbers are being overlooked.

EDUCATIONAL PROGRAMS AND SERVICES

Early Intervention/Preschool

During the late 1960s, it became widely recognized that children who are deaf or hard of hearing and their families must have access to educational efforts before the normal school-entry age. Early intervention can take advantage of the critical period of language development (see Chapter 5). Most early-intervention programs emphasize parental involvement in the educational process. Programs are typically carried out through home visits by a clinician, parental visits to the clinic/demonstration home, or a combination thereof (see Chapter 8). After this type of early home-based training, the child may be placed in a variety of preschool and later primary-/secondary educational settings. Federal legislation now mandates that children and their families receive services from time of identification of a hearing loss and that annual plans be developed based on the needs of the individual child and family.

School Placement Options

It is a mistake to think of the educational options for children who are deaf or hard of hearing as being limited to segregated vs. integrated placement. In general, the most common types of programs for children with hearing impairment may be classified as follows:

1. *Residential schools.* In most such programs a majority of students reside in the school. However, in areas accessible to large populations, substantial numbers of children live at home and commute daily. The pattern is for children within commuting distance to attend on a day basis, with those living farther away staying at school at least during weekdays. Most classes are self-contained. Most residential schools have cooperative programs with local public schools for integrated education for some of their students.

2. *Day schools.* These programs are established in some of the larger metropolitan areas in separate schools for children who are deaf, to which the students commute daily. Students with normal hearing do not attend these schools.

3. *Day classes.* Day-class programs have traditionally been differentiated from day schools in that the latter refer to classes for the hearing impaired in a public school building where the majority of students are hearing. Classroom instruction

may range from completely self-contained classes for the children with hearing impairment, to children spending most of their time in a regular classroom. In the past, children having some hearing and better oral communication skills were integrated. Now many programs, especially at the secondary level, utilize manual interpreters in regular classes thereby enabling many children with profound deafness to attend.

4. *Resource rooms*.   Most resource rooms are planned so that children spend the majority of their day in regular classes, returning to the teacher of the hearing-impaired for special attention, usually in language and in academic areas of concern. Whereas day-class programs typically contain several classes with homogeneous groupings of children with hearing impairment, there may be only one or two resource rooms in a building with the teacher providing individualized services to children who vary in age, hearing loss, and academic achievement.

5. *Itinerant programs*.   Under this type of program, a child attends regular classes full time and receives service on an "itinerant" basis periodically. This may vary from daily to weekly lessons, depending on a child's needs. In these situations one teacher might work with children from several schools.

Educational Placement, Public Law 94-142, and the Least Restrictive Environment

The educational placement of children who are deaf or hard of hearing has undergone steady change since World War II. Fifty years ago, the deaf were educated almost exclusively either in residential schools for the deaf or in day schools for the deaf. For children who were hard of hearing there were only two options: placement in a school for the deaf, or integration with children with normal hearing, without support services at the local school district level.

During the second half of the 20th century, there has been a clear trend toward accommodation of children who are deaf or hard of hearing in public school settings (Moores, 1992; Moores & Kluwin, 1986). Several reasons for this trend can be identified. First was the post-war "baby boom" that tremendously increased the school-age population and, by extension, the numbers of children who were deaf or hard of hearing. Second, the United States was becoming much more urbanized and suburbanized, with clusterings of population, making it more feasible to provide services to children with low-incidence conditions. Third, the rubella epidemic of the mid-1960s doubled the number of children who were deaf or hard of hearing born in approximately a two-year period. State legislators were not willing to build expensive residential facilities for what was seen as a temporary increase in the number of children requiring special services. Local education districts were expected to accommodate this increase in numbers. By 1972, only half of children who were deaf or hard of hearing were enrolled in residential schools (Moores, 1991).

The passage of the previously noted Public Law 94-142, the Education of All Handicapped Children Act of 1975, reinforced the trend toward inclusion. The major goal of PL 94-142 was to assure that all disabled children from ages 3 through 21 receive appropriate special educational services. In 1986, PL 99-457 was enacted,

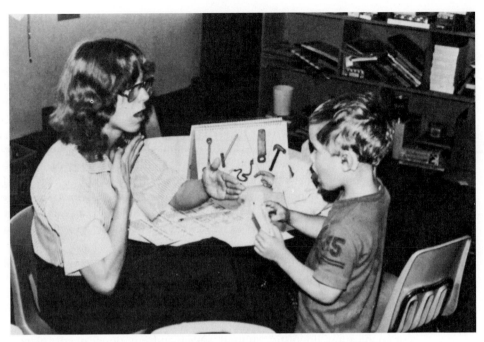

Therapy conducted outside the classroom for mainstreamed children.

which basically mandates these same services to children from birth through two years of age (see Chapter 8). In order to meet this goal, states are mandated to develop plans by which children must be served. As a result of a series of court decisions, the impetus has been to develop appropriate educational programs for those children demonstrating the most severe disabilities and children who previously have not received special services. Much of the activity has also been related to the concept of "least restrictive environment (LRE)," that is, the idea that it is preferable to educate handicapped children (to use the original terminology) together with non-handicapped children to the greatest extent possible. The latest data available indicate that in 1992 only 22% of children who were deaf or hard of hearing were enrolled in residential schools.

The trends toward education in local school settings has been influenced by what has been classified in special education variously as the Regular Education Initiative, Total Inclusion, or Mainstreaming (Moores, 1993). Although there has been some concern that the concept of LRE may apply differently to children who are deaf or hard of hearing—especially children who are deaf—than to some other categories of disability, this has been tied with the mainstreaming movement. Until recently, mainstreaming consisted essentially of moving children classified as having mild mental retardation out of special classes and back into regular classrooms. Essentially, these are children who never should have been segregated in the first place (Kirk, 1975).

In terms of school placement there has been considerable confusion over the interpretation and implications of the concept of least restrictive environment for the education of children who are deaf. In general, while experts have been aware of improvements in education of deaf children in the past, a consensus also exists that major adjustments must be made quickly if we are to serve more adequately the needs of Americans who are deaf. This concern led to the establishment of the Commission on Education of the Deaf, under the Education of the Deaf Act of 1986, to study the quality of education of the deaf. The report of the Commission (1988), *Toward Equality: Education of the Deaf*, concluded that education of persons who were deaf was characterized by inappropriate priorities and inadequate resources. The Report noted that "Parents, deaf consumers, and professional personnel of all persuasions have, with almost total unanimity, cited LRE as the issue that most thwarts their attempts to provide an appropriate education for children who are deaf" (p. x). The Report itself contained a large number of recommendations. The topic of school placement generated eight recommendations, the most for any category in the Report. The recommendations, as numbered in the Report (pp. xvi–xvii) were:

1. The Department of Education should provide guidelines and technical assistance to state and local educational agencies and parents to ensure that an individualized education program for a child who is deaf takes into consideration the following: severity of hearing loss and the potential for using residual hearing; academic level and learning style; communicative needs and the preferred mode of communication; linguistic, cultural, social, and emotional needs; placement preference; individual motivation; and family support.

2. The Department of Education should refocus the least restrictive environment concept by emphasizing appropriateness over least restrictive environment.

3. The Department of Education should issue a policy statement to permit consideration in placement decisions of curriculum content and methods of curricular delivery required by the nature or severity of the child's handicapping conditions.

4. The Department of Education should issue guidelines and standards by which school officials and parents can, in selecting the least restrictive environment, consider potential harmful effects on the child or on the quality of services which the child needs.

5. The Department of Education should publish in the Federal Register a policy interpretation that removal from the regular classroom does not require compelling evidence.

6. The Department of Education should monitor states to ensure that they maintain and nurture center schools as placement options as required by law.

7. The Department of Education should monitor states to ensure the availability and appropriateness of integrative programs for students in center schools.

8. The Department of Education should issue a policy statement requiring that school personnel inform parents of all options in the continuum of alternative placements during each individualized education program conference.

In their entirety, the recommendations of the Commission challenge the philosophical premise that LRE is the "core value" of special education. DuBow (1989) has argued that the U.S. Department of Education, with its primary emphasis on LRE, turned a congressional preference into a requirement and that this emphasis is contrary to both legislative intent, and judicial interpretations of the Act. The Commission's emphasis on appropriateness over LRE, its support for center schools, its demand for individualized educational programs, and its argument that removal from the regular classroom does *not* require compelling evidence that such removal is necessary all call for a refocus of the least restrictive environment concept.

For children receiving services, the question of segregation and integrated placement (mainstreaming) cannot be answered adequately, because the characteristics of the children in different settings are variable. As long ago as 1977, Karchmer and Trybus reported that nearly ⅔ of the children in residential schools were classified as profoundly deaf (91-dB loss or greater in the better ear) as contrasted to only 18% of children in integrated programs. In addition, the percentage of postlingually deafened children was three times as great in integrated programs (13% to 4%). Karchmer and Trybus continued:

> The integrated programs enroll the highest proportion of children from high income families (i.e., over $20,000 annually) and the lowest proportion of very low income families (under $5,000 annually). . . . Children in integrated programs have the highest proportion of college educated fathers (36%) while children in day schools have the lowest (19%). (p. 3)

Karchmer and Trybus (1977) summarized their data as follows:

> This is where mainstreaming is at the present time. It will be interesting and of critical importance to trace the changes in this picture over the next few years under the influence of PL 94-142. For the present, however, it is clear that the integrated programs are generally serving a group of hearing impaired children who are very different on many educationally critical dimensions from those children who attend other types of special educational programs. (p. 3)

In the ensuing years, the situation has become much more complex as residential school enrollment has continued to decline. In a study of 21 public school programs for children who are deaf or hard of hearing and 7 residential schools for the deaf, Moores (1991) concluded that there were greater differences among public-school programs themselves than between residential and public schools. In general, the greatest differences were between large multi-district suburban programs and large urban programs. The suburban programs tended to offer a wide variety of options to children with mild, moderate, severe, and profound hearing losses. Placement ranged from integration with support services in neighborhood schools to self-contained classes for the deaf. Instructional options ranged from oral-aural to American Sign Language. Trained audiologists, counselors, and psychologists were on the staff, and interpreters were available for extra-curricular activities. The large urban programs studied had experienced significant enrollment declines over the previous 10 years. The range of placement and communication options was much more limited. Family income was low and many of the programs did not provide services to the hard-of-hearing. There was a lack of personnel trained to conduct psychological, audiological, speech and language, and educational evaluations. In sum, the residential schools and the suburban programs tended to have sufficient resources, but the programs located in large cities did not, and the situation for children who were deaf or hard of hearing in these settings had reached crisis proportions. We may state that in general, residential schools serve predominantly students who are deaf, and tend to have satisfactory resources; suburban programs serve students who are deaf and hard of hearing and tend to have satisfactory resources; and urban programs serve deaf students and generally do not have satisfactory resources.

Work that has concentrated solely on children who are hard of hearing also indicates that developments since enactment of PL 94-142 in 1975 have been mixed at best. For example, Ross stated in 1977, "Although physically present in the mainstream, they [children who are hard of hearing] have been, more often than not, if one can forgive the cliche, simply drowning there" (p. 5). In a similar vein, Davis (1977) noted that the hard of hearing are the most "mainstreamed" of all children with disabilities, but that they have not received the special help they need:

> The result of these facts is such that few educators point with pride toward the results of mainstreaming, or inclusion, as they are demonstrated in the achievements of hard of hearing children. For one thing very little is known about the children's educational achievements, the types of problems they face in regular classrooms, their acceptance or non-acceptance by normally hearing peers, the relation between the support services offered them and their achievements, or the extent of those support services in the average school system. . . . It is painfully evident that, for the hard of hearing, at least, mainstreaming is a very mixed blessing when the children are not provided with special services. (p. 13)

Given the previously cited figures from Ross (1990) and Schildroth and Hotto (1993), it is clear that most children who are hard of hearing continue to be "mainstreamed," but without appropriate educational services.

Individual and Family Plans

At this point, before considering student characteristics, per se, it would be helpful to consider one major impact of PL 94-142 and subsequent federal legislation; that is, the emphasis on the individual child that is part of the legal mandate. PL 94-142 represented significant breakthroughs in three important areas: a free, appropriate public education (FAPE) for all handicapped/disabled children; education in the least restrictive environment (LRE); and an individual education plan (IEP) for each child, to be updated on an annual basis. The IEP is developed for any given youngster by a cross-disciplinary group of professionals and the child's parents to document annual goals, short-term objectives, special needs, and mechanisms for measuring progress. If parents do not agree with a particular IEP recommendation, due-process safeguards are built into the system.

The enactment of PL 99-457 in 1986 not only extended services to infants, but also expanded the scope of services to include families. This legislation recognizes the essential importance of the family of the disabled child as the basic unit to be served. In place of the IEP, it calls for an individualized *family* services plan (IFSP) that not only considers the child, but also addresses the family's strengths and needs as they relate to the child with a disability within the family. A statement of the major outcomes to be achieved for both the infant and the family, as well as specific specialized services to be provided, are all part of the IFSP.

STUDENT CHARACTERISTICS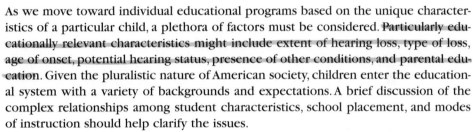

As we move toward individual educational programs based on the unique characteristics of a particular child, a plethora of factors must be considered. Particularly educationally relevant characteristics might include extent of hearing loss, type of loss, age of onset, potential hearing status, presence of other conditions, and parental education. Given the pluralistic nature of American society, children enter the educational system with a variety of backgrounds and expectations. A brief discussion of the complex relationships among student characteristics, school placement, and modes of instruction should help clarify the issues.

First is the complex issue of racial/ethnic status. Approximately 40% of children enrolled in programs for the deaf are classified as minority; approximately 61% are White, 17% are African American, 15% are Hispanic, 4% are Asian/Pacific, with the remainder classified as "Other." The percentages are higher for minority children than those reported for the general school-age population, a situation that was noted for African American children in 1978 by Moores and Oden, who reported that: (a) there was a higher rate of acquired hearing loss in African American children because of gaps in medical services; (b) there was a scarcity of professionals in the field; (c) there were few early identification programs and preschool services; and (d) there was a tendency to inappropriately classify African American children who are deaf as deaf/retarded.

Schildroth (1989) pointed out that "minority children" actually constituted the majority in programs for children who were deaf or hard of hearing in our three most populous states as early as 1985, when they accounted for 61% of enrollment in California, 52% in Texas, and 51% in New York. The overall percentage of minority children in programs for the deaf or hard of hearing increased from 33% in 1985 to 39% in 1992 (Schildroth & Hotto, 1993).

The increase in minority enrollment has not been uniform. In fact, there was a 10% decline in the number of African American children who were deaf in programs for the deaf and hard of hearing from 1985 to 1992, as contrasted to significant increases in Hispanic and Asian/Pacific enrollment. Schildroth and Hotto highlighted this change by noting that in 1985 in programs for the deaf and hard of hearing there were 1.6 African American, non-Hispanic children for every Hispanic child; by 1992 this ratio had dwindled to 1.1 to 1.

There is a great need for a substantially increased number of minority professionals to work with children having hearing impairment. At the same time, there is an equally great need for all professionals to develop a sensitivity toward the multicultural nature of American society. This is especially true of hearing and speech specialists working with children whose reference group may employ a dialect or language different from that of the specialist, with distinctions in phonology, morphology, syntax, semantics, and even social and pragmatic functions of language. Any program of audiologic habilitation or rehabilitation must take such considerations into account to be successful.

Table 7.1 provides some information on the diversity of children who are deaf or hard of hearing in four different settings. The categories "Residential School" and "Day School" are identical to those presented earlier in this chapter. "Local, Integrated" refers to children receiving services on an itinerant basis, and "Local, Not Integrated" includes students in resource rooms and self-contained classes. First, as might be expected, children in residential schools tend to have the lowest percentage (11%) of children with less than severe hearing losses, as opposed to 62% of children in integrated local settings. Moving from residential schools, to separate day schools, to separate classes within schools with children with normal hearing, to integration within regular classrooms, we find a logical decrease in the percentage of children with severe and profound hearing losses.

The primary mode of instruction also follows a sequence that might be predicted on the basis of hearing loss, with auditory/oral-only instruction increasing from 4% of children in residential schools to 60% in integrated settings. There seems to be a good interaction among hearing loss, academic placement, and mode of instruction. The data presented by age complicate the situation somewhat. Half of residential-school students are 14 or older as compared to 25% or less in the other three settings. This indicates that there is some move toward residential-school settings as children grow older. Perhaps many parents are not as willing to enroll young children in residential schools as they are when the children mature into adolescence.

A final factor that requires some discussion is placement by ethnic status. Quite briefly, White students are proportionately more likely to attend residential schools or be in local integrated settings than they are to attend day schools or be in local, not integrated settings. Day schools are predominantly found in large cities, with relatively low White representation, as are local, non-integrated classes. Enrollment of African American children, who constitute 17% of all enrollments, seems to be consistent across categories, but with somewhat lower enrollment in integrated settings. The greatest discrepancy is found with Hispanic children, who account for only 10% of residential students and 26% of day-school students. A variety of reasons may be offered for this. The most relevant explanation might be that the Hispanic American population is predominantly urban, with heavy concentrations in California and Texas. These two states enroll approximately 10,000 children in programs for the deaf and hard of hearing, somewhat more than 20% of the total national enrollment. More than 4000 of the 7500 Hispanic children in programs for the deaf and hard of hearing in the United States are in California and Texas (A. Schildroth, Personal Communication, 1994). Since California and Texas have a total of only three residen-

TABLE 7.1 *Selected Characteristics of Deaf and Hard-of-Hearing Children in Four Different Placements*

	Residential School	Day School	Local, Not Integrated	Local, Integrated
Degree of Loss				
Less than Severe	11%	18%	36%	62%
Severe/Profound	89%	82%	64%	38%
Primary Instruction Method				
Auditory/Oral	4%	23%	25%	60%
Sign and Speech	92%	72%	72%	38%
Sign Only	4%	5%	2%	<1%
Other	<1%	<1%	1%	1%
Age				
Under 14	50%	79%	81%	75%
14 or Older	50%	21%	19%	25%
Ethnic Status				
White	65%	47%	51%	62%
African American	20%	21%	22%	15%
Hispanic	10%	26%	19%	17%
Asian/Pacific	3%	3%	5%	4%
Other	3%	3%	2%	2%

Adapted from: Schildroth, A., and Hotto, S. 1993. Annual Survey of Hearing Impaired Children and Youth. *American Annals of the Deaf,* 138, 163–171.

tial schools for the deaf, most of their deaf and hard-of-hearing population may be found in day schools and local programs. This includes Hispanics, who constitute the largest ethnic enrollment in the two states.

ACADEMIC ACHIEVEMENT

As in other areas, the academic problems of children who are deaf have been documented much more extensively than those of the hard of hearing. In general, children of normal intelligence who are deaf suffer from severe academic retardation caused primarily by difficulties in understanding and expressing standard English. Their achievement, then, tends to be highest in areas with relatively little reliance on English skills and lowest in areas highly dependent on English. Thus, in typical achievement-test batteries, scores on subtests like arithmetic computation, spelling, and punctuation are relatively high. On the other hand, scores on subtests requiring proficiency in English (e.g., reading comprehension, science, and word meaning) are relatively low.

Although arithmetic computation scores of students with hearing impairment are relatively high compared to scores for paragraph meaning, they are far below what should be achieved. Thus, an average 17-year-old should achieve at the 12th-grade level. Yet 17-year-olds who are deaf or hard of hearing are up to eight years behind their peers in reading, and five years in math. Figure 7.1 illustrates these comparisons. It should be noted that the slight drop in achievement among 17-year-old students with hearing impairment may be attributed, in part, to the fact that some of the most capable students may have already graduated before administration of the test.

Although academic achievement of students with hearing impairment is low, compared to standards set by students with normal hearing, there are some indications of improvement over time. Norms for children who are deaf or hard of hearing were developed on the sixth edition of the Stanford Achievement Test in 1974, on the seventh edition in 1983, and on the eighth edition in 1990 (Holt, Traxler, & Allen, 1992). Achievement on the average seems to peak around fourth-grade level in reading comprehension and seventh grade in math computation. However, children who are deaf or hard of hearing appear to have achieved at higher levels in 1990 than in 1983, which in turn, was higher than in 1974. Roughly, a 10-year-old was at the same level of achievement in 1990 as a 12-year-old in 1974. So, despite tremendous continuing problems, improvements have been made.

As might be expected, there have been different patterns of achievement. Holt, et al. (1992) reported median reading-comprehension grade-equivalent scores at age 17 of 3.8 for children with profound losses, 4.5 with severe losses, and 5.4 with less than severe losses. By ethnicity, at age 17 White children who were deaf or hard of hearing had median reading comprehension grade equivalents of 5.4; African American children scores at age 18 (grade 3.6) were higher than at 17. This was not true for White and Hispanic children, suggesting different retention patterns. In terms of school placement, 17-year-old children in local integrated settings read at grade 5.7, compared to 3.8 in day and residential school settings and 2.8 in local non-integrated settings. Holt, et al. were careful to point out that the higher achievement of children in integrated settings could not be attributed to placement, per se, because a majority of these children had less than severe hearing losses and tended to come from families of higher socio-economic status.

In summary, measurable progress in academic achievement among school-age children who are deaf or hard of hearing has occurred over the past two decades, but overall performance is still dramatically below that of the school-age population of children with normal hearing as a whole. Much remains to be done to further improve the academic achievement of children with hearing losses.

ORAL, TOTAL-COMMUNICATION, AND AMERICAN SIGN LANGUAGE PROGRAMS

Historically, children with hearing impairment have been educated using either an oral, a manual, or a total communication approach. The oral approach emphasizes the use of speech, hearing, and speechreading to communicate, while the manual method utilizes a form of signs (see Chapter 4). Total communication involves the use of speech, hearing, speechreading, and manual communication in combination.

With the exception of the move to integrate children who are deaf or hard of hearing with peers with normal hearing, the greatest trend in education of children with hearing impairment since the late 1960s has been a massive shift from oral-only

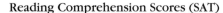

Reading Comprehension Scores (SAT)

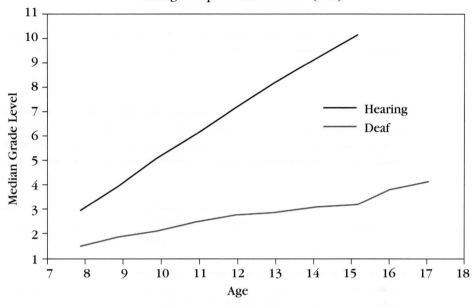

Mathematics Computation Scores (SAT)

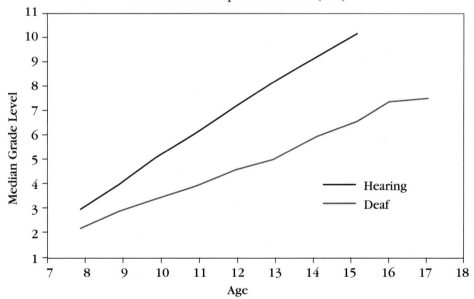

Figure 7.1 Median Stanford Achievement Test (SAT) scores for the 1990 population. *Top panel* shows reading comprehension levels as a function of age in years for both children with normal hearing and children with hearing loss. *Bottom panel* shows mathematics-computation scores for the same two groups.

From P.A. deVilliers. (1992). Educational implications of deafness: Language and literacy. In R. D. Eavey & J. O. Klein (Eds.). *Hearing loss in childhood: A primer, Report of the 102nd Ross conference on pediatric research*. Columbus, OH: Ross Laboratories.

instruction—especially in the preschool and elementary grades—to combined oral-manual instruction, or total communication. Most of the research in the area has been conducted with children having severe to profound losses. Therefore, the extent to which results can be generalized to the entire hearing-impaired population is unclear.

In the 1960s, a move away from oral-only education began to gain momentum based on several empirical findings. First, a growing body of research showed that children who were deaf and had parents who were deaf demonstrated superior academic achievement and English skills compared to children who were deaf and had parents with normal hearing, with oral-aural skills being equivalent. These results seriously challenged traditional beliefs that manual communication would detract from speech, speechreading, use of residual hearing, academic achievement, and acquisition of English. In contrast, it seemed to facilitate English, academic achievement, and speechreading, while having little or no effect on speech or use of residual hearing. Second, the claims of Soviet educators that use of fingerspelling improved language and academic skills received wide attention. Third, educators in the United States were frustrated over the apparent short-comings of the oral-only techniques in use, a frustration that was intensified by the failure of so many of the preschool programs established in the 1950s and 1960s to document any lasting benefits. In fact, the deaf with parents who were also deaf exhibited higher English and academic achievement without preschool than did children with deafness who had parents with normal hearing, and also had intensive preschool experience.

The shift in communication modes was strongly substantiated by the results of a study by Jordan, Gustason, and Rosen (1976), who reported that total communication was used in a majority of programs for the deaf by 1975. The term *total communication* (TC) was used to describe the use of all types of communication: speech, speechreading, residual hearing, fingerspelling, signs, and print. From 1968 to 1975, 302 programs had changed from oral-only methods to some form of simultaneous oral-manual instruction, while only five had changed from oral-manual to oral-only. A followup investigation (Jordan, Gustason, & Rosen, 1979) revealed a continuation of the trend over a 10-year period from 1968 to 1978. During that time 481 programs discontinued oral-only instruction while 538 turned to total communication. At every level—preschool, elementary, junior high, and senior high—total communication was emphasized in a majority of programs. One interesting sidelight is the finding by Jordan, et al. that more than 30% of programs reporting some form of mainstreaming provided sign interpreters in the regular classrooms.

At present, many programs are developing more flexibility toward children's communication needs. Thus, more and more programs are providing options depending on the needs of a particular child at a particular period of time. For example, in a large number of programs classified as total communication programs, some students receive oral-only instruction.

In a five-year evaluation of preschool programs for the severely hearing impaired, Moores and associates (Moores, 1985; Moores, Weiss, & Goodwin, 1978) found that the most successful program implemented cognitive academic and simultaneous oral-manual components from the beginning. Evidence suggested that it was harmful to delay either cognitive-academic training or use of manual communication. Children

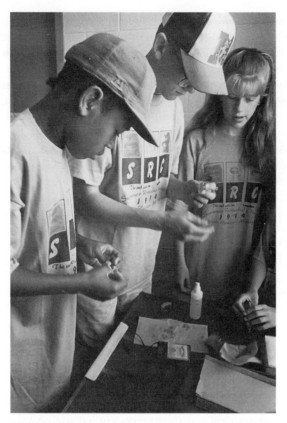

Children check the batteries of their hearing aids at the start of each day.

who did not receive such training and communication at an early age did not catch up by eight years of age. In fact, in some cases, the gap widened. The least beneficial approach for the children studied included an aural-only methodology within a traditional, socially-oriented nursery school framework. In contrast, the most beneficial approach incorporated aural-oral-manual components with a wide degree of flexibility, depending upon the needs of the individual child.

In spite of documented improvements, including the use of different communication systems, more placement options, early intervention programs, qualitative improvements in individual hearing aids, and so forth, there is not reason for sanguinity over either the current situation or projections for the near future. Large numbers of deaf adolescents still posses minimal speech, linguistic, academic, and vocational skills. Progress has been incremental, with no real qualitative breakthroughs, with the possible exception of the expansion of postsecondary programs.

The emergence of total communication programs raised a number of issues. First, since it is clear that many children who are deaf or hard of hearing perform adequately without recourse to manual communication, a need exists to develop an effective way to determine whether total communication or an oral-only approach is the most appropriate for a given child. Philosophically, this represents a break from previous approaches, in which the superiority of one method or another was argued for all children. Concern with the education of a particular child at a particular stage of development may move educators away from simplistic either/or dichotomies.

Recently, interest has been growing in the use of American Sign Language (ASL) in the home and classroom. Historically, most total-communication programs used invented sign systems—which we may think of collectively as manual codes on English—designed to coordinate spoken and signed English. Although these systems borrowed heavily from ASL vocabulary, there were clear distinctions (see Chapter 4). ASL is a full language with its own vocabulary, word order, and mechanisms for forming words congruent with the use of three-dimensional space. Body movement and facial expression are important grammatical components. Manual codes on English, as the term implies, are attempts to represent English. Affixes were invented to signify bound morphemes of English (e.g., -*ly*, -*ment*, -*s*, -*ed*) and the hand shapes of some ASL signs were modified to represent English sound or spelling (e.g., a basic sign for *to be* or *existence* may be signed with an *i* hand shape for *is* and an *r* hand shape for *are*.

Educators in support of manual codes of English reason that a system based on spoken English can be learned more easily by parents and relatives with normal hearing, that it can integrate speech and sign, and that it provides a bridge for access to English print.

Critics of manual codes on English argue that a full-blown natural language, ASL, is already available and that the invented manual codes are awkward, inconsistent, and—ultimately—unworkable.

In a three-day seminar at Hofstra University, a group of educators, administrators, and researchers addressed issues related to the educational use of ASL (Walworth, Moores, & O'Rourke, 1992). Although all participants supported the use of ASL, two quite distinct approaches were identified. One, which has been designated as the bilingual or ASL-only approach, would have communication with children with hearing impairment concentrate almost exclusively on ASL, especially with younger children. Hearing parents and siblings would be taught ASL, and ASL fluency would be stressed. Manual codes on English and combined manual/oral communication would not be employed. Speech training and auditory training, when appropriate, would be separate. English would be learned after ASL was mastered, through print. In sum, ASL would be the primary language and English would be acquired as a second language. This position was represented by Marlon Kuntze, Marie Phillip, and Samuel Supalla.

A second approach, represented by Frank Bowe, Donald Moores, and David Stewart, called for the use of both ASL and manual codes of English and abundant use of code switching. It was argued that manual codes of English are more awkward and less natural than ASL, but that they served a function, just as written codes of English do. Our writing system has only 26 letters and we have to resort to such devises as capitalization, quotations marks, commas, colons, etc. to represent English; but the system is functional. Also, there were concerns about trying to teach English directly through reading and writing. There are millions of hearing Americans who started school with mastery of spoken English but who never achieved functional literacy.

The problems of acquiring English through print would seem to be even more significant for children with substantial hearing losses.

As shown in Table 7.1, the percentage of children taught through sign alone is relatively low; 4% of residential-school enrollment and 5% of day-school enrollment. These numbers will probably grow substantially in the years to come, given the increased interest in ASL and the strong attachment of the deaf community to the language.

POST-SECONDARY EDUCATION

There has been a virtual revolution in post-secondary educational opportunities since the 1960s. Gallaudet University, established in 1864, was the only formal post-secondary program for the deaf for almost 100 years. It was not until after World War II that the university, then Gallaudet College, officially accepted students who were hard of hearing. During the 1960s, the federal government established the National Technical Institute for the Deaf, as a part of the Rochester (NY) Institute of Technology, as well as three federally funded regional vocational-technical programs. Another cluster of programs developed out of federal legislation which specified that states were obligated to spend significant portions of federal money in support of vocational education to provide training for the disabled. The growth was so rapid that 102 post-secondary programs for students who were deaf or hard of hearing were identified in 1983, and 125 in 1990 (Rawlings, Karchmer, Decaro, & Allen, 1991). The programs offer a wide range of support services, including interpreting, note-taking, counseling, and speech and hearing services. For complete information, the reader is referred to *College and Career Programs for Deaf Students* (8th ed; Rawlings, et al., 1991).

SUMMARY

Educational options for children who are deaf or hard of hearing do not follow a clear pattern. For children with severe to profound hearing losses, great strides have been made in recent years. Thus, more children now have a wide range of placement options available, from residential schools to self-contained classrooms, to resource rooms, to services from an itinerant professional. Emotionally charged debates over the use of manual communication also appear to be on the wane, with a range of program options available in most settings. Evidence is accumulating to suggest that academic achievement of this population is higher than in the past. Although many problems continue to exist, significant improvements have been made in recent years in the education of students who are deaf. A major concern, however, lies with a significant lack of services to many minority children.

The educational situation for those classified as hard of hearing also provides less cause for optimism. As discussed previously, a minority of these children presently receive special educational services. There is no clear understanding of their linguistic, social, or academic problems or needs. In addition, only limited funding has been available to school districts to provide special services to the hard of hearing. As a result, the more obvious needs of children who are deaf have received priority (Davis, 1990). The mandates of PL 94-142 and the more recent PL 99-457 have not by themselves had the desired impact. The laws stipulate that special attention be given to children not currently served and that all children must have an individualized education program (IEP/IFSP). If, indeed, the intent of the laws is carried out, children who are hard of hearing will begin to receive the attention often denied them in the past. This has not happened to the extent that is needed.

RECOMMENDED READINGS

Kluwin, T., Moores, D., & Gaustad, M. (Eds.). (1992). *Toward effective public school programs for deaf students*. New York: Teachers College Press.

Meadow, K. (1980). *Deafness and child development*. Berkeley, CA: University of California Press.

Moores, D. (1996). *Educating the deaf: Psychology, principles and practices*. (4th ed.). Boston: Houghton Mifflin.

Moores, D., & Meadow-Orlans, K. (Eds.). (1990). *Educational and developmental aspects of deafness*. Washington, DC: Gallaudet University Press.

Paul, P., & Quigley, S. (1990). *Education and deafness*. White Plains, NY: Longman.

Roeser, R., & Downs, M. (Eds.). (1988). *Auditory disorders in school children*. (2nd ed.). New York: Thieme-Stratton.

Ross, M., Brackett, D., & Maxon, A. (1991). *Assessment and management of mainstreamed hearing-impaired children*. Austin, TX: Pro-Ed.

NATIONAL ORGANIZATIONS

Alexander Graham Bell Association for the Deaf, 3417 Volta Place, N.W.. Washington, DC 20007

American Deafness and Rehabilitation Association, P. O. Box #251554, Little Rock, AR 72225

American Society for Deaf Children, East 10th & Tahlequah, Sulphur, OK 73086

Conference of Educational Administrators Serving the Deaf, Iowa School for the Deaf, 1600 South Highway 275, Council Bluffs, IA 51503

Convention of American Instructors of the Deaf, P. O. Box #9887, Rochester, NY 14623-0887

National Association of the Deaf, 814 Thayer Avenue, Silver Spring, MD 20910-4500

Self Help for Hard of Hearing People, 7800 Wisconsin Avenue, Bethesda, MD 20814

JOURNALS

American Annals of the Deaf, DES-PAS #6, 800 Florida Avenue, N.E., Washington, DC 20002

Journal of the American Deafness and Rehabilitation Association, P. O. Box #251554, Little Rock, AR 72225

Perspectives in Education and Deafness, Gallaudet University Pre-College Programs, 800 Florida Avenue, N.E., Washington, DC 20002

SHHH, 7800 Wisconsin Avenue, Bethesda, MD 20814

Volta Review, 3417 Volta Place, N.W., Washington, DC 20007.

REFERENCES

Bienenstock, M., & Vernon, M. (1994). Classification by the states of deaf and hard of hearing students. *American Annals of the Deaf, 139*(1), 128-131.

Chaves, T., & Solar, I. (1974). Pedro Ponce de Leon, first teacher of the deaf. *Sign Language Studies, 5*, 48-63.

Commission on Education of the Deaf. (1988). *Toward equality in education of the deaf.* Washington, DC: U. S. Government Printing Office.

Davis, J. (Ed.). (1980). *Our forgotten children: Hard of hearing pupils in the schools.* (2nd ed.). Minneapolis: University of Minnesota.

DuBow, S. (1989). Into the turbulent mainstream. *Journal of Law and Education, 18, 2*, 215-228.

Holt, J., Traxler, C., & Allen, T. (1992). *Interpreting the scores: A user's guide to the 8th Edition Stanford Achievement Test for Educations of Deaf and Hard of Hearing Students* (Technical Report 92-1). Washington, DC: Gallaudet Research Institute.

Jordan, I., Gustason, G., & Rosen, R. (1976). Current communication trends of programs for the deaf. *American Annals of the Deaf, 121*, 527-531.

Jordan, I., Gustason, G., & Rosen, R. (1979). An update on communication trends of programs for the deaf. *American Annals of the Deaf, 124*, 350-357.

Karchmer, M., & Trybus, R. (1977). Who are the deaf children in "mainstream" programs? Washington, DC: Gallaudet College of Demographic Studies, Series R, No. 4.

Kirk, S. (August, 1975). Labelling, categorizing and mainstreaming. Paper presented at International Conference of Special Education, Kent, England.

Moores, D. (1985). A longitudinal evaluation of early intervention programs for the deaf. In K. Nelson (Ed.), *Children's language* (pp. 159-186). Englewood Cliffs, NJ: Erlbaum.

Moores, D. (1996). *Educating the deaf: Psychology, principles, and practices.* (4th ed.). Boston: Houghton Mifflin.

Moores, D. (1992). An historical perspective on school placement. In T. Kluwin, D. Moores, & M. Gaustad (Eds.). *Toward Effective Public School Programs for Deaf Students.* (pp. 7-29). New York: Teachers College Press.

Moores, D. (1991). *Dissemination of a model to create least restrictive environments for deaf students*. (Project No. 84133, Grant No. G008720128). Final Report for National Institute on Disability and Rehabilitation Research. Washington, DC.

Moores, D. (1993). Total inclusion/Zero reject models in general education. *American Annals of the Deaf, 138*(3), 251.

Moores, D., & Kluwin, T. (1986). Issues in school placement. In A. Schildroth & M. Karchmer (Eds.). *Deaf children in america* (pp. 105-124). New York: College-Hill Press.

Moores, D., & Oden, C. (1978). Educational needs of Black deaf children. *American Annals of the Deaf, 122*, 313-318.

Moores, D., Weiss, K., & Goodwin, M. (1978). Early intervention programs for hearing impaired children. *American Annals of the Deaf, 123*(8), 925-936.

Rawlings, B., Karchmer, M., Decaro, J., & Allen, T. (1991). *College and Career Programs for Deaf Students*. Washington, DC: Gallaudet University; and Rochester, NY: National Technical Institute for the Deaf.

Rosen, M., Clark, G., & Kivitz, M. (Eds.). (1976). *The history of mental retardation*. Baltimore, MD: University Park Press.

Ross, M. (1977). Definitions and descriptions. In J. Davis (Ed.), *Our forgotten children: Hard of hearing pupils in the schools*. (pp. 5-19). Minneapolis: University of Minnesota.

Ross, M. (1990). Definitions and descriptions. In J. Davis (Ed.), *Our forgotten children: Hard of hearing pupils in the schools*. (2nd ed.; pp. 3-18). Washington, DC: U. S. Department of Education.

Seguin, E. (1866). *Idiocy and its treatment by the physiological method*. New York: Wilbur Ward.

Schildroth, A. (1989). Educational Placement of Hearing Impaired Students. Gallaudet Research Institute Symposium, Washington, DC, May.

Schildroth, A., & Hotto, S. (1993). Annual Survey of Hearing Impaired Children Youth: 1991-1992 School Year. *American Annals of the Deaf, 138*(2), 163-171.

Walworth, M., Moores, D., & O'Rourke, T. (Eds.). (1992). *A Free Hand: Enfranchising the education of deaf children*. Silver Spring, MD: T. J. Publishers.

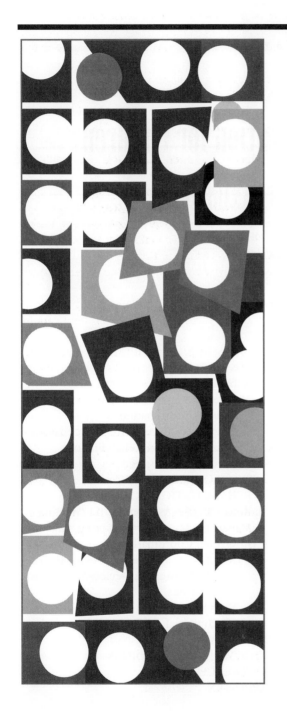

PART TWO

Comprehensive Approaches to Audiologic Rehabilitation

Audiologic Rehabilitation for Children

ASSESSMENT AND MANAGEMENT

MARY PAT MOELLER
SUSAN WATKINS
RONALD L. SCHOW

Contents

INTRODUCTION

This chapter will provide a comprehensive discussion of audiologic rehabilitation for children as provided at two major levels: (a) parent-infant and preschool, and (b) the school years. Before specific components that constitute the rehabilitation process are addressed, however, the reader will get a brief overview of prevalence and service-delivery statistics, applicable definitions and terms, a general profile of the client, typical rehabilitation settings at various age levels, and the identification/assessment process.

PREVALENCE OF LOSS AND LEVEL OF SERVICE

Of all audiologic rehabilitation efforts, those focusing on the child are probably the most frequently applied. While numbers vary depending on the criteria used, it is commonly reported that there are approximately 50,000 youngsters who are deaf in the United States' educational system (about 1 in every 1000 children) and that about 94% of them receive special services (*American Annals of the Deaf*, 1994; Northern & Downs, 1991). Under-reporting problems, however, suggest that this number represents only 2/3 of the total number of children in school who are deaf. According to the US Department of Education (1994), only about 61,000 children with all degrees of hearing impairment were served in public schools during the 1992–93 school year. It appears the great bulk of these children were deaf, since a high percentage of them are being served and there is a much poorer rate of service for the hard of hearing as compared to the deaf.

Ross, Brackett, and Maxon (1991) estimated that there are 16–30 times more children who are hard-of-hearing than profoundly impaired. This estimate would suggest that 1–2 million youngsters are hard of hearing. The estimate of around 1 million school-age youngsters who are hard of hearing (with unilateral and bilateral losses) is supported by some data (Lundeen, 1991). The 2 million estimate also has support (Eagles, Wishik, Doerfler, Melnick, & Levine, 1963; Pugh, 1994). Inclusion of the younger population (0–5 years) could put the total at over 3 million children with hearing loss.

Shepherd, Davis, Gorga, and Stelmachowicz (1981) studied hearing impairment in Iowa and found a relatively constant rate of mild to moderate sensorineural and mixed losses in school children from grades K–12. These impairments included about 2/3 bilateral and 1/3 unilateral losses. About 13% of the children presented some additional disability such as non-correctable visual problems, mental retardation, or motor coordination difficulties. These sensorineural losses did not include youngsters with high-frequency losses limited to 4000 Hz and above, nor did it include conductive losses of 10 dB or more found on the most recent audiogram of another group. These high-frequency and conductive losses affect about four times as many as the sensorineural losses do and although they may be transient or have limited impact, they indicate that several million children not included in some estimates are at risk for hearing difficulties. Jerger (1980) confirmed this general estimate when he reported that 2 1/2 million youngsters from birth to six years old suffer seriously from otitis media (which often causes conductive loss). These numbers are in line with estimates in the Rand Report (1974) that 8–13 million children in the United States need services in a substantial way, if those with unilateral and conductive losses are included.

The level of services (the percentage of youngsters receiving rehabilitation help) reported by Shepherd, et al. (1981) for youngsters having sensorineural and mixed losses varies by the degree of loss. Specifically, there is only a 27% level of service for the mildest losses, but up to a 92% level for the worst losses. Although Iowa was then considered to have exemplary services (70 school audiologists, 500 speech-language pathologists, 100 teachers of the hearing impaired) for its school-age children with hearing impairment, the state was found to be serving only 46% of all such youngsters with some kind of special placement or itinerant service. Further, slightly less than 50% of the overall sensorineural/mixed group was amplified. These data indicate a clear need to address, in a more comprehensive fashion, the needs of children with hearing impairments of all types and degrees.

TERMS/DEFINITIONS

As noted in Chapter 1, a rigid distinction between habilitation and rehabilitation is not being made in this book. Although some prefer to use the word *habilitation* when dealing with children having prelingual hearing impairments, we use the term *audiologic rehabilitation* because of its generic usage in the profession.

Audiologic rehabilitation for the child may be viewed best as an advocacy, in which the rehabilitation professional works with the parents and the child to identify needs in relation to the hearing loss and subsequently arranges to help meet those needs. Needs resulting from hearing loss are detailed in the chapters on amplification (Chapter 2), speech/language communication (Chapter 5), psychosocial (Chapter 6), and educational issues (Chapter 7)—all of which are contained in the first section of this book. Audiologic rehabilitation (AR) includes both assessment and management (see discussion in Chapter 1). While all these AR needs are important, they should be approached differently for various children, depending, among other variables, upon the degree and time of onset of the hearing loss and the age of the child. Consequently, in order to be meaningful, a discussion of audiologic rehabilitation should be seen in the context of a profile of possible clients. The following section specifically focuses on severity and type of hearing loss, age of child, and other disabilities.

PROFILE OF THE CLIENT

Hearing Loss

Deafness categories for children include *congenital* (present at birth), *prelingual* (onset before three to five years), and *postlingual* (onset at or after age five).

Youngsters with congenital deafness should generally be served through early-intervention programs, which include parent-infant and preschool programs. As soon as the loss is identified (preferably by one year of age or before) the parent-infant program should start. Preschool programming typically begins when the child is at least two and one-half years of age and may run concurrently with parent-infant programming. Ideally, children continue with such programs until AR services are provided in connection with school placement. Youngsters with prelingual deafness, with onset after birth, will generally receive similar treatment. Children with postlingual deafness, however, will most likely be served only in the schools.

A variety of children who are hard of hearing also participate in audiologic rehabilitation. Youngsters with milder losses are sometimes identified early and receive AR through early intervention. Other youngsters with slight or mild losses are not identified and/or do not receive assistance until after they start school. Indeed, some losses are progressive and reach significant dimensions only as the child gets older. One type of slight/mild loss involves middle-ear infections, which result in conductive hearing problems. Frequently, such losses are of a transient nature, but in other cases they persist over a long period and require rehabilitation assistance. These conductive problems can have an educational impact on children even if the loss is only on the order of 15 dB HL (Northern & Downs, 1991).

Since many more children are hard of hearing than are deaf, most AR work should be performed for the child who is hard of hearing (although audiologic rehabilitation should not be neglected with either group). Involvement with children who are deaf may be more intensive because of the greater problems caused by the severity of the hearing loss. The child with more pronounced hearing loss tends to experience more language, speech, and educational difficulties, and more remedial efforts will, therefore, be necessary (see Table 1.2; Chapter 7; Allen, 1986). In this chapter we describe the various types of rehabilitative efforts, without precisely distinguishing between service models for children who are deaf and those for children who are hard of hearing. Although this approach involves some loss of specificity, it is necessary in order to avoid excessive duplication. There is, naturally, much in common in AR services regardless of the degree of hearing loss or the mode of communication. Thus, the reader must selectively apply AR techniques consistent with the individual child's needs.

Age

If the assumption is made that children become adults somewhere between 18 and 21 years of age, graduation from high school provides a natural line of demarcation between childhood and adulthood. In that case, we may separate the years from birth to 18 into two basic divisions: those before school years (0–5) and the school years themselves (5–18). In addition, we may make a number of other subdivisions, including the years of infancy and toddlerhood (0–3), the preschool years (3–5), and the kindergarten, grade-school, junior-high, and high-school years (5–18).

In this chapter, we use the two-way division (0–5 and school years), since hearing-impaired children generally undergo a major adjustment of rehabilitation services when they enter regular school programming. Before that, audiologic rehabilitation includes parent-infant and preschool programs. When kindergarten begins, the school personnel will generally take over rehabilitation responsibilities from the early-intervention/preschool professional. These age ranges are general; consequently, some children progress through intervention programs more quickly than others. Services are not time-locked, but sequential, depending on the child's progress.

Other Disabling Conditions

Youngsters with hearing impairment often have other disabling conditions such as visual impairments, motor handicaps, or retardation. As noted earlier, 13% of all students in Iowa with hearing impairment have additional disabilities (Shepherd, et al., 1981). The percentage could be even higher, on the order of 26–30%, based on data from national surveys of young children with hearing impairment (SKI-HI Institute, 1994; see also Chapter 7). Improvements in medical science have resulted in the survival of more children with multiple disabilities. This underscores the need for a multidisciplinary approach to rehabilitation in which important professionals coordinate all services to ensure integrated treatment of the child. (See Chapter 11, Case 1, for an example in working with such a youngster.)

REHABILITATION SETTINGS AND PROVIDERS

AR settings and providers are determined to a great extent by the child's age, the severity of the hearing loss, and the presence of other handicapping conditions. Typically, services start as family-centered programs in the home coordinated by a parent advisor, and progress through preschool programs up through the formal school years. Throughout the rehabilitation process, the services of many professional disciplines are called upon in addition to continued strong parental involvement. Figure 8.1 contains an overview of the AR process as it relates to the roles of clinical audiologists, educators, and medical personnel.

IDENTIFICATION/ASSESSMENT PROCEDURES WITH CHILDREN

Early identification of children with hearing impairment or who are at risk for hearing impairment is critical for successful rehabilitation. Further, proper diagnosis requires precise and appropriate screening and assessment instruments, administered, scored, and interpreted by skilled professionals. The following sections will present prevailing trends in these areas as well as implications for amplification and the overall AR process.

Early Identification

As indicated previously, audiologic rehabilitation personnel are frequently involved in early identification of hearing loss. Naturally, early audiologic rehabilitation efforts cannot be initiated until the presence of hearing loss is known. The status of these

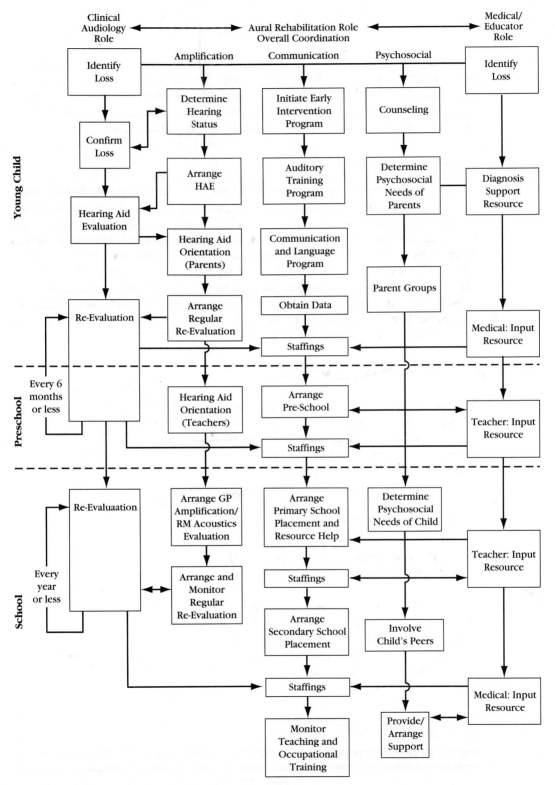

Figure 8.1 An overview of the AR process.

identification efforts is in a stage of rapid development and refinement, and methods are constantly being updated (White, Maxon, & Behrens, 1992). For example, universal hearing screening through use of two diagnostic tests has recently been recommended by the *Joint Committee on Infant Hearing* (1994). When universal screening is not available, high-risk registers (though only 50% effective) are considered the next best approach when used in connection with the birth and hospital stay of newborn children. In this approach, children with a high risk of hearing impairment are identified based on 10 risk factors, including (a) family history, (b) in utero infections such as rubella or cytomegalovirus, (c) anomalies of head or face, (d) low birthweight, (e) hyperbilirubinemia requiring transfusion, (f) ototoxic medications, (g) meningitis, (h) low Apgar scores, (i) mechanical ventilation of five days or longer signifying severe asphyxia, and (j) findings associated with a syndrome. Either the mother will check a maternal questionnaire indicating the presence of these high-risk factors or the mother and physician will note high-risk factors on the birth certificate. A list of high-risk infants can be extracted from the form or from the birth certificate by computer and be sent to the sponsoring agency for follow-up screening. About 15–20% of all infants are designated as being at high risk as a result of these processes (Watkins & Clark, 1993; Mahoney, 1984). Once children with a high risk are identified, diagnostic screening is used to determine whether or not a hearing loss actually exists. When it is established that a loss exists, early intervention efforts can begin.

Diagnostic screening procedures which can identify youngsters at an early age include two physiological methods used in the newborn nursery, auditory brainstem response (ABR), and otoacoustic emissions (OAE). With these techniques it is possible to determine if the baby's responses are consistent with those seen in youngsters with normal hearing. When responses are not normal, the child is rescheduled for full audiological diagnostic testing. This retest should occur preferably by three months of age, but not later than six months. The advantage of this early hospital screening is that no other occasion or place prompts such universal participation until the child enters school, when it is too late to be looking for congenital hearing loss.

Beyond these early screening efforts, some hearing losses in very young children are identified by physicians. Usually such identification is based upon the report of alert parents who notice that their child does not respond appropriately to sound or fails to develop speech and language at the expected time. When organized screening or high-risk programs are not available, attentive physicians and parents are the major sources for hearing-loss identification. The dimensions of the loss can subsequently be established through testing in an audiology clinic.

School Screening

Most children with severe hearing losses and some with milder losses are identified before they enter school. A number of children, however are not identified until they reach school age. Nearly all schools in the United States conduct a pure-tone hearing screening program beginning with kindergarten children or first-graders. Although the specifics of these programs vary, a good model has been recommended by the

American Speech-Language-Hearing Association (ASHA, 1985). Guidelines have also been published for the use of immittance audiometry in school screening (ASHA, 1990). Most children identified in school hearing-conservation programs demonstrate conductive hearing loss. The rehabilitation efforts, therefore, involve coordination with parents, medical practitioners, and teachers. Some children with previously unidentified sensorineural losses may also be identified in these school programs. In such cases, medical referral is indicated to clarify the medical aspects of the loss, followed by audiologic rehabilitation assistance provided by educational audiologists or other personnel.

Medical and Audiologic Assessment

Before audiologic rehabilitation is initiated, the child should undergo a medical examination as well as a basic hearing assessment. Complete, definitive results are not always available on very young children. When the child is old enough, results from such assessments should include information on both ears, giving: (a) otoscopic findings, (b) degree and configuration of loss, (c) type of loss and cause, (d) clarity of hearing (speech identification), (e) most comfortable level (MCL), and (f) threshold of discomfort (TD). Functional skills in the areas of academic achievement, language, and amplification systems should also be evaluated (Erber & Alencewicz, 1976; Roush & Matkin, 1994). Sometimes there is a tendency to omit certain aspects of testing, as, for example, speech recognition on youngsters with severe to profound losses, and sometimes there is a failure to consider hearing-aid insertion gain measures at all frequencies and at varying input levels.

Medical clearance becomes necessary when decisions about amplification are made. After initial hearing-aid fitting, regular assessments should take place even for children with sensorineural losses, since temporary conductive loss may occur and complicate the hearing situation, especially in young children (Ross & Tomassetti, 1988). Audiologic data should be obtained on a regular basis so that, if necessary, amplification or other dimensions of the rehabilitation program can be changed. In the early and preschool years, children should be seen for audiologic assessment at least every six months. After that they should be clinically tested at least once a year.

ASPECTS OF AUDIOLOGIC REHABILITATION: EARLY INTERVENTION/PARENT-INFANT AND PRESCHOOL

Rehabilitation Assessment

With children, the extensive rehabilitative assessments that generally precede management (see model in Chapter 1) are integrated with management more than with adult clients. Thus, we outline here an ongoing assessment approach to the audiologic rehabilitation of the young hearing-impaired child, beginning at the confirmation of the loss and continuing through the child's school years. Throughout the audiologic rehabilitation process, the dimensions and implications of the child's disability require constant diagnostic scrutiny. As suggested in the AR model (Chapter 1), the rehabilitation assessment includes (a) consideration of communication status, (b) associated variables, including psychosocial and educational issues, (c) related physical conditions and management landmarks, and (d) attitudes, especially of parents, toward management.

Management

Overall Coordination. FAMILY-CENTERED PRACTICES–AN ASSESSMENT AND INTERVENTION FRAMEWORK. In recent years there has been an increasing appreciation for the central role family relationships play in a child's development (Andrews & Andrews, 1986; Dunst, 1985; Fitzgerald & Fischer, 1987; Bailey, 1987). Many professionals contend that the young child cannot be effectively evaluated or instructed apart from the ecological system of the family (Bailey & Simeonsson, 1986). There is recognition that developmental influences are bidirectional: the infant's responses affect the family and the family's responses affect the infant. Recognition of the importance of these relationships on the child's development has led to interventions that focus on the child within the family system.

These concepts are not necessarily new to the field of audiologic rehabilitation. It has long been recognized in early-intervention programs for children with hearing impairment that parents are in the best position to provide models of language and auditory stimulation for their child throughout daily routines. In the 1970s, several home demonstration programs were established to guide parents of infants who are deaf in the early stimulation of language. These programs recognized the importance of capitalizing on optimal periods for language acquisition, and the value of taking advantage of the natural parent/child interactions of daily living to develop language and auditory skills. Model demonstration home programs were established in Nashville at the Bill Wilkerson Hearing and Speech Center, at the Central Institute for the Deaf in St. Louis, and at the Lexington School for the Deaf in New York. Another highly successful parent/infant program, the SKI-HI Model (Watkins & Clark, 1993), began in Utah in 1972. This program focused on the training of parent advisors who could provide home-based services to families of young deaf and hard of hearing children. Through its preparation of trainers model, the SKI-HI program developed a network of parent educators that has spanned 45 states and numerous rural communities. The John Tracy Clinic provided outreach guidance to parents through its correspondence courses. During this era, Dr. David Luterman developed an early-intervention program that focused primarily on the support needs of the family. Another unique program that evolved in the early 1970s was the Infant Hearing Resource in Portland, Oregon, which has played a major role in personnel preparation (both preservice and inservice) for parent infant intervention.

These forerunner programs continue to excel today. They have been joined by additional model programs. A text entitled *Infants and Toddlers with Hearing Loss: Family Centered Assessment and Intervention* (Roush & Matkin, 1994) describes these various model programs. A commonality of the majority of the models described in this text is their evolution over the years from an emphasis on child-centered practices to an emphasis on family-centered practices.

In the 1970s and 1980s, it was not uncommon for parent-infant programs to focus *primarily* on the needs of the child. Certainly, parent support was given in many ways, but the priority goals of early intervention dealt with child needs. Family members were actively involved in bringing about changes in the child's development. Parent advisors modeled activities that the parents could use to enhance their child's auditory, speech, and language skills. Parents were taught ways to interact with the child to enhance language learning. Professionals were seen as the "experts," who often were in the position of primary decision makers in the management of the child's audiologic rehabilitation program.

With the passage of PL 99-457 (now included in PL 101-476), emphasis on early-intervention programs for all children with special needs has shifted toward family-centered care. Two primary features characterize family-centered programs: (a) an emphasis on *family support* as a primary intervention goal, and (b) the expectation that families may select their level of involvement in decision making, program planning, and services (Winton & Bailey, 1994). Winton and Bailey describe family-centered programs as being willing "to develop a collaborative relationship with each family and to provide services in accordance with family values and priorities" (p. 24). Programs that are family centered recognize the central role that relationships play in development. Professionals respect the expertise and perspectives of families, and seek to establish balanced partnerships with parents. They employ naturalistic strategies and build relationships that lead to identification of family strengths and priorities (Dunst, 1985; Winton & Bailey, 1994; Harrison, 1994; Moeller & Condon, 1994).

A review of the literature reveals considerable theoretical support for family-centered practices in the field of audiologic rehabilitation.

CONSEQUENCES OF STRESS. Considerable evidence exists that familial stress has a negative impact on child development. Stress can alter the emotional availability of a parent and affect the caregiver style (Brofenbrenner, 1974). The period following diagnosis of a child's hearing loss is known to be stressful for parents with normal hearing. Quittner and Steck (1989) documented a high prevalence of stress in such parents of children who are deaf in their interviews of over 1000 families. Schlesinger and Acree (1984) identified a subset of parents of children with deafness who experienced little relief from stress over time. These parents reported that they felt *chronically powerless* to change their situation. In these families, the researchers found long-term negative consequences on the language and academic achievement of the children who are deaf in comparison to families where the parents felt empowered. Greenstein (1975) found that the affective state of the parent correlated more with the child's language acquisition than did technical aspects of the parental language input. White (1984) reported that maternal emotional states were reflected in mother's language expectations and interactional styles, which exerted long-term effects on the child. Prendergast (1994) found that hearing mothers who were "engaged" with their children who are deaf were better able to provide nurturing language input than parents who were "nonengaged." Collectively, these results point to the importance of programmatic components that promote the psychosocial health and well being of the family.

Greenberg (1983), in fact, documented the efficacy of a family-centered early-intervention program. His program, which included counseling and parent support groups, was successful in reducing familial stress in comparison to a group of families that received minimal intervention. Bailey (1987) noted that *support* is critical to family functioning. He added that families typically prefer informal sources of support and that it is the familial *perception* of support that is fundamental. In other words, a family may appear to have few support systems, but they may perceive themselves to be well supported. It is incumbent upon professionals to identify the family's perception of needs.

PARENT/CHILD LANGUAGE INTERACTIONS. Further justification for family-centered practices comes from the literature on parent/child interaction. The rate of language acquisition in young children has been found to be positively correlated with the extent to which parent language is contingent upon or responsive to the child's verbal and/or nonverbal behavior. (Barnes, Gutfreund, Satterly, & Wells, 1983; Masur, 1982; Tomasello & Farrar, 1986). Directiveness on the part of parents is negatively related to language development in children (Tomasello, Manle, & Kruger, 1986; Tomasello & Todd, 1983). Yet mothers with normal hearing have been found to be more intrusive, directive, and controlling of topics with their deaf children than mothers and children who both have normal hearing (Meadow, Greenberg, Erting, & Carmichael, 1981; Wedell-Monning & Lumley, 1980). Some evidence indicates that this trend can be reversed with family-centered training and support (Greenberg, Calderon, & Kusche, 1984; Luetke-Stahlman & Moeller, 1990). Several authors have also identified problems that parents with normal hearing have when signing to their children enrolled in total communication programs (Moeller & Luetke-Stahlman, 1990; Swisher & Thompson, 1985; Bornstein, Saulnier, & Hamilton, 1980). These authors have emphasized the need for family-centered sign training that is tailored to meet the communicative needs of parents and young children.

OPTIMAL PERIODS FOR LANGUAGE LEARNING. A final justification for family-centered practice comes from the recognition of infancy as an optimal and critical period for language learning (Boothroyd, 1982; Northern & Downs, 1991; Pinker, 1994). The goal is to capitalize, through early intervention and guidance of the child's primary interactants, on this important stage of development throughout routine interactions. Early amplification and intervention can lead to positive gains in speech and language in young children with hearing loss.

SUPPORT FROM EFFICACY STUDIES. Studies suggest that early intervention is effective in reducing the consequences of deafness on child language acquisition, and that significant language gains can result from training parents to be primary interventionists with infants (Herzog, 1985; Clark, 1994). Most professionals are strongly committed to the notion that parent training through early-intervention programs is effective and critical for children with hearing loss. However, objective documentation of the efficacy of early intervention is limited. Some of the most comprehensive efficacy data have come from a series of studies completed by the SKI-HI program in Utah.

Objective testing results on a large number of children enrolled in SKI-HI programs revealed that, on the average, these children make better language gains than would be predicted by maturation alone. They also consistently outdistance the performance of children who did not receive early intervention (Strong, et al., 1994). Moeller (1993) recently completed a longitudinal study of children with moderate to severe hearing losses, who were enrolled in a family-focused auditory-oral early-intervention program. Seven of the 10 subjects enrolled in this study made language gains in response to quality programming that allowed the children to enter kindergarten with language skills that approximated their chronological age. Appropriate amplification, parent guidance, and language intervention were highly effective in allowing these children who were hard of hearing to close the gap between their chronological and language ages prior to school entry. Table 8.1 summarizes additional findings from selected studies that explored the efficacy of early intervention for children with hearing impairment.

In the case of children in total communication programs, the role of the family is also critical. If family members do not receive early instruction so they can implement sign in the home, the child receives very inconsistent exposure to language input, and patterns of ineffective communication in the family can take root. Schick and Moeller (1992) reported on some positive language and literacy outcomes for children who were deaf and who received consistent input with total communication in the home from an early age.

The implications of these collective findings are clear. Environmental influences can have a significant impact on the child's development. Alleviation of stress in the family system will contribute to positive interactions and to a healthy language environment. Rehabilitative efforts that facilitate a nurturing interaction style between parent and child are likely to have long-term positive consequences for the child. Child-centered programs that fail to address the needs of the family system are likely to be of limited success.

SHIFTING ROLES IN THE AUDIOLOGIC REHABILITATION PROGRAM. As early-intervention programs work to implement PL 99-457, many are finding the need for program modification and reconceptualization of professional roles. Bernstein and Morrison (1992) surveyed 134 programs for children with hearing impairment and identified a lack of readiness in most programs to provide the comprehensive services required by the law. Brinker, Frazier, and Baxter (1992) stressed the need for programs to examine how family-focused care can best be approached with disadvantaged families. Winton and Bailey (1994) noted the lack of professional training for working with infants and families as a barrier to overcome in implementing family centered practices.

One of the most dramatic role shifts occurring in audiologic rehabilitation as a result of family centered practice goals is that decision-making authority is to rest with family members. Professionals are challenged to help parents gain the skills and knowledge to be effective advocates and decision-makers for their child. Previously, professionals made many of the decisions regarding the habilitative management of the child. Now professionals are being challenged to work as partners with families in assessment, management, and decision making. So, for example, in the parent

TABLE 8.1 *Summary of Selected Research on Efficacy of Early Intervention Programs for the Hearing Impaired*

Subjects	Results	Reference
30 deaf children enrolled in early intervention (EI) prior to age 2, followed until 40 months	Children enrolled prior to 16 months showed greater language competency than later enrollees: Their mothers were less coercive, more sensitive and accepting of the child.	Greenstein, J. (1975). *Methods of fostering language development in deaf infants. Final Report.* Bureau of Education for the Handicapped (DHEW/OE), Washington, DC. BBB00581.
33 H-I children receiving EI prior to 30 months as compared to 27 identified after 30 months and not yet treated	Group receiving early intervention was significantly better in use of residual hearing, auditory development, receptive and expressive language and parent involvement.	Clark, T. C. (1979). Language development through home intervention for infant H-I children. Unpublished doctoral dissertation. University of North Carolina.
24 deaf children in 2 groups:12 experimental (enrolled in comprehensive EI program) 12 control/comparison (enrolled in sporadic services)	Experimentals showed advanced communicative skills; mothers interacted in a more beneficial style and were more relaxed than controls: Parents experienced reduction of stress.	Greenberg, M., Calderon, and Kusche (1984). Early intervention using simultaneous communication with deaf infants: The effect on communication development. *Child Development,* 55 (2),607–616.
46 children who had completed the SKI-HI program and who were 6–13 years of age as matched with 46 children who had not received treatment	Home-intervention children were significantly higher than non-enrolled children on receptive and expressive language, academic achievement, speech and social-emotional skills—showing lasting effects.	Watkins, S. (1988). *Long-term effects of home intervention with h-i children. AAD 132 (4),* 267–271.
118 severe to profoundly H-I children in Ontario; ages 3, 4, and 5 followed for longitudinal evaluation	Study failed to obtain evidence of lasting gains associated with EI in infancy, intensified programming or direct instruction of parents. However, *qualitative* aspects of programming and parent instruction were not considered. The authors noted that general practice may not represent "best preactice" and may need to improve before objectives are achieved on a broad scale.	Musselman, C., Wilson, A., and Lindsay, P. (1988). *Effects of early intervention on hearing impaired children. Exceptional Children,* 55 (3), 222–228.

TABLE 8.1 *continued*

Subjects	Results	Reference
Evaluated effect of age of initial intervention on H-I children's academic, social-emotional and speech development	Early intervention was not associated with improved performance on any dependent measure.	Weisel, Amatzia (1990). Early intervention programs for hearing impaired children—evaluation of outcomes. *Early Child Development and Care, 41,* 77–87.
47 families of deaf children enrolled in a collaborative EI program designed to assist them in decision making (Project DEIP)	In contrast to families enrolled in a traditional EI program, project DEIP families selected intervention courses that were maintained successfully over time. Increased parental satisfaction with choice, and decrease in due process hearings were documented.	Moeller, M., Confal, K., and Hixson, P. (1990). The Efficacy of Speech-Language Pathology Interevntion: Hearing Impaired Children. *Seminars in Speech and Language,* 11 (4), 227–241.
1,934 H-I children from 97 sites of SKI-HI outreach home intervention program	1. SKI-HI children showed higher rates of development during intervention than prior to and greater gains in language than predicted by maturation alone. 2. SKI-HI children show enhanced auditory, communication and vocabulary skills and full-time hearing aid use. 3. SKI-HI parents were better able to manage hearing loss, communicated meaningfully with their children, and promoted cognitive development. 4. SKI-HI children were identified earlier than national norms and acquired services promptly ($\bar{x}$ age 19.9 months). 5. McConnel (1974) reported 20.8 months average language gains in 27.8 months of intervention in 94 preschoolers. SKI-HI demonstrated month for month gains.	Strong, Carol, J. and Clark, Thomas C. (1992). *Project SKI-HI outreach programming for hearing impaired infants and families: recertification statement, questions, responses, and approval.* Research in Education, January 1992. Department of Education, Washington, DC. EDD00001.

TABLE 8.1 *continued*

Subjects	Results	Reference
Site visitation and interviews of 23 well-established programs for HI-examined for compliance with P.L. 99-457	States interviewed complied with 99-457. At considerable expense they developed parent/infant component, increased staff development, added space, developed interagency networks. They reported increased prevalence of multi-handicapped and minority students, yet had few minority staff. Increased use of ASL observed.	Nober, E. and Nober, L. (1992). *New and Innovative Educational Directions for Young HI Children in the U.S.* Paper presented at the Annual CEC Convention, Baltimore, MD. ED 346705.
5,178 Children enrolled in project SKI-HI.	Children made one month of language gain for every month of intervention. The rate of language development during intervention was nearly twice the rate of development prior to intervention.	Strong, Clark, Barringer, Walden, and Williams (1992).
10 pre-school children with moderately severe hearing losses followed longitudinally.	7 of the 10 children attained language syntax skills commensurate with hearing peers by kindergarten entry. Learning rates allowed the children to overcome early delays. The children had optimal amplification.	Donaghy, K., M. P., and Carney, A. (1994). *Auditory, language and phonological skills in hard-of-hearing preschoolers.* ASHA Convention, New Orleans, LA.

advisor-family partnership, the parent advisor relies on family members to direct the thrust of the services. The young child's needs are expressed as part of the family's concerns. Family members know the child's likes, dislikes, time schedules, favorite toys and activities, food preferences, and many other matters that the parent advisor can't be expected to know. One mother stated, "The advisor I worked with was wise enough to know that no one knows my child better than I do. She respected my suggestions and opinions as much as I respected hers" (Glover, Watkins, Pittman, Johnson, & Barringer, 1996; p. 323). As the parent advisor-family partnership develops and as respect and trust mature, the parent advisor has the opportunity to help family members explore their feelings, clarify their concerns and desires for the child, and see and appreciate the child's unique skills and strengths. Other examples of collaborative decision-making with parents are contained in Chapter 11 (see Case 2).

A second major shift in service delivery influences the roles of the AR clinician. In order to meet comprehensive family and child needs, professionals must employ transdisciplinary teamwork. No one discipline has all the knowledge and expertise to adequately address the comprehensive nature of most cases. The AR clinician in a parent-advisor role has a particularly critical role on the team. Because the parent advisor has frequent contact with the family in their home (e.g. one to two times per week), this professional is often in a good position to gain a full understanding of the family's strengths and priorities, and to work with the parent to implement strategies to achieve these priorities. The parent advisor may also serve in a role of case coordination with the assistance of a Services Coordinator.

The parent advisor/AR clinician can and should draw upon the resources of a community-based team of professionals, depending on the needs that present themselves. Parent advisors need to cultivate the skills for collaborative consultation and teamwork in order to effectively serve families. Idol, Paolucci-Whitcomb, and Nevin (1986) state, "Collaborative consultation is an interactive process that enables teams of people with diverse expertise to generate creative solutions to mutually defined problems. The outcome is enhanced and altered from the original solutions that any team member would produce independently" (p. 9).

IMPLICATIONS OF FAMILY-CENTERED INTERVENTION FOR ASSESSMENT PRACTICES. Extensive and ongoing assessment of a child's needs is fundamental to pediatric audiologic rehabilitation (see model in Chapter 1). Assessment is critical for determining priority intervention needs, determining outcomes, and ascertaining the most efficacious approaches. Assessment practices have been expanded in some of the following ways as a result of early intervention mandates:

1. Ongoing assessment by a transdisciplinary team leads to the development of an *Individual Family Services Plan* (IFSP). The IFSP is like a road map for intervention, and it requires a broadened approach to assessment. The IFSP process requires that the AR team describe the infant's present levels of development across several domains (e.g. physical/motor, cognitive, speech/language, psychosocial, and self-help). Importantly, the IFSP process also requires that professionals identify the family's strengths and needs that are related to the development of the infant (Harrison, 1994). In addition, the document must outline the major outcomes that are

expected for the child *and* the family. This broadened focus on family issues requires modification of traditional child-centered assessment approaches. In many states, service coordinators assist team members in identifying family needs (which can be as encompassing as housing or financial support) and in coordinating the various professional disciplines working with the child. The AR specialist serves as a vital member of this professional team and has significant roles in identifying intervention priorities for the child and the parents. The AR clinician should be particularly attuned to identifying informal sources of support that the family values.

2. Professionals should observe and understand family interactions and needs before advising and instructing (Moeller & Condon, 1994). In earlier years, the audiologic rehabilitation specialist might start intervention without a thorough understanding of how the family and child interact. Clinicians would begin with session one advising parents on techniques for interaction with their child who is deaf. Current practices dictate the need to observe the interactions between the parents and child to determine strengths that exist that can be built upon. In most cases, parents have discovered effective and nurturing ways to interact with their babies. When professionals recognize those strengths in interactions and point them out, the parent may recognize, "Oh, I *do* have some skills to meet the challenges ahead." On the other hand, parents have reported a loss of confidence in their abilities when professionals begin to "teach" them how to interact (Moeller & Condon, 1994). The implication for assessment is the need to be a good observer, who respects the expertise and strategies of the family members. Rather than "expert advice-giver," the AR clinician acts more like a good listener and observer and, later, as a coach.

3. Clinicians need to evaluate the child within the ecological system of the family (Dunst, 1985; Ensher, 1989; Sparks, 1989). In order to involve family members in the assessment process, it is necessary for the AR clinician to select ecologically valid assessment procedures. Ecologically valid assessments include naturalistic contexts, involve focus on child and parent interactions, and recruit the perspectives and observations of significant individuals in the family system. Many tools have recently become available that support the AR clinician in implementing ecologically valid assessments (Stredler-Brown & Yoshinaga-Itano, 1994; Moeller & Condon, 1994).

4. Clinicians must respect the decision-making authority of the family (Bailey, 1987). This premise is particularly relevant to the process of determining the optimal mode of communication for a child with hearing impairment. The process of making this important decision should be one of collaborative problem solving between the family and clinicians (Moeller & Condon, 1994; Moeller, Coufal, & Hixson, 1990). Bailey (1987) notes, "problem-solving is an important skill in any professional, yet it can be counterproductive if applied too early in a goal-setting endeavor, especially if done for the clients rather than with them" (p. 64). The question as to what communication system/mode is best for a family (i.e., oral, total communication, American Sign Language, Cued Speech, Bilingualism-American Sign Language, or signed English) needs to be discussed from the outset and throughout the early intervention period. Parents need to be given objective information on their choices, and on strategies that appear to be most successful for their young child. The Boys Town National Research Hospital has implemented a program called the Diagnostic Early Intervention Project

(DEIP), which is dedicated to helping parents learn and objectively discover what approaches work best for the child and family before deciding on modes or placements (Moeller & Condon, 1994; Moeller, Coufal, & Hixson, 1990). Figure 8.2 shows a schematic model of the stages in the DEIP process. Within this process, there is an openness between the clinician and family to explore options on a continuum and determine objectively which option will best meet the presenting needs. The team and parents collect objective data on family concerns, audiological variables (learning rate in auditory training, amplification success), communication variables (rate of phonological learning, rate of language development), learning variables (play and cognition, learning styles), and medical/genetic issues (presence of additional disabilities) to aid in decision making. Each child and family is unique, with an individualized profile of strengths and needs. Thus, the team avoids a "one size fits all" approach, and rather explores various approaches to determine the "best fit" that will lead to communicative success.

The SKI-HI program also has an excellent home-based program to enable families to make appropriate communication methodology choices. A series of discussions is available for the parent advisor and family to use as they explore different communication methodology options. The discussions include information about the various methodologies as well as suggested activities and supplemental readings. Parent advisors and family members together observe, document, explore, and discuss a variety of child and family factors that are important to consider as they make methodology choices. After a communication methodology decision has been reached, SKI-HI programming resources are available in all communication methodology areas (including Bilingualism) that will promote the child's and family's communication interaction in that methodology.

TEAM STAFFINGS. The specific intervention priorities for a particular family are determined as part of the IFSP process. The clinician and parent will regularly monitor the infant's progress by collecting data in such areas as hearing-aid usage and adjustment, auditory development, vocabulary growth, receptive and expressive language accomplishments, and phonological development. With such information as a basis, team staffings can be held every three to six months to discuss progress monitoring and adjust strategies as needed. At the staffings, perspectives can be shared from other disciplines, such as psychology, pediatrics, audiology, education, as well as other professions involved with the family. The goals of the staffings are to tailor programs to meet the needs of individual children and families.

IMPLICATIONS OF FAMILY-CENTERED CARE FOR INTERVENTION. Family centered parent-infant programs, then, focus on family members as the primary interventionists. The audiologic rehabilitation specialist provides guidance and coaching to the family in several key content areas: (a) fitting and adjustment of amplification and assistive devices; (b) auditory learning (use of residual hearing); and (c) techniques for optimizing communicative development (speech, language, signing, cognitive, and preliteracy skills). Another vital content area for the program is helping the family meet their support

DEIP Management Schedule

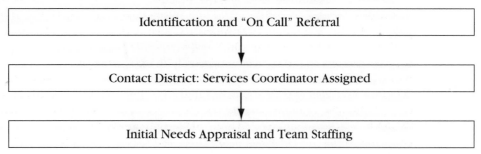

DEIP Management Schedule

| Identification and "On Call" Referral |
| Contact District: Services Coordinator Assigned |
| Initial Needs Appraisal and Team Staffing |

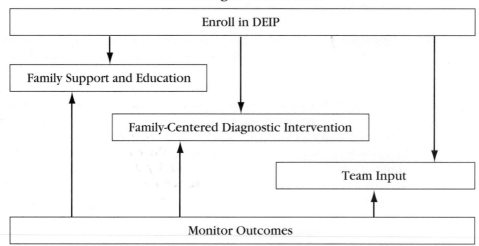

DEIP Management Schedule

| Enroll in DEIP |
| Family Support and Education |
| Family-Centered Diagnostic Intervention |
| Team Input |
| Monitor Outcomes |

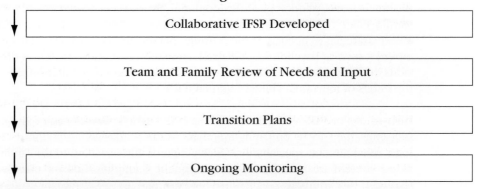

DEIP Management Schedule

| Collaborative IFSP Developed |
| Team and Family Review of Needs and Input |
| Transition Plans |
| Ongoing Monitoring |

Figure 8.2 Diagnostic early-intervention project model

Moeller, Coufal, & Hixson (1990)

needs and providing activities that promote psychosocial well-being. Once the child is of preschool age (around three years old), services typically shift to center-based models where the child attends a preschool. These services are commonly provided in a self-contained program for children who are deaf and hard of hearing, in a reverse-integrated preschool deaf program, in a special-needs multi-categorical classroom, or in a regular preschool program with support services from an AR specialist. Wherever the service delivery or whatever the model, family-centered practices continue to be vital. Families learn at the parent-infant level to be knowledgeable advocates for their children. They become intricately involved in impacting on the child's success. It would be a mistake to "graduate" the child into a center-based program and minimize the contributions family members can make. Instead, programs should continue to address family needs, family support, and family guidance into the preschool years. In the next sections we describe approaches in each of the key content areas at the parent-infant and preschool levels.

Amplification/Assistive Device Issues. HEARING-AID FITTING. Once preliminary medical and audiologic findings are available on the child, the selection of amplification, when appropriate, becomes an early goal in the rehabilitative program. Many experts agree that hearing aids are extremely important tools in early-intervention programs in helping children develop their residual hearing and their speech and language abilities (e.g., Ross, Bracket, & Maxon, 1991). Unfortunately, as previously noted, many youngsters with hearing impairment do not typically use amplification (Matkin, 1984; Shepherd, et al., 1981); consequently, the efforts of the audiologic rehabilitationist may need to be directed toward achieving that goal. The hearing-aid fitting will be performed by an audiologist who may also be providing other rehabilitative services (see Figure 8.1). If the AR therapist does not perform the fitting, he or she will want to review its adequacy. In recent years, the focus in fitting children has been to move away from procedures based on threshold to those focusing more on how the amplified-speech range fits into the child's usable hearing range. The Desired Sensation Level (DSL) method is an example of this latter approach and is reviewed in Chapter 2. Although hearing-aid fitting is a first priority, other assistive amplification devices should also be considered, such as auditory training equipment for the older child.

TYPE AND ARRANGEMENT OF AID. The type of aid (ear-level or body) and the arrangement (monaural, binaural, or other special fitting, such as a direct input feature or integrated FM capability) need careful attention and review in the AR process.

Behind-the-ear (BTE) aids are used by most children from infancy through the teenage years (Bentler, 1993). A 1990 survey indicated that 84% of audiologists recommend BTE aids for children two years of age or younger while the remainder fit body aids all or part of the time (Schow, et al., 1993). Ear-level instruments allow a binaural advantage and the elimination of clothing noise, but sometimes they are subject to severe feedback problems. According to several authorities (Matkin 1984; Ross, et al., 1991) body-type aids should be reserved for use with youngsters having such feedback problems or with certain children having profound impairments, infants and toddlers with small pinnas or congenital atresia, or children with major motor deficits who cannot manage aids by themselves. However, some experts report a strong preference for body aids when fitted on young children with severe and profound losses (Madell, 1984). Some children, especially teenagers, use in-the-ear/canal aids. While requiring special adjustment, these are feasible for use by certain individuals. Curran (1985) found that in-the-ear (ITE) aids when used were recommended for 13- to 18-year-olds with mild hearing losses.

If an ear-level aid is utilized, evidence should justify the selection of the ear(s) to be aided and the reasons for a monaural or binaural fitting. (See a discussion of these factors in Chapter 2, which covers hearing-aid fitting procedures, and in Ross, et al., 1991.) From a rehabilitative standpoint, binaural fittings are nearly always the rule, since children with hearing impairment require every educational advantage possible. Unfortunately, the minority of hearing-impaired children with bilateral losses are using binaural aids. Various reports place this minority at somewhere between 20% and 40% (Shepard, et al., 1981; Bentler, 1993). Even after a careful analysis to eliminate the children with bilateral losses who were not candidates for a second aid, Matkin (1984) found that only 38% of the children who could use two aids were doing so.

If children are found to have little usable residual hearing or serious progressive loss, cochlear implants may be considered (see Chapter 2). Promising results with children who have been implanted are leading to an increased use of these implants, which have now been used on well over 3000 children between the ages of 2 and 17 years since the FDA approved such use beginning in June 1990. Implant device surgery is very expensive, and when children are implanted, extensive audiologic rehabilitation follow-up is needed.

HEARING-AID FEATURES. Several features of the hearing aid should be specified in the assessment/fitting process. These include: (a) frequency response, (b) gain, (c) saturation sound pressure level (SSPL), (d) battery to be used, and (e) provision of a telephone switch and/or direct audio input. The last item is generally advisable for youngsters with hearing impairment since they may be placed in a situation or use equipment where induction-loop amplification is utilized, necessitating reception to come through the telephone mode. In the hearing-aid assessment, the audiologist will specify the type of instrument to be procured along with the desired features of the aids.

Ling (1989) recommended that children with profound hearing impairment should have amplification that provides some gain below 300 Hz so that they can hear suprasegmental information (intensity, duration, pitch, stress, rhythm) and some important vowel formants. He cautioned that the amount of gain at 200–300 Hz should be 30–40 dB less than that provided at 2000–3000 Hz, to avoid masking effects of low-frequency environmental noise.

After the fitting process just described, the child should be seen again by the clinical audiologist. The AR provider should encourage such hearing-aid rechecks and ask the audiologist to provide the following information at both hearing-aid rechecks and periodic reassessments.

1. *Earmold fit and gain setting of aid.* With very young or fast-growing children, the earmold will need to be changed frequently to ensure a well-fitting mold and to provide adequate gain without feedback. Turning the gain down will help eliminate the feedback, but it is an unacceptable long-term solution. The therapist should not rely entirely on the clinical audiologist or the dispenser for this assessment, but should personally monitor the earmold condition on each rehabilitation visit. In some situations, the audiologic rehabilitationist is trained to make ear impressions. This can be a valuable asset to the program, especially considering the frequency of mold changes in an adequate program (see Table 8.2).

2. *Sound-field assessment of hearing aid.* Testing the child in a sound field, with his or her own hearing aid(s) at the normal use setting as well as other settings, gives practical information about the performance of the amplification. Sound-field data usually include unaided and aided findings on speech-reception threshold, speech recognition, warble tone thresholds, and thresholds of discomfort. Unfortunately, Matkin (1984) found that many clinics do very little aided testing with young children.

3. *Real-ear measures.* More precise information on aided results can be obtained with real-ear measures, which provide more accurate and complete information roughly equivalent to sound-field thresholds (see Chapter 2). Real-ear measures can be made with and without the aid in place, and at different input levels above threshold. They make it possible to evaluate benefit from the aid thoroughly without requiring more than passive cooperation from the child. Although the equipment to conduct these measurements is expensive, more and more audiologists are making this service available to their clients. Recent survey results show that approximately one-half of USA audiologists now use real-ear measures at some time during the assessment and fitting process (Schow, et al., 1993).

4. *Electroacoustic assessment of aid.* An electroacoustic check of the hearing aid should provide information on the frequency response, the gain, the SSPL, and the distortion of the instrument (see Chapter 2 for a description of this process). These data can help uncover inadequacies in the amplification that can otherwise be devastating to the child's progress in the rehabilitation program. Electroacoustic checks are particularly helpful in the case of distortions, which are not found in the sound-field or real-ear tests, and when biologic listening checks do not reveal a distortion problem. Additional information that may come from the electroacoustic assessment includes the degree of nonlinearity of the gain control (each notch on the control usually will not produce an equal increment of gain) and the instrument's internal signal-to-noise ratio (S/N). This is also called *equivalent input noise* (Ln).

5. *Five-sound test of aid.* In connection with hearing-aid adjustment, it may be helpful for the AR therapist to use the five-sound test described by Ling (1989). According to Ling, the sounds /u/, /a/, /i/, /ʃ/, and /s/ can be used to determine the effectiveness of an aid. With the infant, visually reinforced audiometry can be used to determine if the child can hear these sounds. Older children can simply indicate they hear the sounds. According to Ling, if the child has measurable residual hearing up to 1000 Hz, she should be able to hear all three vowel sounds when they are spoken in a quiet voice at a distance of five yards. If the child has measurable hearing up to 2000

TABLE 8.2 *Average Months per Set of Earmolds for Children Whose Molds Were Replaced at the First Evidence Of Feedback Difficulty[a]*

	Average Months per Mold	
Degree of Loss	<2 ½-year-old child *(N=25)*	2 ½-to 5-year old child *(N=27)*
Mild (30–55 dB)	3.0	5.2
Moderate (56–75 dB)	2.7	4.1
Severe (76–90 dB)	2.5	5.6
Profound (91–110 dB)	2.0	4.6

Reprinted by permission: SKI-HI data.

[a]Also included are average loss and gain values for children in total project (N=52) with properly fitting molds. Mean loss pure tone average (PTA), 75dB; mean aided loss, 44 dB; mean gain, 31 dB.

or 4000 Hz, she should be able to hear the /ʃ/ and /s/ sounds, respectively, at a distance of one to two yards. Ling indicates that a sixth sound, /m/, can also be helpful in measuring the presence of audition in the range around 250 Hz. Either the five- or six-sound test can also facilitate adjustment of the aid's frequency response.

HEARING-AID ORIENTATION. It is helpful for parents, teachers, school personnel, and other involved professionals to be knowledgeable about the auditory mechanism and hearing. This information can be provided in home visits, in clinic counseling sessions, in parent groups, and through inservice training in the school setting. The following subjects could be discussed:

1. Function, anatomy, and measurement of hearing.
2. Type of loss and effect on child; need for hearing aid.
3. Parts and function of hearing aid.
4. Care, placement, and volume setting of hearing aid.
5. Daily listening checks and earmold checks; troubleshooting of malfunctioning aid.
6. Obtaining loaner hearing aids, batteries, hearing aid parts, new earmolds, repairs.

Abundant printed material is available for use in giving such instruction (see Chapter 2, and "Resource Materials" in Chapter 13). Both parents and professionals may need several exposures to certain aspects of the presentation. Thus, studies have shown that parents often complain that they were never instructed about hearing-aid use, even though dealers and clinical audiologists claim to have given such instruction (Blair, Wright, & Pollard, 1981; Gaeth & Lounsbury, 1966).

The benefit of hearing-aid use may not be readily obvious to parents, especially in cases where auditory communication is minimal. The purposes of hearing-aid use may include some or all of the following: verbal communication, signal or warning function, and environmental awareness (Ramsdell, 1978). Parents must recognize why their child is wearing an aid, since with younger children, parents have the major responsibility for maintaining the aid and ensuring that it is used regularly. If parents

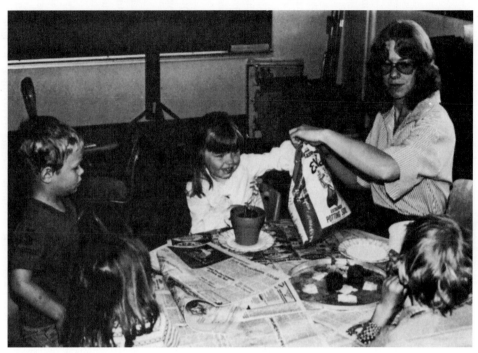

Preschool Classroom of hearing-impaired youngsters.

understand hearing aids, they will be encouraged to help their child form good habits of use.

The aid will be more acceptable to the child when it functions properly, but the procedures for obtaining hearing-aid accessories, repairs, or loaners will vary with local conditions. The AR provider should be aware of these conditions in order to be an effective resource person.

Communication Rehabilitation. AUDITORY LEARNING: PARENT-INFANT AND PRESCHOOL LEVELS. There are many natural opportunities in the home setting for exposing the child to sound. Once the child is fitted with appropriate amplification, the parents and clinician work to provide meaningful and frequent auditory experiences to encourage the child to rely on his or her residual hearing. For many children, systematic introduction to sounds during the early years will have a positive impact on language learning. Effective stimulation of residual hearing is critical to the development of spoken communication (Erber, 1982; Ling, 1976; Ling, 1978; Boothroyd, 1982). Early auditory-learning training should consist of observing and promoting the child's listening experiences in many meaningful daily activities. As Marlowe (1984) recommended, the clinician should "stress listening to people sounds rather than environmental sounds unless the latter are incorporated in meaningful experiences" (p. 6).

A variety of materials have been developed that describe auditory skill development. Erber (1982) developed a particularly useful model that distinguishes between

TABLE 8.3 Auditory Skill Development Sequence

Auditory Skills	Child's Behavior	Stimulation Skills
1. Attending/Detection	Child attends to environmental sounds and voices. Child attends to distinct speech sounds.	Use auditory clues, show child sources of sound. Focus on highly communicative sounds (e.g. food preparation; bath noises; hearing name called).
2. Recognizing	Child recognizes objects and events from their sounds.	Point out sounds and reinforce child's recognition of sources. Allow sound to be child's first source of information. Contrive opportunities for child to respond to meaningful sounds and associate them with sources.
3. Locating	Child locates sound sources in space.	Create localization opportunities and reinforce all child attempts to localize. Recognize that localization gives clues to the sound's source and meaning. Involve child in social games like "hide and seek" to develop localization.
4. Distances and Levels	Child locates sound sources at increased distances and above and below.	Create opportunities for child to hear sounds above, below, and at distances; reinforce child's responses. Use distance listening games to help child tune "selective attention" to sound.
5. Environmental Discrimination, Identification, and Comprehension	Child discriminates, identifies, and comprehends environmental sounds.	Repeatedly stimulate the child with meaningful environmental sounds and reinforce child's discrimination, identification, and comprehension of sounds. Tie these sounds to natural communication routines.
6. Vocal Discrimination, Identification, and Comprehension	Child discriminates, identifies, and comprehends gross vocal sounds, words, and phrases.	Provide natural opportunities for child to discriminate, identify, and comprehend onomatopoeic sounds, words, and phrases. Present contrasting verbal signals within playful social routines.
7. Speech Discrimination, Identification, and Comprehension	Child discriminates, identifies, and comprehends fine speech sounds: vowels, then consonants.	Provide stimulation of vowel, then consonant sounds in meaningful words and situations. Create opportunities for child to demonstrate discrimination, identification, and comprehension of these words.

levels of detection, discrimination, identification, and comprehension (a complete discussion of Erber's model is contained in Chapter 3). Table 8.3 contains a related description of a sequence of listening skills and techniques parents can use to develop these skills. Parents need not see these as discrete, sequential stages; however, it is helpful for them to be aware of a general hierarchy and that some skills will develop later than others. Detailed suggestions for how to help an infant or a preschool child develop auditory skills can be found in Watkins and Clark (1993); Erber (1982); Hasenstab and Horner (1982); Cole (1992); Ling and Ling (1978); and Stein, Benner, Hoversten, McGinnis, and Thies (1980).

Teachers and clinicians in the preschool setting can also take advantage of natural opportunities to encourage the children to rely on their residual hearing. It is common for clinicians in preschool settings to integrate auditory challenges throughout curriculum lessons. Rather than specifying a "listening lesson" or "listening time," clinicians integrate auditory learning as a process that pervades all activities. This can be challenging in a total communication program, where the focus is on visual learning. Clinicians in TC settings need to make a conscious effort to provide realistic auditory challenges to the child that support other communicative goals. Erber's (1982) concept of adaptive auditory skill development is very useful at the preschool level. This concept implies that a clinician constantly is monitoring a child's level of success with a particular auditory contrast or task, and adjusting the task as necessary to bring about successive approximation to the goal.

An innovative auditory development curriculum for the preschool and school-age level recently has been developed by an interdisciplinary team at the University of Miami and the Dade County Public Schools Model Program. This unique program (entitled the Miami CHATS curriculum) is a comprehensive curriculum, that integrates goals for cochlear implant, hearing aid, or tactile aid users. The goals of the curriculum are to provide professionals with a systematic guide to the integration of sensory aids to facilitate the ability of the child with hearing impairment to produce and comprehend oral communication (Vergara, 1994).

It is important for AR clinicians to fit auditory-skill development within a conceptual model of speech and language learning. For many children with hearing loss, the auditory channel is viable for language learning, given appropriate amplification and stimulation. Boothroyd (1982) and Ling (1976) stress the primacy of the auditory channel for speech and language learning. Throughout the course of development, the AR clinician should closely integrate listening goals with those of speech and language learning. For example, a preschool child learning to discriminate temporal patterns should also be working on production of the appropriate number of syllables in simple word approximations. The child learning to detect sounds should have opportunities to answer in a socially appropriate manner when his or her name is called. A child with residual hearing benefits from auditory-based correction when a speech error is made. Ling (1976) stresses the importance of helping the child establish an auditory-feedback loop. That is, auditory skills need to develop to the point where the child can self-monitor his speech productions through audition. These goals are realistic for many children with appropriate amplification. Language, audition, and phonological acquisition are intricately related processes, that should be addressed in an integrated fashion. Rather than "auditory training" the notion is "auditory learning" or "auditory communication" (Cole, 1992). For some children, progress toward auditory goals will be slow, due to limitations of residual hearing. Alternative sensory communication devices may be considered by the team in these cases.

Documentation of learning rates in audition is useful in selecting intervention approaches and in ascertaining the need for additional sensory aids. Dillon and his colleagues described a Goal Attainment Scaling Procedure used with adults to ascertain the efficacy of various devices or approaches (Dillon, et al., 1991). Moeller (1993) adapted this approach for use with infants and preschoolers. The scaling approach allows the AR clinician to systematically track the child's progress across different goals and situations. Table 8.4 illustrates an example of this procedural adaptation. It is also relevant for the AR clinician to carefully monitor changes in a child's phonological development. Substantive changes in vocal and phonological behaviors are often indicators of auditory learning. Oller (1983) cites the onset of true babbling as a critical benchmark, typically observed from 7–10 months of age in normally developing infants. Often, the babbling stage is delayed in children who are deaf (Oller & Eilers, 1988).

COMMUNICATION/LANGUAGE STIMULATION: PARENT-INFANT.   At the same time that auditory-skill development is being initiated in the home, the clinician helps parents build upon their communication strategies with the child. Effective interaction between parent and child is fundamental to the process of language acquisition. The communicative interaction between the child and family members is a primary focus of parent-infant rehabilitation.

When parents and professionals team together in a partnership, intervention can proceed in a fashion of joint discovery (Schuyler & Rushmer, 1987; Moeller & Condon, 1994). During home intervention sessions, the child is engaged in stimulating activities, and the parent and clinician actively monitor the child's responses and adjust techniques as necessary. Family members also receive guidance, information, and support during home visits. The SKI-HI home visit program (see Figure 8.3) is an excellent example of a model that includes a comprehensive management approach.

When the home is the primary intervention setting, the parent advisor and parent use the natural environment and daily events as the milieu for teaching. As much as possible, parents, siblings, and other significant persons in the child's life are encouraged to be "in the driver's seat" in the intervention sessions. Instead of bringing an adult-directed lesson plan with demonstration activities, the parent advisor and parent take advantage of natural interaction situations to practice the provision of nurturing input for the child. For example, a parent advisor might take advantage of the siblings' affinity for a "ring around the rosy" game to emphasize the skill of sound detection for the deaf toddler. A toddler's feeding time can become an ideal time for reinforcing prelinguistic communicative signals and strengthening turn taking. Reinforcing toddler games and toys can also be introduced to encourage language and thinking, but they should not be the primary focus. Parents are supported when language- and auditory-intervention schemes can fit into the rhythm and habits of their daily lives. Parents may need help to discover that it is their "all-day-long"

TABLE 8.4 *Examples of Goal Attainment Scaling with Infant Auditory Goals from IFSP*

Auditory Goals from IFSP

A. Child will respond meaningfully to common environmental sounds.
B. Child will spontaneously alert when name is called.
C. Child will respond with appropriate action to simple, functional commands.
D. Child will respond to functional phrases in distracting environments.
E. Child will wear hearing aids full waking hours.

Specific Goal Accomplishment

Goal	A	B	C	D	E	Comments 3/93
Always						E-hearing aid use is problem at day care
Most of the Time	✓				✓	microwave, door knock, bath water garage opener, dog
Half of the Time			✓			Come here, no no, stop, yeah!!!
Occasionally		✓		✓		Needs to be in listening set
Never						

Taking the *primary listening situations* from the IFSP goals, rate the child's current responses in the targeted listening environments (See attached example).

Child responds to

	Sounds at Home		Calling Name		Functional Phrases		Functional Phrases		Wears Hearing Aids	
	Alert	I.D.	Close	Distant	1 to 1	Group	DayCare	Church	Home	Sitter
Always										
Most of the Time										
Half of the Time										
Occasionally										
Never										
Not Applicable										

Proposed by Moeller, BTNRH (1993)
×-×-× = 3/93   •—•—• = 9/93

routine interactions with the child that build language skills (Simmons-Martin & Rossi, 1990), not structured "sit-down" therapy activities. Language and auditory intervention strategies need to fit within the context of natural, positive parenting.

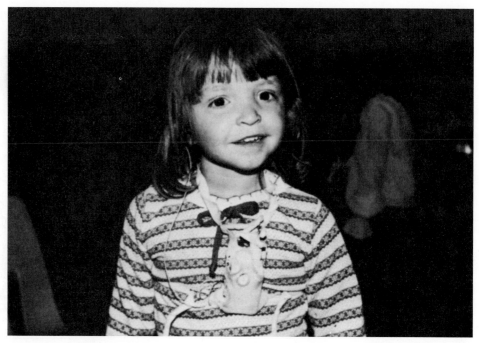

A preschool child equipped with amplifcation for classroom.

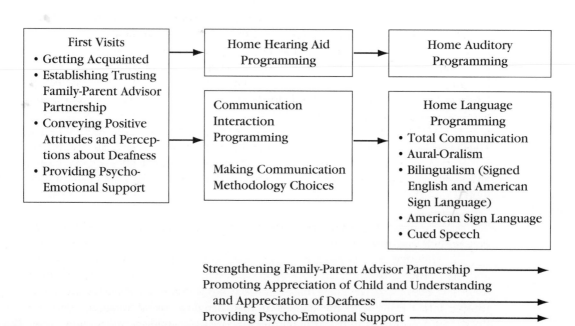

First Visits	Home Hearing Aid Programming	Home Auditory Programming
• Getting Acquainted • Establishing Trusting Family-Parent Advisor Partnership • Conveying Positive Attitudes and Perceptions about Deafness • Providing Psycho-Emotional Support	Communication Interaction Programming Making Communication Methodology Choices	Home Language Programming • Total Communication • Aural-Oralism • Bilingualism (Signed English and American Sign Language) • American Sign Language • Cued Speech

Strengthening Family-Parent Advisor Partnership —————▶
Promoting Appreciation of Child and Understanding
    and Appreciation of Deafness —————————▶
Providing Psycho-Emotional Support ———————▶

Figure 8.3 SKI-HI home visit programming.

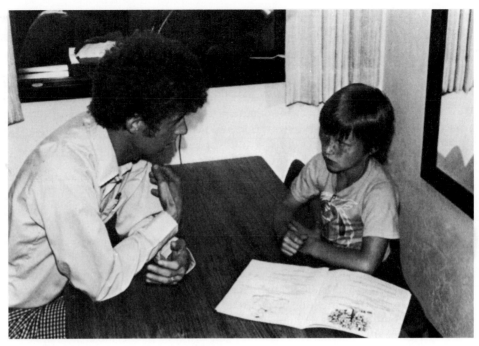

Individual therapy combining attention to language acquisition and auditory training.

A primary focus of the intervention program is promoting nurturing and effective interactions between the parents and the infant. Although mothers of children who are deaf have been described as being overly controlling in interactions with their children, there are many examples in clinical practice of parents who interact in highly facilitative ways with their infants who are deaf and hard of hearing. Perhaps family-centered practices will result in different characterizations of maternal and paternal styles. Some parents will need direct guidance to develop facilitative styles with their infants. However, the parent advisor should not assume this to be the case. There may be many strengths that can be built upon in the parent-child interaction.

During home intervention sessions, the parents and parent advisor work together to implement nondirective language stimulation approaches. Some primary techniques include:

1.   Ensuring that family members recognize the infant or toddler's prelinguistic communication signals (e.g. gestures, vocalizations, eye gaze, cries, points, etc.).

2.   Helping parents interpret communication signals as conversational "turns" and then provide semantically appropriate responses, such as comments or expansions. For example, if the child reaches for the bottle and vocalizes, does the parent recognize that this was a complex signal? How does the parent respond? Optimally, the parent will interpret the child's intention and put the child's idea into words (e.g., "Oh, you want more milk. Here's your bottle.").

3. Facilitating the establishment of conversational turn-taking between primary interactants and the child. Are family members following the child's interest and conversational lead? How does the child respond when family members follow his lead? What activities promote extended turn-taking?

4. Helping parents consider the need to contrive developmentally appropriate opportunities for the child to respond to auditory stimuli in the environment. When the child responds to meaningful sounds, how does the family react? Do they comment on the child's observation and give the sound a name? Do they take the child to the sound and reinforce that it is the source of the sound?

5. Guiding the parents in taking advantage of everyday occurrences to expose the child to relevant language concepts. What language concepts occur naturally and are of interest to the child? What is the child curious about? Primary language targets become evident from observing typical interactions and also from following the child's interest lead.

6. Guiding family members to provide the words for what a child is trying to express (Cole, 1992). This involves helping family members to be accurate interpreters of the child's message and then providing the verbal model for that message.

7. Helping family members develop positive ways to secure and maintain the child's visual attention. Joint attention on objects is positively correlated with vocabulary acquisition in young children (Tomasello & Farrar, 1986). Some evidence suggests that hearing mothers may not always use the most facilitative strategies for securing joint attention on objects (Prendergast, 1994). Deaf mothers of children who are deaf have been observed to implement effective strategies in this regard. Further study of approaches by parents who are deaf would provide useful input for working with parents with normal hearing.

8. Helping family members use parallel talk strategies that describe what the child is doing, seeing or thinking while experiencing an event (Cole, 1992).

9. Guiding parents in strategies for encouraging cognitive and sensorimotor play skills within communicative routines. Parents should learn to encourage the early pretend skills of the toddler, mapping language onto these accomplishments.

A comprehensive summary of methods for establishing effective parent/child communication is included in Table 8.5.

Several resources are useful in helping family members implement an indirect language-stimulation approach. One was developed at the Hanen Early Language Resource Centre in Toronto for children with speech and language delay. The program provides inservice training to professionals and distributes a parent guidebook entitled, *It Takes Two to Talk* (Manolson, 1985). This program can be very useful to clinicians in encouraging developmentally appropriate interactions with infants. Curricular materials for guiding parents and professional training are also available from the Infant Hearing Resource (Parent/Infant Communication, Schuyler & Ruschmer, 1987) and from Project SKI-HI (Watkins & Clark, 1993).

For those children who begin to use signs, families are in need of access to sign classes and materials. Two videocassette family sign programs for families of young children are currently available. One was produced by the SKI-HI Institute and is avail-

TABLE 8.5 *Some Methods for Parents to Establish Effective Communication with Their Child Who is Deaf or Hard-of-Hearing*

Identify the child's early use of signals and respond interactively	Understand the importance of early communication and how babies learn to communicate
	Identify child's early communication
	Respond to child's early communication
	Use interactive turn-taking
	Respond appropriately to child's cry
	Encourage smiling and laughing in early interactions
	Give child choices
	Utilize daily routines for communication
Optimize daily communication in the home	Minimize distracting noises
	Get close to child and on child's level
	Establish eye contact and direct conversation to child
	Provide a safe, stimulating communication environment
	Communicate frequently with child each day
Optimize parent communication with child in early interactions	Understand how parents communicate to babies and young children
	Increase the "back and forth" exchanges in turn-taking
	Encourage vocalization in communicative interactions
	Use touch and gestures in communicative interactions
	Use facial expressions and intonation in communicative interactions
	Interact with child about meaningful hear-and-now experiences; make an experience book

Source: The SKI-HI Model: A Resource Manual for Family-Centered Home-Based Programming for Infants, Toddlers, and Pre-School Children with Hearing Impairments (S. Watkins and T. Clark, 1993, p. 262) Used with permission.

able from Home Oriented Program Essentials, 55 East 100 North, Suite 203, Logan, UT 84321. A more recent program is currently being developed at Boys Town National Research Hospital (Moeller & Schick, 1993). This video program entitled, *Sign With Me: A Family Sign Program* (SWM) focuses on the sign communication needs of parents of children who are deaf, ages birth through three years. SWM is available from Boys Town Press, 13603 Flanagan Blvd., Boys Town, NE 68010 402-498-6511. It includes focus on signing skills, parenting principles and language-stimulation strategies. It is being produced in both American Sign Language and Manually Coded English versions. Parents receive supplemental workbooks with the videotapes that provide additional guidance in parenting principles and language stimulation techniques. This program specifically targets helping parents develop a signing style that is consistent with a visual equivalent of motherese. The tapes also include comprehension tests, using a variety of sign models, including children.

Families involved in signing programs often desire and benefit from opportunities to learn about deaf culture. Furthermore, many parents are seeking resources and support for learning American Sign Language (ASL). The SKI-HI Institute is currently developing and researching Deaf Mentor Programming, which enables family members to learn American Sign Language and to learn about deaf culture. The program utilizes the services of adults who are deaf as mentors and models of the language and culture of the deaf. These Deaf Mentors make regular visits to the home, interact with the child using ASL, show family members how to use ASL, and help the family understand and appreciate deafness and deaf culture. Meanwhile, the family continues to receive visits from a parent advisor who focuses on helping the parents promote English acquisition in the young child who is deaf. In this way, the family and child use both English and ASL and participate comfortably in both the hearing and deaf worlds. A variety of Deaf Mentor materials are currently being developed at the SKI-HI Institute, including guides for teaching families ASL, information on deaf culture, and Deaf Mentor Program operation guides. An array of data is also being obtained on the children and families receiving Deaf Mentor Programming. These data are being compared with data on children who are not receiving bilingual-bicultural programming. Data on program operation, service satisfaction from persons involved in the program, and cost effectiveness are also being obtained.

Hatfield and Humes (1994) also describe a parent-infant program that has incorporated a bilingual-bicultural model, and Busch and Halpin (1994) describe an approach to incorporating deaf culture into the early-intervention program. Presently some controversy exists as to whether parents and programs should implement ASL or Manually Coded English, or both (bilingualism) at the early intervention level. Many professionals and deaf persons stress the importance of considering the natural ways that American Sign Language, a visual-spatial language, is organized and the potential advantages this language organization may have for the young learner who is deaf (Fischer, 1994; Johnson, Liddell, & Erting, 1989). Some professionals stress the importance of children having early access to visual English, especially for the development of early listening skills. Perhaps "bilingualism" provides the best of both worlds. Parents and other family members with normal hearing are able to use English, their natural language, in a visual way (signed English) *and* are also able to learn and use the natural language of persons who are deaf, American Sign Language.

No matter what approach is taken, parents with normal hearing need considerable support to develop good communication with their children who are deaf through the visual mode. According to Moeller, Schick, and Williams, 1994, emphasis needs to be placed on:

1. Developing a lexicon that allows parents to sign simple, conversational phrases to the young child.
2. Developing fluency and prosody in their signing, following principles of visual motherese, used by parents and children, both of whom are deaf.
3. Developing parents' ability to understand a range of signers, including children.
4. Developing parents' ability to sign at a level more complex and diverse than the child's, and participate in contingent, nondirective interactions with the child.
5. Learning to tell stories in an animated, fluent fashion.
6. Maintaining the child's visual attention.

7. Involving parents and extended family members in signing consistently throughout daily interaction.

8. Learning about deaf culture.

COMMUNICATION/LANGUAGE STIMULATION: PRESCHOOL LEVEL. At the preschool level, communication intervention typically occurs in a classroom setting. Between three and five years of age, children benefit from opportunities to socialize with other children, and to develop cognitive, social, and language skills that will support them in future academic pursuits. Although programs typically become center-based at the preschool level, the role of the family remains foundational. Quality preschool programs ensure the continued and substantive involvement of family members in the child's program into the preschool years. Many preschool programs continue to provide home visitation to ensure the link between home and school.

Each child's language program is guided by a thorough analysis of communication strengths, emergent behaviors and priority needs. These are integrated into an Individual Educational Plan (IEP), which becomes the road map for accomplishing language changes. These child-specific goals, however, need to be integrated into a curricular scheme. During the preschool years, children are *active constructors of meaning* in the process of learning (Wells, 1981). They rapidly gain information and language experience through immersion in the world of information around them. A goal of the preschool program for children who are deaf or hard of hearing is to provide opportunities for active learning and experiences, through which the child's knowledge base can be expanded. This language knowledge base will be a critical tool for success in literacy during the school age years.

Regardless of the specific preschool setting (e.g., public school or private; self-contained or mainstreamed) we have found a number of "best practices" that are supportive of children who are deaf or hard of hearing at this level. Some of the "best practice" concepts follow.

1. Children should be regarded as *active* learners, not passive recipients of information. They bring to any learning task past experiences, assumptions, and perceptions that can contribute to the learning. Children's experiential bases should be exploited in learning opportunities. Not only should preschool children be physically active in manipulating materials, they should be encouraged to be mentally active. This can happen through provision of choices, teacher-guided questioning, and opportunities to solve problems (Moeller & Carney, 1993). For example, during a recent snack activity in a preschool classroom, the teacher contrived the need to step away from the snack table and left one of the preschoolers "in charge" of passing out cookies, crackers, and various juices. His problem was to find out what each child wanted from the choices available. Another example of an active learning lesson was an activity where the children experimented with the effects of different pencil sharpeners on their pencils. They learned about relative speeds when comparing how long the manual sharpener took in relation to the electric sharpener. Provision of choices, opportunities to make comparisons, and discussions of solutions to

problems result in active learning and considerable dialogue. Cognitive and language skills, then, are emphasized in an integrated fashion.

2.   Children who are deaf or hard of hearing typically need a systematic approach to vocabulary development. Because they are not able to "overhear," they often miss experiential knowledge and vocabulary that is critical to fully understanding their experiences. A major goal of the preschool program is to strengthen word knowledge and the mapping of language upon experiences. The work of Yoshinaga-Itano and Downey (1986) is very relevant to this goal. They describe a schema-based approach to vocabulary development. Schemata are defined as "organized representations of a person's knowledge about some concept, action or event." In a schema-based approach, a teacher or clinician helps the child understand and appreciate networks of information. The goal is helping the child see how this concept or word relates to information he or she already knows, or how the concept links to other familiar concepts. In a schema-based approach, the teacher is less concerned about teaching specific content, and is more concerned with helping the child form concepts through making appropriate associations. For example, learning specific names for each Halloween item may not be as relevant as learning that Halloween is a holiday that is celebrated, just as Christmas, birthdays, and Passover are celebrated. Celebrations involve parties and customs. In a schema-based content approach, the clinician aids the child in forming concepts and associative networks by presenting information in a way that make the connections clear. Yoshinaga-Itano and Downey (1986) also point out that children who are deaf may learn only the prototypical or stereotypical notion of a word. It is useful for clinicians to provide experiences that help children expand their notion of a word. For example, children in one preschool prepared eggs in different ways for two weeks at snack time. They learned the function of an egg timer one day by contrasting the outcomes when it was used instead of ignored. They contrasted steps in preparation for scrambled vs. hard-boiled eggs vs. omelets. They interviewed classmates on their preferences for the various forms of eggs. The point is that when children have problems to solve and opportunities to manipulate concepts, language and thinking are a natural outgrowth. The schema-based approach is a useful conceptualization for the development of vocabulary in children with hearing impairment.

3.   The function of language is to serve as a tool that children use to access information about the world around them. Question discourse should be a priority goal with children who are deaf or hard of hearing. One of the most frequent verbalizations of a four-year–old child is "Why?" Children who are deaf or hard of hearing are equally curious, but may not have accomplished the verbal skills to pose questions to secure information. In some cases, children who communicate by sign have had limited exposure to question discourse, especially if families with normal hearing are not regularly signing questions around them. Because question-asking is such a useful tool for acquiring information, we believe that language lessons in the classroom should specifically target this skill. In one preschool, the AR specialist (who was providing collaborative consultation to the teacher of the deaf) arrived each day at a designated time with the "question basket." This was an attractive picnic basket which always contained something unusual or interesting for the children to use. Each time

she would arrive, the children would start to ask questions, because they could anticipate that there would be a novel outcome to the activity. By repeating the routine of the "question basket," children could build on previous question routines and learn new ones. Cumulative language experiences can be very useful for expanding a child's repertoire. In the beginning, the children would simply ask "what" or "who" when the basket was shown. With modeling and guidance, they learned to make educated guesses or to ask for clues (Is it heavy? big? small? a toy? an animal?). Many times the clinician brought an object whose function was not clear. This prompted questions like, "What's that for?" One time the object was a small bulb syringe that was used to blow up balloon animals. This prompted the children to ask about its function and about what the clinician was going to make. The inclusion of a few defective balloons led to "Why?" and "What's wrong?" questions. The clinician and teacher teamed up to contrive opportunities to obligate important language functions. The children looked forward to the question basket and there was excellent carryover of the question-asking skills to other parts of the daily routine (e.g., show-and-tell time; recall time after play).

4.   Question comprehension is also a priority goal, so that children can benefit from teacher-guided questioning. In quality preschool programs, many teachers provide learning centers, where collaborative exploration occurs among learners. Children's ability to understand teacher's questions and the observations of others helps promote their thinking and concept organization. A preschool discourse model developed by Blank, Rose, and Berlin (1978) is valuable in guiding children in responding to language demands of increasing cognitive abstraction. Moeller and Carney (1993) documented the efficacy of this preschool discourse model with preschool children who are deaf. This discourse model incorporates four distinct levels of cognitive abstraction. At the simplest level, children use language that matches their immediate perception (e.g., What is this?). At the next level, children are given language demands that require them to selectively analyze their perceptions (e.g., What is happening? How are these different?). At the third level, children must use language to distance from their immediate perceptions and reorder the way they are thinking about an object or event (e.g., What will happen next?). At the most abstract level, children reason about their perceptions (e.g., What made that happen? What would you do?). In the preschool program described by Moeller and Carney (1993), adults gave children opportunities to consider questions at a manageable level, as well as opportunities to stretch their language and thinking to the next level of abstraction. The skills involved in the discourse model appear in children with normal hearing of between four and six years of age. Some of the children who were deaf were able to achieve age-appropriate responses following systematic intervention with this model. Importantly, these types of skills help prepare children for the language and literacy demands of elementary school programs. A complete listing of preschool discourse demands at each of these levels may be found in Blank, et al. (1978).

5.   Quality preschool programs for children who are deaf or hard of hearing implement developmentally appropriate practices. Children with hearing loss are considered *children first*, and their special needs are integrated into quality early child-

hood practices. The National Association for the Education of Young Children has published guidelines for "developmentally appropriate practices" with young children (Bredekamp, 1987). These guidelines (described in Table 8.6) should be considered as foundational for any preschool program serving deaf and hard of hearing children.

6. Quality preschool programs recognize that language (whether oral, signed, or written) is a tool for conveying meanings and for communicating purposefully. Language "lessons," then, need to be integrated in pragmatically appropriate contexts that have communicative value.

7. Many preschool programs use thematic units to encourage language development. Units can be a useful way to present content with topical links (as described above) and to give a child repeated and organized exposure to a topic. Themes selected should be developmentally appropriate, interesting, and relevant to the child's communicative needs. Themes should promote the integration of content learning (facts, lexical items, and concepts) and process learning (self-expression, critical and creative thinking, planning and decision-making, and internal behavioral controls) (Kostelnik, et al., 1991). Moeller and Carney (1993) provided additional guidelines for selection of unit themes.

8. Opportunities for exploration through play should be provided regularly. Children learn cognitive, social, and language skills through play exploration. Adults can provide a support role that helps children map language into their play experiences. Moeller and Carney (1993) describe a cognitively-oriented program, where children learn to verbally plan what they will play. Adults then act as play supporters and "instigators of problems." At the end of play, children are given guided opportunities to recall or review what they have done in play. This process, adapted from the High Scope Educational Research Foundation (Hohmann, Banet, & Weikart, 1979), is effective in helping children mediate their play experiences with language and develop personal narrative skills. Children should be encouraged to develop in both symbolic and constructional play areas. Westby (1980) provides comprehensive guidelines for the development of play that include related language accomplishments. Children with hearing impairment may encounter difficulty at more advanced cooperative play stages, when interactive language is critical to the success of the play. Westby's guidelines help clinicians prepare children for these latter stages.

9. Children benefit in many ways from exposure to quality children's literature. Storytelling should be a daily curricular component. Exposure to stories helps children expand upon event knowledge (scripts), develop a notion of story grammar, and prepare for future literacy tasks. There are many indications in the literature that children who are read to with regularity at home become the most literate (Snow, 1983). Parents should be actively involved in the storytelling program. The *Sign With Me* curriculum described above includes storytelling demonstration tapes called "Read with Me" for signing parents.

10. Children at the preschool level benefit from exposure to early literacy opportunities. These include reading books and being read to, demonstrating knowledge about books (e.g., book handling, reading pictures, recognizing environmental print), beginning to recognize simple print forms, being exposed to functional uses of print, and having opportunities to explore with written symbols.

TABLE 8.6 *Guidlines for Developmentally Appropriate Practices*

1. The clinician or teacher prepares the learning environment and plans activities to promote discoveries and exploration.

2. Content and strategies presented are age appropriate.

3. Curriculum techniques are adjusted to respond to children's learning style, personality, or cultural background.

4. Child-initiated, but adult-supported play is primary vehicle of encouraging developmental growth in all domains.

5. Developmental and learning domains are integrated within the curriculum (e.g. motor, social, language, cognitive, emotional).

6. Learning materials are concrete, real, and relevant to the experiences of young children.

7 Learning materials are presented at various developmental levels to interest and challenge children. They are non-sexist and reflect cultural diversity.

8. Play materials allow for sensorimotor, symbolic, and constructive play.

9. Adults are responsive and comforting. They encourage independence and treat children with respect and dignity.

10. Adults use discipline techniques that guide children to learn self-control, redirect children to use more acceptable behaviors to resolve conflict, and remind children of rules.

Adapted from Bredekamp, 1987.

SPEECH STIMULATION: PARENT-INFANT AND PRESCHOOL. We believe that children in parent-infant programs should not receive formal speech training, which typically involves drill and correction. Instead, we believe parents and professionals should be aware of the general sequence in which speech sounds emerge and then provide extensive modeling of speech at a level that encourages children to move to the next stage of development. An excellent source on speech development for children who are deaf or hard of hearing is *Speech and the Hearing Impaired Child* (Ling, 1976). Another useful source, by Cole (1992), is *Listening and Talking: A Guide to Promoting Spoken Language in Young Hearing-Impaired Children.*

Oller (1983) has identified stages in normally-developing infants' vocal development, that are useful to consider. From birth to two months, infants are in a *phonation stage*, where they produce comfort sounds that may be precursors to vowel production. At this stage, syllables with consonants or vowels are rare. Infants enter a *cooing stage* during the two-to-three month period. They produce comfort sounds often articulated in the back of the oral cavity. These are not well formed, mature syllabic productions. Next is the expansion stage (four to six months). Infants at this stage produce various new sound types, like raspberries, squeals, growls, yells, whispers, and isolated vowel-like sounds. Mature syllables are not yet evident, although some marginal babbling may be seen. The next stage is considered to be a developmental landmark, and is called the *canonical stage* (7–10 months). At this point, infants produce well-formed, reduplicated syllables like /mamama/ or /dadada/. This is considered to be a critical stage, as these syllables function as phonetic building blocks of words. Non-reduplicated canonical utterances (e.g., /bi/, /ada/, /imi/) are also seen frequently at this stage. The period of 11–12 months brings about the variegated babbling stage. Here, infants systematically produce utterances with differing consonantal or vocalic elements. Useful clinical systems for transcribing and studying infant vocalizations have been described by Carney (1991) and by Stoel-Gammon and Cooper (1984).

In most cases, infants who are deaf or hard of hearing spontaneously produce some vocalizations. Parents should encourage the child to develop an abundance of vocalizations by being responsive to the child's vocal attempts (Ling, 1989). Parents can respond by smiling, moving closer to the child, interpreting the vocal attempt communicatively, and imitating the child (Cole, 1992).

Parents can also encourage the child's initial vocalizations by providing animated models of vocalizing during active play with the child. For example, as the child is being gently bounced on the parent's knee, the parent can say /up-up-up/. Vocalizations like /a-boo; a-boo/ would be appropriate during a peek-a-boo game. Parents should be encouraged to respond warmly to reinforce any early accidental vocalizations. At the expansion and canonical babbling stages, parents can reinforce the child's vocal exploration by imitating and modelling interesting auditory patterns. The parent can say, "You said up-up-up! Let's ride horsey up-up-up the hill." For the older infant, new sounds can be imitated and then repeated in syllable chains and then used in simple words ("/ha-ha-ha/—yes, that is HOT!").

Parents should encourage the infant's development of early suprasegmental aspects of speech. Breath control can be developed through playful duration games, where the child is encouraged to vocalize long or short sounds (e.g., vocalizing /u:/ while the sand pours out of a container). Intensity and pitch control can be developed in play where the child is encouraged to make soft and loud (e.g., whisper while the baby doll sleeps; make a loud voice to wake her up), and high and low sounds. Speech rhythms can be learned by encouraging the child to participate in play activities in which speech tempos are produced slowly and quickly (e.g., during a horsey-back ride, the movement and the sound can be contrasted from slow to fast repetitions).

At the preschool level, children often benefit from a goal-oriented approach to speech development. This process begins with a comprehensive analysis of the child's speech-production skills to determine appropriate intervention targets. This might include a phonologically-based assessment (e.g., Test of Phonology; Bankson-Bernthal, 1990), an articulation test, or a procedure specifically designed for deaf and hard of hearing students (Ling, 1976). The decision about which type of assessment to use depends on the diagnostic questions of the clinician and the skill level and residual hearing of the child. For some children who are hard of hearing, for example, a developmental phonological process approach can be very useful. Whatever tools are chosen, the clinician should be well informed about the typical characteristics of speech in children with hearing loss. A comprehensive appraisal of speech should include assessment of: (a) functional auditory skills; (b) phonetic level skills; (c) phonological skills; (d) suprasegmental and vocal behaviors; (e) stimulability for sound production or emergence of skills; and (f) speech intelligibility. Often an oral mechanism assessment is valuable. In our opinion, the speech assessment should not rely solely on imitative productions, but should examine spontaneous productions and extent of carryover, as well.

A thorough discussion of the many speech-training approaches is beyond the scope of this chapter. The reader is referred to Osberger (1983) and to Chapter 5 of this book for a discussion of various speech management approaches. Some concepts that are common to recommended speech training approaches with children with hearing impairment are worthy of mention:

1.   The speech training program should exploit the use of residual hearing to the fullest extent possible. Auditory and speech development should be closely integrated in this process.

2.   Adult expectations can have a significant impact on a child's development of speech. In the classroom and at home, children benefit from regular encouragement to rely on speech to the best of their abilities. This should not be implemented to the degree that it interferes with communication. However, adults need to recognize the value of regular, brief practice opportunities in natural contexts (Ling, 1976) and the value of high expectations.

3.   Many programs find that collaborative consultation models work well for integrating speech into the classroom. The speech/language clinician or AR clinician works closely with the preschool classroom teacher to determine how speech intervention targets can be incorporated naturally in classroom activities. Consultants can assist the teacher in maintaining appropriate and challenging expectations for speech and auditory skill development in the classroom. Although individual speech intervention is often valuable, there may be problems with generalization and carryover if speech is not emphasized in natural routines and contexts. A collaborative team approach can be very effective in accomplishing the goal of generalization of speech skills.

4.   For some children with limited or no residual hearing, speech acquisition can be difficult and tedious. It is essential that the AR clinician provide intervention goals that are achievable and functional, and that they be presented in fun, motivating lessons that are supportive of the child.

5.   Speech development should always be viewed within the broader context of communication. Osberger (1983) stresses the importance of ensuring speech generalization and carryover. Carotta, Carney, and Dettman (1990) discussed a systematic plan for carryover of speech targets that involved the gradual inclusion of the target in increasingly abstract/cognitively demanding contexts. Using the preschool discourse model of Blank, Rose, and Berlin (1978), they proposed a series of activities that took the child through a progression from cognitively simple to cognitively challenging language contexts. For example, if the child was working on a vowel like /au/, the sound would be included in phonologically based activities in the following manner:

a.   Matching perception (simplest level of abstraction)

Name objects seen in a bag (cow, mouse, towel)

b.   Selective analysis of perception

Name something that is . . . (attentive to one or two categorical characteristics).

Example:Name an animal (cow, mouse)

Example:Name something little and brown (mouse)

c. Reordering perception

Identify similarities–How are a cow and a mouse the same?

d. Reasoning about perception

Forming a solution from another person's perspective

The man saw a nail sticking out of the house—what should he do? (pound the nail; sit down and pout)

Carotta's contribution is valuable in many respects. Often, speech-training materials are simple from a language/cognitive viewpoint. They require labelling of pictures or creating simple ideas from pictured stimuli. Children may have difficulty with carryover of speech skills when tasks are abstract and demand a lot of their mental attention. Carotta, et al. (1990) suggest that training materials incorporate increasingly complex cognitive/linguistic materials to help children generalize. At the same time, the child is working on materials useful for language and cognitive development. When the child is ready, approaches that integrate several levels of goals are both useful and expedient.

Psychosocial Aspects. During the early years of the child's life, the psychosocial aspects of the hearing deficit are, for a great part, related to the parents as the primary caregivers and teachers. Parenthood is a great challenge for all fathers and mothers. The added responsibility of having a child with hearing impairment enhances this challenge in various degrees and ways.

NEEDS OF PARENTS. Psychosocial support is vital for the parents of infants with hearing impairment. Thus, many writers have discussed the importance of psychological assistance (see Chapter 6; Moses, 1985; Phillips, 1987). For instance, Lillie (1969) commented:

> The birth of a child does not automatically turn two human beings into understanding and informed parents. Nor does the birth of a hearing handicapped child mean that his parents are endowed with all the understanding and acceptance necessary for them to help their child develop into a whole person. Those parents need guidance. (p. 2)

Mindel and Vernon (1987) wrote: "unless parents' emotional needs are attended to, the programs for young hearing handicapped children have limited benefit." (p. 23)

During the child's early years, the parent advisor is often the key person in enabling families to understand hearing loss and deal creatively and positively with the child. Because over 90% of children who are deaf or hard of hearing have parents with normal hearing, these parents typically have had little or no experience with deafness (Johnson, Liddell, & Erting, 1989). Although family members may not know much about deafness, they have hopes and dreams for their child, and they have many concerns and questions. Often family members are confused and surprised by the variety of emotions they experience by having a family member who is deaf or hard of hearing. The competent parent advisor is able to listen to family members sensitively and with more care, interact with them, and provide needed support, information, and skills.

One of the most valuable contributions the parent advisor can make to the family is to gently and gradually help the family understand and appreciate deafness. Rather than perceiving deafness as a "pathology," a "problem," or "something to be feared," parent advisors can help families to see deafness as a unique human experience that may include linguistic and cultural aspects. Perhaps the very best way for families to understand and appreciate deafness is to interact with deaf persons themselves. The Deaf Mentor Program at the SKI-HI Institute provides the opportunity for families to interact regularly with adults who are deaf (Deaf Mentors).

Of course, the process of understanding and appreciating deafness and the situation of having a child who is deaf is gradual. For most parents with normal hearing the initial reaction to the diagnosis of deafness incudes shock, denial, and confusion. Parents have wished for and expected a "normal" child. Now their dreams are shattered, and they feel devastated and helpless. The shock has numbed them into a state of immobility. They are unable to assimilate what information is given them, as they are not functioning in a normal manner. It has been reported that sometimes after learning the diagnosis for the first time, parents are utterly and literally lost, unable even to locate their cars in the parking lot (Luterman, 1987).

After the initial shock, denial, and confusion stage, some parents experience anger, depression, and guilt: "Why me?" Luterman (1987) noted:

> Anger comes from a violation of expectations. Parents have many expectations about their unborn children, not the least of which is that they will be normal. When they find that the child does not hear normally and cannot be cured, they feel cheated and wonder why they were singled out. (p. 42)

Anger also results from loss of control of personal freedom. Parents may experience a kind of aesthetic disavowal of the child with hearing impairment as they envision the restrictions the child may impose on their plans for the future. Anger also results from not knowing how to help the child. In addition to anger, parents often experience strong guilt feelings, manifested by overindulging the child who has hearing impairment, or placing excessive demands on him. If these findings of guilt and despair are not resolved, parents begin an unending search for a "magic cure" by a doctor who will deny the difficulty, or the "best" school.

This period of anger, depression, and guilt can be followed by a time of withdrawal, solitude, and introspection. As parents learn about deafness and interact with persons who are deaf, they come to see that these people reside, work, produce, and lead normal lives in society. Grant (1987) remarked that arrival at this stage does not preclude continued problems and adjustments. On the contrary, as new crises surface, as new programs, new medical problems arise, parents may go through additional emotional adjustments.

Gradually, most parents come to see that their child has a future and they begin to accept the disability. Acceptance of the disability leads the parents back to the feelings they were experiencing toward their child before the diagnosis of deafness. The duration of each stage depends upon the parents. Some stages may pass in a matter of minutes, others may last for months or years, and, as indicated, the parents may re-experience some of the stages later in their lives. Generally, however, parents go through the stages just described. (See Chapter 6 for additional detail. There, this period is divided into five stages–denial, anger, frustration, mourning, and constructive coping.)

SUPPORT FOR PARENTS. It is the responsibility of the parent advisor first and foremost to convey positive attitudes and perceptions about deafness to family members. Deaf adults (mentors) are invaluable in enabling families to understand and appreciate deafness. For parents experiencing the stages of grief described above, the parent advisor will want to sensitively help the parents deal with these stages. The parent advisor will not want to hurry parents through the stages or encourage avoidance of them; rather, parents should be skillfully, but gently, helped to progress from one stage to the next. The following discussion offers some suggestions as to how this may be accomplished. (See also case examples, Chapter 11.)

During the first stage, which is characterized by confusion and denial, the parent advisor/audiologic rehabilitationist establishes contact with the family. This is done immediately after the diagnosis of a hearing loss. The professional's role is to offer emotional support and realistic hope. The parent advisor explains programs that will involve all family members and how these programs will help the child who is deaf or hard of hearing.

During the next stage, anger and depression, the parent advisor may erroneously try to counteract the parents' emotions by helping them feel less depressed. At this period, the parent advisor needs to exhibit genuine understanding and good listening skills rather than attempt to talk the parents out of their feelings (Moses, 1985).

The effective parent advisor contributes greatly to the third stage, that of quietude and introspection. It is during this time that parents usually open up and ask questions about the future of their child, educational considerations, and society's perception of them and of their youngster. Perhaps the most important contribution the parent advisor can make during this stage is to plan with the parents constructive activities for family members that help the child's listening, communicative, and language abilities. When the parents see the child responding, growing, and learning, acceptance occurs. They realize they have a child who can be taught and loved just like any other child.

CONSULTATION BETWEEN PSYCHOLOGIST AND AR THERAPIST. Some parents do not move easily through the stages just outlined. On the way they may have problems: unrealistic expectations for the child, overprotection, rejection, or confusion over conflicting information about educational methods. They may have problems with general child-rearing practices, such as discipline and sibling rivalry. The parent advisor may need special help from psychologists or social workers in dealing with these problems. Sessions can be set up between the parent advisor and the psychologist or social worker for this purpose. The psychologist or social worker can offer suggestions that can in turn be tried by the parent advisor in the home or discussed with the family as appropriate. For parents who want psychological counseling, the AR therapist should act as facilitator and ensure such therapy is arranged.

SUPPORT-GROUP MEETINGS.   Another invaluable way of giving psychosocial support to parents is to arrange parent group meetings. "There is probably no greater gift that a professional can give to families than to provide them with a support group. Groups are marvelous vehicles for learning and emotional support" (Luterman, 1987, p. 113). Support group meetings are part of many early-intervention programs. Often eight or nine meetings are held, once a week, with a psychologist or social worker in charge. The first part of each meeting often consists of a presentation by a professional. Such topics as "Language Development," "Communication Methods," "Development of Self-Concept," and "Making the Home Environment Responsive" can be discussed. The last part of each meeting is devoted to group interaction. Luterman (1987) described the benefits of support group interactions: (a) They enable members to recognize the universality of their feelings; members come to appreciate that others in the group have similar feelings; (b) they give participants the opportunity to help one another; and (c) they become a powerful vehicle for imparting information.

Parents are great sources of help and comfort to other parents. In attending support-group meetings we have been constantly impressed with the amount of help and moral support parents give each other. Inclusion of adults who are deaf in support groups is highly recommended. Such adults can describe their experiences of being deaf and answer questions about deafness that professionals with normal hearing simply cannot do.

NEEDS OF AND SUPPORT FOR THE CHILD.   Successful resolution of parental anxieties, warm acceptance of the child who is deaf, and establishment of communication with the child promote normal psychosocial development. However, the child may also present social, emotional, or psychological problems. Consequently, the therapist must have a knowledge of what to expect from the child with hearing impairment in these developmental areas.

Development scales established by Vincent, et al. (1986) and others enable professionals to know what behaviors a child should exhibit at a particular age (see Materials Lists in Chapter 13). The audiologic rehabilitationist observes the child's behaviors and determines what age levels they typify. In addition to developmental scales, the therapist should arrange for appropriate developmental and psychosocial assessments for the child. These tests should be administered by competent psychologists who are familiar with hearing-impaired children. According to Davis (1977), this may be difficult since "most psychologists receive little or no training in testing or working with hearing-impaired children" (p. 36). (See Chapter 6 for suggestions on how to resolve this dilemma.)

If the child is lagging in a specific area, the audiologic rehabilitationist can seek help from other professionals such as child-development specialists, psychologists, social workers, occupational and physical therapists, pediatricians, and nurses.

ASPECTS OF AUDIOLOGIC REHABILITATION: SCHOOL YEARS

Rehabilitation Assessment/IEP Meeting

PL 94-142 stipulates that primary- and secondary-school placements must be based on assessments of the child, which are reviewed in an individualized educational program (IEP) meeting (see Chapter 7). The IEP meetings serve to develop, review, or revise annual educational program goals for the student. The AR therapist is responsible for completing an appropriate assessment prior to the IEP meeting. The AR therapist working with the school-age student may be an educational audiologist, an educator of the hearing-impaired, a speech/language clinician, or some other professional charged with the responsibility of coordinating components of the child's educational support services. Assessment of the school-age child includes the four general areas described in the AR model presented in Chapter 1:

1. Communication status, including audiologic and amplification issues, receptive and expressive language, and social communication skills.
2. Associated variables of academic achievement, psychosocial adaptation, and prevocational and vocational skills.
3. Related medical or physical conditions.
4. Attitudes and goals of parents and child.

In many cases, multi-disciplinary input is valuable in gaining a comprehensive understanding of student needs. Assessment guidelines are available in Ross, Bracket, and Maxon, 1982; Moeller, 1988; Ross, 1990; and Alpiner and McCarthy, 1993. Consistent with the goal of ecologically-valid assessment practices, it is useful to include a classroom observation and/or teacher questionnaires regarding the student's performance in that setting. As the section on communication rehabilitation stresses, classroom communication behaviors are unique and complex. Many standardized tests do not reflect the kinds of language skills that are required in the classroom setting. Therefore, observations in that setting and teacher impressions offer invaluable insights for the IEP. The SIFTER (Screening Instrument for Targeting Educational Risk) (Anderson, 1989) is an example of an efficient tool for recruiting teachers' impressions of the student's performance in relation to her peers. A member of the assessment team or a representative of the team who is familiar with the results of the assessment (often the audiologic rehabilitationist) must attend the IEP meeting along with the teacher, parents and child, as appropriate. Based on the educational recommendations from the child's IEP, the AR therapist proceeds to arrange for or provide the needed services. Excellent guidelines for comprehensive service provision were recently published by the National Association for State Directors of Special Education. You can obtain these guidelines, developed by the deaf initiatives project, by writing: Deaf Guidelines Document, c/o National Association of State Directors of Special Education, 1800 Diagonal Road, Suite 320, Alexandria, VA 22314.

Management

Overall Coordination. As a part of the overall coordination, the therapist is responsible for maximizing the child's learning environment (classroom), assisting in securing ancillary services, promoting development of social skills, and arranging for special college preparation or occupational training. If the primary educational programming is delivered by someone other than the AR therapist (e.g., the teacher), the therapist needs to assume a supporting role and assist the teacher in these areas.

CHILD LEARNING ENVIRONMENT (CLASSROOM MANAGEMENT). School placement alternatives are necessary so that the best educational setting can be selected. For the older child, additional placement options are available beyond those listed for the preschool child. Thus, the range of options includes: (a) residential school placement; (b) day school or day classes for the hearing impaired; (c) resource rooms where the child with hearing impairment learns communication skills and is integrated into regular classrooms for less language-oriented subjects, such as math and physical education; (d) integration into public schools with ancillary services like speech therapy; and (e) team-taught combined classes of normal and hearing-impaired youngsters. (See Johnson, 1987, and Chapter 7 on School Placement Alternatives for a discussion of these options.)

The audiologic rehabilitationist is responsible for informing the child's teachers of the conditions that will optimize learning; that is, seating, lighting, visual aids, and reduction of classroom noises. Helpful guides for teachers who have children with hearing impairment in their classrooms have been written (Birch, 1975; Davis, 1977; Gildston, 1973; see also Appendix 8A). In addition, the therapist should ensure that an appropriate student-teacher ratio is maintained. Flint (1971) suggested that a class size for students with hearing impairment must not exceed seven, stressing that a class size of five or less greatly improves learning. It is estimated that one pupil with hearing impairment adds the equivalent of three pupils with normal hearing to regular classes in terms of demand on a teacher's time (Rafferty, 1970).

The AR therapist should also promote home and school coordination. Cooperation can be facilitated by regular conferences between parents and teachers, periodic visits to the home by the teacher, notes, newsletters, and special student work sent home to the parents, telephone conversations, and allowing parents to participate in classroom activities.

ANCILLARY SERVICES. The therapist may also need to help set up ancillary services required for the hearing-impaired child. Services like otologic assessments and treatment; occupational or physical therapy; medical exams and treatment; social services; and neurologic, ophthalmologic, and psychological services are important components of the welfare of a child with hearing impairment (Rafferty, 1970). Finally, secondary students with hearing impairment in public school programs may require the services of notetakers or interpreters.

DEVELOPMENT OF SOCIAL SKILLS.   In a study of 40 mainstreamed students with hearing impairment, Davis, Elfenbein, Schum, and Bentler (1986) found a high incidence of social problems, including peer acceptance difficulties. Over 50% of the students with hearing impairment expressed concerns with peer relations, in contrast to 16% of similar concerns expressed by hearing students. The authors stressed the need for increased attention by school programs to the development of positive self esteem and social interactions in students with hearing impairment. The AR clinician should monitor the social adjustment of the student with hearing impairment and make appropriate referrals as needed. The school counselor or other mental health professional can be supportive in addressing the social integration of the student. Refinement of social language skills can also be supportive of this goal area.

OCCUPATIONAL OR COLLEGE PREPARATION.   Secondary students with hearing impairment need special help in occupational training. Even though the majority of jobs need no more than a high school diploma, it is necessary to provide vocational training and occupational guidance for those high-school students who want to enter the work force. Likewise, college preparation courses and guidance counseling are needed for those who desire a college education (BOL, 1977).

Amplification/Assistive Device Issues.   If children obtain their hearing aids during the early-intervention period and go through the adjustment and orientation steps described earlier in this chapter, they have a good start on dealing with amplification concerns. However, this area requires a continued focus, since new amplification needs or problems may arise when children enter school. Regular hearing-aid reassessment at six-month to one-year intervals and daily monitoring of the aid by school personnel should occur. Unfortunately, such regular monitoring is often neglected. Therefore, audiologic rehabilitation personnel need to be vigilant in this area (Bess & Logan, 1984). The major deficit for these children is their impaired hearing. Therefore, the most obvious management is to restore as much of that hearing through amplification devices and excellent acoustic listening conditions as possible. In this manner, we may remove the need for some therapy that would otherwise be required.

HEARING AIDS.   Some children with hearing impairment are not identified until they reach school, and some of them receive their first amplification attention at this time. As indicated in the section on early intervention, when children with hearing losses are identified, they should also be evaluated medically and audiologically. After specific assessment information has been obtained, the way is cleared for carefully evaluating the place of amplification in the overall management program. Children with mild or more serious losses in the speech frequencies should proceed with a hearing-aid assessment, and additional audiologic rehabilitation can assist them in hearing-aid orientation aspects, as described previously.

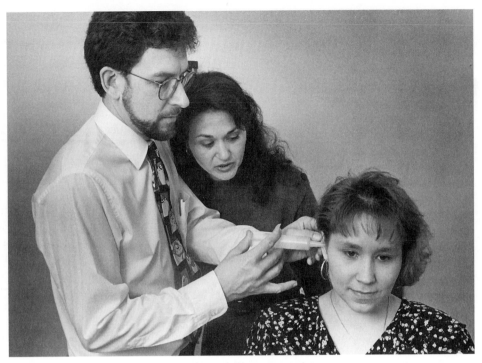

A clinician involved in taking an earmold impression.

Children with slight losses, high-frequency losses, or chronic conductive losses present a more difficult problem in terms of amplification. A careful assessment of such children's language and speech status and a report on their ability to function in the classroom will help determine whether they can function successfully without amplification. Preferential seating can provide some help, but this is, at best, an imperfect and perhaps only temporary solution. Some have recommended fitting hearing aids on children with chronic conductive losses and have shown that it is a feasible alternative (Mathiesen, 1985; Northern & Downs, 1991). Another possible solution is temporary use of FM amplification devices until the hearing problems are resolved. Such units may also be used for children with slight sensorineural losses. However, when a hearing aid can be fitted comfortably, it is generally better to fit children with sensorineural losses with aid(s) while they are younger. As they get older, they tend to become more concerned about the unfortunate social stigma associated with amplification devices. In contrast, children who use amplification from an early age know how much it can help them and are less likely to part company with it as they get older. Nevertheless, getting children to use their hearing aid(s) on a regular basis may be one of the greatest challenges faced by the AR therapist.

Teachers and parents and, later, the child himself can provide information on how regularly the hearing aid is used. The therapist should seek out this information and try to modify behavior when necessary (Hanners & Sitton, 1974). Young children will often respond to methods like public charting of their daily hearing-aid use. The child can be made responsible for the charting. Older children should understand the purpose for amplification. When they are old enough, therefore, they need to receive the same instruction and information about their hearing loss as their parents were given previously. (See Amplification/Assistive Devices under Early Intervention in this chapter.)

Full-time use of an aid is preferable because the child is less likely to forget or lose the instrument. With older children, however, it is sometimes unrealistic. In the case of mild loss, the aid may provide little, if any, benefit in many play or recreational circumstances. The teenager, therefore, may elect not to use the aid during these times. The audiologic rehabilitationist may help the young person identify the situations where the aid should be used.

As the child gets older, she can begin to assume the responsibility for the care and management of the hearing aid. At that point, the AR therapist should teach the child about hearing aid function, repair, and use (see Chapter 2). Maintenance of children's hearing aids is often neglected, as shown in a series of studies starting with Gaeth and Lounsbury (1966). These writers found that approximately half the hearing aids in their study were not in working order and parents were generally ill informed about the rudiments of aid care. Unfortunately, that situation has not improved appreciably as reflected in subsequent studies, nearly all of which have shown 50% poor function among children's aids (Bess, 1977; Blair, et al., 1981; Zink, 1972; Schow, et al., 1993b). Furthermore, school programs have been similarly negligent about maintaining children's aids (Rawlings & Trybus, 1978; Sinclair, Bess, & Riggs, 1981) even though some projects have demonstrated that children's aids may be substantially improved by regular maintenance (Hoverstein, 1981; Kemker, McConnell, Logan, & Green, 1979).

In cases where the child's management skills are deficient due to age or length of experience with the aid, help and instruction should be provided (see Hoverstein [1981] for suggestions).

Assistive Listening Devices/Classroom Acoustics. Other aspects of amplification that become important in the school years include use of classroom amplification systems and the concern for quiet classroom environments. While no knowledgeable person would dispute the importance of quiet conditions for persons with hearing impairment, there has been some controversy about whether school-age youngsters should use educational (FM) auditory systems instead of personal hearing aids. Data from nearly 1900 classrooms for the hearing impaired suggest that about 1/3 of these children use personal hearing aids. Most students in these classes, therefore, use other amplification arrangements. Specifically, 1/4 use FM systems, another 1/3 use a combination of FM and personal aids, while the remainder (1/12) use loop or desk amplification systems (Sinclair & Freeman, 1981).

Personal hearing aids have improved appreciably over the past years so they now provide good fidelity, cosmetic appeal, and even a built-in FM system in some cases (see Chapter 2). In addition, they allow good student-to-student communication and self-monitoring by the child, and in small groups they provide satisfactory amplification for teacher-to-student communication purposes.

Consequently, personal hearing aids may be a reasonable choice in small classes made up entirely of children with hearing impairment when there is excellent acoustic treatment. However, whenever the class is large enough or noisy enough to create adverse signal-to-noise ratios, or when a child is mainstreamed, personal hearing aids (without a special FM circuit) present a major disadvantage. Specifically, when a person using a personal aid is not close to the speaker, the speaker's voice will not be as loud nor will the signal-to-noise ratio be as favorable as when a microphone can be placed close to the speaker. (See Case 3, Chapter 11.)

Chapter 2 contains a description of the different types of classroom amplification equipment in use. *FM radio-frequency* systems, used almost exclusively now, allow teacher and students more freedom and flexibility than other systems. Personal systems are used in the majority of cases but increasingly more classrooms are being outfitted with sound field systems wherein between two and four loudspeakers allow all students in the classroom to benefit from an improved auditory signal (Berg, 1993; Flexer, 1993). These sound-field systems have the advantage that they provide improved listening to students with hearing impairment without any stigma, which may be associated with using special equipment that they alone must wear. Personal FM systems may also be used with hearing aids by direct audio hookup and by induction loop transmission. The older forms of classroom amplification, the *standard* or *hard-wire* systems, and *induction loop amplification* (ILA) systems, are still used for some special applications. One other device is the *infrared system*, which utilizes light rays for transmission. The infrared system is usable in auditoriums and in many public buildings and for personal use and TV watching by some persons with hearing impairment.

The audiologic rehabilitationist must be knowledgeable about the various types of equipment and must be able to instruct others in daily operation and monitoring. Occasionally, AR professionals will also be asked to recommend the best arrangement for a particular setting. More frequently, they will simply be responsible for regularly evaluating, or getting someone else to evaluate, the function of existing systems. Several sources (Bess & Logan, 1984; Ross, 1987) contain thorough discussions of factors that should be considered when evaluating amplification equipment. Suffice it to say that attention should be given to: (a) electroacoustic considerations, (b) auditory self-monitoring capability of the units, (c) child-to-child communication potential, (d) signal-to-noise ratios, (e) binaural reception, and (f) simplicity and stability of operation.

OTHER ASSISTIVE DEVICES. It is important that the youngster with hearing impairment be introduced to other available accessory devices which can be useful in a variety of situations. Such devices include amplifiers for telephone, television, and radio; decoders for television; signal devices for doorbells and alarm clocks; and so forth. These devices are described in Chapter 2. In addition, therapy materials are available to help in familiarization (Castle, 1984).

SOUND TREATMENT. Well-functioning group amplifying systems will be more effective if used in an acoustically treated environment. In this regard, youngsters with hearing impairment with sensorineural losses will have more serious difficulties than the child with normal hearing when noise is present (Ross & Giolas, 1971). When all sounds are amplified, it is important to avoid excessive reverberation in the amplified environment. Reverberation occurs when reflected sound is present and added to the original sound. In an unbounded space (anechoic chamber) there is no reverberation. A sound occurs, moves through space, and is absorbed. However, in the usual listening environment like a classroom, sound hits various hard surfaces as it fans out in all directions, and it is reflected back. Consequently, not only the original unreflected sound, but a variety of reflected versions of the sound are present at once. This results in less distinct signals since signals are "smeared" in the time domain.

Reverberation Time (RT) is a measure of how long it takes before a sound is reduced by 60 dB once it is turned off. In an anechoic chamber, RT is near 0 seconds. In a typical classroom it is around 1.2 seconds. However, in a sound-treated classroom, one with carpets, acoustical tile, and solid-core doors, the RT can be on the order of 0.4 seconds. Finitzo-Heiber and Tillman (1978) showed the effect of RT and environmental signal-to-noise (S/N) ratio. The S/N ratio is a measure of how loud the desired signal (such as a teacher's voice) might be, compared to other random classroom noise. A +12 dB S/N ratio is considered acceptable for children with hearing impairment while +6 S/N and 0 S/N ratios are more typical of ordinary classrooms. As seen in Table 8.7, the speech identification of both children with normal hearing and children with hearing impairment is adversely affected when S/N ratios are poorer and RTs are increased. The performance of the child who is hard of hearing is more adversely affected by poor conditions than it is for children with normal hearing.

In the ordinary classroom, noise levels tend to be about 60 dBA, but in an open classroom they rise to 70 dBA. Gyms and cafeterias have noise levels of 70–90 dBA, with high amounts of reverberation. A carpeted classroom with five students and a teacher generates about 40–45 dBA of random noise. According to Finitzo-Heiber (1981), since voices at close range average 60–65 dBA, the S/N ratio in sound-treated classrooms may be +20 dB if the listener is close to the teacher. If the listener is farther away from the teacher, the signal will get weaker and the S/N ratio will be poorer. In view of poor performance by youngsters who are hard of hearing in noisy conditions (see Table 8.7), it is recommended that class noise levels be 45 dBA for gym and arts/crafts classes, but 30–35 dBA in the classrooms where these students spend most of their time (Bess & McConnell, 1981). Others have suggested that noise levels of about 50 dBA may be more feasible (Berg, 1986; Gengel, 1971). This would allow minimally acceptable S/N ratios of + 15–20 dB. Reverberation times are easier to reduce than noise levels. Thus, carpeting, acoustical tile, and even commercially available foam sheets may be placed in classrooms to help absorb noise. A feasible goal may be to reduce the RT to 0.3–0.4 seconds. In addition, provisions should be made to keep the child with hearing impairment close to the speaker (teacher). This can be accomplished through use of group amplification (FM) equipment, since the location of the microphone is, in effect, the position at which listening occurs. Extensive rationale and methods for providing sound treatment are available elsewhere (Berg, 1986).

TABLE 8.7 *Mean Word Identification Scores of Normal-Hearing and Hearing-Impaired Children under a High-Fidelity (Loudspeaker) and through an Ear-Level Hearing Aid Condition for Various Combinations of Reverberation and S/N Ratios*

Reverberation Time (RT) Sec	S/N Ratio in dB	Mean Word Identification Score (%)		
		Normal Group (PTA =0–10 dB)	Hearing Impaired Group (PTA=35–55 dB)	
		Loudspeaker	Loudspeaker	Hearing Aid
0.4	+12	83	69	60
	+6	71	55	52
	0	48	29	28
1.2	+12	69	50	41
	+6	54	40	27
	0	30	15	11

Adapted from "Room Acoustics' Effects on Monosyllabic Word Discrimination Ability for Normal and Hearing Impaired Children" by T. Finitzo-Heiber and T. Tillman, 1978, *Journal of Speech and Hearing Research, 21*, pp. 440–458.

To summarize, the audiologic rehabilitationist plays a crucial role in providing and encouraging both routine and extensive checks of individual and group amplifying systems and in obtaining adequate sound treatment in the educational setting.

Communication Rehabilitation. Many deaf and hard of hearing students are presently being served in public school settings, where audiologic rehabilitation specialists work to ensure a well-coordinated support service program. Two commonplace occurrences can be barriers to successful education of these students in regular education settings:

1. Classroom educators and administrators often underestimate the impact of the child's language problems on academic performance. Because the child who is hard of hearing, for example, may speak well on the surface and carry on conversations effectively, the teacher assumes that the child's language is "intact." Teachers may focus on whether or not the child can "hear" the instruction rather than whether or not the child can effectively process and understand the language of instruction. Blair, Peterson, and Viehweg (1985) documented significant lags in achievement of students with mild hearing impairment by the fourth grade when compared to their grade-mates with normal hearing. Although their subjects' scores on reading comprehension were close to a fourth-grade level, their peers were averaging a sixth-grade level performance. The problems of the student who is hard of hearing are often subtle, yet very significant. Teachers need to become aware of common language weaknesses that will interfere with academic development unless addressed.

2. Too often, support services are provided in a fragmented fashion. Due to time constraints, inadequate time is often available for teamwork among support service providers (like the AR clinician) and the classroom teacher. In the worst-case

scenario, the support professional is working on isolated language skills that bear little resemblance to the language demands the child is facing in the classroom. The goal is for all facets of the child's program to be closely integrated. This requires frequent communication and teamwork among the professionals serving the child. Parents should also be included in this team approach. The AR clinician who is well informed about the student's language abilities (strengths and weaknesses) in the classroom will be able to select priority goals that dovetail with the curricular demands the student is facing. The focus should be on building language skills to support academic success. This may include focus on attentional, problem solving and study skills.

LANGUAGE IN THE SCHOOL YEARS. Child language research has traditionally focused on grammatical and lexical attainments of the preschool years. As investigators have broadened the age range and scope of their inquiries, much has been discovered about the language achievements unique to the school-age years. Contrary to traditional beliefs that language acquisition was fairly complete by age seven, significant developmental changes have been documented in school-age students in discourse skills, pragmatic abilities, figurative language and metalinguistic skills (Miller, 1990; Nelson, 1984; Nippold, 1988; Stephens, 1988; Wallach & Miller, 1988). The fact that language continues to mature into the school years is obvious when one observes the young elementary student trying to deliver the punchline of a joke, or trying to relay the plot of a movie. These social language functions require the language user to understand shades of meaning and make sophisticated inferences about listener needs in organizing information relay. Such skills are still being acquired and refined by the school-age student. These language issues are relevant to management of the school-age student with hearing loss (Moeller, 1991). Many of these students are educated in regular classroom settings. An appreciation for the language demands placed on school-age learners is very germane to AR planning for school-age students.

Westby (1985) describes the preschool years as a time when children are "learning to talk." That is, children are acquiring the pragmatic phonological, grammatical, and morphological rules that are necessary for conveying their basic needs and desires. But school-age children are in the process of "talking to learn." That is, they are learning to use language to monitor and reflect on their past experiences and to plan, reason, and predict (Westby, 1985). This transition toward use of cognitive-linguistic functions like verbal reasoning, narrative, and prediction, is critical to the process of literacy attainment (Wallach & Miller, 1988; Westby, 1985) and classroom functioning. AR clinicians need to prioritize the language skills that support literacy attainment.

AN EXPANDED MODEL OF LANGUAGE PROCESSING. Miller (1990) proposed a two-level model of language processes. She defined level one (early developing) processes as the basic rules of semantics, syntax/morphology, phonology, and pragmatics. Level II (school-age) processes include three primary areas of development: (1) metalinguistic awareness, (2) discourse knowledge, and (3) higher level pragmatics (Miller, 1990).

Metalinguistic abilities allow a language user to reflect on language as an object of study (Wallach & Miller, 1988). Kamhi (1987) described metalinguistic achievements that progress through several stages: (a) learning to repair communicative breakdowns (which includes a metacognitive awareness of miscommunication), (b) making stylistic adjustments to accommodate the listener (involving ability to manipulate/change the language form), (c) making judgments about the accuracy/correctness of meanings or forms, (d) analyzing words into units (as in phonics), (e) learning to use humor (puns, riddles) and rhymes, and (f) comprehension and use of figurative language (e.g., metaphor, irony, parody).

Metalinguistic skills support literate language functions and are critical to classroom performance. Children who have metalinguistic skills can think about language to the degree that they can make reasonable predictions about the meaning of unknown words in a reading passage or conversation (Miller, 1990). Children can essentially "read between the lines" or make inferences, while reading, about how characters might react to certain events.

Discourse knowledge is important for effective conversational participation. During the school day, students interact with a wide range of conversational partners in different contexts. They converse with peers, which requires colloquial forms and stylistic modifications of language to fit the current "cultural" rules of the peer group. Students also converse with teachers and others in authority, requiring use of polite conventions or a more formal language register. Instructional discourse involves classroom-level dialogues, interaction with print, and independent information seeking. Each situation requires a different set of language rules. This means that students must acquire a considerable amount of linguistic flexibility.

Many times, the AR clinician provides individualized intervention with hearing-impaired students in a face-to-face, social discourse setting. This type of discourse is typically relaxed and colloquial, pertains to shared background between partners, and has frequent opportunity for repairing or correcting misunderstandings (Miller, 1990; Westby, 1985). Yet in a classroom context, students are required to process lengthy input with less opportunity for repair, and often the topics are divorced from the immediate context or shared experience (decontextualized). As the school years progress, topics become increasingly decontextualized and dependent on processing of linguistic information (Westby, 1985). Perhaps most challenging for the student with hearing impairment is the need to participate in conversations that shift among many speakers in a classroom. Furthermore, they must follow conversational rules in the classroom that are often implicit, or conveyed through subtle cues (Kretschmer, 1990).

Classroom discourse also includes *print* discourse, which comes in various forms. Narrative texts involve storytelling, whereas expository texts (like classroom textbooks) include factual accounts designed to impart knowledge. Students must gain the skills for both comprehending and using print. The AR therapist must be sensitive to differences in oral and written narratives (e.g., the style of written narrative is typically more formal and uses more compacted grammatical structures). The AR therapist may want to focus on strengthening oral narration to prepare the student for written discourse tasks. If a student has a theme to write, emphasis can be placed on building an oral narrative, brainstorming concepts for a theme through discussion, providing visual organizers so the student can make necessary concept associations, and then putting ideas into writing.

The third area described by Miller (1990) as a Level II process is called *higher order pragmatics*. She describes school-age students as maturing in two primary areas in this category: (a) learning to communicate intentions in an indirect manner (e.g., "Gimme a drink" gradually evolves to the adult, polite form, "Would it be too much trouble to get me a drink while you are up?"), and (b) learning to provide just the right amount of information to a listener. These skills require perspective-taking and an ability to infer what the listener needs to know. Again, the importance of cognitive-linguistic skills is evident. As students become more sophisticated in their conversational participation, they become attuned to both cultural rules and to listener needs. A good conversationalist "fine-tunes" to the reactions and needs of the listener. The ability to predict accurately the needs and perspective of another is related to conversational participation as well as comprehension of print. Knowledge of character traits and ability to identify with logical reactions to events supports story comprehension (Westby, 1985).

AR specialists need to gain an appreciation for these cognitive-linguistic attainments of the school years, if therapy is to be integrated within the framework of academic development. Functionalistic or pragmatically-motivated language intervention perspectives are relevant to developing language support for academics (Wallach & Miller, 1988). Functionalistic perspectives of language development maintain that language use cannot be separated from meaningful social context and that communicative need or purpose dictates the selection of grammatical and lexical forms. For example, if a student needs to tell a story in class about two peers involved in an accident, the student must select structures that support reference specification to keep the two girls straight for the listener (e.g., "the older girl" vs. "the younger girl with the braids," instead of nonspecific terms like "she"). Cohesive devices must be selected to give the listener the temporal sequence (e.g., "later that night;" "when they came home"). Students typically develop their narrative organization to the point where they can link their ideas logically to avoid unnecessary redundancy.

Clinicians can sometimes fall in the trap of working on grammatical skills in isolation, because this or that skill was identified as a weakness on a test. We feel that clinicians need to carefully consider as priorities the types of rules and content that will support higher-level language functions that are often required in the classroom setting. Emphasis on cohesive devices, using specific references, learning to organize thoughts in a narrative are all examples of skills that will support narrative development and literate language functions. For example, students are routinely asked to use oral and/or written language for such functions as providing explanations and reasons, making comparisons and contrasts, persuading others to a point of view, and providing descriptions or definitions (Bereiter & Engleman, 1966). Often, language must be used to solve verbal problems (e.g., How did the United States respond to the crash of the stock market?; Compare Bush's and Reagan's economic plans; If a train was travelling at X miles per hour, how long . . . ?). These language functions require not only verbal reasoning skills, but also the ability to narrate efficiently. We believe that these language skills should be a priority focus in audiologic rehabilitation.

Students with hearing impairment are often delayed in their comprehension and use of these cohesive ties (DeVilliers, 1988), which can affect both story comprehension and information relay. These higher-order expressive language processes are essential for literacy attainment, yet are often ignored in traditional assessment batteries.

CLASSROOM LISTENING ROLES. It is particularly relevant for the AR specialist to consider the characteristics of classrooms related to *listener* roles. Auditory skill development should not focus on isolated listening activities. Rather, auditory skills should be developed in an integrative fashion, with particular attention to classroom listening demands. Again, the goal is to help the student gain the necessary skills for success in the classroom. Estimates indicate that students spend more than 60% of instructional time in listening (Goodland, 1983). Much of teachers' discourse serves to impart information and is often organized into continuous discourse units. Shifts in speaker and topic are common (Nelson, 1984). Traditional speech recognition measures may tell us little about the readiness of a child with hearing impairment to cope with these types of listening requirements. Nelson (in press) describes classroom behaviors that are essential for classroom participation and comprehension. These include such skills as responding to the teacher's signals of task reorienting, recognizing when one has not understood, reading the teacher's moods and attitudes appropriately, shifting attention to others during their turns, and making comments relevant to the previous discourse contributions.

In examining the issue of classroom listening behaviors, it is also important to consider the role of cognitive-linguistic skills. Schwartz and McKinley (1984) identify two specific types of listening that are commonly required in later elementary and secondary classrooms. *Discriminative* listening involves listening for specific information. This includes cognitive-linguistic processes like identifying the main ideas in a lecture or story, finding relevant details, following directions, relating examples to global concepts, or recognizing a speaker's organization. *Evaluative* or *critical* listening involves judgment of fact vs. opinion, detection of bias or prejudice, drawing inferences, and evaluating arguments. These holistic processes represent a student's operationalizing of cognitive, linguistic, *and* auditory skills to negotiate meaning. Yet, test batteries and auditory training sequences typically focus on isolated, discrete auditory skills. Such results may not reflect the educational significance of the problem because they are divorced from functionalistic contexts and tasks. It is useful for AR specialists to consider higher-level processes when interpreting test or training outcomes. A recently published test, The Listening Test, from Linguasystems, is useful in this regard.

ISSUES IN INTERVENTION: WORLD KNOWLEDGE. There has been an increasing appreciation over the past several years for the contributions *word* and *world* knowledge make in literacy attainment. Vocabulary skills along with critical-thinking skills (e.g., making logical predictions and inferences, and applying verbal reasoning and problem solving skills) are critical to the processes of comprehending discourse, reading and academic texts.

Professionals have often pointed to vocabulary delays of students with hearing impairment as the major problem to overcome in developing literacy skills. This has led to strategies such as pre-teaching words out of context or memorizing lists of classroom vocabulary. However, the problem is broader than just lexical or word understanding. Students' *world-knowledge* and *word-knowledge networks* (schemata) in conjunction with critical-thinking skills play a significant role in literacy attainment. World knowledge is defined by Milosky (1990) as "the knowledge gained from experience, from interacting with others, with the objects, events and situations in life" (p. 1). Children's knowledge of events and experienced scripts (action sequences in long term memory) has considerable influence on their vocabulary acquisition. When new words are encountered, their meaning is processed or negotiated in reference to this fund of world knowledge. When people hear a word like "boot" in a conversation, their previous experiences influence the possible interpretations they will make. For example, an audiologist might hypothesize "FM connector to hearing aids," "method of starting a computer" or "galoshes" when hearing the word "boot." Some processing theories suggest that listeners activate from their lexicon only the relevant possibilities (based on rapid processing of context, situation, traits of the person, etc.) and try to make the incoming information relevant to what they already know (Garrod & Sanford, 1983; Waltz & Pollack, 1985).

When students acquire new words, it is hypothesized that the words are stored in memory in an organized fashion in relation to this world knowledge base (Pearson, 1983). New knowledge is stored in terms of worldly experiences, scripts, main organizing ideas, and key concepts, not just specific facts. Too often, vocabulary-intervention approaches focus on memorization of specific, isolated facts. This approach fails to respect that knowledge structures or schemata guide language and text comprehension (Kail & Leonard, 1986; Yoshinaga-Itano & Downey, 1986).

As noted earlier in this chapter, students benefit from a schema-based approach to vocabulary development. The same concepts noted for preschool-age children can be applied at a more complex level to school-age students. World knowledge "maps" or schema in memory guide a person's comprehension of conversation and text. Schemata are highly flexible and constantly changing as new meanings are encountered (Yoshinaga-Itano & Downey, 1986). For example, upon overhearing the word "Leonardo" several years ago, most listeners would assume from their world knowledge that the topic was the artist, da Vinci. Today, the hypothesis may shift to "Teenage Mutant Ninja Turtles," depending on the listener's experiences with cartoons. Memorizing words in isolation does not support the flexible process of integrating new concepts into an existing conceptual framework.

World knowledge networks also guide readers' interpretation of the meaning of written text. Consider the following passage from a fourth grade reader: "Singing happily, Bonita finished her chores." (Already, readers will find themselves making inferences or reading between the lines based on world knowledge. For example, readers may predict that the young woman is hispanic, and that she enjoys housework or is anticipating a pleasant event.) "Lightheartedly she went up to her room. She had changed into her baseball uniform when she heard her father's footsteps in the hall. She poked her head out the door. 'What is it daddy?' she called out. Mr. Valdez never came back to the ranch house so early unless something was wrong." (Good readers have made many additional inferences that are essential for understanding the relationships and events in the story. Readers have assumed from minor cues that there is a problem on the ranch and that Bonita's mood may change.) This brief passage illustrates that readers actively interact with text, by recruiting world knowledge and by making logical inferences and assumptions. Vocabulary programs must be organized in such a way that the student learns to recruit knowledge networks in order to make appropriate inferences and "read between the lines" to access meaning.

Thus, vocabulary deficits of persons with hearing impairment need to be considered in terms of broader competencies. It is not sufficient to ask, "Does the student know this word?" Rather, AR specialists should consider questions like, "Does the student's world-knowledge base support active processing of meaning in context? Is the student able to associate new information with existing concepts? Does the student see the connection between this information and other established networks of meaning?" The AR therapist should be in close communication with the teacher about concepts and lexical items that are critical to understanding main content objectives from the curriculum. Integration of efforts will make the best use of the student's limited time for learning.

Psychosocial. ADJUSTMENTS FOR MILD LOSSES/AUDITORY-LANGUAGE PROCESSING PROBLEMS. Children with mild hearing problems (i.e., mild sensorineural loss, conductive loss) and those with Central Auditory Processing Disorders (CAPD) may require communication rehabilitation along with children who demonstrate more pronounced losses. Although the language-related problems may be minimized in the case of milder losses, they are apt to be present and require attention (Northern and Downs, 1991). A careful multidisciplinary assessment of the child's difficulties should be conducted consisting of reports from teachers, parents, the child, and others in addition to observation and diagnostic testing.

Most authorities agree that CAPD or auditory-language processing deficits involve a variety of difficulties either in one or all areas of (a) detection, (b) interpretation, or (c) categorization. Such difficulties may involve a peripheral, central, or general cognitive problem, or a combination thereof (Katz, Stecker, & Henderson, 1992). Katz, et al. and others have raised the question of whether children suspected of having auditory-language processing problems are primarily language-disabled or primarily poor auditory processors. These authors urged a synthesis of views. In a simple model, they suggested that sometimes there is a greater problem with language processing and a lesser problem with lower order auditory processing. In other cases, the reverse is true. At yet other times, there may be a more equal problem in the two areas.

One approach in a diagnostic workup on such a child involves an emphasis on both thorough assessment of language skills and on a variety of auditory tasks (Butler, 1983). However, Butler's approach puts most emphasis on informal, practical assessment and management (see Table 8.8 for various functional deficits to be informally evaluated, as suggested by Chermak and Musiek, 1992). Assessment may also involve

TABLE 8.8 *Management of Central Auditory Processiong Disorders*

Functional Deficit	Strategies	Techniques
Distractibility/inattention	Increase signal-to-noise ratio	ALD/FM system; acoustic modifications preferential seating
Poor memory	Metalanguage	Chunking, verbal chaining, mnemonics, rehearsal, paraphrasing, summarizing
	Right hemisphere activation	Imagery, drawing
	External aids	Notebooks, calendars
Restricted vocabulary	Improve closure	Contextual derivation of word meaning
Cognitive inflex—predominantly analytic or predominantly conceptual	Diversify cognitive style	Top-down (deductive) and bottom-up (inductive) processing, inferential reasoning, questioning, critical thinking
Poor listening comprehension	Induce formal schema to aid organization, integration, and prediction	Recognize and explain connectives (additives; causal; adversative; temporal) and patterns of parallelism and correlative pairs (not only/but also; neither/nor)
	Maximize visual and auditory summation	Substitutions for notetaking
Reading, spelling, and listening problems	Enhance multisensory integration	Phonemic analysis and segmentation
Maladaptive behaviors (passive, hyperactive, impulsive)	Assertiveness and cognitive behavior modification	Self-control, self-monitoring, self-evaluation, self-instruction, problem solving
Poor motivation	Attribution retraining: internal locus of control	Failure confrontation, attribution to factors under control

Source: Chermak and Musiek, 1992.

a more formal battery of tests or a combination of formal and informal procedures (Smoski, et al., 1992; Musiek & Chermak, 1994). (Many diagnostic tools have been developed for this purpose; see Chapter 13, List of Resources and Materials.) Regardless of the assessment approach used, the ability to diagnose these difficulties is not yet as exact as we would like it to be.

Useful assistance can probably be rendered by identifying the specific difficulties the child experiences as determined from a list such as seen in Table 8.8. After identifying unusual auditory behaviors, the therapist may assist teachers, parents, and children in becoming more aware of, and hence avoiding, situations that contribute to the child's difficulties. Chermak and Musiek (1992) provided some useful suggestions for therapy with these youngsters.

SUMMARY

This chapter has provided an introduction to the process of audiologic rehabilitation at two distinct levels: the early intervention level and school-age service levels. Although services in these settings are provided by a variety of personnel and in various communication modes, one professional—the parent advisor or the AR therapist—often assumes the important roles of coordinating service provision and serving as an advocate for children and families. This chapter has emphasized the critical importance of family-centered practice and the role of the family throughout the child's educational program. Audiologic rehabilitation services throughout the child's life focus on four major areas: (a) appropriate assessment and selection of intervention priorities, including amplification and communication systems; (b) overall coordination and integration of services within a model of language and literacy attainment; (c) communication rehabilitation; and (d) psychosocial support for the child and family. At the school-age level, the importance of integrated service delivery that considers the unique communicative demands of the classroom setting has been emphasized. Rehabilitation presents challenges to parents, children, and therapists. Nevertheless, if proper attention is given to all of these aspects, prospects for effective management may be very good. If the problems of the child with hearing impairment are underestimated or neglected, the student may experience long-term negative consequences on language, literacy, and social-skill attainment. Aggressive and early management of children who are deaf or hard of hearing through audiologic rehabilitation is important.

RECOMMENDED READINGS

American Speech-Language-Hearing Association (1993). *Guidelines for audiology serivces in the schools. Asha, 35, (suppl. 10) pp. 24–32.*

Bess, F., & McConnell, F. (1981). *Audiology, education and the hearing-impaired child.* St. Louis: C. V. Mosby Co.

Boothroyd, A. (1982). *Hearing impairments in young children.* Englewood Cliffs, NJ: Prentice Hall.

Watkins, S. and Clark, T. C. (1993). *SKI*HI resource manual: Family-centered, home-based programming for infants, toddlers, and preschool-aged children with hearing impairment.* Logan, UT: HOPE, Inc.

Cole, E. B. (1992). *Listening and Talking: A guide to promoting spoken language in young hearing impaired children.* Washington, DC: Alexander Graham Bell Association for the Deaf.

Ling, D. (1989). *Foundations of spoken language in hearing impaired children.* Washington, DC: Alexander Graham Bell Association for the Deaf.

Pugh, G. (1994). *Deaf and hard of hearing students: Educational service guidelines.* NASDSE, Alexandria, VA.

Roush, J., & Matkin, N. D. (1994). *Infants and toddlers with hearing loss.* Baltimore: York Press, Inc.

REFERENCES

Allen, T. E. (1986). Patterns of academic achievement among hearing impaired students; 1974–1983. In A. N. Schildroth and M. A. Karchmer (Eds.), *Deaf children in America* (pp. 161–206). San Diego: College-Hill Press.

Alpiner, J. G., & McCarthy, P. A. (1993). *Rehabilitative audiology: Children and adults.* Baltimore: Williams & Wilkins.

American Annals of the Deaf. (1994). Annual survey of hearing-impaired children and youth. *American Annals of the Deaf, 139*(2), 239–243.

Andrews, J., & Andrews, M. (1986). A family based systemic model for speech-language services. *Seminars in Speech and Language, 7*(4), 359–365.

Anderson, K. L. (1989). Speech perception and the hard-of-hearing child. *Educational Audiology Monograph, 1,* 15–29.

ASHA–American Speech and Hearing Association. (1985). *Guidelines for identification audiometry. Asha, 28,* 49–52.

ASHA–American Speech-Language-Hearing Association (1989). Guidelines for audiologic screening of newborn infants who are at risk for hearing impairment. *Asha, 31,* 89–92.

ASHA–American Speech-Language-Hearing Association (1989). *Specifications for audiometers* (ANSI S3.6-1989). New York: Acoustical Society of America.

ASHA–American Speech and Hearing Association (1990). Guidelines for screening for hearing impairments and middle ear disorders. *Asha, 32*(Suppl. 2), 17–24.

ASHA–American Speech-Language-Hearing Association (1993). Guidelines for audiology services in the schools. *Asha, 35*(Suppl. 10), 24–32.

Bailey, D. B., & Simeonsson, R. J. (1986). Design issues in family impact evaluations. In L. Bickman and D. L. Weatherford (Eds.), *Evaluating Early Intervention Programs for Severely Handicapped Children and Their Families.* Austin, TX: Pro-Ed.

Bailey, D. J. (1987). Collaborative goal setting with families: Resolving differences in values and priorities for service. *Topics in Early Childhood Education, 7*(2), 59–71.

Bankson, N. W., & Bernthal, J. E. (1990). *Bankson-Bernthal test of phonology.* San Antonio, TX: Special Press, Inc.

Barnes, S., Gutfreund, M., Satterly, D., & Wells, G. (1983). Characteristics of adult speech which predict children's language development. *Journal of Child Language, 10,* 65–84.

Bentler, R. A. (1993). Amplification for the hearing-impaired child. In J. G. Alpiner and P. A. McCarthy (Eds.), *Rehabilitative audiology: Children and adults.* Baltimore: Williams and Wilkins.

Bereiter, C., & Engelmann, S. (1966). *Teaching disadvantaged children in the preschool.* Englewood Cliffs, NJ: Prentice Hall.

Berg, F. S. (1986). Classroom acoustics and signal transmission. In F. Berg, et al. (Eds.), *Educational audiology for the hard of hearing child* (pp. 157–180). Orlando, FL: Grune and Stratton.

Berg, F. S. (1993). *Acoustics and sound systems in schools*. San Diego: Singular.

Bernstein, M., & Morrison, M. (1992). Are We Ready for PL99-457? *AAD, 137*(1), 7–13.

Bess, F. H., Logan, S.A. (1984).Amplification in the educational setting. In F. Bess & J. Jerger (Eds.), *Pediatric audiology* (pp. 147–176). San Diego: College-Hill Press.

Birch, J. (1975). *Hearing impaired children in the mainstream*. Reston, VA: Council for Exceptional Children.

Blair, J., Petersen, M., & Viehweg, S., (1985).The effects of mild sensorineural hearing loss on academic performance of young school-age children. *Volta Review, 87*(2), 87–93.

Blair, J., Wright, K., & Pollard, G. (1981). Parental understanding of their children's hearing aids. *Volta Review, 83*, 375–382.

Blank, M., Rose, S., & Berlin, L. (1978). *The language of learning: The preschool years* (pp. 8–21). New York: Grune & Stratton.

BOL Statistics. (1977). *Education attainment of workers, special labor force report 209.* USDL Bureau of Labor Statistics. Washington, DC: U.S. Government Printing Office.

Boothroyd, A. (1982). *Hearing impairments in young children*. Englewood Cliffs, NJ: PrenticeHall.

Bornstein, H., Saulnier, K., & Hamilton, L. (1980). Signed English:A first evaluation. *American Annals of the Deaf, 125*, 467–481.

Bredekamp, S. (1987). *Developmentally appropriate practice in early childhood programs serving children from birth through age 8*, (expanded ed.). Washington, DC: National Association for the Education of Young Children.

Brinker, R., Frazier, W., & Baxter, A. (1992). Maintaining involvement of inner city families in EI programs through a program of incentives: Looking beyond family systems to social systems. *OSERS News in Print. Winter, 4*(1), 9–19.

Bronfenbrenner, U. (1974). *Is early intervention effective? A report on longitudinal evaluations of preschool programs* (vol. II). (Department of Health, Education and Welfare, Office of Human Development, Office of Child Development, Children's Bureau, Department of Health, Education, and Welfare Publication No. OHD-76-30020). Washington, DC: U.S. Government Printing Office.

Busch, C., & Halpin, K. (1992). Incorporating deaf culture into early intervention. In B. Schick & M. P. Moeller (Eds.), *Proceedings of the Seventh Annual Conference on Issues in Language and Deafness*. Omaha, NE: Boys Town National Research Hospital, 117–125.

Carney, A.E., (1991). Vocal development in hearing-impaired infants. *Journal of the Acoustical Society of America, 90*, 2296 (A).

Carotta, C., Carney,A. E., & Dettman, D., (1990).Assessment and analysis of speech production in hearing-impaired children. *Asha, 32*, 59 (A).

Castle, D. (1984). *Telephone training for hearing-impaired persons: Amplified telephones, TDD's, codes.* Washington, DC: Alexander Graham Bell Association for the Deaf.

Chermak, G. D., & Musiek, F. E. (1992). Managing central auditory processing disorders in children and youth. *American Journal of Audiology,* 61-65.

Clark, T. (1994) SKI-HI: Applications for home-based intervention. In J. Roush & N. D. Matkin (Eds.), *Infants and toddlers with hearing loss* (pp. 237-252). Baltimore: York Press, Inc.

Cole, E. B. (1992). *Listening and Talking: A guide to promoting spoken language in young hearing impaired children.* Washington, DC: Alexander Graham Bell Association for the Deaf.

Curran, J. R. (1985). ITE aids for children: Survey of attitudes and practices of audiologists. *Hearing Instruments, 36*(4), 20-25.

Davis, J. (1990). Personnel and service. In J. Davis (Ed.), *Our forgotten children: Hard of hearing pupils in the school* (2nd. ed.). Washington, DC: Self Help for the Hard of Hearing.

Davis, J., Elfenbein, J., Schum, R., & Bentler, R. (1986). Effects of mild and moderate hearing impairments on language, educational, and psychosocial behavior of children. *JSHR: 51*(1), 53-63.

deVilliers, P. (1988). Assessing English syntax in hearing-impaired children: Eliciting production in pragmatically-motivated situations [Monograph]. *Journal of the Academy of Rehabilitative Audiology, 21* (suppl.), 41-71.

Dillon, H., Koritschoner, E., Battaglia, J., Lovegrove, R., Ginis, J., Mavrias, G., Carnie, L., Ray, P., Forsythe, L., Towers, E., Goulias, H., & Macaskill, F. (1991). Rehabilitation effectiveness I: Assessing the needs of clients entering a national hearing rehabilitation program. *Australian Journal of Audiology, 13*, 55-65.

Dunst, C. J. (1985). Rethinking early intervention. *Analysis and Intervention in Developmental Disabilities, 5*, 165-201.

Eagles, E., Wishik, S., Doetfler, L., Melnick, W., & Levine, H. (1963). Hearing sensitivity and related factors in children [Special Monograph]. *Laryngoscope,* 1-95.

Ensher, G. L. (1989). The first three years: Special education perspectives on assessment and intervention. *Topics in Language Disorders, 10*(1), 80-90.

Erber, N. P. (1982). *Auditory training.* Washington, DC: Alexander Graham Bell Association for the deaf.

Erber, N. P., & Alencewicz, C.M. (1976). Audiological evaluation of deaf children. *Journal of Speech and Hearing Disorders, 41*, 256-267.

Finitzo-Heiber, T. (1981). Classroom acoustics. In R. Roeser & M. Downs (Eds.), *Auditory disorders in school children* (pp. 250-262). New York: Thieme-Stratton.

Finitzo-Heiber, T., & Tillman, T. (1978). Room acoustics' effects on monosyllabic word discrimination ability for normal and hearing impaired children. *Journal of Speech and Hearing Research, 21*, 440-458.

Fischer, S.D. (1994). Critical periods: Critical issues. In B. Schick, & M. P. Moeller, *Proceedings of the 7th Annual Conference on Issues in Language and*

Deafness. The use of sign language in educational settings: Current concepts and controversies (pp. 1–12). Omaha, NE: Boys Town National Research Hospital.

Fitzgerald, M. T., & Fischer, R. M. (1987). A family involvement model for hearing-impaired infants. *Topics in Language Disorders, 7,* 1–19.

Flexer, C. (1993). Management of hearing in an educational setting. In J. G. Alpiner and P. A. McCarthy (Eds.), *Rehabilitative Audiology: Children and Adults* (2nd ed.). Baltimore: Williams and Wilkins, 176–210.

Flint, W. (1971). Literacy: The keystone for providing more opportunities for deaf children. *Proceedings of the Forty-Fifth Meeting of the Convention of American Instructors for the Deaf.*

Gaeth, J., & Lounsbury, E. (1966). Hearing aids and children in elementary schools. *Journal of Speech and Hearing Disorders, 31,* 283–289.

Garrod, S., & Sanford, A. (1983). Topic dependent effects in language processing. In G. Flores d'Areais & R. Jarvella (Eds.), *The process of language understanding.* New York: John Wiley and Sons.

Gengel, R. (1971). Acceptable speech-to-noise ratios for aided speech discrimination by the hearing impaired. *Journal of Audiological Research, 11,* 219–222.

Glover, B., Watkins, S., Pittman, P., Johnson, D., & Barringer, D. G. (1994). SKI-HI home intervention for families with infants, toddlers, and preschool children who are deaf or hard of hearing. *Infant-Toddler Intervention: The Transdisciplinary Journal, 4*(4), 319–332.

Goodland, J. (1983). *A place called school. Prospects for the future.* New York: McGraw-Hill.

Grant, J. (1987). *The hearing impaired: Birth to six.* Boston: College Hill Press.

Greenberg, M. (1983). Family stress and child competence: The effects of early intervention for families with deaf infants. *American Annals of the Deaf, 128,* 407–417.

Greenberg, M., Calderon, R., & Kusche, C. (1984). Early intervention using simultaneous communication with deaf infants: The effect on communication development. *Child Development, 55*(2), 607–616.

Greenstein, J. (1975). *Methods of fostering language development in deaf infants. Final Report.* Bureau of Education for the Handicapped (DHEW/OE), Washington, DC. BBB000581.

Hanners, B. A., & Sitton, A. B. (1974). Ear to hear: A daily hearing aid monitor program. *Volta Review, 76,* 530–536.

Harrison, M. F. (1994). Preparing the Individualized Family Service Plan: An illustrative case. In J. Roush & N. D. Matkin (Eds.). *Infants and toddlers with hearing loss,* (pp. 113–132). Baltimore: York Press, Inc.

Hasenstab, M. S., & Horner, J. S. (1982). *Comprehensive intervention with hearing impaired infants and preschool children.* Rockville, MD: Aspen Systems.

Hatfield, N., & Humes, K. (1992). Developing a bilingual-bicultural parent-infant program: Challenges, compromises and controversies. In B. Schick & M. P. Moeller (Eds.), *Proceedings of the Seventh Annual Conference on Issues in*

Language and Deafness. Omaha, NE: Boys Town National Research Hospital.

Herzog, J. E. (1985). A study of the effectiveness of early intervention for hearing handicapped children. *Dissertation Abstracts International*, 46, 121A.

Hohmann, M., Banet, B., & Weikart, D. (1979). *Young children in action*. Ypsilanti, MI: High/Scope Press.

Hoverstein, G. (1981). A public school audiology program: Amplification maintenance, auditory management, and inservice education. In F. Bess, et al. (Eds.), *Amplification in education*. Washington, DC: Alexander Graham Bell Association for the Deaf.

Idol, L., Paolucci-Whitcomb, P., & Nevin, A. (1986). *Collaborative consultation*. Rockville, MD: Aspen.

Jerger, J. (1980). Dissenting report: Mass impedance screening. *Annals of Otology, Rhinology, and Laryngology*, 89(Suppl. 69), 21–22.

Johnson, C. D. (1987). Educational management of the hearing impaired child. In J. G. Alpiner and P. A. McCarthy (Eds.), *Rehabilitative audiology: Children and adults* (2nd ed.). Baltimore: Williams and Wilkins (pp. 241–268).

Johnson, R., Liddell, S., & Erting, C. (1989). *Unlocking the curriculum: Principles for achieving access in deaf education*. Gallaudet Research Institute Working Paper 89-3. Washington, DC: Gallaudet University.

Joint Committee on Infant Hearing. (1994). Position statement. *Audiology today*. 6(6), 6–9.

Kail, R., & Leonard, L. (1986). Word-finding abilities in language-impaired children [Monograph 25]. *Asha Monographs*, Rockville, MD: Asha.

Kamhi, A. (1987). Metalinguistic ability in language-impaired children. *Topics in Language Disorders*, 7(2), 1–13.

Kostelnik, M., Howe, D., Payne, K., Rohde, B., Spalding, G., Stein, L., & Whitbeck, D. (1991). *Teaching young children using themes*. Glenview, IL: Good Year Books.

Kretschmer, R. (March, 1990). Classroom discourse: How regular classrooms are organized, implications for mainstreaming hearing handicapped children. Paper presented at the meeting of the Nebraska Educators of the Hearing Impaired Conference, Lincoln, NE.

Lillie, S. M. (1969). *Management of deafness in infants and very young children through their parents*. Address at the 47th Annual International Convention, Council for Exceptional Children, Denver.

Ling, D. (1989). Foundations of spoken language in hearing impaired children. Washington, DC: Alexander Graham Bell Association for the Deaf.

Ling, D. (1978). Auditory coding and recoding: An analysis of auditory training procedures for hearing-impaired children. In M. Ross & T. Giolas (Eds.), *Auditory management of hearing-impaired children: Principles and prerequisites for intervention* (pp. 181–218). Austin, TX: Pro-Ed.

Ling, D. (1976). *Speech and the hearing impaired child: Theory and practice*. Washington, DC: Alexander Graham Bell Association for the Deaf.

Ling, D. (1976). *Speech for the deaf child*. Washington, DC: Alexander Graham Bell Association for the Deaf.

Ling, D., & Ling, A. (1978). *Audiologic habilitation: The foundations of verbal learning in hearing-impaired children*. Washington, DC: Alexander Graham Bell Association for the Deaf.

Lundeen, (1991) Prevalence of hearing impairment among school children. *Language, Speech and Hearing Services in Schools, 22*, 269–271.

Luterman, D. (1987). *Deafness in the family*. San Diego: College-Hill Press.

Madell, R. (1984). Audiological management of the hearing-impaired child in the mainstream setting. In J. Northern & W. Perkins (Eds.), *Seminars in Hearing, 5*, 353–365.

Manolson, A., (1985). *It takes two to talk* (2nd ed.). Toronto: Hanen Early Language Resource Centre.

Marlowe, J. A.. (1984). The auditory approach to communication development for the infant with hearing loss. In W. Perkins (Ed.), *Current therapy of communication disorders: Hearing disorders* (pp. 3–9). New York: Thieme-Stratton.

Masur, E. F. (1982). Mothers' responses to infants' object-related gestures; Influences on lexical development. *Journal of Child Language, 9*, 23–30.

Mathiesen, C. J. (1985). *Hearing aid applications in young children with recurrent otitis media*. Unpublished master's thesis, Idaho State University.

Matkin, N.D. (1984). Wearable amplification: A litany of persisting problems. In J. Jerger (Ed.), *Pediatric audiology: Current trends* (pp. 125–145). San Diego: College-Hill Press.

Meadow, K., Greenberg, M., Erting, C., & Carmichael, H. (1981). Interactions of deaf mothers and deaf preschool children: Comparisons with three other groups of deaf and hearing dyads. *American Annals of the Deaf, 126*, 454–468.

Miller, L. (1990). The roles of language and learning in the development of literacy. *Topics in Language Disorders, 10*(2), 1–25.

Milosky, L. (1990). The role of world knowledge in language comprehension and language intervention. *Topics in Language Disorders, 10*(3), 1–13.

Mindel, E. D., & Vernon, M. (1987). *They grow in silence: The deaf child and his family* (2nd ed.). Silver Spring, MD: National Association of the Deaf.

Moeller, M. P. (1988). Language assessment strategies [Monograph Supplement]. *Journal of the Academy of Rehabilitative Audiology. 21*, 73–99.

Moeller, M. P. (1991). Current issues and challenges in language development and the hearing impaired child. In J. A. Feigin & P. G. Stelmachowicz (Eds.), *Pediatric Amplification: Proceedings of the 1991 National Conference.* Omaha, NE: Boys Town National Research Hospital.

Moeller, M. P. (September, 1993a). Auditory learning: Efficacy and validation issues. Paper presented at the 1993 Conference on Developments in Pediatric Audiology: Assessment and Amplification. Omaha, NE: Boys Town National Research Hospital.

Moeller, M. P. (September, 1993b). Research on home use of FM systems: Impact on language. Paper presented at the 1993 Conference on Developments in Pediatric Audiology: Assessment and Amplification. Omaha, NE: Boys Town National Research Hospital.

Moeller, M. P., & Carney, A. E. (1993). Assessment and intervention with preschool hearing-impaired children. In J. Alpiner & P. McCarthy (Eds.), *Rehabilitative audiology: Children and adults* (2nd ed.), 106–136. Baltimore: Williams & Wilkins.

Moeller, M. P., & Condon, M.-C. (1994). D.E.I.P.: A collaborative problem-solving approach to early intervention. In J. Roush & N. D. Matkin (Eds.), *Infants and toddlers with hearing loss*, (pp. 163–194). Baltimore: York Press, Inc.

Moeller, M. P., Coufal, K., & Hixson, P. (1990). The efficacy of speech-language intervention: Hearing impaired children. *Seminars in Speech and Language*, *11*(4), 227–241.

Moeller, M. P., & Luetke-Stahlman, B. (1990). Parents' use of Signing Exact English: A descriptive analysis. *Journal of Speech & Hearing Disorders*, *55*, 327–338.

Moeller, M. P., Schick, B., & Williams, K. T. (1994). Sign with me: A family sign program. In B. Schick & M. P. Moeller (Eds.), *Proceedings of the Seventh Annual Conference on Issues in Language and Deafness*. Omaha, NE: Boys Town National Research Hospital.

Moses, K. L. (1985). Infant deafness and parental grief: Psychosocial early intervention. In F. Powell, et al. (Eds.), *Education of the hearing impaired child*, (pp. 85–102). San Diego: College-Hill Press.

Nelson, N. (1984). Beyond information processing: The language of teachers and textbooks. In G. P. Wallach & K. G. Butler (Eds.), *Language learning disabilities in school-age children*, (pp. 154–178). Baltimore: Williams and Wilkins.

Nelson, N. (1988). *Planning individualized speech and language intervention program* (2nd ed.). Tucson, AZ: Communication Skills Builders.

Nippold, M. (Ed.) (1988). *Later language development: Ages nine through nineteen*. Boston: College-Hill Press.

Northern, J., & Downs, M. (1991). *Hearing in children* (4th ed.). Baltimore: Williams & Wilkins.

Oller, D. K. (1983). Infant babbling as a manifestation of the capacity for speech. In S. E. Gerber & G. T. Mencher (Eds.), *The development of auditory behavior*, (pp. 221–236). New York: Grune & Stratton.

Oller, D. K., & Eilers, R. E. (1988). The role of audition in infant babbling. *Child Development*, *59*, 441–449.

Osberger, M. J. (1983). Development and evaluation of some speech training procedures for hearing-impaired children. In I. Hochberg, H. J. Levitt, & M. J. Osberger (Eds.), *Speech of the hearing impaired-Research, training and personnel preparation*. Austin, TX: Pro-Ed.

Parent Infant Communication. (1995) Infant Hearing Resource Staff. (3rd ed.) Portland, OR

Pearson, P. (1982). A primer for schema theory. In R. E. Krestschmer (Ed.), Reading and the hearing-impaired individual. *Volta Review*, *84*(5), 25–35.

Phillips, A. L. (1987). Working with parents. A story of personal and professional growth. In D. Atkins (Ed.), Families and their hearing-impaired children. *Volta Review*, *89*(5), 131–146.

Pinker, S. (1994). *The language instinct.* New York: William Morrow.

Prendergast, S. (1994). Maternal manual communication and deaf toddler gaze in play: A comparison of dyads with deaf and hearing mothers. In B. Schick & M. P. Moeller (Eds.), *Proceedings of the Seventh Annual Conference on Issues in Language and Deafness.* Omaha, NE: Boys Town National Research Hospital.

Pugh, G. (1994). Deaf and hard of hearing students: Educational service guidelines. NASDSE, Alexandria, VA.

Quittner, A., & Steck, J. (November, 1989). Impact of hearing loss on child development and family adjustment. Paper presented at the meeting of the American Speech-Language-Hearing Association, St. Louis, MO.

Rafferty, M. (1970). *Report of the study committee on state wide planning for the education of the deaf and severely hard of hearing in California state schools.* Sacramento: California State Department of Education.

Ramsdell, D. (1978). The psychology of the hard-of-hearing and the deafened adult. In H. Davis & R. Silverman (Eds.), *Hearing and deafness* (4th ed., pp. 499–510). New York: Holt, Rinehart & Winston.

Rand Report. (1974). *Improving services to handicapped children.* Santa Monica, CA: The Rand Corporation.

Ross, M. (1987). Classroom amplification. In W. Hodgson & P. Skinner (Eds.), *Hearing aid assessment and use in audiologic habilitation* (3rd ed., pp. 231–265). Baltimore: Williams & Wilkins.

Ross, M. (1990). *Hearing-impaired children in the mainstream.* Parkton, MD: York Press.

Ross, M., Brackett, D., & Maxon, A. (1991). *Assessment and management of mainstreamed hearing-impaired children: Principles and practices.* Austin, TX: Pro-Ed.

Ross, M., & Giolas, T. (1971). Effects of three classroom listening conditions on speech intelligibility. *American Annals of the Deaf, 116,* 580-584.

Ross, M., & Tomassetti, C. (1987). Hearing aid selection for preverbal hearing-impaired children. In M. C. Pollack (Ed.), *Amplification for the hearing impaired* (3rd ed., pp. 213-253). New York: Grune & Stratton.

Roush, J., & Matkin, N. D. (1994). *Infants and toddlers with hearing loss.* Baltimore: York Press.

Schick, B., & Moeller, M. P. (1992) What is learnable in MCE? *Journal of Applied Psycholinguistics, 13,* 313–340.

Schlesinger, H., & Acree, M. (1984). Antecedents to achievement and adjustment in deaf adolescents: A longitudinal study of deaf children. In G. B. Anderson & D. Watson (Eds.). *The habilitation and rehabilitation of deaf adolescents* (pp. 48–61). Washington, DC: The National Academy of Gallaudet College.

Schow, R. L., Balsara, N. R., Smedley, T. C., & Whitcomb, C. J. (1993a). Audiologic Rehabilitation by ASHA Audiologists: 1980-1990. *American Journal of Audiology. 2*(3), 28–37.

Schow, R. L., Maxwell, S. A., Crookston, G J., & Newman, M. T. (1993b). How well do adults take care of their hearing instruments? *Hearing Instruments, 44*(3), 16–20.

Schuyler, V., & Rushmer, N. (1987). *Parent infant habilitation: A comprehensive approach to working with hearing-impaired infants and toddlers and their families*. Portland: IHR Publications.

Schwartz, L., & McKinley, N. (1984). *Daily communication strategies for the language disordered adolescent*. Eau Claire, WI: Thinking Publications.

Shepherd, N., Davis, J., Gorga, M., & Stelmachowicz, P. (1981). Characteristics of hearing impaired children in the public schools: Part I-Demographic data. *Journal of Speech and Hearing Disorders, 46*, 123–129.

Simmons-Martin, A. A., & Rossi, K. G. (1990). *Parents and teachers: Partners in language development*. Washington, DC: Alexander Graham Bell Association for the Deaf.

Sinclair, J. S., & Freeman, B. A. (1981). The status of classroom amplification in American education. In F. Bess, et al. (Eds.), *Amplification in education*. Washington, DC: Alexander Graham Bell Association for the Deaf.

SKI-HI Institute (1994). *SKI-HI 1992–1993 national data report*. Logan UT: Utah State University, SKI-HI Institute.

Snow, C. E. (1983). Literacy and language: Relationships during the preschool years. *Harvard Educational Review, 53*(2), 165–189.

Sparks, S. M. (1989). Assessment and intervention with at-risk infants and toddlers: Guidelines for the speech-language pathologist. *Topics in Language Disorders., 10*(1), 43–56.

Stein, D., Benner, G., Hoversten, G., McGinnis, M., & Thies, T. (1980). *Auditory skills curriculum*. North Hollywood, CA: Foreworks.

Stephens, M. I. (1988). Pragmatics. In M. Nippold (Ed.), *Later language development* (pp. 247–263). Boston: College-Hill Press.

Stoel-Gammon, C. & Cooper, J. A. (1984). Patterns of early lexical and phonological development. *Child Language, 11*, 247–271.

Stredler-Brown, A., & Yoshinago-Itano, C. (1994). A multidisciplinary evaluation tool. In J. Roush & N. D. Matkin (Eds.), *Infants and toddlers with hearing loss*, (pp. 133–162). Baltimore: York Press.

Strong, C. J., Clark, T. C., Barringer, D. G., Walden, B. E., & Williams, S. A. (1992). *SKI-HI home-based programming for children with hearing impairments: Demographics, child identification, and program effectiveness*. Logan, UT: HOPE, Inc.

Strong, C. J., Clark, T. C., Johnson, D., Watkins, S., Barringer, D. G., & Walden, B. E. (1994). SKI-HI home-based programming for children who are deaf or hard of hearing: Recent research findings. *Infant-Toddler Intervention: The Transdisciplinary Journal, 4*(1), 25–36.

Swisher, V., & Thompson, M. (1985). Mothers learning simultaneous communication: The dimensions of the task. *American Annals of the Deaf, 130*, 212–217.

Tomasello, M., & Farrar, M. J. (1986). Joint attention and early language. *Child Development, 57*, 1454–1463.

Tomasello, M., Mannle, S., & Kruger, A. (1986). The linguistic environment of one to two year old twins. *Development Psychology, 22*, 169–176.

Tomasello, M., & Todd, J. (1983). Joint attention and lexical acquisition style. *First Language, 4*, 197–212.

U.S. Department of Education (1994). *Sixteenth Annual Report to Congress on the Implementation of the Individuals with Disabilities Education Act.* Washington, DC: Author.

Vergara, K. C. & Miskiel, L. (1994). *CHATS: The Miami cochlear implant, auditory and tactile skills curriculum.* Intelligent Hearing Systems. Miami, FL.

Vincent, L., Davis, J., Brown, P., Broome, K., Funkhouser, K., Miller, J., & Gruenewald, L. (1986). *Parent inventory of child development in non-school environment.* Madison: University of Wisconsin, Department of Rehabilitation Psychology and Special Education.

Wallach, G., & Miller, L. (1988). *Language intervention and academic success.* Boston: College-Hill Press.

Waltz, D., & Pollack, J. (1985). Massively parallel parsing: A strongly interactive model of natural language interpretation. *Cognitive Science, 9*, 51–74.

Watkins, S. (1984). *Longitudinal study on the effects of home intervention on hearing impaired children.* Unpublished doctoral dissertation, Utah State University.

Watkins, S., & Clark, T. C. (1993). *SKI*HI resource manual: Family-centered, home-based programming for infants, toddlers, and preschool-aged children with hearing impairment.* Logan, UT: HOPE, Inc.

Watkins, S., & Parlin, M. (1987). SKI-HI 1986–87 national data report. Logan, UT: Utah State University, SKI-HI Institute.

Wedell-Monnig, J., & Lumley, J. (1980). Child deafness and mother-child interaction. *Child Development, 51*, 766–774.

Wells, G. (1981). *Learning Through Interaction.* New York: Cambridge University Press.

Westby, C. (1985). Learning to talk—talking to learn: Oral- literate language differences. In C. S. Simon (Ed.), *Communication skills and classroom success* (pp. 181–219). San Diego, CA: College-Hill Press.

Westby, C. (1980). Assessment of cognitive and language abilities through play. *Language Speech and Hearing Services in the Schools, 3*(11), 154–163.

White, S. (1984). Antecedents of language functioning in the deaf: Implications for early intervention. Project Summary. UDDOE, EDD0001.

White, K. R., Maxon, A. B., & Behrens, T. R. (1992) Neonatal hearing screening using evoked otoacoustic emissions: The Rhode Island Hearing Assessment Project. In Bess, F. H. & Hall, J. W. (eds.) *Screening children for auditory function.* Nashville, Bill Wilkerson Center Press. pp. 207–214.

Winton, P. J., & Bailey, D. B., Jr. (1994). Becoming family centered strategies for self-examination. In J. Roush & N. D. Matkin (Eds.), *Infants and toddlers with hearing loss* (pp. 23–42). Baltimore: York Press.

Yoshinaga-Itano, C., & Downey, D. (1986). A hearing-impaired child's acquisition of schemata: Something's missing. *Topics in Language Disorders, 7*(1), 45–57.

Appendix Eight A

General Suggestions for the Child with Hearing Impairment in the Regular Classroom

1. The child with hearing impairment should be encouraged to watch the teacher whenever he is talking to the class.
2. The teacher should use natural gestures when they complement, not substitute for speech.
3. Whenever reports are given or during class meetings, have children stand in the front of the class so the child who is hard of hearing can see lips.
4. During class discussions, let the child who is hard of hearing turn around and face the class so he can see the lips of the reciter.
5. To help the child follow instructions accurately, assignments should be written on the board so she can copy them in a notebook.
6. Like other children with sensory defects, the child with impaired hearing needs individual attention. The teacher must be alert to every opportunity to provide individual help to fill gaps stemming from the child's hearing defect.
7. Ask the child with hearing impairment if he understands after an extensive explanation of arithmetic problems or class discussion. Write key words of an idea or lesson on the chalkboard or slip of paper.
8. Enlist class cooperation in understanding the problem of the child with hearing impairment. Designate a student to be her helper in assignments, someone who notes that she is on the right page and doing the right exercise. However, do not let the child with hearing impairment become too dependent on her "helper."
9. The child with impaired hearing should be seated no further than five to eight feet from the teacher. He should be allowed to shift his seat in order to follow the change in routine. This position will enable him to see the teacher's face and to hear her voice more easily.
10. If the child's hearing impairment involves only one ear or if the impairment is greater in one ear than the other, seat the child in the front with the poorer ear toward the noisy classroom and the better ear turned to the teacher or primary signal. When both ears have the same loss, center placement is recommended.
11. Seat the child with hearing impairment away from the heating/cooling systems, hallways, playground noise, etc.
12. If a choice of teachers is possible, the child with a hearing loss should be placed with the teacher who enunciates clearly. Distinct articulation is more helpful than a raised voice.
13. The child with hearing impairment should be carefully watched to be sure she is not withdrawing from the group or that she is not suffering a personality change as a result of her hearing impairment. Make her feel like "one of the gang."

14. Be natural with the child who is hard of hearing. He will appreciate it if he knows you are considerate of his disability.

15. In the lower grades, watch particularly that the student with hearing impairment does her part and is not favored or babied.

16. Use visual aids in your presentation of lessons. Visual aids provide the hearing impaired with the association necessary for learning new things.

17. Encourage the child with hearing impairment to accept his disability and inspire him to make the most of it. Maintain his confidence in you so he will report any difficulty.

18. Parents should know the truth about their child's achievement. If marking is lenient because of the disability, the parents should know that the child is not necessarily equaling the achievement of a child with normal hearing.

19. Students with hearing impairment need special encouragement when they pass from elementary to junior-high school and later into senior high. The pace is swifter. There is much more discussion. Pupils report to five or more teachers instead of one.

20. As the youngster with hearing impairment approaches the age of 16, be especially watchful. She may want to give up. Explain that she needs much preparation to enjoy a life of success and happiness.

How to Help a Child with Hearing Impairment Use Speechreading Skills More Effectively

1. Don't stand with your back to the window while talking (shadow and glare make it difficult to see your lips).

2. Stand still and in a place with a normal amount of light on your face while speaking.

3. Keep your hand and books down from your face while speaking.

4. Don't talk while writing on the chalkboard.

5. Be sure you have the child's attention before you give assignments or announcements.

6. Speak naturally. Do not exaggerate or overemphasize. It is to be expected that it will be more difficult to hold the attention of the child who is hard of hearing. Never forget that the hearing-impaired get fatigued sooner than other children because they not only have to use their eyes on all written and printed work, but also have to watch the lips.

7. Particular care must be used in dictating spelling. Use the words in sentences to show which of two similar words is meant (i.e., "Meet me after school" and "Give the dog some meat"). Thirteen words look like "meat" when spoken, such as been, bead, and beet. The word "king" shows little or no lip movement. Context of the sentence gives the child the clue to the right word. Have the child who is hard of hearing say the words to himself before a mirror as he studies his spelling lesson.

8. If the child who is hard of hearing misunderstands, restate the question in a different way. Chances are you are using words with visual images that are

difficult to speechread. Be patient and never skip her. Be sure that things are understood before you move ahead.

How to Help the Child with Hearing Impairment Use Speech Skills More Effectively

1. A severe hearing impairment that lasts over a period of time tends to result in a dull, monotonous voice and inaccurate enunciation. Therefore, a child with such hearing loss should be encouraged to speak clearly. Keeping the child "speech conscious" will help her resist the usual damage to the voice that a severe hearing impairment produces. Do not let the child get the habit of shaking her head or speaking indistinctly instead of answering in complete sentences.

2. Encourage him to participate in musical activities. This will stimulate his residual hearing and add rhythm to his speech.

3. Since a hearing impairment affects the language processes, the child should be encouraged to compensate by a more active interest in all language activities: reading, spelling, original language, etc.

4. If the young child who is hard of hearing is poor in reading, chances are he needs basic phonics to improve both reading and speech.

5. Teach the child to use the dictionary with skill, to learn the pronunciation system so he can pronounce new words.

6. Build up her vocabulary by assigning supplementary materials.

7. Give him a chance to read ahead on the subject to be discussed. Make sure he is familiar with the vocabulary so he can follow along better.

8. Praise and encourage the hearing-impaired child, where justified, to give her a feeling of success, which she needs in order to build up her confidence in her speaking abilities.

Audiologic Rehabilitation for Adults

ASSESSMENT AND MANAGEMENT

JEROME G. ALPINER

DEAN C. GARSTECKI

Contents

INTRODUCTION

The vast majority of persons who are hearing impaired in the United States are adults who have acquired hearing loss due to etiologies such as illness, accident, noise exposure, and the aging process (Santore, Tulko, & Kearney, 1983; Christensen, 1994). Most of these individuals have maintained some residual hearing which enables them to communicate. The effect of hearing loss on these adults varies greatly depending on time and circumstances of loss as well as extent of loss. Many persons with hearing loss benefit from audiologic rehabilitation (AR) procedures which include evaluation and use of sensory aids, communication training (speechreading, auditory training, compensatory and repair strategies), and counseling. *Hearing-loss management* is another way of describing the AR process that is designed to empower these individuals through a multidisciplinary approach. Innovative new forms of amplification represent the most significant recent development in AR. These now afford the person with hearing loss the opportunity to communicate more effectively than ever before, particularly in conjunction with other rehabilitation measures.

Profile of the Adult Client

Although the age of 65 is often considered the beginning of "old age," hearing loss due to aging may occur well before. The present chapter deals primarily with those adults who could be classified as hard of hearing and who experience hearing-related problems during their working years. (Chapter 10 focuses on the special problems of the adult elderly in the retirement years.) A fair amount of what is said here applies to the adult with either congenital or acquired deafness.

Management of adults with hearing loss must be planned in terms of concomitant problems in social, familial, and vocational relationships. Hearing loss in adults usually develops gradually, and the progression of loss is slow; that is, the hearing impairment "sneaks up." Ordinarily, the higher frequencies diminish first, so the person hears speech but does not always understand clearly what is said. In the early stages, the person with hearing impairment often blames others for mumbling or not speaking sufficiently loud. Ultimately, these situations lead to frustrations and tensions due to breakdown in the communication process. Soon difficulties begin to emerge with spouses, children, employers, and friends. Although these persons may suspect a hearing problem, this suggestion may not be accepted or understood by the person with hearing impairment. A hearing problem is often not easily accepted because it involves the acknowledgment of a physical disability. Consequently, audiologic rehabilitation becomes an appropriate therapeutic consideration to help minimize problem areas.

To describe how patients may react upon recognizing the presence of hearing loss, a case study of one 50-year-old male client is presented. This man has a moderate bilateral sensorineural loss of hearing with a greater deficit in the higher frequencies. Ability to understand speech is 80% in quiet and 64% in noise. It was determined, after medical examination, that the cause of the hearing loss was unknown. The physician referred the patient back to the center where he had been seen previously, for speechreading therapy, a hearing aid assessment, and other audiologic rehabilitation. The loss was of mild to moderate severity at that time and the patient did not want a hearing aid. During the previous five years, the client had married and purchased his own business. He reported that he was having both family and business difficulties with regard to communication. He stated that he did not want to take the time to involve himself in the rehabilitation process. After considerable conversation and counseling, however, he admitted that he had to do something or his marital and business difficulties would increase. He agreed to amplification on a trial basis; he would not agree to other audiologic rehabilitation procedures. He stated that he just did not have time if his business was to succeed. He was willing to return for three post–hearing-aid follow-up sessions. His attitude is not unique (he probably fits into Attitude Type II as discussed in Chapter 1 and later in this chapter).

It is not always easy for individuals to accept the limitations of a sensory system that once functioned normally. Acceptance, however, is a requisite to engaging in hearing-aid evaluation and rehabilitation. Until the person with hearing impairment fully realizes the problem, there will be a tendency to shy away from rehabilitation. Thus, hearing loss represents more than a set of numerical measures. There is also a psychological factor. It may be easier for some adults to withdraw socially from the mainstream than to accept hearing aids or hearing therapy. This profile may help increase our awareness of the complexities involved in providing audiologic rehabilitation.

Rehabilitation Settings

Adults with hearing impairment seek rehabilitative care when they experience the need for better use of their residual hearing and/or amplification. They also may seek care to improve their social or vocational communication skills, or to increase their ability to manage hearing-loss–related problems. Rehabilitative care is delivered in a variety of settings. Some are full-service centers staffed by communication specialists. Others are limited-service centers staffed by audiologists or major centers including university speech and hearing clinics, community hearing societies, hospitals, otologic clinics, senior citizen centers, vocational rehabilitation offices, audiology private practices, and hearing-aid sales offices.

University Programs. The first adult audiologic rehabilitation centers were provided in university training programs that served World War II veterans with hearing loss. The focus was directed toward improvement of the adult's communication skills through use of appropriate amplification and communication training, with counseling and education of adults with hearing impairment, and their families and significant others.

This early model continues to influence present-day programs. When hearing-loss management goes beyond the fitting of a hearing aid at Northwestern University Hearing Clinics, for example, faculty and students provide a comprehensive program of hearing care. First consideration is given to optimizing sensory capability through use of personal amplification systems used alone and in conjunction with assistive listening devices. Communication skills are assessed and treated through use of speech stimuli presented in various linguistic contexts (i.e., syllables, words, sentences, short stories, and running dialogue) under auditory, visual, or combined auditory-visual presentation modes. This information is used to develop a profile of speech-processing ability which, when used in conjunction with self-report information and an assessment of communication strategies, defines overall communication capabilities and identifies areas of concern to address in management. Finally, instrumental, informational, and emotional adjustment counseling needs are identified and addressed in personalized and group activities. Participation in this program is generally considered to be long-term, that is, 8 to 10 weekly sessions. Those individuals who merely want orientation in the four key areas (new hearing aid use, assistive devices, legal rights under the Americans with Disabilities Act [ADA], and communication hints) are invited to participate in a four-week series of one-hour, small-group sessions (Garstecki & Erler, 1994).

Military. Various audiologic rehabilitation programs are available for current and former military personnel in military and Veterans Administration Medical Centers. Programs range from one-time, one-hour hearing-aid orientation sessions after hearing-aid fitting, to comprehensive programs meeting over a period of several weeks. Both individual and group sessions may be conducted depending on the philosophy of the facility.

Areas of rehabilitation covered may include counseling, self-assessment inventories, hearing-aid orientation, communication and assertiveness training, or visual and auditory training. Significant others, usually spouses, may be included in audiologic rehabilitation. The length of time devoted to the entire process depends on the resources available.

Community Centers and Agencies. Community hearing societies, such as those in San Francisco, Chicago, Milwaukee, New York, and other large cities, provide rehabilitation settings where participants are usually highly motivated and well directed toward management of their problems. In one of these programs, two 6-hour sessions are provided on successive weekends. Concentrated programs draw people with a high interest in improving their ability to compensate for their loss. Attrition is reduced under this concentrated meeting format as compared to when sessions are spread over longer periods of time.

Vocational rehabilitation offices provide adults whose hearing is impaired with access to a network of assessment and management services often important for optimizing their potential for gainful employment, and for helping them function as contributing members of a community.

Private Practice Audiologists and Hearing Instrument Specialists. With some exceptions, services offered by audiologists in private practice who are affiliated with otologic medical groups often do not extend beyond the fitting of a hearing aid, orientation to its use, and counseling regarding management of hearing problems. The advantage of services provided in such a setting is that otologic and audiologic needs, often including the fitting of a hearing aid, can be met in one place. For most adults with hearing impairment, this service satisfies all their rehabilitative needs. Others, however, have additional concerns related to knowing how to deal effectively with their hearing loss. Once the hearing impaired know they have a hearing loss, they usually want to learn how to compensate effectively for the problems such a loss creates.

Almost half of those dispensing hearing aids are audiologists while the remainder are hearing-instrument specialists in sales offices (Cranmer-Briskey, 1994); therefore, salespeople in these latter settings play a critical part in the rehabilitation process. Hearing-instrument specialists provide hearing aids and associated devices, and assist in initial adjustment to hearing-aid use. They also provide supplies and services to keep the aid in working order. Few such specialists are trained to provide other rehabilitative services. However, as more audiologists dispense hearing aids, comprehensive audiologic rehabilitation service will be provided.

Consumer Groups. An emerging hearing-rehabilitation source may be found in such groups as the Self-Help for Hard of Hearing People, Inc. (SHHH) and the Association of Late Deafened Adults (ALDA) (see Chapter 13, Resources and Materials List—Adults/Elderly). SHHH has existed since 1979 and has a nationwide network of support groups for all persons who are hard of hearing. ALDA was formed in 1987 and focuses on late-deafened adults whose deafness was acquired during adolescence or later. These people share the experience of becoming deaf after having had normal hearing as a child. SHHH and ALDA can be described as self-help, social, outreach, and advocacy groups. Each publishes a periodical and sponsors an annual convention. Local chapters hold monthly social activities and other special events. Wanting to increase public awareness of the problems associated with hearing loss, members of these organizations first successfully spearheaded solutions to such problems as use of public telephones by hearing-aid wearers and installation of group amplification systems in theaters, churches, lecture halls, and other public meeting places. Later they took a major role in passage of the ADA. Consumer groups provide a vehicle by which adults with hearing impairment can improve their ability to self-manage their problems. However, in some instances, important questions have gone unanswered, been incorrectly answered, or been answered from experience rather than from a data-base, thereby creating more problems than originally existed. The value of the rehabilitative service provided in consumer group settings often relates to the quality of input from professional hearing health-care consultants.

REHABILITATION ASSESSMENT

Procedures used in audiometric and self-report assessment of potential rehabilitation program participants are described in this section. *Hearing impairment* refers to limitations in hearing ability, while *hearing disability* and/or *handicap* refers to the primary and secondary effects of these limitations on everyday life.

While we have extensive audiometric methods for measuring hearing impairment, recent monographs edited by Schow and Smedley (1990) and Newman and Jacobsen (1993) have brought new attention to the use of self-report techniques to measure not only impairment but its primary and secondary consequences as well. The need to combine audiometric measures with self-report assessment for determining hearing impairment and its consequences is a priority for clinicians and researchers involved in hearing-loss management. Fortunately, an ever-increasing number of audiologists in the United States is giving greater attention to these self-report instruments. Schow, et al. (1993) reported that self-assessment use by ASHA audiologists had increased from 18% in 1980 to 37% by 1990.

Assessment of the consequences of hearing loss is important in the audiologic rehabilitation process for several reasons. First, there is a need to obtain information that will help one understand the hearing loss and communication consequences of hearing impairment. Second, an assessment of the psychological consequences of the hearing loss is needed. Emotional and psychological problems may be more detrimental to the well-being of the individual in a way that goes beyond the organics of the loss and the effect on communication. Client input is helpful in dealing with this aspect of audiologic rehabilitation. Third, there is a chance to change or manipulate circumstances in the family, work, or social environment, and self-report helps clarify the impact of hearing loss in those areas. Finally, it is important to assess the effectiveness of audiologic rehabilitation. Self-report procedures can be used both pre- and post-therapy, thereby allowing a measure of improvement in communication function and emotional, social, and vocational well being. It is expected that efforts in both audiometric and self-report assessment will continue to expand and improve in order to provide more adequate information about hearing loss and its consequences.

Audiometric Impairment Assessment

The audiometric assessment assists in two areas: (a) diagnosis and (b) rehabilitation. The basic diagnostic test battery consists of pure-tone air and bone-conduction audiometry, speech threshold tests, speech-recognition tests, immittance, and measures of tolerance. The basic audiometric battery results indicate whether a hearing loss exists, the degree and type of loss, and if the loss is likely to be remedied medically or surgically, or compensated for through amplification. A variety of test procedures may be added to the standard assessment battery to differentiate cochlear from retrocochlear problems, determine vestibular function, assess middle-ear function, and measure central auditory-processing ability.

The standard diagnostic battery, followed by hearing-aid fitting and hearing-aid orientation (HAO), will generally address most audiologic rehabilitation needs. However, sometimes there is a need to go beyond and develop relevant goals and activities for improving communication skills or addressing secondary consequences of the loss. In these cases we can extend the audiometric test battery to include identification of those circumstances under which speech-recognition ability changes. For example, test materials might be selected to help determine patterns of word recognition difficulty. The California Consonant Test (Owens & Schubert, 1977) has been found to be sensitive to the phonemic confusions demonstrated by individuals with high-frequency sensorineural hearing loss (Schwartz & Surr, 1979). The results of such tests are helpful in designing management programs for adults who demonstrate phonemic confusions (see Chapter 3).

Since everyday conversation requires comprehension of contextualized speech, it may be of interest to measure the sentence-recognition ability of an adult with hearing impairment. Monosyllabic words provide phonemic and semantic cues to their perception, and sentences provide syntactic and temporal cues. While the resolving power of sentence tests is lower than that of word tests, sentence recognition tests provide useful information for purposes of assessment and management. Sentence materials used for this purpose include CID Everyday Speech Sentences (as found in Davis & Silverman, 1970), Synthetic Sentence Identification (SSI) (Jerger, Speaks, & Trammell, 1968), and Speech Perception in Noise (SPIN) test materials (Kalikow, Stevens, & Elliott, 1977).

The CID Everyday Sentence Lists are well suited for use with persons who are deaf and can be used in the presence of competing noise for those who are hard of hearing. They enjoy continued use as part of the standard protocol for testing the deaf at the National Technical Institute for the Deaf (NTID). SPIN test results provide a realistic estimate of speech-recognition ability for persons who are hard of hearing since they incorporate noisy listening conditions. SSI materials also have been shown to be useful in simulating noisy conversational conditions for purposes of hearing-aid fitting.

In addition to varying types of presentation conditions (quiet or noise background), consideration should be given to other test materials. Erber (1971), Garstecki (1980), and others have suggested that since everyday message perception involves simultaneous processing of auditory and visual speech information, communication skills should be evaluated using materials presented in a way that utilizes both visual and auditory information. This would involve speechreading testing in conjunction with auditory recognition tests (Garstecki & Erler, 1996).

Self-Report: Primary and Secondary Effects of Loss

As explained in Chapter 1, the primary effect of hearing loss is on verbal forms of communication (called *disability* by the World Health Organization [WHO, 1980]). Secondary consequences from hearing loss (called *handicap* by the WHO) typically include psychosocial, vocational, and educational issues. A loss of hearing is measured easily in terms of decibels on an audiometric grid or percent correct on a speech-recognition test, thereby yielding numerical indicators of the amount of hearing impairment. Unfortunately, these numbers are not indicators of the day-to-day consequences which may be manifest by hearing impairment. We know from experience, for example, that two individuals with the same numerical hearing loss may encounter entirely different problems as a result of their hearing loss. A case history interview is one way of obtaining information on the day-to-day effects resulting from a hearing deficit on a given person.

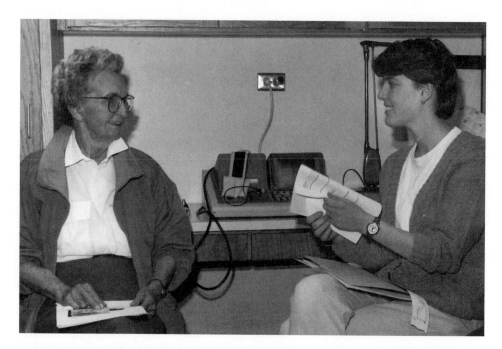

A case history is obtained from the individual prior to audiometric assessment.

Case History. Some audiologists prefer to have case history information before seeing the client. Others use an interview technique, since there are times when a
client's responses should be further explored. The interview form is useful for eliciting information on general topics, such as the nature and onset of the problem,
whether or not hearing is changing, the kinds of situations in which communication
difficulties are experienced, the history of hearing-aid use, and a general case history
(see Figure 9.1). The history, along with the audiogram, provides the clinician with an
initial impression of the client.

Other Forms of Self-Report. Within the past 30 years, significant efforts have
been made to assess hearing consequences beyond the traditional case history.
Alternate approaches used for assessment are discussed in the section that follows
and their role in audiologic rehabilitation is explained. Most of these instruments
involve self-report by questionnaire. Such questionnaires have been used in an abbreviated form for screening purposes to select rehabilitation candidates, or in longer
versions to explore a small number of consequences resulting from the hearing problem, or in very comprehensive instruments that explore multiple (up to 22) dimensions of the hearing loss.

    Schow and Gatehouse (1990) summarized a variety of fundamental concerns
related to self-report, including the need to consider different hearing domains (e.g.,

Case History Form

Adult Case History

Audiology

Date _____

Referral Source _____

Physician _____

Informan _____

Name _____ Birth date _____ Age _____

Address _____ Phone _____

(Street)   (City)   (State)   (Zip)

Occupation (if retired, former occupation) _____

Send reports to: _____

_____

Nature and onset of problem:_____

_____

Other evaluations (when, where) _____

Does your hearing seem to be getting worse? _____

Does your hearing fluctuate? _____ Is one ear better than the other? _____

Client reports difficulty with hearing in:

       Groups _____ Individuals _____

       Distance_____

       Telephone: RE _____ LE _____ Both _____

       Radio and TV_____

       Direction of sound _____

       Does hearing loss interfere with work?_____

Ever worn a hearing aid? _____ When? _____ How long? _____

Who recommended an aid? _____ Attitude toward use _____

Complaints _____

Present aid: Make _____ Model _____ Receiver _____ Ear _____

Any bias toward a particular type or make of hearing aid?_____

Special training in aural rehabilitation _____

Medical History

History of hearing loss in family_____

Middle ear infections _____

Ear surgery _____

Other serious diseases or illnesses_____

_____

Concussion _____

Vertigo _____

Tinnitus _____

Nausea _____

Drug therapy _____

Noise exposure_____

Other factors that might have contributed to loss _____

Latest medical examination_____

Figure 9.1 Speech and Hearing Center.

369

hearing impairment, disability, handicap) in test design and use, a detailed listing of about 20 instruments used in self-report of hearing, specific applications for which self-report may be used, and a variety of psychometric issues which need careful attention.

They also summarized the various kinds of information assessed in connection with self-report inventories. These focus areas include both primary and secondary effects of hearing loss.

1. Speech communication: general speech; estimates of communication ability in various settings: home, work, social, one-on-one, small and large groups.
2. Speech communication: special; while listening to TV, a telephone; with and without visual cues; and while in adverse listening situations.
3. Emotional reactions/feelings, behaviors, and attitudes about hearing impairment and hearing aids including response to auditory failure, acceptance of loss.
4. Reactions and behaviors of others/societal feedback including vocational consequences with reference to the hearing loss.
5. Nonspeech communications; door and phone bell, warnings, traffic, localization.
6. Other related symptoms; fluctuating hearing loss, reactions to tinnitus and limited tolerance for loud sounds.

Erdman (1993) further underscored the importance of self-report in measuring the primary and secondary effects of hearing loss. She pointed out that self-report instruments are easy and inexpensive to use. They can be used for a wide variety of purposes, with different populations, and are non-invasive and non-threatening. These factors account for their wide popularity for hearing and other concerns. By assessing the psychosocial and other consequences of hearing loss using self-report, AR clinicians can much more adequately addr369ess audiologic rehabilitation. They can measure not only communication difficulties which may require amplification but also other concerns like tinnitus and dizziness, which may be measured with self-report. These instruments can also promote systematic followup to identify effective and ineffective management. This includes outcome measures to determine whether hearing aids are adequate and/or if other rehabilitation efforts have been successful.

A variety of efforts have been made to assess the psychosocial results of hearing loss. At first, pure tones provided the basis of these measures. One of the earliest attempts involved the use of pure-tone and speech-recognition information to derive a Social Adequacy Index (Davis, 1948). Similarly, the American Medical Association and the American-Speech-Language-Hearing Association (ASHA) at one time suggested that the handicapping consequences of hearing loss can be estimated from pure-tone findings (Colodzin, et al., 1981). By 1990, however, the emphasis had shifted from exclusively audiometric tests to more frequent use of self-report along with audiometric findings, as noted in a survey of ASHA audiologists (see Table 9.1). The instruments most used in the USA will be described and examples of items or one form of

TABLE 9.1 *Respondents to Various Adult* Self-Assessment Questionnaires as Reported in 1990 Survey*

	1990 N=140**	
Questionnaires	N	%
HHS	34	24
Denver	32	23
HPI	21	15
SAC/SOAC	19	14
CPHI	14	10
Other	27***	19

* Questionnaires used exclusively for the elderly are discussed in Chapter 10 and thus excluded from this table.

** Of 469 responding clinically active ASHA audiologists, these 140 (33%) were the only ones who reported use of such questionnaires.

*** 21 of these were a unique, informal, in-house form.

the questionnaire will be found in the appendices of this chapter. Several other instruments will also be described here and may be found elsewhere (Alpiner & Schow, 1993).

Screening for Identification of Loss and Selection of Rehabilitation Candidates. During the 1960s and early 1970s, several brief, self-report screening-type scales were introduced for use in national interview surveys, including the Rating Scale for Each Ear (RSEE) and the Health, Education, and Welfare Expanded Hearing Ability Scale (HEW-EHAS)—sometimes called the Gallaudet Scale (Schein, Gentile, & Haase, 1970). These two scales were used as substitutes for pure-tone testing to estimate prevalence of hearing loss. The RSEE with its generic reference to hearing troubles may especially be viewed as more related to an estimate of hearing impairment rather than the consequences of it.

SELF-ASSESSMENT OF COMMUNICATION (SAC) AND THE SIGNIFICANT OTHER ASSESSMENT OF COMMUNICATION (SOAC). These are two companion questionnaires for screening primary communication difficulty and secondary emotional and social consequences. They were developed by Schow and Nerbonne (1982). The SAC (see Appendix Nine A) has 10 items and allows rating on a five-point continuum indicating a range of difficulty from *little* to *great*. Items are used to assess communication difficulties in various situations, the clients' emotional feelings about their handicap, and the clients' perception of how their hearing is viewed by others (societal response). The SOAC (see Appendix Nine A) contains the same 10 items, except now the behaviors are rated by a significant other, such as a spouse. Both questionnaires have a variety of psychometric data available on them and continue to enjoy support on a national basis (ASHA, 1992). These questionnaires are used in conjunction with pure-tone screening at health fairs and in other settings where adults are having their hearing tested and being referred for audiologic rehabilitation. Schow (1991) has shown how a protocol including SAC/SOAC will provide a reasonable strategy for identifying referrals.

NEW SCREENING INSTRUMENTS. A new tool which includes self assessment, plus visual and auditory aptitude, is the Alpiner-Meline Aural Rehabilitation (AMAR) Screening Scale (Alpiner, Meline, & Cotton, 1991). Using this scale, individuals are classified into one of three rankings: No Need, Questionable Need, or Absolute Need. It is quick and efficient to administer and helps to determine whether or not more comprehensive assessment is necessary for planning audiologic rehabilitation. Another recently developed questionnaire is the Hearing Handicap Inventory for Adults (HHIA, and HHIA-S) (Newman, et al., 1991). The HHIA is a modification of an instrument used in screening programs for senior citizens, the Hearing Handicap Inventory for the Elderly (see Chapter 10).

Rehabilitation Assessment Inventories. More detailed inventories of disability were developed throughout the world during the 1960s and 1970s, including the Hearing Handicap Scale (USA), the Hearing Measurement Scale (Australia), the Denver Scale (USA), and the Social Hearing Handicap Index (Denmark) (Alpiner, et al., 1974; Ewertsen & Birk-Nielsen, 1973; High, Fairbanks, & Glorig, 1964; Noble & Atherley, 1970). Two of these enjoy wide continued use in the USA and are described in more detail below.

THE HEARING HANDICAP SCALE (HHS). The HHS was the first major self-assessment inventory of this type (High, et al., 1964). The HHS consists of 20 formalized questions with a five-point closed-set answering arrangement. Two forms of the test are available (a nice and unusual feature in self-report), both assessing four content areas: speech perception, localization, telephone communication, and noise situations. The HHS has been used widely since its introduction and, as indicated in Table 9.1, enjoys continued popularity. Schow and Tannahill (1977) proposed a range of hearing handicap categories allowing for interpretation of HHS scores in measuring the effect of hearing loss on everyday communication activities. (The HHS [Form A] is found in Appendix 9B.)

THE DENVER SCALE OF COMMUNICATION FUNCTION (DSCF) (ALPINER, ET AL., 1974). The DSCF was originally designed to measure pre- and post-audiologic rehabilitation therapy, or attitudes and feelings pre- and post-hearing aid selection. The scale allows adults whose hearing is impaired to be compared with themselves, not with their therapy counterparts or any norm. The DSCF allows a client to judge himself in communication function using a semantic differential-type continuum for each of 25 separate items. A profile form is used for plotting client responses (see Figure 9.2). The form allows seven responses ranging from "agree" to "disagree," and includes a "midpoint." The 25 questions within the questionnaire have been grouped into four categories: family communicative situations (items 1–4); client's personal feelings (items 5–9); perception about social-vocational situations

Profile Form for the Denver Scale of Communication Function

Client _____ Case # _____ Sex _____ Age _____

Preservice administration _____ Postservice administration _____
(date) (date)

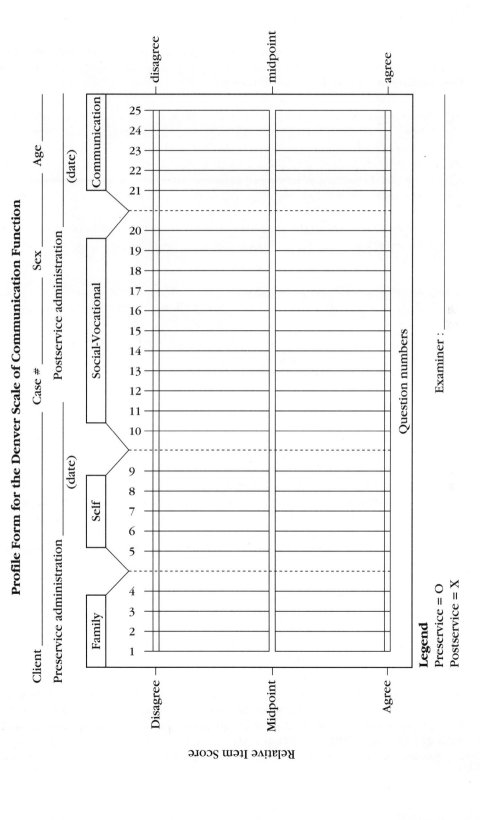

Examiner : _____

Legend
Preservice = O
Postservice = X

Figure 9.2 Profile form.

From J. Alpiner, W. Chevrette, G. Glascoe, M. Metz, & B. Olsen (1974). *The Denver Scale of Communication Function.* Denver, CO: University of Denver.

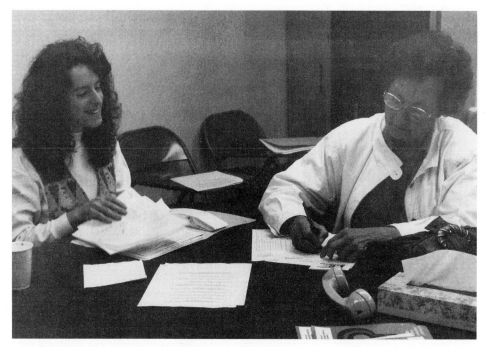

An adult with hearing loss completes a self-report form to provide valuable information concerning her hearing status.

(items 10–20); and client's general communication experience (items 21–25) (see original questions in Appendix Nine C). Schow and Nerbonne (1980) modified the original Denver Scale of Communication Function into the Quantified Denver Scale (QDS). The QDS yields an estimate of disability that allows comparison of scores with other persons having similar or different losses. Recently, a shortened version of the QDS was shown to have adequate test characteristics when used either as a screening instrument or as an intervention assessment instrument. It was not as well suited as some other instruments for use with the elderly, however (Mulrow, et al., 1990).

By the late 1970s, a new flurry of activity in hearing self-report had begun, which has continued into the 1980s and 1990s. Specifically, Sanders (1975) designed scales for special situations like vocational and home environments. At about that time, other scales were developed for special populations, including two for nursing-home residents (these are discussed in Chapter 10). Jerger and Jerger (1979) proposed a method involving visual and auditory tasks for quantifying auditory handicap (QUAH), and in 1983 another scale was published by McCarthy and Alpiner (1983), the M-A Scale. In Denmark, a new handicap scale was proposed by Salomon and Parving (1985). With so many new instruments, some, including the three mentioned above, have received limited use (see Table 9.1) and only preliminary psychometric development. Nevertheless, one of the most promising of these is the M-A Scale, which, like SAC and SOAC, incorporates a companion scale for assessing significant others.

THE M-A SCALE OF HEARING HANDICAP. This scale assesses the secondary consequences of adult hearing loss: psychological, social, and vocational. It is administered to both the individual with hearing loss and a significant other in the client's environment, usually a spouse. The following important findings emerged in the initial M-A study for audiologic rehabilitation:

1. Individuals with hearing impairment may fail to accept, understand, or deal with hearing problems while members of the family are keenly aware of the handicapping effects.
2. Some family members are unable to recognize, understand, or deal with the individual's hearing impairment.
3. The person with hearing loss and her family members often fail to agree on what are the problem areas.

Diagnostic Comprehensive Inventories

HEARING PERFORMANCE INVENTORY (HPI). This was the first of two major detailed comprehensive questionnaires and was developed by Giolas, Owens, Lamb, and Schubert (1979) and subsequently revised several times into shorter versions (Lamb, Owens, Schubert, & Giolas, 1984). Considerable psychometric work has been devoted to this instrument (e.g., Demorest & Walden, 1984; Gatehouse, 1990). The HPI consists of six sections: (a) understanding speech; (b) intensity; (c) response to auditory failure; (d) social; (e) personal; and (f) occupational. Figure 9.3 shows the response form. Examples of items from the HPI follow:

1. You are watching your favorite news program on television. Can you understand the news reporter when her voice is loud enough for you?
2. Does your hearing problem interfere with helping or instructing others on the job?
3. Does your hearing problem tend to make you feel nervous or tense?

COMMUNICATION PROFILE FOR THE HEARING IMPAIRED (CPHI). A detailed inventory, CPHI was designed by Demorest and Erdman (1987). It is a psychometrically rigorous self-assessment instrument that was standardized on 433 active-duty personnel at Walter Reed Army Medical Center. The majority of these individuals reportedly demonstrated noise-induced, high-frequency, sensorineural hearing loss bilaterally. They were predominantly males, ranging in age from 20–70 years. A detailed report of the demographic characteristics of standardizing group members is provided by Demorest and Erdman (1987). Because standardizing group composition was representative of only a narrow segment of the adult population with impaired hearing, there is some question about the appropriateness of applying CPHI response data to individuals who do not match the characteristics of the standardizing group. In order for CPHI response data to be meaningfully interpreted, results must be judged against the performance of a comparable target group (Garstecki & Erler, 1995a, b).

Hearing Performance Inventory (Revised Form)

Name _____

Address _____

Age _____ Date _____

Phone _____

Test Location _____

Sex _____ Marital Status _____

Employed _____

Education _____

Hearing aid wearer: Yes ☐ No ☐

Prior audiologic rehabilitation course experience? _____

If Yes, when? _____

	Practically Always	Frequently	About Half the Time	Occasionally	Almost Never	Does Not Apply		Practically Always	Frequently	About Half the Time	Occasionally	Almost Never	Does Not Apply
1.	☐	☐	☐	☐	☐	☐	46.	☐	☐	☐	☐	☐	☐
2.	☐	☐	☐	☐	☐	☐	47.	☐	☐	☐	☐	☐	☐
3.	☐	☐	☐	☐	☐	☐	48.	☐	☐	☐	☐	☐	☐
4.	☐	☐	☐	☐	☐	☐	*49.	☐	☐	☐	☐	☐	☐
5.	☐	☐	☐	☐	☐	☐	50.	☐	☐	☐	☐	☐	☐
6.	☐	☐	☐	☐	☐	☐	51.	☐	☐	☐	☐	☐	☐
7.	☐	☐	☐	☐	☐	☐	52.	☐	☐	☐	☐	☐	☐
8.	☐	☐	☐	☐	☐	☐	53.	☐	☐	☐	☐	☐	☐
9.	☐	☐	☐	☐	☐	☐	54.	☐	☐	☐	☐	☐	☐
10.	☐	☐	☐	☐	☐	☐	55.	☐	☐	☐	☐	☐	☐
11.	☐	☐	☐	☐	☐	☐	56.	☐	☐	☐	☐	☐	☐
12.	☐	☐	☐	☐	☐	☐	57.	☐	☐	☐	☐	☐	☐
13.	☐	☐	☐	☐	☐	☐	58.	☐	☐	☐	☐	☐	☐
14.	☐	☐	☐	☐	☐	☐	59.	☐	☐	☐	☐	☐	☐
15.	☐	☐	☐	☐	☐	☐	60.	☐	☐	☐	☐	☐	☐
*16.	☐	☐	☐	☐	☐	☐	61.	☐	☐	☐	☐	☐	☐
17.	☐	☐	☐	☐	☐	☐	*62.	☐	☐	☐	☐	☐	☐
18.	☐	☐	☐	☐	☐	☐	63.	☐	☐	☐	☐	☐	☐
19.	☐	☐	☐	☐	☐	☐	64.	☐	☐	☐	☐	☐	☐
20.	☐	☐	☐	☐	☐	☐	65.	☐	☐	☐	☐	☐	☐
21.	☐	☐	☐	☐	☐	☐	66.	☐	☐	☐	☐	☐	☐
*22.	☐	☐	☐	☐	☐	☐	67.	☐	☐	☐	☐	☐	☐
23.	☐	☐	☐	☐	☐	☐	*68.	☐	☐	☐	☐	☐	☐
24.	☐	☐	☐	☐	☐	☐	69.	☐	☐	☐	☐	☐	☐
25.	☐	☐	☐	☐	☐	☐	70.	☐	☐	☐	☐	☐	☐
26.	☐	☐	☐	☐	☐	☐	71.	☐	☐	☐	☐	☐	☐
*27.	☐	☐	☐	☐	☐	☐	*72.	☐	☐	☐	☐	☐	☐
28.	☐	☐	☐	☐	☐	☐	73.	☐	☐	☐	☐	☐	☐
*29.	☐	☐	☐	☐	☐	☐	74.	☐	☐	☐	☐	☐	☐
30.	☐	☐	☐	☐	☐	☐	75.	☐	☐	☐	☐	☐	☐
31.	☐	☐	☐	☐	☐	☐	76.	☐	☐	☐	☐	☐	☐
*32.	☐	☐	☐	☐	☐	☐	*77.	☐	☐	☐	☐	☐	☐
33.	☐	☐	☐	☐	☐	☐	*78.	☐	☐	☐	☐	☐	☐
34.	☐	☐	☐	☐	☐	☐	79.	☐	☐	☐	☐	☐	☐
35.	☐	☐	☐	☐	☐	☐	80.	☐	☐	☐	☐	☐	☐
36.	☐	☐	☐	☐	☐	☐	81.	☐	☐	☐	☐	☐	☐
37.	☐	☐	☐	☐	☐	☐	82.	☐	☐	☐	☐	☐	☐
38.	☐	☐	☐	☐	☐	☐	83.	☐	☐	☐	☐	☐	☐
*39.	☐	☐	☐	☐	☐	☐	84.	☐	☐	☐	☐	☐	☐
40.	☐	☐	☐	☐	☐	☐	85.	☐	☐	☐	☐	☐	☐
41.	☐	☐	☐	☐	☐	☐	*86.	☐	☐	☐	☐	☐	☐
*42.	☐	☐	☐	☐	☐	☐	87.	☐	☐	☐	☐	☐	☐
43.	☐	☐	☐	☐	☐	☐	88.	☐	☐	☐	☐	☐	☐
44.	☐	☐	☐	☐	☐	☐	89.	☐	☐	☐	☐	☐	☐
45.	☐	☐	☐	☐	☐	☐	90.	☐	☐	☐	☐	☐	☐

*Items to be reversed before scoring.

Figure 9.3 Hearing Performance Inventory—Revised Form.

From S. W. Lamb, E. Owens, E. D. Schubert, & T. G. Giolas (1984). *Hearing Performance Inventory—Revised Form*. San Diego: College-Hill Press.

The CPHI contains 145 items and 22 scales in four categories: Communication Performance (plus a Communication Importance component for this category only), Communication Environment, Communication Strategies, and Personal Adjustment. Each category contains subsets of topically focused items. Responses to each item are rated on a five-point Likert scale of frequency, agreement, or importance. Detailed information relating to scale composition and item analyses is reported by Demorest and Erdman (1986). The following are examples of items:

1. One way I get people to repeat what they said is by ignoring them.
2. I feel threatened by many communication situations due to difficulty hearing.
3. The difficulties I have with my hearing restrict my social and personal life.

Outcome Measures. Many of the previously described instruments have been used in global assessments measuring the effects of hearing-aid use or after other forms of rehabilitation. A number of specific tools to check hearing-aid outcome have also been introduced. The first of these was the Hearing Problem Inventory (HPI-A) (Hutton, 1980), which includes 51 items. Another, the Hearing Aid Performance Inventory (HAPI), was proposed shortly thereafter. As described by Walden, Demorest, and Hepler (1984), this inventory has 64 items which probe into four situations confronted by the hearing-aid user. These include noisy situations, quiet situations, situations with reduced signal information, and situations with non-speech stimuli. More recently, some additional questionnaires have been proposed by Cox and her associates for measuring benefit from hearing aids. These include the Profile of Hearing Aid Benefit (PHAB), which is a 66-item inventory, and the Intelligibility Rating Improvement Scale (IRIS), which has 47 items (Cox, et al., 1991). A shortened version of the PHAB, called the APHAB, has also recently been proposed (see Chapter 2). Finally, there have been questionnaires designed for use with persons using hearing aids who have severe and profound losses (Owens & Raggio, 1988; Kaplan, Bally, & Brandt, 1990) and for persons using cochlear implants (Rihkanen, 1990).

Concerns about Existing Questionnaires. Despite their acceptance and use, the psychometric properties of many self-report scales remain undefined. And as we look back on more than 30 years of effort in hearing self-report there are few, if any, perfect instruments. For example, one major development in the last few years has been increased care in differentiating the different domains of hearing (primary and secondary consequences, or WHO disability and handicap). Yet several of the instruments with the most psychometric development have been misnamed and/or they have confused the measurement among the different domains of hearing. Noble (1994) has recently discussed the confusion in this area within the HPI, the CPHI, and the HHIA (HHIE). He also describes many other problems such as the difficulty of moving from the needs found in young military personnel to people retired or living alone, and expresses a well-founded concern about the sheer size of a device with 145 items. This underscores concerns expressed by others over the limited effort that has been directed toward study of individual scale items or comparison of results across different target populations (Demorest & Erdman, 1986, 1994; Garstecki &

Erler, 1995). Yet Erdman (1994) urges the development of even more self-report instruments along with continued refinement of the ones in use.

Recent Promising Developments in Self-report. Once we recognize that so far we have no perfect self-report instruments, even among the few with the most intensive psychometric effort, it is possible to recognize that much progress has still been made in refinement of this unique method, which shows great promise for use in audiologic rehabilitation. As the self-report procedures in use are refined and improved they will pave the way for some better tools in the future. And even with relatively simple unrefined instruments, much has been accomplished. For example, beginning in 1980, researchers in the United Kingdom began gathering data through the use of an open-ended problems questionnaire (Stephens, 1980; Barcham & Stephens, 1980; Tyler, et al., 1983). Patients simply made a list of hearing difficulties and placed them in order of importance with the biggest difficulties first. From this questionnaire, Stephens has derived useful strategies for dealing with hearing impairment, such as helping persons with TV, door, and phone problems with relevant assistive devices, even when they do not opt for personally worn hearing aids.

Now, concerted international effort has produced two new instruments: the Gothenburg Profile (Ringdahl, et al., 1993) used in Sweden and Germany and the Hearing Disability and Handicap Scale (HDHS). The HDHS scale involves the joint efforts of researchers in Canada, Wales, and Australia (Hetu, et al., 1994) and both English and French forms are available. There are 20 items with half in the disability and half in the handicap domains (see Appendix Nine D). Factor analysis is being used to insure that separate domains are being measured, and validity and reliability data are also being gathered. Duplicate forms of 10 items may eventually emerge, making this an extremely useful, practical instrument.

Various options for self-report are now available to the audiologist engaged in audiologic rehabilitation. The successful use of any assessment tool (auditory or self-report) depends on the skill and experience of the audiologist who administers it. With careful interpretation, however, many of these self-assessment tools, along with audiometric data, can be very useful in rehabilitation planning.

Summary Profile of Assessment for Rehabilitation Planning

A communication profile provides a means of recording speech-processing skills across a range of stimuli (e.g., syllable recognition to comprehension of interpersonal dialogue) and alternate reception modalities (e.g., auditory-only, visual-only, and combined auditory-visual modalities) (Garstecki & Erler, 1996). One approach used with individuals who are deaf at the National Technical Institute for the Deaf was described by Sims (1985). This profile incorporated results from word recognition measures, speechreading measures, manual communication skill, simultaneous spoken and signed language skill, and written English comprehension. Considering such information in the design of treatment programs helps define isolated and interacting factors that may contribute to communication handicap.

After gathering audiometric and self-report data and summarizing these in a pro-file, the audiologist is in a position to determine the need for audiologic rehabilitation and how to approach the management of problems. There is no formula or guaranteed indicator of the need for audiologic rehabilitation. It is the audiologist and the hearing-impaired adult who decide whether or not to embark on such an effort, and it is the audiologist's responsibility to facilitate the design and implement a client-centered program based on client goals and needs.

Goldstein and Stephens (1981) developed a model of the rehabilitative process that incorporates instrumental and non-instrumental components while also considering sequencing and interaction of various procedures. The model is depicted as a computer flow-chart (see Chapter 1 and Figure 9.4). As one reads from left to right, each column in the figure is another presentation of the same process, only depicted in greater detail. Thus, the assessment component considers four areas. Attitude toward or acceptance of the hearing-loss conditions and expectations which interact favorably with the prospects for rehabilitation are viewed as critical ingredients feeding into the management process. Data gathered and stored in assessments are reviewed, analyzed, and integrated into decisions on the sequence of events, devices or procedures, and goals to be incorporated into a management plan. Also, amplifying device, sensory aid, and warning system need and use are considered. Communication strategies are developed. The role of ancillary professionals is reviewed. Finally, communication training is provided, consisting of providing information, building communication skills, successful use of an amplification system, and counseling.

This model clearly demonstrates that audiologic rehabilitation is a broad, interrelated series of events. It is a dynamic process, not merely audiologic assessment, hearing-aid fitting, and speechreading instruction.

To determine the need for audiologic rehabilitation, consideration should be given to:

1. *Communication Status*: measurement of auditory, visual, and other communication skills. This could include finding out if the adult with hearing impairment experiences difficulty understanding speech without or with speechreading cues, understanding low-intensity speech presented in a noise background, etc. Client input through self-report helps provide significant information regarding his/her communication abilities.

2. *Associated Variables*: variables that potentially influence communication status are weighed. These include social, emotional, vocational, family, and educational issues.

3. *Related Conditions*: physical, mental, and other related conditions are considered.

4. *Attitude*: Goldstein and Stephens indicated that the nature and sequencing of treatment, as well as the degree of success, depend on four attitude types:

    Attitude Type I: The patient has a strongly positive attitude toward hearing aids and audiological care. Both auditory and psychological factors are amenable to therapeutic solutions.

(Enter through Diagnostic-Identification Process)			
Assessment (CARA)	Communication Status	(I-A, B)	Auditory Visual Language Manual Communication Strategies Previous Rehabilitation Overall
	Associated Variables	(II-B)	Psychological Sociological Vocational Educational
	Related Conditions		Mobility Upper Limb Audiologic Pathilogy
	Attitude	(II-D)	Type I Type II Type III Type IV
Management (PACO)	Psychosocial/Counseling	(II-A, B, D)	Interpretation Information Counseling/Guidance Acceptance Understanding Expectation

	Amplification (Instrumental)	(I-C)	Hearing Aid Fitting
			Cochlear Implants
			Assistive Devices
			  Assistive Listening
			  Alerting/Warning
			Tactile
			Communication
			Instruction/Orientation

	Communication Training	(II-B, C; III-A, V)	Goals Philosophy Tactics Skill Building
	Overall Coordination (Ancillary)	(II-B, C, E; III-C, IV)	Vocational Educational Social Work Medicine
(Discharge)			

Note: This model is consistent with the Goldstein/Stephens (1981) model and the ASHA position statement on definitions and competencies in Audiologic rehabilitation (ASHA, 1984). The numbers and letters in parentheses refer to the ASHA statement related to the procedures listed.

Figure 9.4 Audiologic rehabilitation model as used in this text.

Attitude Type II: The patient has an essentially positive attitude toward hearing aids and audiologic rehabilitation, but some complications are present. The patient may have earlier had a negative therapy experience or social, educational, or vocational factors which preclude the use of simple solutions. Also included in this group are clients with difficult-to-fit audiometric configurations, or mild impairment for which both the client and the audiologist want assurance of benefit to warrant the cost of treatment. About 2/3 to 3/4 of clients fitted with hearing aids fit into Type I, the remainder into Type II.

Attitude Type III: The patient has a fundamentally negative attitude although there exists a shred of cooperative intent. The negative attitude towards hearing aids may arise from a variety of situations and comes in many forms. It may reflect the stigma of a hearing aid or a generalized inability to cope with change in status.

Attitude Type IV: The patient belongs to a small group who reject hearing aids and the entire rehabilitation process. A total discharge from the therapy process is likely, but a last-ditch effort to salvage a thread of management potential should be attempted.

THE MANAGEMENT PROCESS

Psychosocial and Counseling Rehabilitation

A critical component of an adult's rehabilitation program is that which encompasses provision of professional advice, mutual exchange of ideas and opinions, and discussions and deliberations on matters relating to personal management of hearing loss. Adults with hearing impairment want to talk with someone about the way they feel about problems at home, on the job, and in interpersonal communication situations (Frankel, 1981). Professionals may provide information relating to the nature of hearing loss, its consequences, and its treatment. There may be a need for clarification of attitudes and ideas and for assistance in emotional adjustment to hearing loss.

Wylde (1982) described important areas to address in the counseling process (see Table 9.2). Counseling topics can be categorized in terms of those addressing the need for general information concerning hearing loss management, information regarding acceptance and adjustment to sensory aids and other rehabilitation strategies, and information and support in emotional adjustment to hearing loss.

Informational counseling is cognitively-based assistance. It is instruction, guidance, and expert advice. For example, helping someone to develop appropriate strategies to use in managing difficult communication situations is an informal counseling experience. Providing an individual with information on hearing loss, medical treatment, sensory aids and assistive devices, communication with hearing-impaired individuals, conservation of residual hearing, community services available for individuals with impaired hearing, and the legal rights of individuals with hearing impairment would be considered informational counseling.

TABLE 9.2 *Counseling Areas for Audiologists*

Informational	Rational Acceptance Adjustment	Emotional Acceptance/Adjustment

Hearing Loss
  Description
  Comparison with normal
  Cause
	Hearing Loss
	  Permanency
	  Need for treatment
	  Need for additional testing
		Effect of hearing loss on self
		  Feelings
		  Attitude
		  Image

Anatomy/function of ear	Need for hearing aid(s)	Ability to communicate Ability to work

Availability of medical assistance	Need to conserve residual
	  hearing
		Effect of hearing loss on
		  relationships

Hearing aids
  Costs
  Where to purchase
  Advantages/disadvantages
  Care/use/function
	Audiologic rehabilitation
	  Need to learn new
	  communication skills
		Family
		  Friends
		  Associates

Availability of other technical
  devices
	Need to improve communication
	  habits
	  Family	

Availability of other services	Friends Work place	

From "The Remediation Process: Psychologic and Counseling Aspects" by M. A. Wylde. In *Handbook of Adult Rehabilitative Audiology*, 2nd ed. (pp. 137–159) by J. G. Alpiner (Ed.), 1982, Baltimore: Williams and Wilkins.

Acceptance/adjustment counseling relates to other assistance or support. It may include activities relating to sensory-aid procurement such as petitioning third-party payers or philanthropic organizations for financial support. It may involve arranging for public transportation to attend clinic sessions. It could involve working with an aide in managing daily living tasks which include wearing and maintaining operation of one's hearing aids.

Emotional adjustment or affective counseling may involve dealing with negative feelings associated with hearing loss or with negative feelings of self-worth. For an elderly individual, emotional-adjustment counseling might emphasize development of a family- or peer-support system. It might involve clarification or validation of personal needs or feelings resulting from hearing loss. It also could focus on defining the roles of family members and peers in communication situations.

Common psychosocial problems of clients with hearing impairment stem from family, vocational, or social situations involving the client's communication, or, more likely, miscommunication. At times, these problems are sufficiently severe to warrant referral to ancillary professionals. The audiologist may be the first person whom clients see with regard to their communication problems. If the audiologist feels uncomfortable about working with clients who appear to demonstrate problems beyond the need to improve communication function, it is recommended that appropriate referral be made to family counselors, social workers, psychologists, or others.

Group counseling sessions may be used effectively to improve communication. There clients often realize for the first time that they are not the only ones experiencing difficulties. Thus, the group situation may improve clients' willingness to discuss their problems openly. Group members may be able to offer each other suggestions for how to cope with specific communication problems (see sample group outline, Chapter 13.)

Problems relating to hearing impairment commonly occur in family communication situations. Clients may feel that their role as a family member has diminished and they are frustrated by an inability to participate effectively in family discussions. Complaints may include the perception that family members have neither the patience nor the courtesy to communicate with them. Family members may feel equally frustrated. Consequently, a vicious cycle can result and, until the cycle is broken, the client may isolate herself from her family. Under such circumstances, it often proves helpful to include family members in management sessions. Family members may reach a better understanding of the difficulties experienced by the client, as well as learn about the ramifications of hearing loss. Finally, this approach may help improve the lines of communication in the family setting.

Clients may also experience difficulties in their vocational role. In this connection it may be necessary for the audiologist, with the client's permission, to contact the client's employer to educate him about hearing loss. A referral to a vocational rehabilitation counselor may also be in order. Vocational rehabilitation counselors are found in all states and their positions are funded by state and federal appropriations. They work with both clients and employers to assess the appropriateness of specific vocations. Counselors will determine whether the client is overemployed, underemployed, or unemployed.

Communication difficulties in social situations are often another major concern. Group situations (meetings, parties, and so forth) and settings with high levels of background noise (e.g., factories, restaurants) may cause serious communication difficulties. These situations can cause the client to withdraw socially and take a less active role in everyday living activities. Participating in an audiologic rehabilitation program may be a first step in reestablishing social relationships. If rewarding, the program may provide the client with the motivation needed to remain in the mainstream.

Essentially, there are two types of risks associated with provision of counseling service. One is the risk of malpractice. The other is the risk of burnout. Malpractice claims may occur when the counseling clinician fails to evaluate properly an individual's counseling needs, provides a substandard counseling service, fails to reveal alternative solutions to concerns raised in counseling sessions, or fails to refer when alternate types of professional services are indicated.

Burnout occurs when the boundaries of a counseling relationship are not clearly specified. Counseling boundaries typically are not verbalized. They often are negotiated non-verbally during the course of a professional relationship. Through clinician feedback, the individual with impaired hearing should come to the realization that while it may be appropriate to discuss job communication problems with the counselor, it may not be appropriate to discuss financial concerns or serious illness. It is within boundaries to discuss what it is like to have impaired hearing. It is outside boundaries to discuss unrelated medical conditions, chronic feelings of unhappiness, or marital instability. If both parties guard against potential risks, the counseling experience can be professionally rewarding for the clinician and vital to the personal future of individuals with impaired hearing.

Amplification/Sensory Aids

Hearing-Aid Orientation (HAO). In addition to counseling during the initial hearing-aid fitting process as described above and in Chapter 2, the client is typically taken through a hearing-aid orientation process. Recent survey data indicate that 76% of ASHA audiologists who perform HAO do so in three individual sessions of about 30 minutes each. Most other audiologists use group sessions or some combination of group and individual sessions to orient the new user (Schow, et al., 1993). It is likely that the individual sessions are most focused on issues related to the hearing aid, with some emphasis on communication strategies, while group sessions were reported to usually have a broader focus. The group time was reported to usually last 30–60 minutes and was divided in the following manner: 34% hearing aids, 21% communication strategies, 14% auditory training, 12% assistive listening devices (ALDs), 11% speechreading, and 9% other areas of concern such as anatomy, types of loss, etc.

One example of an orientation program is at the Department of Veterans Affairs' audiology program in Denver. After completion of the hearing-aid evaluation and selection procedure and prior to the fitting of the aid, the client is given an initial orientation. Topics covered include:

1. Why do you need hearing aids?
2. Do you have communication difficulties:

    a. with family and friends?
    b. at work?
    c. at social gatherings?
    d. at recreational events?
    e. in other situations?

3. Do you have difficulties dealing with loudness, clearness, and frustration?
4. Things that may happen:

    a. You may think people mumble.
    b. You may think people avoid you.
    c. You don't understand all of the words.
    d. It may seem easier to stay home and avoid people.

5. Where do you have problems because of your hearing loss? Name some of these problems.

The above items are used in either individual or group sessions of about one hour. A booklet is given to the client to take home and discuss with significant others.

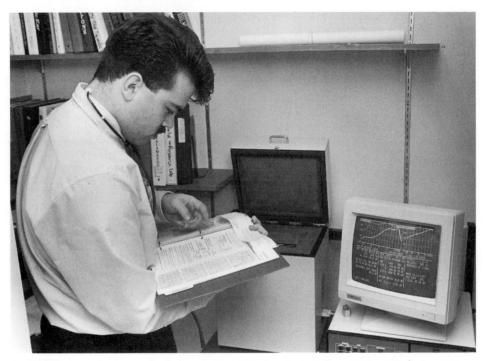

A clinician conducts an electroacoustic analysis of a hearing aid to determine if it meets specifications.

This initial orientation has helped to prepare the client prior to being fitted with hearing aids in three or four weeks.

Key items for presentation to the client before or after fitting include those listed below:

1. An overview of the anatomy and physiology of the auditory system, including a pictorial representation of the ear.
2. The different types of hearing, including conductive and sensorineural, with descriptions of each type.
3. General information about hearing aids, including cost, monaural versus binaural selection, and various modifications.
4. Trouble-shooting, including feedback, "dead" hearing aid, hearing aid going "on and off."
5. General maintenance procedures to ensure proper functioning of the aid.
6. Communication suggestions for members of the family.
7. General overview of audiologic rehabilitation techniques.

Many times a simple maintenance schedule will help prevent problems from occurring.

1. Everyday   a. check to see that no wax is in the earmold
                   b. test the battery
                   c. dust aid off with tissue

2. Every Evening   a. turn aid off, open battery case, and place in dry location

3. Every Year   a. receive a complete hearing test and hearing aid check
                   b. check plastic tubing; replace if necessary
                   c. have earmold checked

4. When Necessary a. replace earmold
                   b. wash earmold with mild soapy water
                   c. change batteries
                   d. have hearing aid cleaned

Below are some questions that may arise after the client is fitted and may therefore be good for discussion purposes during individual or group orientation sessions.

1. Why does my hearing aid amplify background noise?
2. Why do I experience a feeling of fullness in my ear when I wear my aid?
3. Why does my hearing aid whistle?
4. Why do I sound different when I am wearing my aid?
5. What can I do about wind noise?
6. Why does the earmold hurt my ear?
7. Will my aid create further hearing loss?
8. Why do others yell at me when they see that I am wearing an aid?
9. Why can't I understand others better with my aid?

The audiologist should be ready to answer these and other questions during the hearing-aid orientation process.

Even experienced hearing-aid users can often profit from hearing-aid orientation, although the degree of coverage is usually not as extensive as with the person utilizing amplification for the first time. (Further materials may be obtained from the Alexander Graham Bell Association in Washington, DC, or see Chapter 13, Resources.)

Cochlear Implants. Some adults with profound hearing impairment cannot be helped by hearing aids. After many years of experimental research, the cochlear implant is now being consistently used for carefully selected persons who have no other means available to them for auditory communication (see Chapter 2). Audiologic rehabilitation is considered to be very important for persons who have received cochlear implants. Training in speechreading also appears to be significant for improving communication. The procedures used are very similar to those employed in the typical audiologic rehabilitation process (see Chapter 12, Case 4). It is important for cochlear-implant candidates to understand the risks involved in surgery and the physical limitations of available implant systems. These risks and limitations are far outweighed by the benefit experienced by many in improved interpersonal communication with and without the benefit of visual speech cues.

Communication Rehabilitation

When more extensive work is needed beyond counseling and hearing-aid orientation, traditional management for adults has emphasized speechreading and auditory training. Speechreading exercises have typically been based on one of two methods—the analytic (work focusing on small units like syllables) and the synthetic (where the focus is on larger message units like sentences). For the past 15 or 20 years, however, there has been a steady movement away from these formal drillwork exercises in speechreading or auditory training, so they are now offered less frequently than in the past (Walden & Grant, 1993; see AR survey in Chapter 13). Instead, more attention is focused on environmental control training, assertiveness training, and teaching anticipatory and repair communication strategies (Erber & Lind, 1993).

Early pioneers in this more general "progressive" approach were Fleming (1972) and Hardick (1977) who presented their programs in the form of group therapy. Fleming proposed that as her clients discussed their communication problems, they developed improved listening skills. The focus, however, was on developing assertive behavior and personal adjustment to hearing loss. Walden and Grant (1993) suggested that there was little systematic clinical research to support these new methods despite their popularity. They felt that exploring the utility of these newer methods may represent the greatest research need in rehabilitative audiology. They also noted that cochlear implant rehabilitation has promoted some resurgence of the older methods.

More traditional communication rehabilitation programs have been and continue to be available in a few special locations like the National Technical Institute for the Deaf and in some Veterans Hospital settings. For example, the Department of Veterans Affairs Rehabilitative Audiology Desk Reference (1989) lists basic procedures involved in the communication assessment process. These include assessment of the ability to correctly perceive increasingly complex speech stimuli under auditory and combined auditory-visual processing modes. Results from this assessment are incorporated in the design of an individualized communication management program. Such a program might include development or refinement of listening skills, visual communication training, auditory training, counseling, speech conservation, and other individualized special services.

While the more general "progressive" approach is at present more popular, it remains to be seen whether both methods will enjoy continued use, or which will be shown to be the most effective.

Auditory Communication Training Strategies. When auditory communication problems remain after medical or surgical intervention and after the fitting of a hearing aid, sometimes more extensive communication training is indicated. Client interviews, self-reports, and responses to hearing-handicap/disability questionnaires provide information about clients' everyday communication problems that the audiologist may find useful in designing a practical, client-centered program. Experiences encountered by the client can be simulated in such a program, along with instruction on how to apply appropriate strategies to improve success in communication situations. In current clinical practice, adults with hearing impairment generally want to focus on how to improve their everyday communication skills. They are frustrated by the filtering and distorting effect that hearing loss has on message perception. They want immediate solutions to everyday problems.

Such clients are taught the variables which may be altered to improve communication and then helped to work out strategies to improve these variables in their favor. Use of appropriate communication strategies will help ensure success outside the clinic environment. For example, an anticipatory strategy would be to predict problems that may relate to the communication environment and to plan how to circumvent these problems. An example of a repair strategy would be to ask a speaker to repeat a message, using a slower rate or clarifying key information. Finally, an example of an appropriate listening strategy would be to focus on understanding an entire message over understanding of isolated words (Garstecki & Erler, 1996).

Figure 9.5 contains a listening quiz that may be presented to encourage the client to increase awareness of the importance of listening and various other factors involved in successful communication. Answers to all the items are false, according to the author of the quiz. Erber (1988) and Tye-Murray (1994) have contributed important recommendations and materials to help teach various communication skills including anticipatory and repair strategies. Gagne and Erber (1987) have also introduced a device for hearing loss simulation (HELOS) to allow students to experience hearing loss for communication training purposes.

Garstecki (1981) described a feedback approach for auditory communication training which will illustrate a modern approach to the more traditional method. The client's everyday communication situation is analyzed in terms of major parameters, including message and background noise characteristics. Then auditory communication exercises are designed to improve the client's ability to understand messages when the speaker is outside viewing range, as when in another room, or speaking on the telephone, over a public address system, or on a radio broadcast. The exercise materials are selected based on the client's interests and needs (for example, a hardware store manager may be presented with newspaper or magazine articles relating to hardware store items, services, and topics of concern to customers). These listening exercises are accompanied by information and instructions on how to stage-manage the communication situation to the client's benefit. Thus, the adult with hearing impairment learns how to optimize listening conditions, ask appropriate questions, and predict messages from nonverbal and situational cues.

Snell (1994) provided a description of the auditory training methods used at the National Technical Institute for the Deaf (NTID). Training is geared at different levels because some students can identify only spondees, while others do reasonably well in identifying connected discourse. Self-instruction is used in which materials are presented from one of four areas: (a) phonetic feature training which includes 10 lessons of 40 minutes each in "vowel power" or in "consonant crunch," (b) technical vocabulary from other courses, (c) "Sounds of English," which includes exercises in learning the lyrics of contemporary popular music, and (d) "reading and listening," which involves having students read various books while they listen to recordings of these books being read. The difficulty of the training task is regulated by changing speaking rate, length of sentences, male vs. female voices, and levels of competing background

T ☐ F ☐   1. Listening is largely a matter of intelligence.
T ☐ F ☐   2. Speaking is a more important part of the communication process than listening.
T ☐ F ☐   3. Listening requires little energy, it is "easy".
T ☐ F ☐   4. Listening is an automatic, involuntary reflex.
T ☐ F ☐   5. Speakers can command listening to occur within an audience.
T ☐ F ☐   6. Hearing ability significantly determines listening ability.
T ☐ F ☐   7. The speaker is totally responsible for the success of communication.
T ☐ F ☐   8. People listen every day. This daily practice eliminates the need for listening training.
T ☐ F ☐   9. Competence in listening develops naturally.
T ☐ F ☐ 10. When you learned to read, you simultaneously learned to listen.
T ☐ F ☐ 11. Listening is only a matter of understanding the words of the speaker.

Figure 9.5 Listening quiz.

From D. C. Garstecki (1981). Auditory-visual training paradigm for hearing-impaired adults. *Journal of the Academy of Rehabilitative Audiology, 14,* 223–238.

noise. Some of these materials are now available from NTID in the form of videodiscs while others involve technology that allows new materials to be made or accessed via computer on a custom basis. Other similar programs are becoming available commercially, but primarily on an experimental basis. For example, the Iowa Audiovisual Speech Perception Laser Videodisc material which is used for assessing consonant, vowel, and sentence recognition was developed by Tyler, Preece, and Tye-Murray in 1987 and is available for purchase from the 3M Corporation in St. Paul, Minnesota. The Connected Speech Test by Robyn Cox is available through the Memphis University Speech and Hearing Center. There are other videodiscs as well as compact disc recordings that may be of interest in clinical management of hearing loss in adults.

Many methods are available for improving auditory communication. The following considerations should be met in selection of a training program: (a) the client must first be evaluated to determine the level at which training should begin, (b) results should be quantifiable, and (c) instruction should focus on the client's everyday communication problems.

Throughout the training program, individual or group activities may be utilized. The major difference between the two types of activities is that message topics may be more generalized in group instruction; also, some participants will find some levels of group exercise more challenging than others. Role-playing and group discussion are incorporated into the program to facilitate application of new information in a controlled environment before carryover to everyday communication situations.

Auditory-Visual Communication Training. Whenever possible, both auditory and auditory-visual training are incorporated into the rehabilitation program. Progress in one realm often expedites progress in the other during the early stages of management. The purpose of auditory-visual training is to improve the adult's ability to use visual cues to supplement auditory information, as in face-to-face conversation, where the speaker's lip movements, facial expression, body gesture, and the communication setting may complement perceived acoustic cues to message perception. Commonly encountered auditory-visual communication experiences include viewing television programs, theatrical productions, and lectures.

As in auditory communication training, it is important that the client optimize his sensory capabilities through use of a hearing aid. For those who experience vision problems in everyday communication situations, corrective lenses should be used. Hardick, Oyer, and Irion (1970) determined that binocular visual acuity poorer than 20/40 may contribute to visual speech perception or speechreading difficulty. Recent attention to changes in visual contrast sensitivity with age indicates another important area in optimizing the ability of the adult with hearing impairment to succeed in auditory-visual communication.

The organizational approach proposed by Garstecki (1981) for feedback type auditory-communication training applies as well to auditory-visual training, with the exception that the range of message types incorporated in this paradigm de-emphasizes word and syllable information. The baseline measure can be made using videotaped or face-to-face presentations of unrelated sentence materials, such as Utley Lipreading Test sentences or CID sentences, presented at a conversational speech level along with multispeaker babble at a 0-dB SN ratio.

Some of the principles applied in traditional speechreading training are incorporated in auditory-visual communication training, with the addition that materials are presented with voice. Describing the importance of visual cues to communication, Ripley and Cummings (1977) stressed the value of training clients to recognize cues and become aware of body movements and gestures that accompany everyday conversation. For example, a simple shake of the head may indicate negation; clenched fists, anger; and so forth. It is to the client's advantage to become aware of these cues since they may offer a way of gaining additional meaning from a conversation. By heeding the speaker's facial expressions, the listener may gain additional insight into the mood of the conversation and the emotional state of the speaker. Raised eyebrows, a smile or a frown, a puzzled look, or an expression of surprise are just a few of the facial cues that contribute information to communication. A simple exercise can be utilized in therapy to teach awareness of facial expressions; each client may act out certain emotions, with other clients guessing what is meant.

Clients should also be taught to observe environmental cues. This means showing them how to take advantage of cues inherent in specific communication situations. By taking advantage of environmental cues, the client may take an educated guess at the topic of conversation. Role-playing activities can be used in the management situation to practice observation of environmental cues.

It is also helpful to demonstrate to clients with hearing impairment that some cues to message perception are provided by visible lipreading movements. Ripley and Cummings (1977) recommended that, during therapy sessions, groups of sounds be presented that are homophenous in nature, beginning with the most visible and proceeding to the least visible sounds. The order of presentation of homophenous sound groups may vary depending on the viseme scheme used (see Chapter 4). In most programs, /f,v/ and /p,b,m/ are two of the viseme groups considered easiest and presented early on, as suggested by Binnie, Jackson, and Montgomery (1976): These sound groups or visemes are introduced using a traditional, analytic approach. Initially, they are presented in isolation, along with an explanation and demonstration of how they appear on the lips. As a visual aid, it may be helpful to write sounds in common script rather than in phonetics for the client.

In the synthetic approach to speechreading, sounds are incorporated into words and sentences. Thus, visual speech-perception skills can be developed through use of "quick recognition" and "quick identification" exercises (Jeffers & Barley, 1971). In quick-recognition exercises, the client must visually discriminate among three similarly positioned phonemes (e.g., *thin, fin, pin*). Quick-identification exercises provide an opportunity for the client to better understand word homophoneity through consideration of alternate word choices for a single speech movement pattern (e.g., *fat, fad, fan, vat, van, fanned*). By incorporating homophenous words in sentences, the client learns the importance of linguistic cues to message perception.

The current approach to communication rehabilitation focuses on auditory-visual presentation of materials because this is the way clients usually process everyday conversation, and bisensory presentation improves message perception significantly. However, this focus does not preclude utilizing "visual-only" or "auditory-only" approaches to rehabilitation or attempting to improve these modalities independently. In all efforts, however, major emphasis should be placed on improvement of the hearing-impaired client's everyday communication skills.

Case History. While the client who wishes to pursue extensive auditory or auditory-visual communication training is relatively rare, there are a few who need this type of focused work. The following sample case illustrates such an auditory-visual training program. The client was a 39-year-old sales executive who had a severe, bilateral, sensorineural hearing impairment resulting from scarlet fever. His unaided speech reception thresholds were 85 and 95 dB HL for his right and left ears, respectively. Unaided speech recognition scores were 36% and 28%, respectively, for right and left ears. At 60 dB HL, his aided speech recognition was 60% (measured using NU test No. 6 word lists presented in quiet). Interview and HPI self-report results revealed that his greatest difficulties occurred in situations that restricted his stage-managing opportunities, such as when attending a theatrical production, lecture, or church service. He reported problems following one-on-one as well as group conversation, especially when it was impossible to ask for repetition, rephrasing, or further clarification of a message. This client wanted practical advice and immediate solutions to his communication problems.

In consideration of this client's poor auditory-speech recognition ability, regular procedures for establishing baseline-level performance were modified to provide an estimate of auditory-visual sentence perception under a + 6 dB primary-to-competing signal condition (S/N ratio). With a baseline score of 50%, the client was expected to demonstrate improved performance under conditions of greater message redundancy. He attained a score of 100% when stimulus material consisted of short paragraphs with accompanying pictures of related visual background cues. Management goals progressed from this point back toward the baseline condition with materials

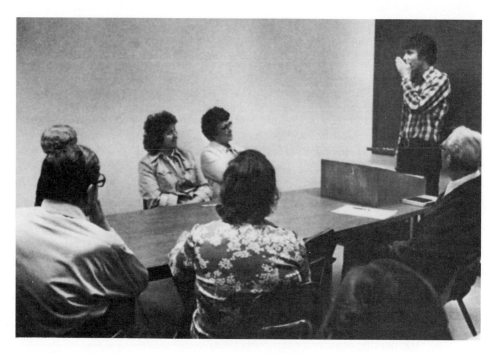

Presenting oral discourse with restricted visual cues.

designed to provide a progressively decreasing amount of linguistic content and situational cues.

Reassessment at the end of an eight-week training program resulted in an improvement from 50% to 90% in the client's ability to perceive unrelated sentences in noise. The client attributed his success to an improvement in his "problem-solving" ability. Problems created in training were resolved through discussion and systematic, logically progressing, message-perception exercises. He more consciously applied what he practiced in training to everyday social and work situations. By developing successful strategies under controlled training conditions, he felt more confident when facing difficult communication situations. This approach worked for this client because he could understand those communication parameters over which he had control and those for which he had to compensate. The management plan was logically organized, and the procedures had direct bearing on the client's immediate communication concerns. Other examples of auditory-visual communication training procedures are provided by Garstecki (1981).

Overall Coordination and General Considerations

Most audiologic rehabilitation involves only amplification fitting and orientation. As noted above, there are some special cases where more comprehensive services, including auditory-visual communication training, are needed. There are also some cases where expanded services beyond what the audiologist can provide are appropriate. The audiologist should consider which, if any, additional rehabilitation procedures should be recommended. The client's condition may call for referral to other professionals such as physicians, psychologists, social workers, vocational counselors, and family counselors. Generally, professionals in other disciplines will refer back to the audiologist directly or work with the client concurrently. Additional procedures may be necessary when dealing with clients who are elderly, deaf, mentally retarded, or with additional physical problems. Often it is desirable to include family members in the therapy session so they may better understand the client's situation.

Some other general considerations are reviewed below under the areas of program design, goals, and format; consumer information; ADA; tinnitus and vertigo; and computer software.

Program Design, Goals, Format. In designing an appropriate rehabilitation program, consideration should be given to the audiologist's approach to the client and the program, management goals, and overall program format. Clients must feel certain that the audiologist understands their problem and has their primary needs in mind in all rehabilitation procedures. The audiologist, in turn, should focus on solutions to major handicapping and remediable problems. Family members, spouses, and close friends should be part of the rehabilitation process. Also, both individual and group management activities should be provided.

Individual therapy permits intensive instruction, focusing only on the client's individual difficulties. When this format is used, fewer sessions may be required to reach the goals established for rehabilitation. Also, one-on-one sessions are sometimes more acceptable to an individual who does not want to or is unable to attend long-term therapy. Oyer (1966) cited several of the advantages afforded by group therapy, including peer evaluation, psychologic support from others with hearing loss, opportunity to compare and contrast individual efforts, and opportunity to perform socially in a practice environment. Finally, economics may promote interest in a group management format.

Program goals should be practically oriented to motivate the adult to succeed. They should serve to inform the client about the dynamics of everyday communication, the communication cycle, and the impact that hearing loss has on this process. Barriers to effective communication should be identified and hints for how to stage-manage difficult situations should be discussed and practiced.

The program should be conducted in a pleasant, comfortable, functional environment. Efforts should be directed toward equipping a management facility in which environmental conditions can be manipulated and controlled to simulate various communication conditions. No helpful data exist regarding the appropriate length for a therapy term. It is not uncommon to find the length of a term dependent on the length of an academic quarter or semester if the setting is a university program. For other agencies, there appears to be no generally accepted time-frame; terms may be three-day concentrated sessions (six hours per day) or training may last 4 to 10 weeks or up to six months (one to one and one-half hours per week). Perhaps the best way to establish the length of a term is to consider the initial goals established.

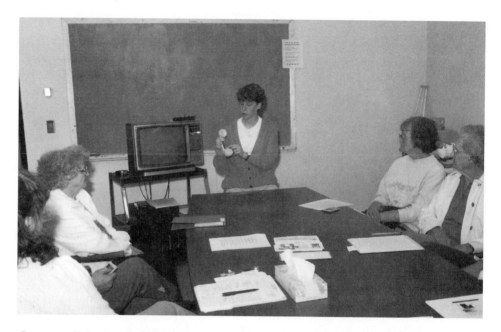

Group audiologic rehabilitation using videotape to reinforce information about ALD's.

Eisenson, Auer, and Irwin (1963) stated that a listener cannot give continuous attention beyond 30–60 minutes. In group sessions, clients seem to realize their maximum benefit in 60–90 minutes.

Consumer Information. The impact consumers have on rehabilitation program design and services to the population of persons with hearing loss at large must be mentioned. When asked what their critical needs were, groups of adults with hearing loss in Iowa City, New York, Duluth, and Galveston reported that they lacked opportunities to learn how to improve their communicative skills. More importantly, professional resources and referral agents lacked information about their needs. Finally, these people wanted quality care from competent health care providers (Davis, 1980; Madell, 1980; Smaldino & Sahli, 1980; Stream & Stream, 1980).

Such voicing of concerns has led to the development of consumer-oriented rehabilitation programs which direct great emphasis on meeting the practical, everyday needs of individuals with hearing impairment. As a result, problems encountered in public meeting places, for example, have received greater attention than in the past, and group amplification systems are increasingly being installed and promoted for use by hearing-impaired individuals.

As mentioned earlier in the chapter, consumer groups have also been formed to raise the public's general level of consciousness about hearing impairment as well as to provide useful information to those concerned about living with hearing loss. For example, Self-Help for Hard of Hearing People, Inc. (SHHH) provides newsletters, periodical publications, national and local meetings, and service programs on topics of general interest to individuals with hearing impairment. Through such actions, consumer groups may complement the efforts of audiologists and other hearing health professionals.

Americans With Disabilities Act (ADA). On July 26, 1990, President George Bush signed the Americans With Disabilities Act into law (PL 101-336). The intent of this new law was to eliminate discrimination against all individuals with disabilities. It provides a standard for addressing discrimination in regard to hearing loss and guarantees equal opportunity for individuals with disabilities in employment, public accommodations, transportation, state and local government services, and telecommunications.

Title I (Employment) protects individuals with disabilities from discrimination in all aspects of employment (EEOC, 1991). Under Title I, employers are allowed to inquire about one's ability to perform job tasks, but may not screen out individuals with hearing disabilities, for example, in an employee-selection process. Employers are expected to make existing facilities and/or equipment accessible and usable. This could include providing a telephone amplifier, interpreter, or visual alerting device for use by an individual with impaired hearing. However, employers do not need to provide accommodations that impose undue hardship or expense.

In the regulations governing Title I, hearing loss is regarded as a potentially disabling condition when it substantially limits one or more of life's major activities, such as telephone communication. Hearing care providers may need to demonstrate to potential employers how a job candidate with impaired hearing may be able to perform essential job functions with or without assistive devices.

Title II (Pubic Services) protects qualified individuals with disabilities from exclusion or denial of services, programs, or activities sponsored by a public entity. A public entity may be defined as any state or local department, agency or other instrumentality of a state or local government, or Amtrak and any commuter rail authority (DOJ, 1991a). Title II guarantees that auxiliary services will be made available to ensure communication access. These services include any means of accessing information through use of telephone technology, telephone relay services, public address systems, transcription services, written notice, and telecaptioning systems. The hearing-care provider has a vital role to play in selecting and fitting devices, and orienting others in their use to accommodate hearing disability.

Title III (Public Accommodations) ensures non-discrimination toward individuals with disabilities in the employment of goods, services, facilities, privileges, advantages, and accommodations of any public entity (DOJ, 1991b). Auxiliary aids and services must be provided unless undue burden would result. Burden is measured by the cost and nature of required action, resources of the providing facility, and size of the business. Hearing-care providers will need to consider the types of assistive devices and related service that would guarantee access to public places.

When this access is granted, public accommodations equipped with audible emergency alarms must provide an alarm signal that exceeds prevailing sound levels by 15 dBA. Alarms having a periodic element, such as a single-stroke bell, must be provided to facilitate perception by an individual with impaired hearing. In addition, public accommodations are required to modify policies and procedures to allow the use of service animals, such as hearing-ear dogs.

Under Title III, telephones must be hearing-aid compatible and allow for a signal intensity increase ranging from 12–18 dBA. Telephones equipped with amplifiers must be identified by appropriate signature. Telephone Devices for the Deaf (TDDs) used with conventional public pay phones must be permanently affixed to the telephone enclosure and identified by the international "telephone communication device for the deaf" symbol. Title III also ensures that no individual is discriminated against because of absence of auxiliary aids and services, unless it can be demonstrated that taking such steps would result in undue hardship.

Title IV (Telecommunications) amends Title II of the Communication Act of 1934 by making a rapid, efficient communication service available to all individuals regardless of hearing ability. Title IV ensures that telecommunication relay services are available that enable a communicatively-disordered individual to communicate in a manner functionally equivalent to that of someone without a disorder (FCC, 1991). Telecommunication relay system providers are responsible for supplying communication assistants (CAs) who meet the specialized needs of individuals with speech or hearing disabilities. Hearing-care providers may play an important role in educating CAs to understand hearing loss, its effects on communication, how to overcome communication problems, and the general influence of hearing loss and deafness on everyday psychosocial functions.

Implementation of the ADA should provide an opportunity to extend the practice of hearing loss management well outside the confines of hearing clinics and beyond instrumental compensation for hearing loss. As the ADA is implemented, it will become increasingly more common for audiologists to carry their practice into the community, interacting with engineers, architects, public transportation officials, employers, assistive device manufacturers and distributors, telecommunication service representatives, businesses serving individuals with hearing disabilities, and attorneys. It is also likely that the hearing care provider will assume the added role of "case worker" in championing the rights of individuals with impaired hearing to access the community and workplace.

Tinnitus and Vertigo. Tinnitus is a condition in which individuals hear noises with varying characteristics. For example, tinnitus has been described as a ringing sound, as crickets chirping, as water rushing, and so forth. The etiologies for tinnitus are numerous, including fluid in the middle ear and tumors along the auditory pathways. Tinnitus questionnaires have been useful in determining the extent of this problem on a client (see Appendix 9E).

Vertigo, in turn, is defined as the sensation of movement. It frequently occurs due to lesions in the inner ear, either auditory or vestibular. Meniere's disease is one of the more common causes of vertigo. Vertigo is common for individuals who have both conductive and sensorineural hearing losses.

It is not uncommon for persons to contact an audiologist because of tinnitus or vertigo, rather than hearing loss. According to a recent survey, 26% of ASHA audiologists were regularly evaluating tinnitus in 1980 and this had increased to 42% in 1990 (Schow, et al., 1993). Often the audiologist will refer the person to a physician for a medical examination and possible dietary or medical management. In other cases, the audiologist may provide counseling to help the client adjust to a condition which may not be medically correctable. Survey data from 1990 show that 23% of ASHA audiologists also may fit a special device for the masking of tinnitus called a tinnitus masker (see Chapter 2) on a patient where tinnitus is very annoying. In addition, some therapy efforts have involved biofeedback training where patients learn they can control heart rate or blood pressure. They are then often able to develop control of the level and annoyance from tinnitus. In any of the above situations, it is helpful if a medical assessment takes place prior to audiologic rehabilitation.

Computer Software.   Use of computer-assisted rehabilitation continues to expand. Many computer programs have been developed for selecting amplification systems and the most appropriate hearing-aid characteristics for a given hearing loss. As noted earlier, the DAVID system for speechreading at NTID is used on a computer-driven laser videodisc interactive system and other laser and compact discs are available for use in rehabilitation (see Chapter 12, Case 3). Smaldino and Smaldino (1994) have reviewed computer applications in rehabilitation planning. They recommend the development of software that is highly flexible, unique to a particular need, and possible for the average clinician to use without being a computer expert. Such systems may open up new horizons in the future of AR.

SUMMARY

This chapter has provided an overview of audiologic rehabilitation procedures for the adult with hearing impairment. A profile of adult clients and the settings in which they may obtain assistance for their hearing impairment has been presented. Medical, audiometric, and non-audiometric procedures have been outlined with regard to assessing communication difficulties and planning for individual rehabilitation needs. Specific rehabilitation procedures have been described, including hearing-aid selection, adjustment, and orientation; listening improvement; and auditory-visual communication therapy. Psychosocial and other aspects of the client with hearing impairment were also discussed with relation to problems that may need attention during the management process. Most adults with hearing impairment can be assisted by a carefully managed AR program which emphasizes the client's individual needs.

RECOMMENDED READINGS

Alpiner, J., & McCarthy, P. (1993). *Rehabilitative audiology: Children and adults* (2nd ed.). Baltimore: Williams & Wilkins.

Erber, N. P. (1993). *Communication and adult hearing loss.* Melbourne, Australia: Clavis.

Gagne, J. P., & Tye-Murray, N. (Eds.). (1994). *Research in audiological rehabilitation: Current trends and future directions.* Academy of Rehabilitative Audiology.

Garstecki, D.C. (1993). Chapter IX. Hearing aid acceptance in adults. In J. G. Clark & F. N. Martin (Eds.), *Effective counseling in audiology: Perspectives and practice.* Englewood Cliffs, NJ: Prentice Hall.

Kaplan, H., Bally, S., & Garretson, C. (1985). *Speechreading: A way to improve understanding.* Washington, DC: Gallaudet College Press.

Rezen, S., & Hausman, C. (1985). *Coping with hearing loss: A guide for adults and their families.* New York: Dembner Books.

Smaldino, J., & Smaldino, S. E. (1993). Computers in hearing rehabilitation. In J. Alpiner & P. McCarthy (Eds.), *Rehabilitative audiology: Children and adults* (2nd ed.). Baltimore: Williams & Wilkins.

REFERENCES

Alpiner, J. G., Chevrette, W., Glascoe, G., Metz, M., & Olsen, B. (1974). *The Denver Scale of Communication Function.* Unpublished study, University of Denver.

Alpiner, J. G., Meline, N. C., & Cotton, A. D. (1991). An aural rehabilitation screening scale: Self assessment, auditory aptitude, and visual aptitude. *Journal of Academy of Rehabilitation Audiology, 24,* 75-83.

Alpiner, J. G., & Roche, V. (1995). Hearing loss and tinnitus. *Geriatric Medicine,* 237-283. Baltimore: Williams & Wilkins.

Alpiner, J. G., & Schow, R. L. (1993). Rehabilitative evaluation of hearing-impaired adults. In J. Alpiner & P. McCarthy (Eds.), *Rehabilitative audiology: Children and adults* (2nd ed.). Baltimore: Williams & Wilkins.

ASHA—American Speech-Language-Hearing Association. (1992). Considerations in screening adults/older persons for handicapping hearing impairments. *Asha, 34*(6), 81-87.

Barcham, L. J., & Stephens, S. D. G. (1980). Use of the open-ended problems questionnaire in auditory rehabilitation. *British Journal of Audiology, 14,* 49-54.

Binnie, C. A., Jackson, P. L., & Montgomery, A. A. (1976). Visual intelligibility of consonants: A lipreading test with implications for aural rehabilitation. *Journal of Speech and Hearing Disorders, 41,* 530-539.

Christensen, R. A. (1994). Hard of hearing prevalence. In R. L. Schow, J. J. Mercaldo, & T. C. Smedley (Eds.) *The Idaho Hearing Survey* (Chap. 2). Pocatello, ID: Idaho State University Press.

Colodzin, L., Del Polito, G., Dickman, D., McLaughlin, R., & Sullivan, R. (1981). On the definition of hearing handicap. ASHA task force on the definition of hearing handicap. *Asha, 23,* 293-297.

Cox, R. M., Gilmore, C., & Alexander, G. C. (1991). Comparison of two questionnaires for patient-assessed hearing aid benefit. *Journal of American Academy of Audiology, 2,* 134-145.

Cranmer-Briskey, K. S. (1994). Today's market numbers set the challenge for next 25 years. *Hearing Instruments, 45,* 5-7.

Davis, H. (1948). The articulation area and the social adequacy index for hearing. *Laryngoscope, 58,* 761-778.

Davis, H., & Silverman, S. R. (1970). *Hearing and deafness.* New York: Holt, Rinehart and Winston.

Davis, J. M. (1980). Advice from some satisfied consumers. *Journal of the Academy of Rehabilitative Audiology, 13,* 122-127.

Demorest, M. E., & Erdman, S.A. (1986). Scale composition and item analysis of the communication profile for the hearing impaired. *Journal of Speech and Hearing Research, 29,* 515-535.

Demorest, M. E., & Erdman, S.A. (1987). Development of the communication profile for the hearing impaired. *Journal of Speech and Hearing Disorders, 52,* 129-143.

Demorest, M. E., & Erdman, S. A. (1994). Research in audiological rehabilitation: The challenges [Monograph.]. In J. P. Gagne & N. Tye-Murray (Eds.), *Research in audiological rehabilitation: Current trends and future directions.* Academy of Rehabilitative Audiology.

Demorest, M. E., & Walden, B. E. (1984). Psychometric principles in the selection, interpretation, and evaluation of communication self-assessment inventories. *Journal of Speech and Hearing Disorders, 49,* 226-240.

Department of Justice (DOJ) (1991a). 28 CFR Part 35: Nondiscrimination on the basis of disability in state and local government services: Final rule. *Federal Register, 56*(144, July 26), 35694-35723.

Department of Justice (DOJ) (1991b). 28 CFR Part 36: Nondiscrimination on the basis of disability by public accommodations and in commercial facilities: Final rule. *Federal Register, 56*(144, July 26), 35544-35604.

Eisenson, J., Auer, I. J., & Irwin, J. V. (1963). *The psychology of communication.* New York: Appleton-Century-Crofts.

Equal Employment Opportunity Commission (EEOC) (1991). 29 CFR Part 1630: Equal employment opportunity for individuals with disabilities: Final rule. *Federal Register, 56*(144, July 26), 35726-35755.

Erber, N. P. (1971). Auditory and audiovisual reception of words in low frequency noise by children with normal hearing and by children with impaired hearing. *Journal of Speech and Hearing Research, 14,* 496-512.

Erber, N. P. (1988). Communication therapy for hearing-impaired adults. Melbourne, Australia: Clavis.

Erber, N. P., & Lind, C. (1993). Communication theory: Theory and practice [Monograph]. In J. P. Gagne & N. Tye-Murray (Eds.), *Research in audiological rehabilitation: Current trends and future directions.* Academy of Rehabilitative Audiology.

Erdman, S. A. (1993). Self-assessment: From research focus to research tool [Monograph]. In J. P. Gagne & N. Tye-Murray (Eds.), *Research in Audiological Rehabilitation: Current Trends and Future Directions.* Academy of Rehabilitative Audiology.

Erdman, S. A. (1993). Counseling hearing impaired adults. In J. Alpiner & P. McCarthy (Eds.), *Rehabilitative audiology: Children and adults* (2nd ed.). Baltimore: Williams & Wilkins.

Ewertson, H., Birk-Nielsen, H. (1973). Social hearing handicap index: Social handicap in relation to hearing impairment. *Audiology*, *12*, 180-187.

Federal Communications Commission (FCC) (1991). 47 CFR Parts 0 and 64: Telecommunications services for hearing and speech disabled: Final rule. *Federal Register*, *56*(148, August 1), 36729-36733.

Fleming, M. (1972). A total approach to communication therapy. *Journal of the Academy of Rehabilitative Audiology*, *5*, 28-31.

Frankel, B. J., Adult onset hearing impairment: social and psychological correlates of adjustment. Doctoral dissertation. The University of Western Ontario, London, Ontario (1981).

Gagne, J. P., & Erber, N. P. (1987). Simulation of sensorineural hearing impairment. *Ear and Hearing*, *8*, 232-243.

Garstecki, D. C. (1980). Alternative approaches to measuring speech discrimination efficiency. In R. R. Rupp & K. G. Stockdall (Eds.), *Speech protocols in audiology* (pp. 119-143). New York: Grune & Stratton.

Garstecki, D. C. (1981). Auditory-visual training paradigm for hearing-impaired adults. *Journal of the Academy of Rehabilitative Audiology*, *14*, 223-238.

Garstecki, D. C., & Erler, S. F. (1995a). Older women and hearing. *American Journal of Audiology*, 4(2), 41-46.

Garstecki, D. C. & Erler, S. F. (1995b). Older adult performance on the communication profile for the hearing impaired. *Journal of Speech and Hearing Research*, 38(6).

Garstecki, D. C. & Erler, S. F. (1996). Hearing loss management in children and adults. In S. E. Gerber & G. T. Mencher (Eds.), *Auditory dysfunction*. Needham Heights, MA: Allyn & Bacon.

Gatehouse, S. (1990). Determinants of self-report disability in older subjects. *Ear and Hearing*, *11*(5), 55-65.

Giolas, T., Owens, E., Lamb, S. H., & Schubert, E. D. (1979). Hearing performance inventory. *Journal of Speech and Hearing Disorders*, *44*, 169-195.

Goldstein, D. P., & Stephens, S. D. G. (1981). Audiological rehabilitation: Management model I. *Audiology*, *20*, 432-452.

Habib, R. G., & Hinchcliffe, R. (1978). Subjective magnitude of auditory impairment. *Audiology*, *17*, 68-76.

Hardick, E. (1977). Aural rehabilitation programs for the aged can be successful. *Journal of the Academy of Rehabilitative Audiology*, *10*, 51-67.

Hardick, E. J., Oyer, H. J., & Irion, P. E. (1970). Lipreading performance as related to measurements of vision. *Journal of Speech and Hearing Research*, *13*, 92-100.

Hétu, R., Stephens, D., Noble, W., Getty, L., Philibert, L., & Désilets (July, 1994). Hearing disability and handicap scale (HDHS): A short questionnaire for clinical use. *Paper presented at the XXII International Congress of Audiology*, Halifax, Nova Scotia.

High, W. S., Fairbanks, G., & Glorig, A. (1964). Scale for self-assessment of hearing handicap. *Journal of Speech and Hearing Disorders, 29,* 215-230.

Hutton, C. L. (1980). Response to a hearing problem inventory. *Journal of the Academy of Rehabilitative Audiology, 13,* 133-154.

Jeffers, J., & Barley, M. (1971). *Speechreading (lipreading).* Springfield, IL: Charles C. Thomas.

Jerger, J., Speaks, C., & Trannell, J. (1968). A new approach to speech audiometry. *Journal of Speech and Hearing Disorders, 33,* 318-328.

Jerger, S., & Jerger, J. (1979). Quantifying auditory handicap: A new approach. *Audiology, 18,* 225-237.

Johnson, D. (1976). Communication characteristics of a young deaf adult population: Techniques for evaluating their communication skills. *American Annals of the Deaf, 12,* 409-424.

Kalikow, D. N., Stevens, K. N., & Elliott, L. L. (1977). Development of a test of speech intelligibility in noise using sentence materials with controlled word predictability. *Journal of the Acoustical Society of America, 61,* 1337-1351.

Kaplan, H., Bally. S., and Brandt, F. D. (1990). Communication strategies, attitudes, and difficulties in the prelingually deaf population. *ASHA Convention Program, 116.*

Lamb, S. W., Owens, E., Schubert, E. D., & Giolas, T. G. (1984). Hearing Performance Inventory. *Hearing Disorders in Adults.* San Diego: College-Hill Press.

A listening guide. (1981). Chicago: Beltone Electronics Corp.

Madell, J. (1980). Self-perceived needs of adults with hearing impairments. *Journal of the Academy of Rehabilitative Audiology, 13,* 116-121.

McCarthy, P. A., & Alpiner, J. G. (1983). An assessment scale of hearing handicap for use in family counseling. *Journal of the Academy of Rehabilitative Audiology, 16,* 156-270.

Mulrow, C. D., Tuley, M. R., & Aguilar, C. (1990). Discriminating and responsiveness abilities of two hearing handicap scales. *Ear and Hearing, 11*(3), 176-180.

Newman, C. W., & Jacobsen G. P. (1993). Self-assessment of hearing. *Seminars in Hearing,* 14(4), 299-384.

Newman, C. W., Weinstein, B. E., Jacobson, G. P., & Hug, G. A. (1991). Test-retest reliability of the hearing handicap inventory for adults. *Ear and Hearing, 12*(5), 355-357.

Noble, W. G. (1978). *Assessment of impaired hearing: A critique and a new method.* New York: Academic Press.

Noble, W. G. (1994). Self-report methodology in hearing disability and handicap assessment. *International Collegium of Rehabilitative Audiology, 8,* 13-18.

Noble, W. G., & Atherley, G. R. C. (1970). The hearing measurement scale: A questionnaire for the assessment of auditory disability. *Journal of Audiological Research, 10,* 229-250.

Owens E., & Raggio, M. W. (1988). *Hearing performance inventory for severe to profound hearing loss.* San Francisco: University of California Press.

Owens, E., & Schubert, E. D. (1977). Development of the California consonant test. *Journal of Speech and Hearing Research, 20,* 463-474.

Oyer, H. J. (1966). *Auditory communication for the hard of hearing.* Englewood Cliffs, NJ: Prentice Hall.

Rihkanen, H. (1990). Subjective benefit of communication aids evaluated by postlingually deaf adults. *British Journal of Audiology, 24,* 161–166.

Ringdahl, A. Eriksson-Mangold, M., and Karlsson, K. (1993) (June) The Gothenburg profile: A self-report inventory for measuring experienced hearing disability and handicap. *International Collegium of Rehabilitative Audiology Newsletter* (6).

Ripley, J., & Cummings, T. (1977). *A guide to teaching beginning lipreading groups.* Unpublished project, University of Denver.

Saloman, G., & Parving, A. (1985). Hearing disability and communication handicap for compensation purposes based on self-assessment and audiometric testing. *Audiology, 24,* 35–145.

Sanders, D. (1975). Hearing aid orientation and counseling. In M. Pollack (Ed.), *Amplification for the hearing impaired* (pp. 323–372). New York: Grune & Stratton.

Santore, F., Tulko, C., & Kearney, A. (1983). Communication therapy for the adult with impaired hearing. *New York League for the Hard of Hearing Rehabilitation Quarterly, 8*(1), 5–7.

Schein, J., Gentile, A., & Haase, K. (1970). Development and evaluation of an expanded hearing loss scale questionnaire. *Vital and Health Statistics, 2,* 37.

Schow, R. L. (1991). Considerations in selecting and validating an adult/elderly hearing screening protocol. *Ear and Hearing, 12*(5), 337–347.

Schow, R. L., Balsara, N. R., Smedley, T. C., & Whitcomb, C. J. (1993). Aural rehabilitation by ASHA audiologists: 1980-1990. *American Journal of Audiology, 2*(3), 28–37.

Schow, R. L., & Gatehouse, S. (1990). Fundamental issues in self-assessment of hearing. *Ear and Hearing, 11*(5, Suppl.), 6–16.

Schow, R. L., & Nerbonne, M. A. (1980). Hearing handicap and Denver scales: Applications, categories, interpretation. *Journal of the Academy of Rehabilitative Audiology, 13,* 66–77.

Schow, R. L., & Nerbonne, M. A. (1982). Communication screening profile: Use with elderly clients. *Ear and Hearing, 3,* 135–147.

Schow, R. L., & Smedley, T. C. (1990). Self-assessment of hearing. *Ear and Hearing, 11*(5, Suppl./Special Issue).

Schow, R. L., & Tannahill, C. (1977). Hearing handicap scores and categories for subjects with normal and impaired hearing sensitivity. *Journal of the American Audiology Society, 3,* 134–139.

Schwartz, D. M., & Surr, R. K. (1979). Three experiments on the California Consonant Test. *Journal of Speech and Hearing Disorders, 44,* 61–72.

Sims, D. G. (1985). Visual and auditory training for adults. In J. Katz (Ed.), *Handbook of clinical audiology* (pp. 565–580). Baltimore: Williams & Wilkins.

Smaldino, J., & Sahli, J. (1980). A litany of needs of hearing-impaired consumers. *Journal of the Academy of Rehabilitative Audiology, 13,* 109–115.

Smaldino, J., & Smaldino, S. E. (1993). Computers in hearing rehabilitation. In J. Alpiner & P. McCarthy (Eds.), *Rehabilitative audiology: Children and adults* (2nd ed.). Baltimore: Williams & Wilkins.

Snell, K. (1994). National Technical Institute for the Deaf. Personal communication.

Stephens, S. D. G. (1980). Evaluating the problems of the hearing impaired. *Audiology, 19,* 205–220.

Stream, R. W., & Stream, K. S. (1980). Focusing on the hearing needs of the elderly. *Journal of the Academy of Rehabilitative Audiology, 13,* 104–108.

Tye-Murray, N. (1994). Communication strategies training [Monograph]. In J. P. Gagne & N. Tye-Murray (Eds.), *Research in Audiological Rehabilitation: Current Trends and Future Directions.* Academy of Rehabilitative Audiology.

Tyler, R. S., Baker, L. J., & Armstrong-Bednall, G. (1983). Difficulties experienced by hearing aid candidates and hearing aid users. *British Journal of Audiology, 17,* 191–201.

Walden, B. E., Demorest, M.E., & Hepler, E. H. (1984). Self-report approach to assessing benefit derived form amplification. *Journal of Speech and Hearing Research, 27,* 49–56.

Walden, B. E., & Grant, K. W. (1993). Research needs in rehabilitative audiology. In J. Alpiner & P. McCarthy (Eds.), *Rehabilitative audiology: Children and adults* (2nd ed.). Baltimore: Williams & Wilkins.

WHO (1980). *International classification of impairments, disabilities, and handicaps: A manual of classification relating to the consequences of disease.* Geneva, Switzerland, World Health Organization, 25–43.

Wylde, M. A. (1982). The remediation process: Psychologic and counseling aspects. In J. G. Alpiner (Ed.), *Handbook of adult rehabilitation audiology* (2nd ed.). Baltimore: Williams & Wilkins.

Appendix Nine A

Self-Assessment of Communication (SAC)

Name_____ Date_____

One of the following five descriptions should be assigned to each of the statements below.
Select a number from 1 to 5 next to each statement (do not answer with *yes* or *no*).

      1) Almost Never (or Never)   4) Frequently (About $3/4$ of the Time)
      2) Occasionally (About $1/4$ of the Time)   5) Practically Always (or Always)
      3) About $1/2$ the Time

Various Communication Situations

Circle Number Below

1. Do you experience communication difficulties when speaking with one other person? (For example, at home, at work, with a waitress, store clerk, spouse, boss, etc.)	1 2 3 4 5
2. Do you experience communication difficulties when conversing with a small group of people? (For example, with friends, family, or co-workers, in meetings or casual conversations, over dinner or while playing cards, etc.)	1 2 3 4 5
3. Do you experience communication difficulties while listening to a large group? (For example, at church or in a civic meeting, in a fraternal or women's club, at an educational lecture, etc.)	1 2 3 4 5
4. Do you experience communication difficulties while participating in various types of entertainment? (For example, movies, TV, radio, plays, night clubs, musical entertainment, etc.)	1 2 3 4 5
5. Do you experience communication difficulties when you are in an unfavorable listening environment? (For example, at a noisy party, where there is background music, when riding in an auto or bus, when someone whispers or talks from across the room, etc.)	1 2 3 4 5
6. Do you experience communication difficulties when using or listening to various communication devices? (For example, telephone, telephone ring, doorbell, public address system, warning signals, alarms, etc.)	1 2 3 4 5

Feelings About Communication

7. Do you feel that difficulty with your hearing limits or hampers your personal or social life?	1 2 3 4 5
8. Do problems or difficulty with your hearing upset you?	1 2 3 4 5

Other People

9. Do others suggest that you have a hearing problem?	1 2 3 4 5
10. Do others leave you out of conversations or become annoyed because of your hearing?	1 2 3 4 5

Raw Score (simply add all numbers above) _____

••Self-assessment of communication (SAC). (From "Communication Screening Profile: Use with Elderly Clients" by R.L. Schow and M.A. Nerbonne, 1982, *Ear and Hearing*, 3, 135-147.)

Significant Other Assessment of Communication (SOAC)

Name_____ Date_____

Form filled out with reference to _____ (client/patient)

Informant's relationship to client/patient _____ (wife, son, friend, etc.)
One of the following five descriptions should be assigned to each of the statements below.
Circle a number from 1 to 5 next to each statement (do not answer with *yes* or *no*).

- 1) Almost Never (or Never)
- 2) Occasionally (About 1/4 of the Time)
- 3) About 1/2 the Time
- 4) Frequently (About 3/4 of the Time)
- 5) Practically Always (or Always)

Various Communication Situations

Circle Number Below

1. Does he/she experience communication difficulties when speaking with one other person? (For example, at home, at work, with a waitress, store clerk, spouse, boss, etc.)	1 2 3 4 5
2. Does he/she experience communication difficulties when conversing with a small group of people? (For example, with friends or family, or co-workers, in meetings or casual conversations, over dinner or while playing cards, etc.)	1 2 3 4 5
3. Does he/she experience communication difficulties while listening to a large group? (For example, at church or civic meeting, in a fraternal or women's club, at an educational lecture, etc.)	1 2 3 4 5
4. Does he/she experience communication difficulties while participating in various types of entertainment? (For example, movies, TV, radio, plays, night clubs, musical entertainment, etc.)	1 2 3 4 5
5. Does he/she experience communication difficulties when you are in an unfavorable listening environment? (For example, at a noisy party, where there is background music, when riding in an auto or bus, when someone whispers or talks from across the room, etc.)	1 2 3 4 5
6. Does he/she experience communication difficulties when using or listening to various communication devices? (For example, telephone, telephone ring, doorbell, public address system, warning signals, alarms, etc.)	1 2 3 4 5

Feelings About Communication

7. Do you feel that difficulty with his/her hearing limits or hampers his/her personal or social life?	1 2 3 4 5
8. Does any problem or difficulty with his/her hearing upset you?	1 2 3 4 5

Other People

9. Do others suggest that he/she has a hearing problem?	1 2 3 4 5
10. Do others leave him/her out of conversations or become annoyed because of his/her hearing?	1 2 3 4 5

Raw Score (simply add all numbers above) _____

**Significant other assessment of communication (SOAC). (From "Communication Screening Profile: Use with Elderly Clients" by R.L. Schow and M.A. Nerbonne, 1982, *Ear and Hearing, 3,* 135-147. Adapted by permission.

Appendix Nine B

Hearing Handicap Scale (Form A)

1. If you are 6 to 12 feet from the loudspeaker of a radio do you understand speech well?
2. Can you carry on a telephone conversation without difficulty?
3. If you are 6 to 12 feet away from a television set, do you understand most of what is said?
4. Can you carry on a conversation with one other person when you are on a noisy street corner?
5. Do you hear all right when you are in a street car, airplane, bus, or train?
6. If there are noises from other voices, typewriters, traffic, music, etc., can you understand when someone speaks to you?
7. Can you understand a person when you are seated beside him and cannot see his face?
8. Can you understand if someone speaks to you while you are chewing crisp foods, such as potato chips or celery?
9. Can you carry on a conversation with one other person when you are in a noisy place, such as a restaurant or at a party?
10. Can you understand if someone speaks to you in a whisper and you cannot see his face?
11. When you talk with a bus driver, waiter, ticket salesman, etc., can you understand all right?
12. Can you carry on a conversation if you are seated across the room from someone who speaks in a normal tone of voice?
13. Can you understand women when they talk?
14. Can you carry on a conversation with one other person when you are out-of-doors and it is reasonably quiet?
15. When you are in a meeting or at a large dinner table, would you know the speaker was talking if you could not see his lips moving?
16. Can you follow the conversation when you are at a large dinner table or in a meeting with a small group?
17. If you are seated under the balcony of a theater or auditorium, can you hear well enough to follow what is going on?
18. When you are in a large formal gathering (a church, lodge, lecture hall, etc.), can you hear what is said when the speaker does not use a microphone?
19. Can you hear the telephone ring when you are in the room where it is located?
20. Can you hear warning signals, such as automobile horns, railway crossing bells, or emergency vehicle sirens?

From "Scale for Self-Assessment of Hearing Handicap" by W.S. High, G. Fairbanks, and A. Glorig, 1964, *Journal of Speech and Hearing Disorders, 29*, pp. 215-230. Reprinted by permission.

Appendix Nine C

Denver Scale of Communication Function

The following questionnaire was designed to evaluate your communication ability as you view it. You are asked to judge or scale each statement in the following manner.

If you judge the statement to be very closely related to either extreme, please place your check mark as follows:

Agree __X__ _____ _____ _____ _____ _____ __X__ Disagree

or

If you judge the statement to be closely related to either end of the scale, please mark as follows:

Agree _____ __X__ _____ _____ _____ __X__ _____ Disagree

or

If you judge the statement to be only slightly related to either end of the scale, please mark as follows:

Agree _____ _____ __X__ _____ __X__ _____ _____ Disagree

or

If you judge the statement to be irrelevant to or unassociated with your communication situation, please mark as follows:

Agree _____ _____ _____ __X__ _____ _____ _____ Disagree

PLEASE NOTE: Mark each statement with only one mark and judge each item separately. You may comment on each statement in the space provided.

If you wish you may simply assign a number for each statement as follows:

Agree _____ _____ _____ _____ _____ _____ _____ Disagree
       1   2   3   4   5   6   7

Number

1. The members of my family are annoyed with my loss of hearing. _____
2. The members of my family sometimes leave me out of conversations or discussions. _____
3. Sometimes my family makes decisions for me because I have a hard time following discussions. _____
4. My family becomes annoyed when I ask them to repeat what was said because I did not hear them. _____
5. I am not an "outgoing" person because I have a hearing loss. _____

6. I now take less of an interest in many things as compared to when I did not have a hearing problem. _____

7. Other people do not realize how frustrated I get when I cannot hear or understand. _____

8. People sometimes avoid me because of my hearing loss. _____

9. I am not a calm person because of my hearing loss. _____

10. I tend to be negative about life in general because of my hearing loss. _____

11. I do not socialize as much as I did before I began to lose my hearing. _____

12. Since I have trouble hearing, I do not like to go places with friends. _____

13. Since I have trouble hearing, I hesitate to meet new people. _____

14. I do not enjoy my job as much as I did before I began to lose my hearing. _____

15. Other people do not understand what it is like to have a hearing loss. _____

16. Because I have difficulty understanding what is said to me, I sometimes answer questions wrong. _____

17. I do not feel relaxed in a communicative situation. _____

18. I don't feel comfortable in most communication situations. _____

19. Conversations in a noisy room prevent me from attempting to communicate with others. _____

20. I am not comfortable having to speak in a group situation. _____

21. In general, I do not find listening relaxing. _____

22. I feel threatened by many communication situations due to difficulty hearing. _____

23. I seldom watch other people's facial expressions when talking to them. _____

24. I hesitate to ask people to repeat if I do not understand them the first time they speak. _____

25. Because I have difficulty understanding what is said to me, I sometimes make comments that do not fit into the conversation. _____

Adapted from *Denver Scale of Communication Function* by J.C. Alpiner, W. Chevrette, G. Glascoe, M. Metz, and B. Olsen, 1974.

Appendix Nine D

Hearing Disability and Handicap Scale

Name: _____

Age: _____

1. In your own opinion, and according to comments made by the people around you, how would you describe your hearing problem?
   - ○ Very severe
   - ○ Severe
   - ○ Moderate
   - ○ Slight

2. How long have you had this hearing problem?
   - ○ Less than a year
   - ○ From one to two years
   - ○ From three to four years
   - ○ More than five

3. Including today's visit, how many appointments have you had at an audiology clinic?
   - ○ Only one
   - ○ two or three
   - ○ four or five
   - ○ More than five

4. What is your main occupation?
   - ○ Paid employment
   - ○ Unemployed
   - ○ Housewife
   - ○ Student
   - ○ Retired
   - ○ Other (specify)

   _____

5. Do you wear hearing aids?
   - ○ No
   - ○ Yes
       - ○ For one ear
       - ○ For two ears
       - ○ Other (specify)

If you have some comments, please write them in the space below:

_____

_____

Indicate, by checking the appropriate box, how often you experience each one of the situations described below. Please answer all of the questions and check only one answer for each.

	Never	Sometimes	Often	Always
1. Do you have difficulty following a conversation normally in any of the following situations: at work, in a bus or car, or when shopping?	O	O	O	O
2. Can you hear the sound of the door opening when you are inside the room?	O	O	O	O
3. Do you worry that people will find out you have a hearing problem?	O	O	O	O
4. Is it difficult for you to ask people to repeat themselves?	O	O	O	O
5. Do you have difficulty hearing what is being said on TV if someone other than you adjusts the volume?	O	O	O	O
6. Can you hear the water boiling in the pan when you are in the kitchen?	O	O	O	O
7. Do you get upset if you give the wrong answer to someone because you have misheard them?	O	O	O	O
8. Does your hearing condition restrict your social or personal life?	O	O	O	O
9. Do you have difficulty hearing what's being said on the radio if someone other than yourself adjusts the volume?	O	O	O	O
10. Do you hear the footsteps of someone coming into the room without seeing them?	O	O	O	O
11. Does it bother or upset you if you are unable to follow a conversation?	O	O	O	O
12. Do you find that you are more tense and tired because of your hearing difficulties?	O	O	O	O
13. Do you have difficulty hearing in a group conversation?	O	O	O	O
14. Can you hear someone ringing the door-bell or knocking on the door?	O	O	O	O

	Never	Sometimes	Often	Always
15. Do people avoid you because of your hearing difficulties?	O	O	O	O
16. At present, would you say you lack self-confidence because of your hearing difficulty?	O	O	O	O
17. Do you find that although you can hear someone speaking, you cannot understand what they are saying?	O	O	O	O
18. Can you hear the telephone ringing from another room?	O	O	O	O
19. Do you ever feel cut off from things because of your hearing difficulty?	O	O	O	O
20. Do you feel your hearing condition has an influence on the relationships you have with your spouse or a person close to you?	O	O	O	O

From Hetu, et al., 1994.

Appendix Nine E

Tinnitus Questionnaire

Tinnitus Questionnaire

Date of Onset: _____ Related to Specific Incident: _____

_____

Tinnitus is   ___ Constant   ___ Intermittent
Tinnitus is   ___ Unilateral   ___ Bilateral

Description of Tinnitus: ____ Ringing ____ Buzzing ____ Hissing
                        ____ Pulsing ____ Popping ____ Wind ____ Roaring
                        ____ Insects ____ Clicking
                        Other: _____

Is The Tinnitus:

1. Masked by Environmental Sounds?   ___Yes   ___No
2. Interfering with Sleep?   ___Yes   ___No
3. Aggravated by Any Stimuli?   ___Yes   ___No
   ___Noise ___Caffeine ___Alcohol ___Other:_____
4. Interfering with Daily Activities?   ___Yes   ___No
5. Handicapping You in Any Way?   ___Yes   ___No
   _____
6. Interfering with Family Relationships?   ___Yes   ___No
Comments:
_____
_____

Subjective Degree of Problem

	Mild		Moderate		Severe
Patient's Impression	1	2	3	4	5
Examiner's Impression	1	2	3	4	5

_____   _____
Date   Examiner

Patient's Name: _____   Age: _____

Audiologic Rehabilitation for Elderly Adults

ASSESSMENT AND MANAGEMENT

JAMES MAURER
RONALD L. SCHOW

Contents

INTRODUCTION

Today there is greater need than ever for providing audiologic rehabilitation services to older persons. Approximately 12.5% of the population in this country is 65 years of age and older. The 1990 U.S. population of 31 million persons of retirement age is projected to increase to 65 million by the year 2030, as medical technology continues to extend our lifespans and the post-World War II "baby boom" becomes the 21st century's "geriatric boom." In 1990, 1 in 35 Americans was 80 or older, and this number could increase to 1 in 12 by 2050 (Taeuber, 1992). Senior adults will continue to live longer and be more active. A major requisite for maintaining and enhancing the quality of their remaining lifespan will be to maintain communication skills. The audiologist plays a pivotal role in providing rehabilitative services specifically tailored to the older person's need to maximize the quality of life during this increased lifespan.

Intervention for hearing loss among older persons is among the most challenging pursuits for clinical audiologists. This chapter addresses that challenge, which includes (a) knowledge about aging clients and the environmental milieu which surrounds them and interacts in unique ways with hearing loss, (b) methods of identifying and assessing the handicapping condition, (c) techniques for rehabilitating amplification needs and receptive communication skills, and (d) counseling strategies aimed at both gaining acceptance of the intervention process and relieving the stress associated with a decline in auditory skills during the later years of life.

PROFILE OF THE CLIENT

In order to provide the senior citizen whose hearing is impaired with appropriate audiologic rehabilitative treatment, the audiologist must understand the factors involved in the aging process that directly relate to the individual's ability and desire to communicate. For no other age group does the environment undergo so many changes as for the aging individual. These changes must be given special consideration when rehabilitation measures are planned and implemented. An individual's lifetime generally pursues a course towards greater growth and development of physical, psychological, and social needs. If changes occur that impede the acquisition or continuance of these needs, the individual may be forced to readjust his lifestyle to accommodate the change. A younger person who draws support from a large reservoir of both internal and external resources readapts to a new situation more readily than an older individual who is more limited in options. As the support system continues to decrease with age, the frequency and severity of significant lifestyle changes, described by Ronch and Van Zanten (1992) and summarized below, continue to increase. Although most aging persons undergo a certain degree of change in every area listed below, their capacity to adapt to these changes is highly individualized, depending upon genetic inheritance, life experiences, past and present environments, and traditional ways of dealing with life.

1. Members of the family of origin—parents, brothers, and sisters—become ill or die.
2. Marital relationship—there is strain due to death or illness of spouse, estrangement due to empty-nest syndrome, pressures due to retirement.
3. Peer group—friends die or become separated by geographical relocation for health, family, or retirement reasons.
4. Occupation—many older people retire.
5. Recreation—becomes scarce due to physical limitations or unavailability of opportunities.
6. Economics—income is reduced by retirement, limited income is tapped by inflation or medical costs not covered by insurance.
7. Physical condition—loss of youth, changes in physiological and biological aspects of the body cause poor health and its emotional consequences.
8. Emotional/sexual life—loss of significant others through death, separation, and reduction in sexual activity due to societal expectations, health, personal preference, or death of partner.

Variables of the Aging Process

The increasing number of lifestyle changes results in a more heterogeneous population than that of any other age group. It is, therefore, impossible to assess accurately the effects of aging based solely on a person's chronological age. Not all individuals of the same age experience aging in the same way. Some people appear youthful well into their 80s, while others manifest old-age behaviors by their early 40s.

The apparent variability of each person's rate and degree of aging, regardless of chronological age, is attributable to the unique interaction of three aspects of the aging process: biological, experiential, and psychosocial. *Biological* aging is determined by genetic programming, which affects cellular deterioration within a predetermined time frame. *Experiential* aging, in turn, is shaped by life forces and the associated environmental insults which contribute to physical deterioration in later life. *Psychosocial* aging reflects maladaptive behaviors and reduced social output when confronted with the radical lifestyle changes of chronological aging (Maurer & Montserrat-Hopple, 1992).

Physical and Mental Health

Most elderly persons are in relatively good health, but as reported by the U.S. Bureau of the Census (1990), approximately 9% of adults 65–69 years old need assistance with their everyday activities, and this increases to 45% for those 85 and over. Only a small proportion of the aging population has physical disabilities so severe as to interfere with successful rehabilitative treatment. In general, the aging process is characteristically manifested by a slowing down or reduction of the bodily systems. According to Brody (1973), a gradual attrition of brain cells in the older individual can significantly affect the neuronal conduction rate. As transmission speed decreases, response time to sensory input increases. Subsequently, an older person may need more time to perceive, process, organize, and react to sensory stimuli than younger individuals. This change can be further exacerbated by gradual deterioration of sensory receptors, a decline in motor coordination, and increased fatiguability. Biochemical changes can lead to metabolic imbalances or endocrine insufficiencies followed by lowered resistance to disease, and increased resistance to healing of injuries.

To some degree, the senior adult is required to adjust to a certain amount of physical disability and reduced activity level. As each new physical problem becomes apparent, and is further reinforced by the inevitable continuance of deterioration, the older person is confronted daily with her own mortality. Realization of the consequences of age can, therefore, significantly affect an individual's attitude towards self-fulfillment. That is why it is difficult to discuss the physical and mental factors contributing to the aging process as separate entities. The interaction between the two is symbionic, with changes in one almost certainly influencing the other. Mental or psychological factors associated with aging have been delineated by Ronch and Van Zanten (1992) as (a) intellectual-cognitive changes and (b) emotional-personality alterations.

Intellectual-Cognitive. Robertson-Thabo (1984) reported that longitudinal studies on intelligence and aging generally do not indicate significant changes in intelligence-test performance until the late years of life. As the author indicated, however, some aging persons decline in some aspects of cognitive functioning, while others do not. Extra-aging factors may well account for individual differences.

Atchley (1972) proposed that intelligence is probably more affected by health than by age. Reduced neural efficiency with its associated latency in response at the central processor may contribute to a gradual decrement in certain aspects of memory, logic, and awareness (Hunter, 1960). Rabbitt (1965) reported that aging individuals had greater difficulty in discriminating between relevant and non-relevant stimuli. This may interfere with the older person's ability to accurately assess sensory input and, subsequently, make appropriate responses. Craik (1977) noted increasing deficits in short-term memory as age increased. While this may mean that it takes longer to learn new materials, it does not necessarily affect the quality of learning.

Emotional-Personality. The aging population has a high incidence of mental illness (Butler, 1975). They account for about 1/4 of all reported suicides in this country (Butler & Lewis, 1977) and the suicidal death rates for older persons have been increasing in recent years (U.S. Department of Health and Human Services, 1993). As senior adults confront lifestyle changes, not all can readily adapt. Concomitant declines in sensory/motor skills and increased risk of illness and injury create a loss of independence and personal control. Feelings of depression, anxiety, and even hostility may cause the individual to withdraw from stress-producing environments and situations. Thus senility, long regarded as the inevitable consequence of growing older, is no longer attributed entirely to biochemical changes associated with aging, nor is it considered entirely unalterable. The influence of hearing impairment, for example, on behaviors otherwise described as "senile" (e.g., inattentiveness, inappropriate responding) may give justifiable cause for a second opinion from a hearing specialist. In fact, recent studies have shown that hearing loss has an adverse effect on quality of life, and on emotional, behavioral, and social well-being. Bess, et al. (1989) found a systematic relationship between hearing loss and functional/psychosocial status in 153 elderly subjects, and that hearing loss accounted for a significant amount of the variation when they controlled for demographic variables like age, number of illnesses, and medication amounts. Mulrow, et al. (1990) found similar results on a sample of 204 elderly males.

Economic Status

Adjustments to radical lifestyle changes are made easier when economic factors are not a concern. A higher income allows greater mobility to seek better health care and to continue supportive social contacts. The affluent, socially active older person is more inclined to compensate for the detrimental effects of age by purchasing necessary medications, eye-glasses, dentures, or hearing aids. Low-income persons, on the other hand, have fewer options.

Retirement is perhaps the primary factor for change in the senior adult's economic status. Loss of employment not only may alter financial security, but may reduce social interaction and erode self-esteem. The percentage of the aging population below the poverty level has been reduced from about 25% in 1970 to about 12% in 1990, but the elderly are more likely to be "near poor" than the younger population, since about 18% of the elderly are in this category (U.S. Department of Health and Human Services, 1993).

Although most older individuals are not considered poor, many live on fixed incomes and have their prime financial asset tied up in the equity of their home. The financial benefit of selling the house is frequently offset by the emotional stress produced by the subsequent loss of neighborhood, territorial familiarity, and security. Because of their attachment to familiar objects, many of the aged fear change and will sacrifice food and medical care rather than give up their environmental surroundings (Ronch & Van Zanten, 1992).

The economic status of senior citizens who live in long-term extended care facilities is usually lower than that of their counterparts who reside in privately owned homes.

Living Environments

Older adults may live independently, with family members, or in some type of health-care facility. Most live in their own residence, while only 15% live with a relative other than their spouse or a non-relative (Taeuber, 1992). Private residences for older persons, particularly of low income, are usually located in heavily populated, noisy, and sometimes dangerous urban areas. Many elderly adults are confined to their homes due to financial and health considerations and are often cared for by their spouses or children. Just over 50% of the aging population live with a spouse and almost 13% live with their children or other relatives. The number living alone rapidly increases with advancing age until 47% are doing so when they are 85 years or over (Taeuber, 1992).

The older individual is likely to require professional health care beyond the capabilities of the family environment. For some, this only may necessitate moving to an apartment complex which provides health care services when needed. Those recently hospitalized who are yet unable to return home may choose to stay temporarily in short-term care facilities designed to provide 24-hour intensive-care services by a professionally trained staff.

Health-care facilities most often associated with the aging population are nursing homes which provide long-term care. Kemper and Murtaugh (1991) estimate that the lifetime risk of institutionalization for those 65 in 1990, based on past rates, would be 43%. About 52% of women versus 33% of men will use a nursing home before they die. In addition, 70% of women who died at 90 had lived in a nursing home. Those in nursing homes represent an older segment of the geriatric population with generally more advanced physical and mental deterioration. Further, they are more socially isolated, with about half having no nearby relatives. Families frequently use nursing homes for those near death and most admissions are short term (3/4 are for less than a year) (Taeuber, 1992).

Hearing Loss and Aging

The prevalence of hearing loss increases as age increases, as reflected by Figure 10.1 and Table 10.1. Almost half the persons in the United States with hearing problems are aged 65 years and older (Ries, 1994). For nursing-home residents and the hospitalized elderly, this figure climbs even higher. Schow and Nerbonne (1980) evaluated 202 nursing-home residents from five facilities and found that 82% of their sample demonstrated pure-tone threshold averages (PTAs) of 26 dB HL or greater, with 48% exhibiting PTAs of at least 40 dB HL.

TABLE 10.1 *Prevalence Rates of Hearing Impairment, per 100 Persons, in the Civilian, Noninstitutionalized Population of the U.S.*

Age Group in Years	Number	Prevalence Rate (%)
3–17	968,000	1.8
18–24	650,000	2.6
25–34	1,659,000	3.4
35–44	2,380,000	6.3
45–54	2,634,000	10.3
55–64	3,275,000	15.4
65–74	4,267,000	23.4
75+	4,462,000	37.7
All	20,295,000	8.6

Note: Rates are based on 1990–91 interview data from the National Center for Health Statistics (Ries, 1994).

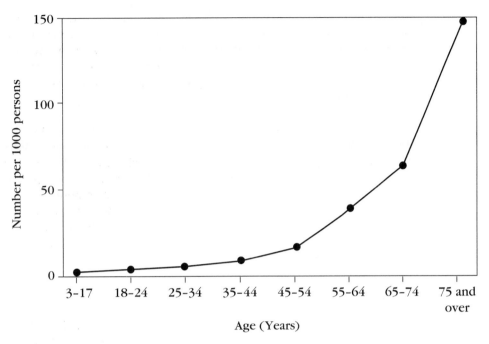

Figure 10.1 Average annual age-specific number of persons three years of age and over who cannot hear and understand normal speech per 1000 persons: United States, 1990–91.

Ries, 1994.

Presbycusis. The aging process is perhaps the most common cause of hearing impairment. This type of deficit, *presbycusis*, was described by Schuknecht (1964) as an accumulation of age-related degenerative changes within the auditory system. In its most common form, presbycusis is a gradual process, initially affecting hearing sensitivity for the higher frequencies of a pure-tone audiogram. During its early stages, most individuals are unaware of the loss, but as the deficit progresses, the ability to understand speech, especially in the presence of background noise, becomes increasingly impaired.

Presbycusis is not the only cause of hearing loss in the geriatric population. Rarely does this type of impairment occur alone based solely on the effects of age. Cumulative effects of such factors as excessive noise exposure, ototoxic drugs, infectious diseases, head trauma, and genetic predisposition must also be considered. When superimposed upon a presbycusic hearing loss, these factors account for the wide variety of audiometric configurations and degrees of severity demonstrated by the aging population.

Phonemic Regression. In some older individuals, presbycusis is characterized by a more severe speech-recognition problem than would be expected on the basis of the pure tone threshold configuration. This phenomenon, referred to as *phonemic regression* (Gaeth, 1948), causes perceptual confusions and distortions of the phonetic elements of speech and may not be overcome by amplification alone. Increasing the intensity of speech is not always helpful, because phonemic regression is generally attributed to a central auditory-processing disorder (CAPD). Gaeth concluded that there is a central auditory origin for phonemic regression when he found little relationship between this condition and age, duration of loss, educational or socioeconomic background, intelligence, or reaction time scores. More recently Jerger, et al., (1990) found that when CAPD could be identified with various tests, these subjects would perceive a greater hearing problem than those without CAPD. When sensorineural pure-tone configurations of equal severity are compared for young and old persons, aging adults generally demonstrate greater difficulty with speech-perception ability than their younger counterparts. However, this difference will not be evident with tests in quiet, only with tests under degraded conditions.

IDENTIFICATION/REHABILITATION ASSESSMENT FOR ELDERLY ADULTS

A continuing need exists for auditory assessment protocols that present a meaningful profile of the older adult with hearing impairment. Loss of hearing sensitivity is only one aspect of a complex set of interacting variables that cumulatively reflect the hearing problems. Because of the increased physical and mental limitations of older adults, the assessment process should focus widely and the four assessment aspects in the model used throughout this book are appropriate with the elderly as with other age groups.

1.   *Communication assessment* should focus on breakdowns the individual is experiencing, thus aiming more realistically at understanding the effects of hearing loss and ultimately arriving at an effective management plan. Measuring these different dimensions of communication and hearing loss can be a formidable undertaking. The heterogeneity of the population defies any semblance of use of standardized testing procedures used with infants, for example. Nonetheless, there is an emerging consensus on many issues which can help guide this process. Included in the assessment should be a combination of conventional audiologic test data with interview and self-assessment responses that are sensitive to communication skills (Weinstein, 1994). Self report may also be helpful in the other areas of assessment.

2.   *Associated variables* include concerns about social, psychological and financial issues. Vocational retirement may lead to a new lifestyle and limited finances, and older people may find themselves socially isolated and restricted to the confines of their homes. The necessary encouragement often provided by family and friends may be restricted or nonexistent. Unlike their affluent peers, the aged poor have fewer options available to them in seeking audiologic rehabilitative assistance. Many cannot afford the necessary medical and clinical services, the purchase of hearing aids, or special amplification devices. Transportation costs can

also be prohibitive, and travel to rehabilitative centers for hearing-aid orientation classes, adjustments, or repairs may be beyond the financial reach of much of this population.

3. *Related conditions* that interact with hearing loss include, among others, health status, activity level, and manual dexterity. Changes in health status have perhaps the most significant effect on an individual's ability to participate actively in remediation. Difficulties with motor coordination, vision, memory, or general health may prohibit an aging person from initiating or sustaining interest in the intervention process. The senior citizen may not be enthusiastic about involvement in audiologic rehabilitation when other disabilities, unrelated to the hearing loss, are life-threatening and cause greater concern. These disabilities are generally more severe among residents in extended health care facilities but can be managed. In a report on 62 nursing home residents who wore amplification, Smith and Fay (1977) concluded that almost 30% required daily assistance from staff due to severe health limitations.

4. *Attitude* is a significant factor. In itself, growing older is not an obstacle to successful participation in an audiologic rehabilitative program. Nor are financial, health, or other limitations always the basis for reluctance to participate. In an investigation of 152 nursing home residents who were both physically and mentally capable of participating in a recommended rehabilitation program, 35% refused all assistance (Alpiner, 1973). Other reports have reinforced this common finding of reluctance to follow recommendations for amplification assistance (Schow, 1982; Weinstein, 1994). Therefore, regardless of associated variables and related conditions, attitude is of crucial importance. Without an optimistic outlook towards the future, the older person's motivation can rapidly decline.

Senior citizens who are in good physical and mental health, financially secure, and socially active often have the free time and desire to get involved in programs that will improve their communicative skills. Similarly, many older persons view a hearing loss as a minor inconvenience, and actively seek assistance so as not to allow the impairment to interfere with their lifestyles. But a number of older people do not want to be a bother to relatives and friends, and some believe that nothing can be done to help them. Some feel that a rehabilitation specialist's time is better spent with younger people, who have more productive years ahead of them to contribute to society. A number of aging individuals refuse rehabilitation because they are reluctant to admit either the presence of a hearing loss or its severity.

The older person with a hearing deficit must come to believe in the importance of utilizing maximum auditory function. This can only be achieved through an environment in which communicative ability is considered essential and rewarding. Thus, a society that values good auditory skills is more likely to encourage its members with hearing impairment to seek rehabilitative treatment. If family, friends, and those who care for the aged demonstrate acceptance of amplification and express positive feelings towards rehabilitation, the older person may learn to accept the same attitudes and come to value the same goals.

Audiologic Testing of Older Persons

Changes in a number of conventional audiologic procedures may be necessary in the assessment of biologically older persons. These include longer-duration tonal presentations, increased delay between tone and word presentations, use of live-voice rather than recorded word lists, greater attention to client fatigue through use of speech-recognition half lists and abbreviated test sessions, employment of assessment items with increased content redundancy, such as sentence tests, and an increased schedule of social reinforcement for responding. Modifications of test stimuli and response modes are particularly critical for the multiply handicapped, such as those with receptive and expressive language problems due to cerebral vascular accidents, Alzheimer's disease, and other chronic brain syndromes, those who have had laryngectomies, and individuals afflicted with psychoses or depression. Even apparently healthy older persons may evidence memory-retrieval difficulties when the quality of the message is degraded (Simon & Pouraghabagher, 1978).

Some older persons require allowances for increased response time during both pure-tone and speech audiometry. In some cases, re-instruction is necessary because of delayed responding, perseverative responses, and even memory-recall failure during the presentation of longer stimuli, such as sentences. Biologically younger aging persons who are in good physical condition may reveal none of these difficulties, in spite of subtle signs of neural depopulation during sensitized and degraded speech testing.

Determining performance skills for messages presented in noise seems to be a fruitful area of assessment for older persons, since one of their chief complaints regarding hearing is difficulty understanding a speaker in the presence of background noise. Propositional or meaningful noise, such as occurs in the background at a luncheon or meeting, is particularly disruptive. Differentiating between peripheral and central factors affecting speech perception would seem to be a worthwhile pursuit in diagnostic testing, since the prognosis for hearing-aid performance is considerably poorer in instances of central auditory involvement (Stach, 1990). Since presbycusis represents a combined sensorineural dysfunction, audiologic test batteries should be designed to separate peripheral and central performance. Stach, Jerger, and Fleming (1985) use Synthetic Sentence Identification (SSI) in testing for CAPD. They also propose that persons with CAPD may need to be fit with special assistive devices that control better for signal-to-noise ratio than do conventional hearing aids.

Young-old persons, those who are biologically younger than their years, seem to be well represented in the caseloads of audiology clinics; however, less mobile, biologically older individuals are measurably less conspicuous. The latter group represents one of the greatest challenges to the field of audiology, not only because of the increased incidence of hearing loss alluded to earlier, but also because they are less prone to do anything about it. They remain an invisible segment of the population unless the audiologist makes a special effort to seek them out. One method for accomplishing this is to conduct hearing screenings in nursing homes, in low-income apartment buildings, or outside the facilities for the elderly in a variety of medical settings, health fairs, or mobile testing vans (McCartney, Maurer, & Sorenson, 1974;

Schow, 1982, 1990). Various programs have been conducted for many years at Portland State University, Idaho State University, and elsewhere with grants from a number of foundations.

Hearing-threshold data, follow-up testing, audiologic rehabilitative services, and self-report measures on a large population of elderly tested at Portland State University provided information that attests to the need for involvement among audiologists and audiologic rehabilitation specialists. The following summary statements reflect data on over 13,000 older persons (65–99 years) whose hearing deficits would be considered communicatively significant within a similar sample of younger persons.

1. Most did not seek professional assistance until the hearing difficulty became moderately impairing.
2. Lack of intervention by any discipline characterized the majority of the group.
3. The most common form of intervention cited among those obtaining assistance was from hearing-aid representatives, with physicians and audiologists in second and third place, respectively.
4. The three most common reasons for not obtaining help were high cost of intervention (medical, prosthetic, etc.), lack of knowledge concerning the service available, and lack of transportation, in that order.
5. Elderly African Americans were three times less likely to seek intervention than elderly Whites with the same hearing loss.
6. The most common complaint in receptive communication was difficulty hearing in noise, the incidence of which increased with each age decade.
7. The most common method of adjustment to stress associated with hearing impairment was denial by projection (i.e., "It's not that I can't hear, it's that the speaker mumbles!").
8. Most older persons judge their own hearing ability in relation to cohorts in their chronological age group; therefore underestimating the severity of the problem (i.e., "My hearing is good . . . [for my age]").

Assessment of Primary and Secondary Effects of Loss

Traditional audiologic measures do not directly address the consequences of hearing loss in daily living activities. An increasing number of assessment instruments have been reported which evaluate attitudes and feelings associated with hearing impairment. However, only a few are specifically in tune with the problems experienced by the aging population.

Widely used self-report measures used for the elderly include the Hearing Handicap Inventory for the Elderly (HHIE) (Ventry & Weinstein, 1982), the Hearing Handicap Scale (HHS), the Denver Scale of Communication Function (DSCF and also the quantified version), and the Self/Significant Other Assessment of Communication (SAC, SOAC). The use of these questionnaires has increased of late (Schow, et al., 1993) and they are recommended for screening or a test battery approach on the elderly (ASHA, 1992; Schow, 1991; Weinstein, 1994). Chapter 9 contains additional information on self report and specific information on HHS, DSCF, and SAC/SOAC. That chapter also contains information on two longer inventories which in most cases will be too lengthy for use with the elderly. However, these longer inventories may in some cases provide useful tools for evaluating various personal adjustment issues such as response to auditory failure, self acceptance, anger, stress, etc. The HHIE (see Appendix 10A), as originally proposed, has 25 items and two subscales, one consisting of social-situational items, while the other items measure emotional responses. It is a reasonable length for the elderly, but was subsequently shortened to a 10-item version, making it more comparable with the 10-item SAC. The SAC has the advantage that it may be used in programs serving both elderly and younger individuals. Both the HHIE and the SAC have been widely employed in screening programs, and psychometric information on them is summarized in recent reports (ASHA, 1992; Weinstein, 1994).

The questionnaires listed above are being used to identify problems related to hearing deficiency and measure changes following intervention. While these instruments have received most use so far, new measuring devices are emerging that will be used in the future (see Chapter 9).

Additional measures specifically designed for nursing home residents are available, such as the Nursing Home Hearing Handicap Index (NHHI) (Schow & Nerbonne, 1977). This assessment features brevity, relevance, and versatility in the sense that two separate test versions are provided, one that can be self-administered and one that permits response by nursing-home staff. The staff assessment thus provides a "reality check" on the older person's self-assessment. (These scales are found in Appendix 10B.) Other tools of this type may be found in McCarthy & Sapp (1994).

There are four primary reasons for using interview questionnaires and self-report measures that reflect the presbycusic with a reasonable degree of validity: (a) they provide a measure of the perceived handicap of the individual in his or her living environment while more objective test scores do not; (b) they open windows for counseling the older adult; (c) they may provide prognostic significance in the sense that particular score values may relate to the person's adaptability to overcome disability; and (d) they may document the success of the audiologic rehabilitation program as a follow-up measure.

ASPECTS OF AUDIOLOGIC MANAGEMENT

Following the rehabilitation-assessment, various forms of audiologic rehabilitation can be undertaken. The management process is presented here in four major sections:

1. *Psychosocial and counseling considerations*, which focus on attitudes among the elderly and methods of adjusting to stress related to hearing difficulties, as well as counseling strategies aimed at reducing the impairment associated with depressed hearing skills.

2. *Amplification intervention*, in which prosthetic devices are fitted and appropriate follow-up is provided.
3. *Communication rehabilitation*, which focuses on factors that contribute to total life satisfaction through social communication and self actualization.
4. *Overall coordination* of the intervention program, which involves appropriate clinical sensitivity and coordination on behalf of hearing-impaired older persons to achieve realistic objectives in audiologic rehabilitation.

As noted in Chapter 1, audiologic rehabilitation is ignored by a large number of persons who need it. Even with those who enter into the process, the simple reality is that most persons who are deaf or hard of hearing, who undergo assessment for their hearing problems, are not evaluated as thoroughly as the recommendations described earlier would prescribe. Further, many of these persons receive only a semblance of the idealized treatment that we summarize in this chapter. By far the majority who receive rehabilitation services do so in connection with obtaining a hearing aid. Therefore, the fitting of amplification and the hearing-aid counseling and orientation which follow are considered key components of audiologic rehabilitation, since only a few persons need more extensive management than this. But hearing-aid dispensing which has no goal other than a sale will be woefully inadequate.

Unfortunately, such narrow, sale-focused, hearing-aid counseling and orientation are often provided in a terribly abbreviated fashion (see the survey of rehabilitation procedures in Chapter 13). Therefore, a number of rehabilitation-oriented audiologists have been proposing methods of counseling and orientation that will be simple and accordingly used by more practitioners (Erdman, 1994; Montgomery, 1994; Radcliffe, 1994). Good amplification follow-up need not be complicated nor go on interminably. Client-centered efforts that focus on real needs and problem solving desired by the user will allow us to achieve effective rehabilitation as soon as the problems are solved.

Instructive and reassuring counseling must surround our efforts to help with amplification. Most orientation programs focus on several important components. These components are typically consistent with the PACO management model used in this text (see Chapter 1). First, they counsel the person about hearing loss and its consequences. Next, they familiarize the client with hearing aids and other assistive devices. They typically include efforts to improve communication through visual attentiveness, repair strategies, and assertiveness. And they focus on specific problems and their solution by involving key associates, family members, and other professionals. Outcome measures that look at use, benefit, and satisfaction can help us document our efforts. Indeed, as will be noted later, such measures are now available to demonstrate how the orientation described above can dramatically improve our efforts at amplifying the hearing of persons who are hearing impaired (Brooks, 1989). Such evidence is extremely important, because there are many unbelievers among those who need our services, and favorable outcome findings are increasingly needed for documentation to those who pay for services.

Psychosocial and Counseling Considerations

The varying degrees of adjustment to hearing loss within the geriatric population reflect the heterogeneity of the group. Lifestyles and subsequent need for oral communication differ widely. Some people are gregarious, socially active, and motivated to listen carefully and to draw from nonverbal cues during difficult communicative situations. In general, these are the biologically younger aging persons, whose attitudes are less resistant to change and who evidence fewer emotional and physical problems. This group is more likely to take hearing deficiencies in stride, require less rehabilitative follow-up, and compensate more successfully in a communicative sense. Others, who may exhibit the same extent of hearing deficiency, but who are not socially outgoing or adept at adjusting to new situations, may demonstrate greater handicap and poorer adjustive behaviors. They also may demonstrate more limited ability to integrate non-auditory stimuli, such as speechreading skills. These individuals tend to appear biologically older and more resigned to the aging process. Consequently, their communicative skills as well as attitudes toward intervention may be severely affected.

The aging individual with a hearing impairment often struggles through communication situations. Frequently, verbal messages are misinterpreted and inappropriate answers are given. Family and friends may attribute the older person's seeming inattentiveness and lack of appropriate social interaction to a number of causes, ranging from indifference to senility, any of which may lead to less and less social interaction between the aging individual and his support system.

When deprived of social interaction due to either a hearing loss and/or the attitudes of those around them, older persons become frustrated and reciprocate by avoiding those environments in which difficulties are encountered (i.e., family gatherings, church, movies, and other social activities previously enjoyed). Such a loss in close interpersonal communication can lead to decreased personal stimulation, resulting in depression and self-depreciation. Thus, many older persons with hearing impairment exhibit what has been described as the "geriapathy syndrome" (Maurer, 1976):

> The individual feels disengaged from group interaction and apathy ensues, the product of the fatigue which sets in from the relentless effort of straining to hear. Frustration, kindled by begging too many pardons, gives way to subterfuges that disguise misunderstandings. The head nods in agreement with a conversation only vaguely interpreted. The voice registers approval of words often void of meaning. The ear strives for some redundancy that will make the message clearer. Finally, acquiescing to fatigue and frustration, thoughts stray from the conversation to mental imageries that are unburdened by the detective hearing mechanism.

In order to deal with the stresses associated with a hearing loss, the aging individual resorts to adjustive behaviors. These behaviors fall into two general categories: (a) those that defend against the problem, and (b) those that offer stress reduction through escape from the problem. While anyone encountering stress may engage in defense and escape behaviors, it is propitious to re-examine these adjustment meth-

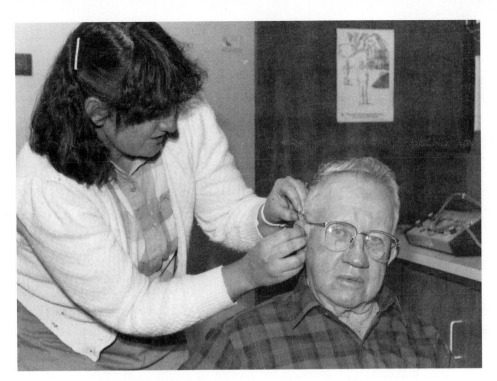

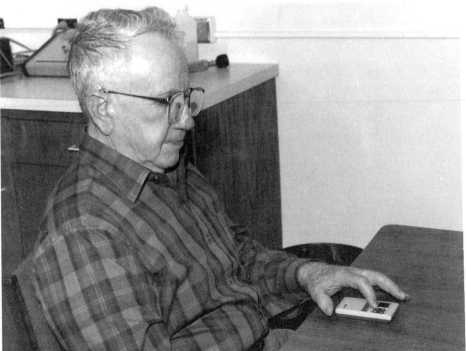

A digital programable BTE hearing aid is placed in the patients ear. The volume can be adjusted with a remote control unit.

defense and escape behaviors, it is propitious to re-examine these adjustment methods as they relate to hearing impairment and aging (Maurer & Rupp, 1979).

Defense Techniques. Elderly persons with hearing impairment resort to a variety of coping mechanisms to handle the challenges presented by their hearing loss. The techniques deemed to defend the patient against any stigma attached to the hearing impairment include attention getting, identification, compensation, rationalization, and projection.

ATTENTION GETTING. This method of adjustment is used to draw attention away from the hearing impairment by diverting concern to some other aspect of behavior or physical deficit. For example, the senior citizen who distracts the listener with a seemingly endless list of complaints, ranging from poor motor coordination to financial hardship, may be masking or devaluating the importance of the hearing impairment. The increased attention given to the older person's acting-out behaviors is reinforcing, and may sidetrack the listener's concern for the auditory problem.

IDENTIFICATION. Older individuals may reduce the stress accompanying a hearing impairment by assuming the identity or attributes of others whom they respect or admire. This defense technique is illustrated by the senior citizen who discounts the limitation of an auditory deficit by espousing the inherited keenness of her father's visual acuity.

COMPENSATION. This method of adjustment is characterized by a substitution of activities to accommodate a hearing loss. Some people compensate successfully, as with the individual who acquires speechreading skills and learns to be more attentive in difficult communicative environments. Others choose to eliminate the aversiveness of difficult-to-hear situations by giving up previously enjoyed pastimes and decreasing social interactions. For the latter group, the hearing disability is not so apparent if difficult listening situations never arise.

RATIONALIZATION. This defense mechanism relieves stress by providing invalid, but nevertheless logical and often socially acceptable reasons for auditory difficulties. For example, an older individual who is unable to hear a lecturer adequately may attribute the missed information to boredom or fatigue.

PROJECTION. Perhaps the most common method of adjustment among aging persons with presbycusic hearing losses is projection. Characteristically, the older individual transfers her auditory difficulties to the behavior of others. This is exemplified by the senior citizen who denies a hearing disability by attributing communication problems to the spouse, who supposedly does not "enunciate clearly."

Escape Techniques. As for defense mechanisms, the escape techniques some elderly individuals with hearing impairment resort to are intended to protect against or help them cope better with their hearing loss. The most common of these behaviors include insulation, negativism, regression, repression, and fantasy.

INSULATION. Stress caused by hearing impairment may be lessened by simply retreating from the problem. Usually, the older person takes no rehabilitative action, showing little concern for possible alternatives and withdrawing completely to the security of the home, where there is less demand for receptive communication.

NEGATIVISM. This method of adjustment is characterized by aggressive, antagonistic behavior. The senior citizen with hearing impairment refuses any assistance towards audiologic rehabilitation, pessimistically offering reasons why treatment is not beneficial or possible to obtain.

REGRESSION. By reverting to past, more dependent behaviors, an older person may effectively escape from the stress associated with a hearing loss. This is illustrated by the senior citizen who, when confronted with a difficult listening situation, turns to her spouse for repetition of the message. By readily assisting, the spouse, in turn, reinforces this dependency, thereby unwittingly encouraging further regressive behaviors, such as the constant need for physical assistance with the hearing aid.

REPRESSION. This escape mechanism enables the individual with hearing impairment to avoid communicative difficulties by inhibiting or forgetting them. For example, the older person who consistently forgets to wear hearing aids cannot be held accountable for misunderstood messages from family and friends, although that same individual never forgets to wear eyeglasses and earrings.

FANTASY. Escape from stress may be achieved by retreating from the adversities of reality into an imagined world where no physical deficits or social pressures exist. For the geriatric patient with hearing impairment, the continual frustration of listening to a confusing environment may lead to such inhibition, and subsequently be replaced by a more reinforcing fantasized world of daydreams.

The previously described adjustment methods are learned in childhood and utilized throughout one's lifetime to deal with the normal stresses of living. However, for the older individual these tension-reducing mechanisms may interfere with effective rehabilitative treatment if the stress-producing stimuli associated with the hearing loss are not recognized and dealt with during intervention.

Amplification

While presbycusis currently is not a medically treatable disorder, the alternative choice—wearable amplification—is not highly regarded among many older persons. The present generation of aging individuals is not far removed from the earlier stigmata of highly visible and clumsy hearing aid devices, unkind associations between deafness and dumbness, and uncharitable jokes about deafness and aging. Other factors which contribute to this vein of reticence include the initial high cost of hearing aids, continued lack of knowledge about the service-delivery system, and frequent lack of transportation to and from clinics and hearing-aid dealerships.

Results of a questionnaire interview survey conducted among a random sample of 153 elderly individuals with hearing impairment who had not purchased hearing aids tend to support this contention. Responding to the question, "What prevents older persons with hearing difficulties from getting help?", 47% of the respondents cited the high cost of appliances as the prime reason, 15% indicated lack of knowledge concerning where to go for assistance and what services were available, 11% attributed lack of transportation as the main problem, while 7% cited pride and vanity as the primary reasons for not seeking help. The remaining 20% described a variety of other problems, including fear of doctors and hearing-aid dealers, lack of awareness of a hearing difficulty, projected determination to "get by" without assistance despite the handicap, and unfavorable reports about hearing aids from relatives and friends (Lundberg, 1979). Older persons tend to tolerate greater hearing impairment than younger persons before seeking audiologic assistance for their problems (Haggard, 1980).

Hearing-Aid Evaluation and Adjustment. Although amplification is worn by individuals of all ages, most people who wear aids are beyond the sixth decade of life. A survey of 15,508 households in the United States revealed that 75% of the hearing-aid wearers were between 60 and 100 years of age, compared with only 25% for persons under age 60 (Broenen, 1983).

Acknowledging the need for amplification represents considerably more than admitting to a sensory deficit within this age group. It represents an acquiescence to the reality of aging, an acknowledgment that another bodily system is failing. As one woman emphatically stated during a hearing-aid counseling session, "Well, I suppose this thing will go along with my dentures, glasses, and support brace. It's getting so it takes me half the morning to make myself *whole!*"

Nonetheless, most older persons can benefit from appropriately tested and fitted hearing aids, and the attitudes concerning amplification are gradually changing. In countries where hearing aids are provided at little or no cost by government programs, such as Denmark and the United Kingdom, evidence suggests that older persons with amplification can achieve life satisfaction benefits near equal to those of younger individuals wearing amplification (Birk-Nielsen, 1974; Brooks, 1989). Contributing to a more positive acceptance of hearing aids are increased miniaturization and versatility of the devices, increased sophistication in hearing-aid selection and fitting techniques including programmable technology, better consumer protection through FDA regulations, and increased professional awareness of the need for adequate rehabilitative follow-up among the aging. Nevertheless, hearing-aid users still express serious concerns, which can be instructive in helping avoid certain pitfalls. Smedley and Schow (1990) summarized a large number of these complaints based on their survey of 490 elderly users. The main groups of complaints fell into four categories: (1) the negative effects of background noise (28%), (2) fitting, comfort and mechanical problems (25%), (3) concerns that the aid provides too little bene-fit (18%), and (4) feelings that the cost of aids, batteries, and repairs is excessive (17%).

Some hearing-aid companies have conceded to the physical limitations of older persons by offering oversize or touch-type volume controls, fool-proof battery com-partments, and fingernail slots for easier removal of in-the-ear hearing aids. Earmold companies now offer "geriatric handles" on their devices and, as seen in Figure 10.2 below, certain manufacturers provide handles on hearing aids. A few hearing-aid man-ufacturers have grown concerned about the special needs of elderly persons in nurs-ing homes and convalescent hospitals, persons whose visual, tactile, neuromuscular, and memory difficulties contraindicate conventional forms of amplification. Therefore, Frye Electronics, for example, designed an inexpensive rechargeable body-type aid that features a large red volume control and accommodates a variety of hear-ing-loss candidates. While the cosmetic-conscious older person may reject the con-cept of a body-worn aid, Smith and Fay (1977) found in a long-term care facility in New York that body aids were more successfully accepted by the elderly than other forms of amplification. Out of 49 satisfied hearing aid users, 35 wore body systems while 14 used ear-level and eyeglass instruments. This finding is consistent with our experience among residents of a convalescent hospital for the aging. The popular aversion to body-aid "visibility" may be a blessing in disguise for nursing-home resi-dents with poor management skills and visual limitations.

Biologically younger old persons generally accept amplification with fewer mis-givings and adjustment problems. Those with physical limitations require substan-tially more assistance. In particular, the success of hearing aids depends to a great extent upon the individual's neurological state and his ability to physically manage the prosthesis. Those with central auditory-processing problems, such as post-stroke victims, often are not good candidates for hearing aids. In some instances,

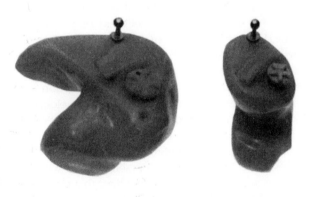

Figure 10.2 In-the-ear (ITE) and canal hearing aids with handles.
Courtesy of Starkey Northwest.

amplification of the speech message may further degrade the older person's ability to process the signal (Jerger & Jerger, 1971). This suprathreshold message distortion may not be apparent from the results of a conventional hearing test, but may be revealed during a comprehensive audiologic assessment. Nonetheless, Kricos, Lesner, Sandridge, and Yanke (1987) endorsed the need to counsel patients with central auditory processing deficits (CAPD) about the benefits and limitations of amplification. Hearing aids may not produce significantly improved speech recognition scores, but may allow centrally impaired persons to maintain what these investigators describe as "more natural auditory contact with the world" (p. 341). Furthermore, Stach (1990) has shown that assistive listening devices (ALDs) may provide some help for these CAPD cases. Certainly, the recommendation for amplification should not be ignored or contraindicated because of neurological impairment without a quantitative assessment of potential benefits during a reasonable trial period with different devices.

A number of modifications in conventional hearing-aid evaluation techniques may be necessary for biologically older persons. First, early fatigue, lengthened reaction time, and a lower frustration threshold may mandate shorter sessions and the need for return visits to complete the evaluation. Although this recourse is often not desirable because of transportation problems, it may be necessary in view of other factors, including variability in performance scores, necessity for additional assessment, and perhaps most crucial, the need for concurrent counseling. Second, conventional word lists, sound-field procedures, real-ear measures, and programmable adjustments may need to be altered or abbreviated due to the older patient's diminishing alertness and fatiguability. Also, during the hearing-aid evaluation, for example, tests for sentence comprehension in cafeteria or propositional noise (intelligible background conversation) may provide a more valid indication of amplification success than monosyllabic word lists. Matthies, Bilger, and Roezckonski (1983) found that the age-related decrement in speech intelligibility in noise tended to disappear over a 90-day period as their subjects gained experience wearing amplification in noise. Third, the number of hearing-aid choices may be restricted by the individual's lack of management skills, or by firmly entrenched attitudes as to what type of instrument will and will not be tolerated. Fourth, the biologically aging segment of the population requires more extensive rehabilitative follow-up, including counseling, supervised orientation, and hearing-aid earmold modifications.

The hearing-aid evaluation process among the elderly may encompass the entire 30- to 60-day trial period offered by the dispenser, often taxing the patience of those whose primary interest is sale closure. However, the clinical audiologist must remain steadfast in terms of ethical responsibilities toward even the slowest clients.

The question of whether aging persons should wear one hearing aid or binaural amplification is an individual one, depending to a great extent upon prosthesis management and financial capabilities that must be weighed against perceived gains in social-receptive skills. An added variable is the attitudinal difference between wearing one instrument, as opposed to two. Thus, it is not uncommon to hear an elderly person comment, "I don't need two of these, do I? I'm not deaf!" Apparently, if one hearing aid represents a milestone in acquiescence to sensorineural aging, two become a millstone! However, life satisfaction is greater for those who can adjust to appropriately fitted binaural amplification. Birk-Nielsen (1974) noted in comparing monaural versus binaural amplification that two aids reduced the amount of social-hearing handicap among older persons. This two-ear advantage includes better speech perception in noise, reduced localized autophony (voice resonance), improved spatial balance and localization, and improved sound quality. Among those who have physical, financial, or cosmetic limitations, or whose quiescent lifestyles fail to support the need for two instruments, the choice of which ear to fit becomes an issue. Considerations that enter into this decision among geriatrics include: (a) earedness for social communication gain in quiet and in noise, (b) severity of arthritic or other physical involvements in the arms and hands as related to prosthesis manipulation, (c) handedness, (d) accustomed ear for telephone use, and (e) lifestyle factors affecting sidedness, such as driving a car or location of bed in a convalescent home. A more exhaustive treatise on the topic of hearing-aid selection is contained in Chapter 2.

Detailed discussions on fitting strategies and the use of audiologic and self report to measure benefit may be found in material prepared by Gatehouse (1994) and Seewald (1994). Both authors provide a glimpse of how methods for hearing-aid fitting may be improved for the elderly in the future, and they also emphasize a relatively recent concern in measuring hearing-aid benefit. Namely, care should be taken to assess benefit after a period of acclimatization following 6–12 weeks of exposure to amplification. Prior to that time, overall improvements are subject to additional change and thus are suspect.

Several methods are available for measuring the perceived benefit of amplification and, indeed, self report has been shown to be useful in dealing with acclimatization issues. The Hearing Handicap Scale, the Hearing Handicap Inventory for the Elderly, and other self-report inventories as discussed in Chapter 9 have been shown to be of value in measuring hearing-aid benefit (Taylor, 1993). Smedley and Schow (1992) used benefit, use, and satisfaction measures including SAC/SOAC and a simple seven-point scale and showed how these may help provide feedback from users of new devices, such as the newer programmable hearing aids. While only a few such questionnaires have received extensive psychometric scrutiny, it is possible to use data from a variety of measures to chart and document change. Brooks, for example, has provided a series of useful reports detailing his efforts to improve hearing-aid services. In one of his reports, Brooks (1989) employed a relatively simple self-report tool of 39 items, The Hearing Assessment Questionnaire, which he used in his own clinic on 758 patients seen over one year's time. Using this on newly fitted patients (along with measurements of hearing-aid use time), he provided one of the most dramatic data sets showing the importance of extensive counseling and hearing-aid orientation that has ever appeared in the professional literature. Brooks's work carefully controlled for age and hearing loss of the clients, as seen in Figure 10.3, and it may be noted that hearing-aid use time for those who are extensively counseled improved dramatically (in some cases by a factor of two).

Counseling the New User. The first two weeks of hearing-aid use are critical. The audiologist should be ready for any problem that might occur between the client, the

(a) Distribution of 758 subjects fitted with NHS BTE hearing aids according to age and hearing loss, and whether (EC) or not (NEC) extra counseling was provided.

| | | Age (Years) | | | | | | | |
| | | ≤60 | | 61–70 | | 71–80 | | ≥81 | |
		EC	NEC	EC	NEC	EC	NEC	EC	NEC
Hearing Loss (dB)	≤40	39	68	53	60	43	57	7	11
	41–50	19	16	23	30	34	49	28	32
	51–60	9	8	7	11	19	25	27	22
	61–70	2	4	2	6	7	11	10	19

(b) Average daily use time for patients having NHS aids supplied without extra counseling, as a function of degree of hearing loss and age when fitted.

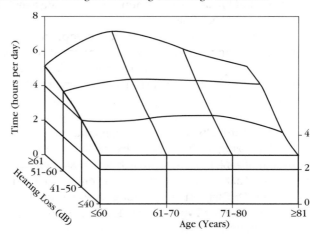

(c) Average daily use time for patients having NHS aids supplied with extra counseling, as a function of degree of hearing loss and age when fitted.

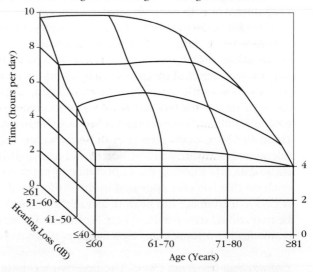

Figure 10.3 Data from Brooks (1989) based on United Kingdom National Health Service (NHS) provision of hearing aids.

amplification system, and the environment. Counseling, either face to face or by telephone, is a continuing commitment that is based on the individual's adjustment needs. As pointed out earlier, the reasons for rejection of amplification devices are infinite, ranging from simple management difficulties to complex attitude adjustment problems. The clinician must allow these reasons to surface early in the trial period before rejection becomes ingrained. Another concept to be aware of during counseling is that rejection usually works in tandem with other age-related deficits. For example, rejection and reduced short-term memory may combine to become counterproductive, as summed up in the statement of an 89-year–old woman who, during a moment of exasperation, announced, "I can never remember which way the battery goes in, and I hear better without this thing, anyway!" Needless to say, she had the battery inserted backwards.

Attention given to the primary complaints of the client, family members, and friends during the pre-intervention phase should be re-addressed during the hearing-aid trial period. Information from a case history illustrates the utility of this concept. The pre-intervention counseling session included the following list of complaints:

1. Difficulty understanding in church.
2. Daughter tired of repeating.
3. Inability to hear whispers, soft sounds.
4. Inability to hear driver on Senior Adult Center bus outings.
5. Difficulty understanding in dining room.
6. Turning TV set up too loud (daughter's complaint).

Consequently, audiologic surveillance during the first two weeks was aimed not only at prosthesis management, but at the environments where difficulties were noted. The above checklist of complaints became an immediate target for intervention. Each problem was investigated and appropriate measures were taken to reduce or eliminate it. For example, once the client was taught to compensate for listening difficulties encountered in church sanctuary, the recommended amplification device became an integral aspect of improved listening. Considered separately from the environment, the hearing aid would have been doomed to failure. Similarly, the over-loud TV volume control was corrected by allowing the daughter to adjust the loudness to a "comfortable" level while the client was seated in her customary chair with her aids turned to half gain. This listening level was subsequently marked on the TV volume control with an easily visible fingernail polish.

Individual Hearing-Aid Orientation. The majority of hearing-aid users receive help with individual rather than a group orientation structure (Schow, et al., 1993). While group sessions have certain advantages which will be discussed later, many are not sufficiently mobile to meet regularly in the group environment. Whenever possible, it is important to have a significant other person in attendance during individual therapy, to facilitate carryover to the residential environment.

A prime example showing the need for extensive orientation is the 10 Step Earmold Insertion Program (Maurer, 1979). Earmold and ITE (in-the-ear) hearing-aid insertion is a common problem among the elderly. Lack of proper insertion may produce feedback and even physical pain. Use of this program among older persons with management problems has been highly successful, as illustrated in Figure 10.4, which also contains the learning curve of the client who prompted the program.

An 83-year–old woman was observed to have difficulty inserting her silhouette earmold, which had been provided, along with her behind-the-ear hearing aid, by a salesman over a year earlier. A peer brought her into the audiology clinic because the woman had discontinued wearing her aid, and the two friends were having problems communicating. An observation of her repeated attempts at inserting the mold in her ear revealed: (a) she was capable of placing the aid appropriately on her ear, (b) having placed the aid, she engaged in trial-and-error attempts at locating the mold and grasping it "where the salesman showed me," (c) her arthritic fingers invariably grasped the mold or tubing improperly or her hand turned so that the mold was at an impractical angle for proper insertion, and (d) her baseline for correct earmold placement in five trials was zero.

The woman acknowledged that she had received a 10-minute instruction following the sale of her aid. However, she had not received additional audiologic rehabilitation. Consequently, her various manipulative behaviors, such as placing the aid on the table, opening the battery compartment, picking up the appliance, putting the mold in her ear, and so on, occurred in no methodical order. Analysis of the hearing aid showed that it was functioning properly and was reasonably appropriate for the client's needs.

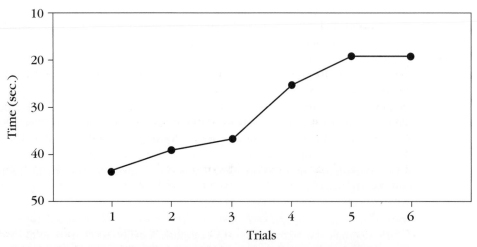

Figure 10.4 Time (seconds) required to achieve criterion over successive trials involving removal of amplification.

From "Aural Rehabilitation for the Aging." [p. 329] by J.F. Maurer. In *Hearing and Hearing Impairment* by L.J. Bradford and W.G. Hardy [Eds], 1979, New York: Grune & Stratton.

A 10-step management program was designed around a time base. The terminal objective was to chain manipulative behaviors to respective stimuli in a serial order so that the complex act of establishing proper use of the prosthesis could be broken into discrete responses. It seemed more effective to work backwards from the point where the aid was operating in the ear (reverse chaining), since previous trials involving getting the mold in the ear had failed. In addition, the probability of error was reduced, with the ear as a starting point; besides, the reinforcement of amplified sound was at a higher rate early in the program when encouragement was most needed. With the exception of the first, each succeeding step was repeated until the behavior was deliberate and proficient. This was accomplished within five trials per step. Since Step 1 provided a relative time base for estimating the terminal proficiency of the chaining program, it was timed and graphed. Social reinforcement was provided with each successful manipulation. It is also noteworthy that emphasis during the first half of the program was primarily tactile, in the sense that stress was placed on how the earmold "feels in the ear" when it is properly seated, how it "feels to the fingers" when it is properly seated, and how it "feels to the fingers" when it is grasped properly. During the second half of the program, visual contact with the prosthesis was emphasized to reinforce the appropriate grasp of the mold and the precision of the chaining process.

Step 1:
Gain turned down—earmold and aid removed—prosthesis placed in box—battery compartment opened.
Step 2:
Gain turned down—earmold loosened by grasp on heel near tubing insert—earmold reinserted—gain turned up.
Step 3:
Gain turned down—earmold partially removed (1/4 inch)—earmold reinserted—gain turned up.
Step 4:
Gain turned down—earmold completely removed from canal (1 inch)—earmold reinserted—gain turned up.
Step 5:
Gain turned down—earmold completely removed—fingers release contact—fingers reestablish contact—earmold reinserted—gain turned up.
Step 6:
Gain turned down—earmold completely removed—hand to lap—hand to aid and fingers reestablish contact with mold—earmold reinserted—gain turned up.
Step 7:
Gain turned down—earmold completely removed—aid removed—visual inspection of finger placement on mold—earmold reinserted—aid replaced—gain turned up.
Step 8:
Gain turned down—earmold completely removed—aid removed—prosthe-

sis placed in box—hand to lap—hand to aid and fingers reestablish contact with mold—earmold reinserted—aid replaced—gain turned up.

Step 9:

Gain turned down—earmold completely removed—aid removed—prosthesis placed in box—battery compartment opened—hand to lap—battery compartment closed—fingers reestablish contact with mold—earmold reinserted—aid replaced—gain turned up.

Step 10:

Gain turned down—earmold completely removed—aid removed—prosthesis placed in box—battery compartment opened—box and prosthesis taken to another room by examiner—patient taken to the other room—battery compartment closed—fingers reestablish contact with mold—earmold reinserted—aid replaced—gain turned up.

It was deemed important to take time to encourage precise grasping of the earmold during the early stages; yet the entire program was completed in less than 30 minutes. Moreover, the length of the second cycle of Step 10, involving replacement of amplification, was found to closely approximate the amount of time required for removal of amplification in Step 1 (about 20 seconds). What appears most significant, however, is that a relatively simple application of behavioral engineering corrected a problem the client had been struggling with for months.

Hearing-Aid Orientation in Groups. Some persons may fit into a group training structure rather than, or in addition to, individual sessions. This will not be feasible for everyone, however, because all do not have attitudes that lend themselves to group interaction; they may prefer meeting times that do not coincide with the group meeting time; or they may simply prefer the individual attention created by a one-on-one situation. But when group sessions are feasible they can be very helpful. Aging individuals are generally understimulated. As noted earlier, their nucleus of cohorts is smaller than in previous years, and the opportunity to participate in a group experience is often welcomed. An important aspect of a small group is the opportunity to share information. In such meetings the audiologist takes the position of group leader and facilitates discussions by (a) bringing out those persons who are reluctant to share their experiences, (b) inhibiting those few who might dominate the group, (c) permitting the discussion topics to surface from the group rather than from the clinician, (d) acting as a resource person when expertise is needed, and, most importantly, (e) acting as a good listener. Achieving homogeneous grouping (i.e., bringing together persons who have similar perceived communication problems, as revealed in self-assessment profiles), when feasible, is desirable.

A recent survey showed the broad focus typically found in these group sessions to be mostly on the use of hearing aids, with successively lesser amounts of attention on communication strategies, auditory training, assistive listening devices (ALDs), and speechreading (see Chapter 13; Schow, et al., 1993). In addition to the ideas on hearing-aid orientation listed in Chapter 9, a good group meeting is one that: (a) is primarily success- rather than problem-oriented, (b) provides an element of entertainment, (c) focuses on no more than three learning objectives, (d) incorpo-

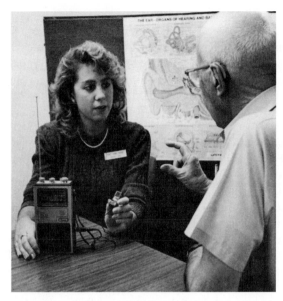

An elderly person learns about a simple assistive listening device system.

rates sharing of ideas in a counseling medium, and (e) culminates with a clear understanding of how each member can take charge of his or her newly acquired learning
through carry-over activities. The clinician may improve group cohesiveness by asking members to contact each other by telephone, the objective being for the person
called to guess who the "mystery caller" is and report on the experience at the next
group meeting.

Additional help in planning group meetings can be found in Chapter 13, which
contains a complete outline for a series of group meetings as prepared by Giolas.

The "Significant Other." The significant other person should understand the prosthetic device, its main components, and the conditions under which it should be
worn; should possess basic trouble-shooting information, and warranty and repair
information; and should be proficient at inserting, removing, and using the instrument. It is helpful to provide a written description of this information, as well as a list
of special resources appropriate to the aging client. This would include the audiologist's phone number, the location and telephone number of a drug store providing
low-cost batteries, special alerting, wake-up, and communication devices available,
information on captioned films for television, if appropriate, and a time schedule for
hearing-aid checks, audiologic rehabilitation meetings, and annual audiologic assessment (see details on the above items in Chapter 2).

Advocacy in Restrictive Environments. The best method for encouraging audiologic rehabilitative assistance from the administration and staff of convalescent hospitals, nursing homes, high-rise facilities for the aging, and senior adult centers is to

offer them something in return. The hearing problems of their clientele rank low when compared to the sleeping, eating, cleaning, entertainment, and other health needs within the facility. Sometimes it is difficult to gain entry into a restrictive environment on the basis of one client who has a hearing impairment and needs carry-over assistance. A workable strategy for overcoming staff resistance is to seek out the activities director and explain that you are working with the client and his/her family. Offer to provide a slide session on hearing and aging as a staff inservice activity aimed at helping the staff understand and manage all clientele with hearing difficulties. Leaving the activities director with this public-service gesture and a copy of your professional credentials removes much of the suspicion associated with the doorstep intervention tactics of some commercial vendors.

A stimulating, solution-oriented talk nearly always produces advocates among residents and staff members—individuals who later may become allies in the rehabilitation plan. A nucleus is formed, and interest is maintained through a recognized need for further education as well as an open communication line to the audiologist's office. Elsewhere we have reported a variety of experiences in providing hearing services for nursing homes (Schow, 1992). In a number of such homes where hearing was tested we found that only 11% of potential hearing-aid candidates were using amplification; another 20% of these responded that they had hearing aids, but were not using them. Therefore, the need for rehabilitation is apparent and residents will be at a disadvantage if it is not provided. A multi-step program is proposed as an effective plan for ensuring that hearing services are available for the hearing impaired in these facilities. This program includes the following:

1. Screening of hearing, as required by federal law, with pure tones, visual inspection, and self- and staff members' assessment of hearing (Nursing Home Hearing Handicap Index).
2. Thorough diagnostic testing for those who fail screening, along with charting of results and informing staff.
3. Selection of amplification candidates, trials with hearing aids or assistive devices, and thorough amplification orientation for those who become permanent users.
4. Inservice to staff, including instruction on the auditory mechanism, the causes and effects of hearing loss in the elderly, the role of the audiologist and facility staff in hearing health care and amplification devices, and encouragement of a communication environment that facilitates interpersonal relationships among residents and staff. (See Maurer & Rupp, [1979] 159–160, and Weinstein [1984b] 267, for specific strategies.)
5. Continued monitoring of and help for all amplification users and affiliated professionals.

Hurvitz, et al. (1987) demonstrated an effective self-paced computer AR program designed to provide communication training to a nursing home population. Their software program covers content related to (a) mechanisms of the ear, (b) audiograms, (c) management of the hearing problem, (d) speechreading, (e) hearing aids, and (f) communication skills training. Short informational paragraphs are presented followed by multiple-choice questions in a user-friendly format. Patients trained with this program showed more knowledge gains than in a conventional group classroom approach. Punch and Weinstein (1994) also recently produced computer-assisted instructional material for assisting clients with hearing problems.

Assistive Listening Devices (ALDs). A seemingly endless number of products and devices are now available for assisting older persons with hearing impairment in a variety of environments. The hearing aid may be looked on as a general purpose device, while ALDs serve a variety of special listening needs, such as telephone listening, TV listening, listening in a large meeting room where one is some distance from the speaker, etc. A number of other listening and speaking devices are available, ranging from simple hardwire amplification systems for use in automobiles to infrared and FM systems for use in nursing homes, churches, and auditoriums (see Chapter 2 for a complete listing of devices).

Communication Rehabilitation

Auditory-visual communication training which emphasizes speechreading and auditory training has been described in Chapter 9 and is appropriate for certain elderly clients. Individual speechreading instruction was deemed appropriate for a 62-year-old woman who had suffered loss of hearing in one ear due to Meniere's disease. Socially active in the community and reluctant to disclose her impairment to others, the woman preferred the privacy of individual therapy. She was an avid bridge player; one activity that satisfied the five ingredients of a good group meeting described earlier consisted of "playing" bridge through a two-way mirror with only visual cues for statements such as "I bid three spades," "I pass," and so forth. The woman improved her ability to speechread the language of her favorite game. This proved fortuitous, since the signs of Meniere's syndrome (roaring tinnitus, vertigo, and nausea) signaled the eventual loss of hearing in her good ear.

Perhaps a greater area of need than speechreading is with respect to general communication training as has been promoted recently by Erber (1987, 1994) and is explained in Chapter 3 of this text. In order for audiologic rehabilitation to be successful for the older person, positive changes must be brought about in the entire social-communicative milieu. The audiologist-counselor, acting in the multiple roles of diagnostician, hearing-aid specialist, audiologic rehabilitation specialist, and gerontologist, becomes an integral part of this milieu.

Problems of audition, including loss of hearing sensitivity, slowing of neural processing of messages, increased difficulty understanding in noise, and deficits in short-term auditory memory storage, interact significantly in the communication process. A peripheral high-frequency hearing loss alters the code of the message received, thereby affecting the content and even influencing the outgoing response:

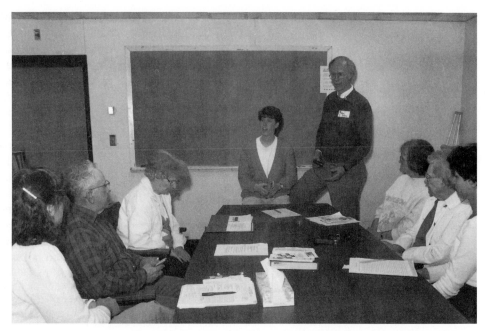

When group sessions are held it is important to provide temporary amplification assistance with ALD's for those participants not yet using hearing aids.

> Mr. Jacobson was helping his grandson paint the family shed. "Gramps," the younger person said, "let's quit for awhile and go get some thinner."
>
> The older man stared in amazement at his grandson. "Go get some dinner? Son, we just had lunch!"

Further, the message-delivery speed of the nightly television newscaster may alter the message code and content for older persons who simply cannot "keep up." As a result, maintaining intellectual currency with events in the world may slip in priority, affecting both general knowledge and the content of conversations with others. Increasing failure to inhibit background conversations and noises while attending to primary messages degrades the code and content to such an extent for some of the elderly that they retreat from these environments. The feedback of earlier communication may be tested severely by lapses in recent memory, not only altering the older person's trust in reality but even leading to a denial of it.

> Mrs. Andrews' chief complaint about her new hearing aid was lack of battery life.
>
> "Are you opening the battery case at night when you're not using the instrument?" the audiologist inquired.
>
> "Heavens no. You didn't tell me to do that!"
>
> "Yes, she did, mother," the daughter chimed in. "Don't you remember? It's even stated in that booklet in your purse."
>
> "Well, this is the first time I've *heard* about it," the older woman retorted.

The critical implication of an auditory impairment on an aging individual is that it affects the lenses through which the client views reality. Thus, when the code and content of messages are altered, feedback is affected so that the client comes to distrust what others say as well as her own interpretation of communicative events. Even continuing accumulation and expression of knowledge may stagnate, as reality is restructured to avoid or escape from the stresses associated with growing older with a hearing impairment. This is reflected in such common disengagement statements as, "I don't go to church anymore," "I've given up on the Senior Adult Center," and ultimately, "Why should I go to lipreading classes and buy a hearing aid that lasts five years? I won't be around that long, anyway."

A prime example of these forces at work in the expressive communication skills of the older person is the case of the person who has undergone laryngectomy. Most individuals who have had total laryngectomy surgery are within the senior adult age group. Most have hearing difficulties, and since esophageal speech generally has reduced intensity and less well defined vowel formants, persons with laryngectomies are less intelligible to peers, who are also likely to be aging and hearing impaired. The esophageal speaker's increased tension and effort aimed at being understood are often undermined by an increase in noise from the tracheostoma, a surgically produced hole in the neck through which the person breathes after the larynx is removed, causing further depreciation in speech intelligibility. For too many, the frustrations arising from failure to communicate lead to extinction of esophageal speech and withdrawal from social situations.

The counselor-audiologist is positioned between the aging client and reality, since the counselor's own communication skills and knowledge are called into play to assist the older person in restructuring the client's lifestyle to ameliorate or compensate for the hearing impairment. Effective communication can still occur, however, when the counselor empathizes or shares common experiences with the aging client.

Sensitivity achieved through listening will have great effect on the outcome of the rehabilitation program. Slower in adapting to change and more fixed in their attitudes than younger persons with hearing impairment, elderly patients demand more professional time for their feelings to surface. In some instances, the audiologist can bring about positive changes by simply permitting the client to register complaints and thereby achieve a more favorable polarity in making decisions:

> "My voice is so different with these aids on," Mrs. Gregory said, shaking her head. "I don't think I can get used to them."
> "Uh-huh."
> "Do I sound like this to others? My voice sounds so gravelly."
> "Hmm."
> "I wonder if I've been talking too loud to people . . . before I got these, I mean." Her eyes brightened. "Well, I certainly keep my voice down now."
> "Uh-huh."
> "I can hear a whisper now . . . in a quiet room. But . . . Oh, the racket when I'm doing dishes! I took them off and put them on the window sill."
> "Uh-huh."

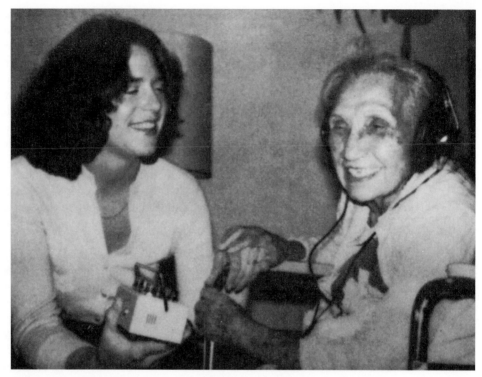

Devices like a hardware auditory trainer can facilitate communication.

"I could hear the clerk in the checkout line yesterday. Heard everything he said . . ."
"Hmm."
"I suppose it's a matter of . . . getting used to them." She nodded her head. "They help . . . they really do."

In other instances, listening to the aging client permits the audiologist to orchestrate necessary changes in lifestyle, thus maintaining the delicate balance between hearing for pleasure and adjusting to the perceived nuisances of a new prosthesis. For some individuals, communicative rehabilitation must concentrate on facilitating non-auditory channels:

Mr. Stanley, a 77-year-old former steamfitter, had suffered a stroke which compounded the communication problems already associated with a severe high-frequency hearing loss. Amplification failed to improve his degraded speech-recognition skills. Individual speechreading training also failed to demonstrate any change in his ability to communicate visually. However, placement in a small-group speechreading program that also emphasized group counseling produced a number of positive changes which cumulatively increased his life satisfaction. His self-tolerance and sense of humor returned as he listened to others openly discuss communicative "failures" with which he could identify. The frequency of his face-watching behavior increased, and despite the lack of progress noted in formal speechreading tests, there was a demonstrable improvement in his social-communicative skills. Moreover, his wife reported that a telephone amplifier had been installed in the home at his request and that her husband was starting to watch television again.

Listening to the elderly client can also effect changes in the audiologist's prescriptive statements:

> One assertive client, returning for her first annual hearing test and hearing-aid check, advised the clinician, "You shouldn't tell people not to wear their aids when sleeping. I sleep on my left side and wear my hearing aid in my right ear so I can hear the doorbell or the telephone ringing. It makes me feel more secure."

Overall Coordination

A well-coordinated rehabilitation program for older persons requires an organized body of knowledge about the clientele. This includes clinical sensitivity toward elderly persons in general, a thorough understanding of the older person in question, and prioritization of this information into a meaningful rehabilitative plan. In too many instances, failure or rejection of hearing amplification during the intervention process is due either to lack of clinical sensitivity toward the client's needs, feelings, and priorities, or to insensitivity toward the population of aging individuals as a group. No segment of the world population of persons with hearing impairment has more living experiences and well-established attitudes than the chronologically aged. To treat longevity lightly in this highly heterogeneous group is to open the door to failure.

Intake information, gleaned through interviews or formal assessment measures, is essential. Specific areas that are particularly useful among older persons are: (a) the hearing deficiencies, including history, duration, and potential site(s) of lesion, as well as both a self-assessment of the hearing problems and assessments by significant other persons; (b) the history of previous attempts at intervention, medical or prosthetic; (c) clinician's knowledge about associated physical or mental difficulties, including arthritis, neuromuscular limitations, visual problems, tinnitus, and memory difficulties; and (d) an assessment of current life satisfaction.

Information on life satisfaction tends to surface during an informal, pre-intervention counseling session. The kinds of questions to be probed include: To what extent do physical, mental, or economic conditions make this individual dependent upon others? What is the current activity level of this person? In what ways does this individual interact with the living environment and extended surroundings? Is the older person motivated to interact more in a social communicative sense? Is life satisfaction limited to vicarious pleasures, such as watching television in solitude, or is the self-imposed isolation a likely consequence of the hearing disability?

The pervading question in this context is: Will the rehabilitation program make a significant, positive impact on the life satisfaction of this older person? A well-developed client profile substantially increases the probability of successful audiologic rehabilitation. Thus, the profile permits an educated focus on current aspects of the older person's lifestyle. It addresses and administers to client needs, rather than those of the clinic or the practitioner. It delineates whether the individual is a candidate for intervention; what particular plan should be tailored to meet the person's needs; what hypothetical objectives and terminal goals might be accomplished; what significant other persons should be involved; and where, when, and under whose auspices the program should be carried out.

Directive, informational counseling that includes "laundry lists" of questions aimed at elderly persons is not well advised. While such an approach may be useful for time-oriented attendants at a hospital nursing station, the salience of the information sampled in this manner may be lost in the undertow of real needs and feelings that surface when the clinician simply listens to the client. Most of the complaints of older persons about their hearing difficulties, for example, are situation specific: "I can't hear in church," "I can't understand the speaker when there are people talking," "I don't watch the news on television, because the announcer talks too fast." Knowledge about such concerns provides for a practical, operational baseline from which positive rehabilitative changes can be measured.

The key to whether significant other persons should be included in the plan and subsequent coordination of the rehabilitation program is the extent of their present contribution toward the elderly individual's life satisfaction. Thus, observing interactions between the older person and others reveals the kind of support they will provide and whether they will be allies during intervention. Perhaps one of the paramount questions the clinician should ask on an intuitive level is whether significant others' support is based on a valid concern for the aging individual, or whether it is irregular or counterproductive. Relatives, friends, and staff members in the geriatric environment can constitute important links in the rehabilitative chain. Others who may act in concert with the audiologist to facilitate adjustive behaviors include members of the professional community who have knowledge about the client, the family support system, and the client's lifestyle. Relevant parties may include members of the clergy, physicians, welfare workers, and leaders of organizations and clubs in which the client holds membership.

SUMMARY

The audiologic rehabilitation specialist has a unique opportunity to provide services to the geriatric population. The complexity of changes occurring in advanced age together with the difficulties encountered due to auditory deficits requires that the audiologist become resourceful and willing to modify established techniques and protocols. The audiologist can significantly contribute to a positive future for persons with impaired hearing who are elderly—one that is more productive and less isolated. Better receptive communication skills may help lessen the stress caused by other disabilities, as well as facilitate social interaction between older persons and their living environments.

The need for specialized training in gerontology among graduate students specializing in speech and hearing sciences becomes increasingly apparent as longevity increases and the population of older persons expands. The current lack of commitment to training in gerontology among graduate programs in the United States must be radically reversed if audiologists are to maintain a leadership role in the care of aging persons with hearing impairment (Nerbonne, Schow, & Hutchinson, 1980; Raiford & Shadden, 1985). Addressing the problems of presbycusis is a professional challenge we must all face together.

RECOMMENDED READINGS

Clark, J. G., & Martin, F.N. (1994). *Effective counseling in audiology: Principles and practice*. Englewood Cliffs, NJ: Prentice Hall.

Mauer, J., & Monserrat-Hopple, M. (1992). Counseling the older adult who is hearing impaired. In R. Hull (Ed.), *Aural rehabilitation* (2nd ed.). San Diego: Singular.

McCarthy, P. and Sapp, J. (1993). Rehabilitative considerations with the geriatric population. In J. Alpiner & P. McCarthy (Eds.), *Rehabilitative audiology: Children and adults* (2nd ed., pp. 331-373). Baltimore: Williams & Wilkins.

Mueller, H. G., & Geoffrey, V. C. (1987). *Communication disorders in aging: Advances in assessment and management*. Washington, DC: Gallaudet University Press.

Ripich, D. (1991). *Handbook of geriatric communication disorders*. Austin, TX: Pro-Ed.

Schow, R., Christensen, J., Hutchinson, J., & Nerbonne, M. (1978). *Communication disorders of the aged*. Baltimore: University Park Press.

Shadden, B. B. (Ed.) (1988). *Perspectives on communication behavior and aging: A source-book for clinicians*. Baltimore: Williams & Wilkins.

Smith, C., & Fay, T. (1977). A program of auditory rehabilitation for aged persons in a chronic disease hospital. *Asha*, *19*, 417-420.

REFERENCES

Alpiner, J. (1973). Aural rehabilitation and the aged client. *Audecibel*, *22*, 102-104.

ASHA-American Speech-Language-Hearing Association. (1992). Considerations in screening adults/older persons for handicapping hearing impairments. *Asha*, *34*(6), 81-87.

Atchley, R. C. (1972). *Social forces in later life*. Belmont, CA: Wadsworth Publishing Company.

Bess, F., Lichtenstein, M., Logan, S., Burger, M., & Nelson, E. (1989). Hearing impairment as a determinant of function in the elderly. *Journal of the American Geriatric Society*, *37*, 123-128.

Birk-Nielsen, H. (1974). Effect of monaural versus binaural hearing and treatment. *Scandinavian Audiology, 3,* 183–187.

Brody, H. (1973). In M. Rockstein & M. Sussman (Eds.), *Development and aging in the nervous system* (pp. 70, 121–133). New York: Academic Press.

Broenen, J. A. (1983). Hearing aid population profile. *Hearing Instruments, 34,* 12–18.

Brooks, D. N. (1989). The effect of attitude on benefit obtained from hearing aids. *British Journal of Audiology, 23,* 3–11.

Edwards, J. N., & Klemmack, D. L. (1973). Correlates of life satisfaction: A re-examination. *Journal of Gerontology, 26,* 497–502.

Erber, N. (1988). *Communication Therapy for Hearing Impaired Adults.* Abbotsford, Victoria, Australia: Clavis Press.

Erber, N., & Lind, C. (1994). Communication Therapy: Theory and practice [Monograph]. In J. P. Gagne and N. Tye-Murray (Eds). *Research in audiological rehabilitation: Current trends and future directions. Journal of the Academy of Rehabilitative Audiology.*

Erdman, S. (1994). Counseling hearing impaired adults. In J. Alpiner & P. McCarthy (Eds.), *Rehabilitative audiology: Children and adults* (2nd ed., pp. 331–373). Baltimore: Williams & Wilkins.

Gaeth, J. (1948). *A study of phonemic regression associated with hearing loss.* Unpublished doctoral dissertation, Northwestern University.

Gatehouse, S. (1994). Components and determinants of hearing aid benefit. *Ear & Hearing, 15,* 30–49.

Haggard, M. P. (1980). Six audiological paradoxes in the provision of hearing aid services. *Excerpta Medica,* 1–14.

Hunter, W. F. (1960). The psychologist works with the aged individual. *Journal of Counseling Psychology, 7,* 120–126.

Hurvitz, J., Goldojorb, M., Walcek, A., & Manna-Levin, K. (November, 1987). *Comparison of two aural rehabilitation methods in a nursing home.* Paper presented at the ASHA National Convention, New Orleans.

Jerger, J., & Jerger, S. (1971). Diagnostic significance of PB word functions. *Archives of Otolaryngology, 93,* 573–580.

Jerger, J., Oliver, T., & Pirozzolo, F. (1990). Speech understanding in the elderly. *Journal of the American Academy of Audiology, 1,* 75–81.

Kemper, P., & Murtaugh, C. (1991). Lifetime use of nursing home care. *New England Journal of Medicine, 324*(9), 595.

Kricos, P., Lesner, S., Sandridge, S., & Yanke, R. (1987). Perceived benefits of amplification as a function of central auditory status in the elderly. *Ear and Hearing, 8,* 337–342.

Lundberg, R. (1979). *Research survey.* Unpublished manuscript, Portland State University.

Matthies, M., Bilger, R., & Roezckowski, C. (1983). SPIN as a predictor of hearing aid use. *Asha, 25*(10), 61.

Maurer, J. F. (1976). Auditory impairment and aging. In B. Jacobs (Ed.), *Working with the impaired elderly* (p. 72). Washington, DC: National Council on the Aging.

Maurer, J. F. (1979). Aural rehabilitation for the aging. In L. J. Bradford & W. G. Hardy (Eds.), *Hearing and hearing impairment* (pp. 319-338). New York: Grune & Stratton.

Maurer, J. F. (1982). The psychosocial aspects of presbycusis. In R. Hull (Ed.), *Rehabilitative audiology* (pp. 271-281). New York: Grune & Stratton.

Maurer, J. F., & Rupp, R. R. (1979). *Hearing and aging: Tactics for intervention.* New York: Grune & Stratton.

McCarthy, P. and Sapp, J. (1993). Rehabilitative considerations with the geriatric population. In J. Alpiner & P. McCarthy (Eds.) *Rehabilitative audiology: Children and adults* (2nd ed., pp. 331-373). Baltimore: Williams & Wilkins.

McCartney, J. H., Maurer, J. F., & Sorenson, F. D. (1974). A mobile audiology service for the elderly: A preliminary report. *Journal of the Academy of Rehabilitative Audiology, 7*(2), 25-35.

Montgomery, A. A. (1994). WATCH: A practical approach to brief auditory rehabilitation. *The Hearing Journal, 47*(10), 10, 53-55.

Mulrow, C., Aquilar, C., Endicott, J., Velez, R., Tuley, M., Charlip, W., & Hill, J. (1990). Association between hearing impairment and the quality of life of elderly individuals. *Journal of the American Geriatric Society, 38,* 45-50.

Nerbonne, N. A., Schow, R. L., & Hutchinson, J. M. (1980). Gerontologic training in communication disorders. *Asha, 22,* 404-408.

Punch, J., & Weinstein, B. (November, 1994). Hearing handicap inventory for the elderly: A multimedia version. Paper presented at the ASHA National Convention, New Orleans.

Rabbitt, P. M. A. (1965). An age decrement in the ability to ignore irrelevant information. *Journal of Gerontology, 20,* 233-238.

Radcliffe, D. (1994). Beyond amplification: Aural rehabilitation for adults. *The Hearing Journal, 47*(10), 13-21.

Raiford, C., & Shadden, B. (1985). Graduate education in gerontology. *Asha, 27*(6), 37-43.

Ries, P. (1994). Prevalence and characteristics of persons with hearing trouble: United States, 1990-91. National Center for Health Statistics. *Vital Health Statistics, 10*(188).

Robertson-Thabo, E. (1984). Psychological changes with aging. In L. Jacobs-Condit (Ed.), *Gerontology and communication disorders* (pp. 73-130). Rockville, MD: American Speech-Language-Hearing Association.

Ronch, J. L. (1992). Who are these aging persons? In R. Hull (Ed.), *Rehabilitative audiology* (pp. 185-213). New York: Grune & Stratton.

Schow, R. L. (1982). Success of hearing aid fitting in nursing home residents. *Ear and Hearing, 3*(3), 173-177.

Schow, R. L. (1992). Hearing assessment and treatment in nursing homes. *Hearing Instruments, 43*(7), 7-11.

Schow, R. L., Balsara, N. R., Smedley, T. C., & Whitcomb, C. J. (1993). Aural rehabilitation by ASHA audiologists; 1980-1990. *American Journal of Audiology, 2*(3), 28-37.

Schow, R. L., & Nerbonne, M. A. (1977). Assessment of hearing handicap by nursing home residents and staff. *Journal of the Academy of Rehabilitative Audiology, 10*(2), 2–9.

Schow, R. L., & Nerbonne, M. A. (1980). Hearing levels among elderly nursing home residents. *Journal of Speech and Hearing Disorders, 45*(1), 124–132.

Schow, R. L., Reese, L., & Smedley, T. C. (1990). Hearing screening in a dental office using self assessment. *Ear and Hearing, 11*(5, Suppl.), 28–40.

Schuknecht, H. F. (1964). Further observations on the pathology of presbycusis. *Archives of Otology, 80*, 369–382.

Seewald, R. (1994). Current issues in hearing aid fitting [Monograph]. In J. P. Gagne and N. Tye-Murray (Eds.), *Research in audiologic rehabilitation: Current trends and future directions. Journal of the Academy of Rehabilitative Audiology.*

Simon, J. R., & Pouraghabagher, A. R. (1978). The effect of aging on the stages of processing in a choice reaction time task. *Journal of Gerontology, 33*, 553–561.

Smith, C. R., & Fay, T. H. (1977). A program of auditory rehabilitation for aged persons in a chronic disease hospital. *Asha, 19*, 417–422.

Smedley, T. C., & Schow, R. L. (1990). Frustrations with hearing aid use: Candid observations from the elderly. *Hearing Journal, 43*(6), 21–27.

Smedley, T. C., & Schow, R. L. (1992). Satisfaction/disability rating for programmable vs. conventional aids. *Hearing Instruments, 43*(11), 34–35.

Stach, B. (1990). Hearing aid amplification and central processing disorder. In R. E. Sandlin (Ed.), *Handbook of hearing aid amplification*, Vol. 2. Boston: College-Hill Press.

Stach, B., Jerger, J., & Fleming, K. (1985). Central presbycusis: A longitudinal case study. *Ear and Hearing, 10*, 304–306.

Stephens, S. D. G., & Goldstein, D. (1983). Auditory rehabilitation in the elderly. In R. Hinchcliffe (Ed.), *Hearing and balance in the elderly* (pp. 201–227). New York: Churchill Livingstone Press.

Taeuber, C. (1992). *Sixty-Five Plus in America.* Washington, DC: U.S. Department of Commerce, Economics and Statistics Administration. Bureau of the Census.

Taylor, K. (1993) Self-perceived and audiometric evaluations of hearing aid benefit in the elderly. *Ear and Hearing, 14*(6), 390–394.

U.S. Bureau of the Census (1990). *The Need for Personal Assistance With Everyday Activities: Recipients and Caregivers*, Current Population Reports, Series P-70, No. 19, Table B. Washington, DC: U.S. Government Printing Office.

U.S. Department of Health and Human Services. (1993). Health Data on Older Americans: United States, 1992. Series 3: Analytic and Epidemiological Studies, No. 27. Yattsville, MD: Publication No. (PHS) 93-1411.

Ventry, I. M., & Weinstein, B. E. (1982). The hearing handicap inventory for the elderly: A new tool. *Ear and Hearing, 3*, 128–134.

Weinstein, B. (1984). Management of hearing impaired elderly. In L. Jacobs-Condit (Ed.), *Gerontology and communication disorders* (pp. 244–279). Rockville, MD: American Speech-Language-Hearing Association.

Weinstein, B. (1994). Presbycusis. In J. Katz (Ed.), *Handbook of Clinical Audiology* (4th Ed.). Baltimore: Williams & Wilkins.

Appendix Ten A

Hearing Handicap Inventory for the Elderly (HHIE)

Instructions The purpose of this scale is to identify the problems your hearing loss may be causing you. Check **YES, SOMETIMES,** or **NO** for each question. **Do not skip a question if you avoid a situation because of your hearing problem**. If you use a hearing aid, please answer the way you hear **without** the aid.

		Yes (4)	Some-times (2)	No (0)
S-1	Does a hearing problem cause you to use the phone less often than you would like?			
E-2	Does a hearing problem cause you to feel embarrassed when meeting new people?			
S-3	Does a hearing problem cause you to avoid groups of people?			
E-4	Does a hearing problem make you irritable?			
E-5	Does a hearing problem cause you to feel frustrated when talking to members of your family?			
S-6	Does a hearing problem cause you difficulty when attending a party?			
E-7	Does a hearing problem cause you to feel "stupid" or "dumb"?			
S-8	Do you have difficulty hearing when someone speaks in a whisper?			
E-9	Do you feel handicapped by a hearing problem?			
S-10	Does a hearing problem cause you difficulty when visiting friends, relatives, or neighbors?			
S-11	Does a hearing problem cause you to attend religious services less often than you would like?			
E-12	Does a hearing problem cause you to be nervous?			
S-13	Does a hearing problem cause you to visit friends, relatives, or neighbors less often than you would like?			

	Yes (4)	Some-times (2)	No (0)
E-14 Does a hearing problem cause you to have arguments with family members?			
S-15 Does a hearing problem cause you difficulty when listening to TV or radio?			
S-16 Does a hearing problem cause you to go shopping less often than you would like?			
E-17 Does any problem or difficulty with your hearing upset you at all?			
E-18 Does a hearing problem cause you to want to be by yourself?			
S-19 Does a hearing problem cause you to talk to family members less often than you would like?			
E-20 Do you feel that any difficulty with your hearing limits or hampers your personal or social life?			
S-21 Does a hearing problem cause you difficulty when in a restaurant with relatives or friends?			
E-22 Does a hearing problem cause you to feel depressed?			
E-23 Does a hearing problem cause you to listen to TV or the radio less often than you would like?			
E-24 Does a hearing problem cause you to feel uncomfortable when talking to friends?			
E-25 Does a hearing problem cause you to feel left out when you are with a group of people?			

Important – Please go back over the questions to make sure you have not skipped any. Remember, Do not skip a question if you avoid a situation because of your hearing problem. Also make sure that you answered the way you hear without a hearing aid.

For Clinicain's Use Only

Total Score: _____   Subtotal E: _____

Subtotal S: _____

From "The Hearing Handicap Inventory for the Elderly: A New Tool" by I. M. Ventry and B.E. Weinstein, 1982, Ear and Hearing, 3, pp.128–134. Reprinted by permission.

Appendix Ten B

Nursing Home Hearing Handicap Index (NHHI): Self-Version for Resident

Circle the appropriate number	Very Often				Almost Never
1. When you are with other people do you wish you could hear better?	5	4	3	2	1
2. Do other people feel you have a hearing problem (when they try to talk to you)?	5	4	3	2	1
3. Do you have trouble hearing another person if there is a radio or TV playing (in the same room)?	5	4	3	2	1
4. Do you have trouble hearing the radio or TV?	5	4	3	2	1
5. (How often) do you feel life would be better if you could hear better?	5	4	3	2	1
6. How often are you embarassed because you don't hear well?	5	4	3	2	1
7. When you are alone do you wish you could hear better?	5	4	3	2	1
8. Do people (tend to) leave you out of conversations because you don't hear well?	5	4	3	2	1
9. (How often) do you withdraw from social activities (in which you ought to participate) because you don't hear well?	5	4	3	2	1
10. Do you say "what" or "pardon me" when people first speak to you?	5	4	3	2	1

Total _____ x 2 = _____

$$-20$$

_____ x 1.25 = _____ %

From "Assessment of Hearing Handicap by Nursing Home Residents and Staff" by R. L. Schow and M. A. Nerbonne, 1977, *Journal of the Academy of Rehabilitative Audiology, 10*, pp.2–12. Reprinted by permission.

Nursing Home Hearing Handicap Index (NHHI): Staff Version

Circle the appropriate number	Very Often				Almost Never
1. When this person is with other people does he/she need to hear better?	5	4	3	2	1
2. Do members of the staff, family and friends make negative comments about this person's hearing?	5	4	3	2	1
3. Does he/she have trouble hearing another person if there is a radio or TV playing in the same room?	5	4	3	2	1
4. When this person is listening to radio or TV does he/she have trouble hearing?	5	4	3	2	1
5. How often do you feel life would be better for this person if he/she could hear better?	5	4	3	2	1
6. How often is he/she embarassed because of not hearing well?	5	4	3	2	1
7. When alone does he/she need to hear the everyday sounds of life better?	5	4	3	2	1
8. Do people tend to leave him/her out of conversations because of not hearing well?	5	4	3	2	1
9. How often does he/she withdraw from social activities in which he/she ought to participate because of not hearing well?	5	4	3	2	1
10. Does he/she say "what" or "pardon me" when people first speak to him/her?	5	4	3	2	1

Total _____ x 2 = _____

-20

_____ x 1.25 = _____ %

From "Assessment of Hearing Handicap by Nursing Home Residents and Staff" by R. L. Schow and M. A. Nerbonne, 1977, *Journal of the Academy of Rehabilitative Audiology, 10*, pp. 2–12. Reprinted by permission.

PART THREE

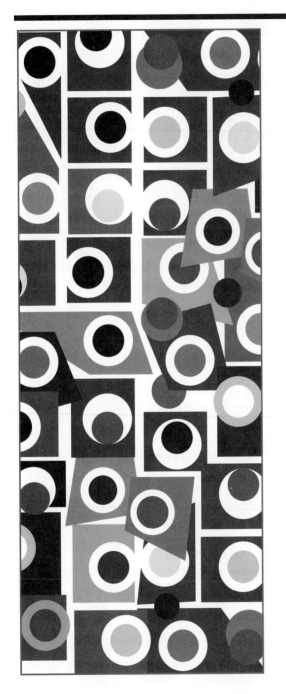

Implementing Audiologic Rehabilitation: Case Studies and Resource Materials

11

Case Studies: Children

MARY PAT MOELLER

Contents

INTRODUCTION

Children with hearing loss represent a heterogeneous group, with highly individual characteristics and needs. Differences in degree of hearing loss, family constellation and resources, medical history, language abilities, school support, and styles of learning contribute to each child's unique profile. The five case examples that follow describe individualized approaches to case management, with process-oriented strategies for problem solution. In each of the cases that follow, two concepts are central to the intervention: (a) clinicians must ascertain intervention priorities through differential diagnosis and careful determination of a child and family's primary needs; and (b) individualized management requires a process of clinical decision making and objective monitoring of the efficacy of intervention (see Chapter 8).

The process of pediatric audiologic rehabilitation is complex and challenging. Parents and clinicians face numerous management decisions early in the course of audiologic rehabilitation. Should the child's rehabilitation focus on auditory/oral development or is a visually-oriented approach needed? If a visual approach is needed, should it be oriented toward American Sign Language or Manually Coded English? What type of amplification will best meet this child's needs? Should sensory communication aids be considered? Will the child's needs be met in an inclusive educational setting, or will a specialized setting better serve this child? Answers to these and other management questions are rarely simple and rarely without controversy. Parents face many of these questions at a time when they are trying to cope with the diagnosis of hearing loss. They deserve objective guidance that is based on thoughtful examination of the child's needs and abilities in light of the options available.

AR service delivery for children is further complicated by the increasing incidence of children with hearing loss who have significant secondary disabilities. These children require sophisticated assessment and management through a team approach. Federal mandates require that early intervention be provided in a family-centered manner (Roush & Matkin, 1994). This has brought about a reconceptualization of the professional's role in the decision making and management process. The goal of empowering family members in the management of the child's needs also requires a diverse and individualized approach, given the wide range of family systems represented in the clinician's caseload. Each of these factors dictates the need for objective, individually tailored approaches and flexible, innovative service delivery models.

The case studies that follow represent five unique concerns that influenced the course of rehabilitative management:

1. Family-centered intervention for a child with multiple disabilities.
2. Clinical decision making: a child with a cochlear implant.
3. Clinical decision making: issues in selection of placement and communication mode.

4. Late identification in a child who was hard of hearing: auditory/linguistic considerations.
5. Diagnostic therapy: a tool for solving complex intervention problems.

In each of the following cases, multidisciplinary service delivery was necessary and advantageous. No one discipline has all the skills and expertise to address the complex nature of the problems that often present themselves. The audiologic rehabilitation specialist needs to cultivate the skills of working as a team member, joining in collaborative consultation with allied professionals and parents. Multidisciplinary perspectives contribute to a holistic understanding of the child's and family's needs.

Although the cases described are based on real persons, names and other biographical facts have been changed to maintain patient confidentiality.

CASE 1—JOEY: FAMILY-CENTERED INTERVENTION: MULTIPLE DISABILITIES

AR specialists working at the parent/infant level are meeting new professional challenges, including the opportunity to work with very young infants in the context of the family system (see Chapter 8). It has been estimated that 33–38% of infants with hearing loss have complex developmental needs resulting from secondary disabilities (Schildroth & Hotto, 1993; Moeller, Coufal, & Hixson, 1990). This case illustrates the importance of transdisciplinary approaches to case management. Overall coordination among various professionals and families is essential in meeting the needs of deaf infants with additional disabilities (Moeller, Coufal, & Hixson, 1990).

Background Information

Joey's profound bilateral sensorineural hearing loss was diagnosed through auditory brainstem response testing when he was 10 months of age. Subsequent behavioral testing demonstrated no response to speech or tonal stimuli at the limits of the equipment. Birth history records revealed heart decelerations from 30 weeks gestation until Joey's birth. An emergency C-section was done at 36 weeks gestation due to fetal distress. Joey required oxygen and remained in the neonatal intensive care unit (NICU) for five days following birth. Discharge diagnoses included hypocalcemia, respiratory distress, cardiac rhythm abnormalities, hyperbilirubinemia, and an abnormal pneumogram. Joey was on a heart monitor for the first seven months of his life. Joey also has a medical history of dizziness and balance problems, myopic astigmatism, poor coordination, and hypotonia.

Joey was delayed in achieving developmental milestones. He sat unsupported at 10 months and walked at 18 months. At four years of age, Joey is not yet toilet trained. The parents began signing to Joey immediately after diagnosis of the hearing loss, and he produced his first sign at 13 months of age. The mother reported that Joey was producing signed phrases up until about 16 to 18 months. At that time, he discontinued use of many of the signs he knew and did not combine signs. Regression in both social and language behaviors was noted by the family.

Previous Rehabilitation

Joey had been served since infancy by a homebound early-intervention program. At two years of age, he was placed in a self-contained toddler and preschool program, where he was served by an educator of the deaf, a speech/language pathologist, and an occupational and physical therapist (OT/PT). Although Joey was learning to cooperate with the routine of his preschool classroom, he demonstrated little evidence of learning from the group setting. He rarely initiated interactions or conversations with others. Although he knew over 100 signs, he rarely used them for functional communication. His attention to communication from others was fleeting. He demonstrated stereotypical and self-stimulatory behaviors. At three and one-half years of age, Joey's family relocated and he was placed in a self-contained public school program for deaf students with support services in speech/language pathology and OT/PT, similar to those of his previous program. Joey's social, behavioral, and attentional difficulties continued in the new school environment. Joey's educational team and parents requested consultation from an AR team due to concerns for his inattention, slow language learning, and atypical behaviors.

A comprehensive, multidisciplinary assessment was initiated in response to the expressed concerns. The communication portion of the evaluation was conducted by a team of AR specialists, who relied on valid instruments relevant to the child's environment and informal observations to analyze Joey's needs. The assessment began with parent interviews. The mother expressed a primary concern that her son may have autism. This child's well-educated parents had taken him to many different professionals in an effort to understand his problems. Experts in "autism" reported that Joey did not show "full-blown" autism syndrome. However, they had not worked with deaf children, and were uncertain how to interpret Joey's behaviors. The mother had read extensively on the subject and was an excellent reporter of her son's unique constellation of behaviors. She indicated that he had extreme fixations with lights and electronic equipment with switches. If left to his own devices, Joey would spend an entire day running and staring at lights or turning a VCR off and on. Although the parents had purchased numerous developmentally appropriate toys, these items did not hold Joey's attention. The mother indicated that Joey did not seem to know how to play with toys.

Joey's mother aptly described her son as socially isolated, preferring to be "in his own world." The family had learned to sign fluently to their son, but few rewards for this effort were forthcoming. Joey's communication remained extremely delayed in comparison to that of his deaf peers at school. The parents faithfully implemented full-time hearing-aid use, which they reported resulted in exacerbation of negative behaviors and self-stimulatory vocalizations. During the initial parent interview, Joey was allowed to play in an attractive playroom with numerous developmentally appropriate toys. Joey spent the entire period fixating on the lights in the room and did not become involved with toys or individuals present.

Formal, structured language testing is often inappropriate with a youngster who has fragile social interactions. The AR specialist found it necessary to identify ecologically valid assessment tools that would provide insights on Joey's communicative skills in a variety of environments. The Communication and Symbolic Behaviors Scales (CSBS) (Wetherby & Prizant, 1993) was an ideal selection in that it makes use of observational contexts that place few demands on the young child. Symbolic play skills and communicative means can be explored with this tool during semi-structured play activities. In addition, the MacArthur Communicative Development Inventory (Dale & Thal, 1993), which is a parent report scale, gave the clinician valuable information on Joey's sign-vocabulary used in the home. Results indicated that Joey used signs and gestures to communicate a small range of language functions (behavioral regulation, commenting, rejecting, and answering). His receptive sign vocabulary of 192 words was roughly equivalent to a 21-month developmental level. He presented as a curious and highly independent youngster. Rather than requesting help with a mechanical toy, for example, he would persist in trying to discover how to operate it.

Joey's warm and supportive home environment was a strength. The family had already learned through discovery various strategies to structure Joey's behavior and attention. They described the need to "Joey-proof" their home. In fact, the parents had become experts in helping their son succeed through environmental structuring. Many family strengths that could be incorporated in the individual family services plan (IFSP) were noted. The family was able to identify many primary needs. Foremost among them was the need for a definitive diagnosis so that appropriate management strategies and expectations could be implemented with Joey. In essence, the parents were "doing all the right things," yet watched as their child remained very delayed and became more difficult to manage. The parents expressed the need for a team to integrate perspectives and to understand their child in the holistic context of the family.

Joey was severely delayed in his symbolic skills, including play. His symbolic play skills at age four were commensurate with a 19–22-month level. His constructional play skills were well in advance of his symbolic play skills. He exhibited difficulty integrating various sensorial inputs. For example, if Joey's hands were involved in sensory exploration activities, he was not able to attend to any other input. Activities in his classroom frequently seemed to cause a "sensory overload" for Joey. When this occurred, he would "tune into" lights or the feel of his shirt and "tune out" the language input around him.

Overall Coordination

Team members from various disciplines made multiple observations of Joey in an effort to make a differential diagnosis and understand his needs. Transdisciplinary team discussion centered on the constellation of major findings of (a) serious delays in symbolic language use (in spite of positive opportunities for language acquisition in the home), (b) history of regression in language and social behaviors, (c) limited social interaction, (d) significant delays in symbolic play with strengths in constructional play, (e) tendencies for obsessions with lights and mechanical objects, and (f) self-stimulatory behaviors. Based on these findings, it was the team consensus that Joey was exhibiting the characteristics of pervasive developmental disorder (PDD) in addition to profound deafness. This diagnosis had important implications for Joey's intervention program. The team psychologist was able to offer many insights into the impact of the two disabilities on behavior, learning, and daily living. He assisted the family in implementing a consistent behavior management program at home.

Communication Rehabilitation Adjustment

Joey's program, which was designed to meet the needs of young children who are deaf, required adaptation in view of Joey's complex needs. AR team members had the opportunity to observe Joey in his school placement and to problem-solve with the school-based intervention team. Observations, and the adaptations and recommended strategies included:

1.   Although Joey could follow the classroom routine, he rarely learned from group lessons. Classroom observation revealed that often the language level of lessons was too complex for Joey. Thus, he failed to pay attention. With team input, the teachers found ways to modify the language requirements for Joey and provide him opportunities for active learning. Less reliance on large group lessons and increased reliance on short, individualized lessons was implemented.

2.   During unstructured play time, Joey wandered around the room. Assessment results suggested a strong need for emphasis on building Joey's symbolic play skills. Modifications included involving adults as play partners and the use of indirect language and play-stimulation methods. All adults encouraged turn-taking interactions in a nondirective manner, by following Joey's lead.

3.   Assistance from a behavioral specialist was implemented at home and at school. Emphasis was placed on reducing time spent with fixations and reducing aggressive behaviors.

4.   Joey's parents were motivated to implement full-time hearing-aid use, and they had accomplished this goal early in the rehabilitation program. However, behavior problems and inappropriate vocalizing escalated greatly when he wore amplification. The team and the parents agreed to remove amplification until other behaviors were brought under control. Amplification would be tried again in the future in the context of the overall behavior program.

5.   A priority for Joey's program was to strengthen the social foundation for language learning. He required indirect playful approaches, where he was motivated to remain in interaction with others and engage in turn-taking. Joey had a

number of strong interest areas that could be capitalized upon in this regard. For example, he loved the feel of socks on his arms and enjoyed pulling socks off and on his arms. This pleasurable activity was built into a social game ritual. The clinician offered Joey several socks and suggested, "Wanna play with the long sock? or the baby sock?" etc. Joey would select the appropriate sock (demonstrating comprehension) and the clinician would then help him put it on. She would then sign, "ready, pull" and would pull the sock off. Joey was so delighted with the outcome he would spontaneously make eye contact and sign "more" to have the game repeat. In examples like this, the AR clinician set up interactions that capitalized on the child's interest and involved social interaction with another person as a mandatory part of the game. Strategies from the Hanen Early Language Resource Centre guide, *It Takes Two to Talk* (Manolsen, 1992) were useful for parent guidance.

6.   As Joey's parents found, structuring the environment was instrumental in helping him succeed. He needed boundaries in wide-open spaces. He learned better in rooms without access to switches. He responded well when his limits were clearly defined and he could be actively engaged in lessons.

Psychosocial/Counseling Aspects

It was critical for the educational and AR teams to consider family needs. In talking with the parents, it was clear that living with Joey 24 hours a day brought many challenges. Sleep disruption was common; going out in public was nearly impossible; controlling driven obsessions was a full-time job. Joey's parents did everything they could to help him. Even so, their rewards came very slowly and in unpredictable ways. It helped for the team to make recommendations that gave consideration to the impact on home life. The parents needed the team to address behavioral issues in a comprehensive and ongoing manner. They also needed a chance to talk to other parents of children like Joey. They needed time away from Joey's problems. They needed practical direction to allow them to cope with today and to be hopeful about tomorrow.

CASE 2—ANN: CLINICAL DECISION MAKING: COCHLEAR IMPLANT

In some cases, successful rehabilitation is dependent on the willingness of the family and the AR specialist to explore and access various options. Objective monitoring of a child's progress can lead a clinician to question the efficacy of the current approach. When this occurs, the clinician and family need to objectively explore alternative routes to accomplish the desired goals. The next case illustrates this important process. The process works most effectively when the parents and clinician can work in a balanced partnership, with each partner willing to experiment in order to determine what works best for the child (Moeller & Condon, 1994).

Background Information

Ann was diagnosed with a moderate to profound, bilateral sensorineural hearing loss at 17 months of age. Pregnancy, birth and developmental history were uneventful, with the exception of speech and language development. Audiologic monitoring during her toddler years demonstrated progression in hearing thresholds to a profound hearing loss. Etiology was unknown.

Ann's parents lived in a rural community. Their school district provided home-bound early-intervention services. The parents elected to educate Ann using an auditory-oral approach. Ann was fitted with powerful, binaural BTE hearing aids at 18 months of age and wore them regularly for her full waking hours. Family members became actively involved in Ann's program and were excellent language stimulation models for her. Objective assessment of Ann's progress at 28 months of age revealed language skills at a 10–12-month level. She was babbling, and produced a few words, intelligible only to family members.

Psychological assessment results indicated that this child had above-average intelligence and was attentive and cooperative. There were no indications of learning difficulties.

Assessment and Monitoring Plan

In spite of many ideal characteristics of Ann's program (i.e., strong family support, an experienced auditory/oral teacher), she continued to progress at a slow rate of development. Objective monitoring of language and auditory progress at 42 months of age revealed communicative skills below an 18-month level. She could not consistently detect the presence of sound and had a restricted phonological repertoire. The parents were concerned that Ann understood very little of what was said to her and that the family rarely understood Ann's spontaneous verbalizations. However, the family was still highly committed to an auditory/verbal approach. The AR clinician discussed with the family the importance of objectively monitoring outcomes over the next several months to determine if program modifications could result in success or whether modality changes were needed. The parents and clinician selected six family-desired goals and set a time frame of six months for their accomplishment. The family and clinician worked steadily toward the achievement of these goals.

Six months later, Ann had made little progress toward achievement of the focus goals. She was experiencing increased communication frustration, as were her parents. The parents and clinician jointly decided to experiment with the same six goals, but to try them in total communication. Within two months' time, Ann had achieved the goals and her parents were cautiously optimistic about her new-found success. Several years later, the parents reflected on the importance their involvement in "experiments" played in helping them see the need for a change in Ann's program. "If you had just told us to make this change," they stated, "we could never have accepted it. It helped us to objectively see how Ann performed so we could base our decision on her needs."

TABLE 11.1 *Longitudinal Language Test Results for Ann as a Function of Chronologic Age (CA)*

	CA:	2:6	3:6	4:6	4:11	6:10
Receptive		10 months	14 months	3:1	4:7*	6:5*
Expressive		12 months	14 months	3:0	4:6*	6:6*
Vocabulary		4 words	18 months	4:1*	5:9*	7:3*
MLU			1.2	3.4	4.9	6.31

*Standard scores were within the average range for her age in comparison to children with normal hearing.

The family devoted themselves to learning sign language and building communication with Ann at home. Ann was involved in a self-contained, cognitively-oriented preschool program for children who were deaf, where total communication was used. Ann made rapid gains in her language skills, as illustrated in the longitudinal test results presented in Table 11.1.

However, Ann's progress in speech and auditory development lagged behind her gains in language. She remained highly unintelligible, had limited functional auditory skills (with conventional hearing aids or with vibrotactile devices) and had some abnormal vocal behaviors typical of children with profound deafness (e.g. glottalizations, pitch breaks). Her parents continued to advocate for her oral skills and requested input on sensory aids that might benefit Ann.

Amplification: Cochlear Implantation

Assessment. Ann's parents were referred to the Cochlear Implant team. Ann underwent a series of pre-implant candidacy assessments. Her parents actively sought information and guidance from multiple sources, including deaf-community members. They explored all sides of the issues and appeared to have realistic expectations when they made the decision to proceed with implantation.

Implementation. Ann underwent surgical implantation of a Nucleus 22 Channel cochlear implant in her left ear at five and one-half years of age. All 22 electrodes were inserted into the cochlea. The audiogram in Figure 11.1 illustrates pre- and post-implant thresholds for Ann.

When the cochlear implant minispeech processor was first mapped six weeks post-surgery, Ann expressed distress and complained that the sound was too loud. Implant team members used a conservative approach over the next several months of implant use, making sure that the sound input was within comfortable limits. Gradual adjustments over time led to an increased dynamic range, and the child adjusted well with no further complaints.

Auditory Training. One month after her hookup, Ann was enrolled in intensive audiologic rehabilitation therapy sessions designed to strengthen her auditory skills through reliance on the cochlear implant. The initial goals of intervention were to increase Ann's skills for detection, discrimination and identification of various parameters of sound,

Audiological Record

Frequency (Hz)

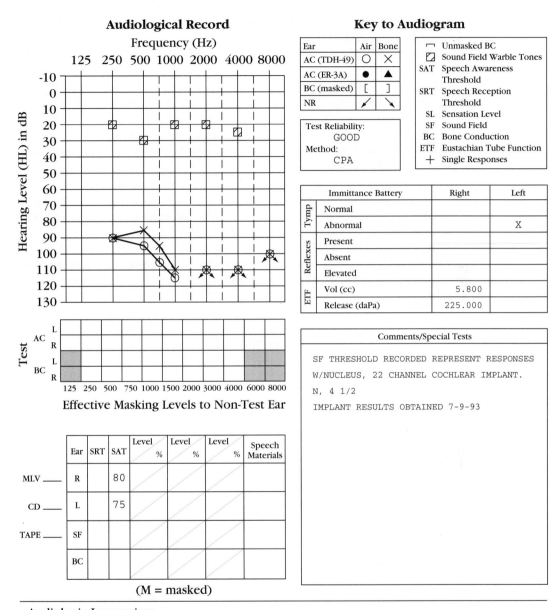

Key to Audiogram

Ear	Air	Bone
AC (TDH-49)	◯	✕
AC (ER-3A)	●	▲
BC (masked)	[	]
NR	↙	↘

Test Reliability:
GOOD
Method:
CPA

⌐	Unmasked BC
▨	Sound Field Warble Tones
SAT	Speech Awareness Threshold
SRT	Speech Reception Threshold
SL	Sensation Level
SF	Sound Field
BC	Bone Conduction
ETF	Eustachian Tube Function
+	Single Responses

	Immittance Battery	Right	Left
Tymp	Normal		
	Abnormal		X
Reflexes	Present		
	Absent		
	Elevated		
ETF	Vol (cc)	5.800	
	Release (daPa)	225.000	

Effective Masking Levels to Non-Test Ear

Comments/Special Tests

SF THRESHOLD RECORDED REPRESENT RESPONSES
W/NUCLEUS, 22 CHANNEL COCHLEAR IMPLANT.
N, 4 1/2
IMPLANT RESULTS OBTAINED 7-9-93

	Ear	SRT	SAT	Level / %	Level / %	Level / %	Speech Materials
MLV ___	R		80				
CD ___	L		75				
TAPE ___	SF						
	BC						

(M = masked)

Audiologic Impression:

Recommendations:

Figure 11.1 Audiological record: Case 2—Ann.

including long/short, continuous/discontinuous, and number of presentations. Both environmental and speech stimuli were used in motivating and pragmatically-appropriate activities. Speech targets included use of appropriate syllable number, appropriate pitch and rate. In addition, the clinician focused on development of fricatives and postvocalic sounds, which were likely audible to Ann with the implant. The cochlear implant team also made visits to Ann's school program to provide inservice, demonstrate strategies, and observe Ann's responses in naturalistic contexts. School visits promoted carryover of intervention goals to the classroom-based program.

Ann's progress with the implant was monitored objectively at six-month intervals. Limited progress was observed 6 months post implant, although the parents reported some changes at home. By 12 months post implant, Ann's auditory and vocal behaviors began to improve. Steady growth in auditory learning, speech acquisition, speechreading, and speech intelligibility were noted over the next year. Changes in Ann's auditory behaviors are summarized in Table 11.2.

Ann was not able to attain any of the skills represented in Table 11.2 prior to implantation. The data indicate that she has made steady and continuous improvement in her auditory skills following implantation and intervention. Improvements in auditory skills have led to concomitant improvements in her speech and spoken language. At

TABLE 11.2 *Changes in Ann's Auditory Behaviors Post Implant*

	Months Post Implant		
	6	12	18
Detection			
GASP phoneme detection	NR	Detects 80% Not voiceless fricatives	98% *not th*
Sound Discrimination			
Change/No change	50%	72%	82%
SCIPS			
1 vs. 3 syllable	38%	62%	94%
1 vs. 2 syllable	44%	100%	81%
2 vs. 2 syllable	50%	81%	100%
1 vs. 1 syllable	44%	88%	100%
Closed-Set Word Recognition			
Spondee Recognition	20%	DNT	90%
Monosyllable-Spondee-Trochee			
Word Pattern Recognition	8%	41%	67%
Stress Patterns	38%	54%	83%
Minimal Pairs	53%	58%	79%
NUCHIPS	28%	34%	56%
Open-Set Word Recognition			
PBK 50			
Word	–	–	10%
Phoneme	–	13%	22%

two years post implant, Ann was able to use speechreading and listening to understand redundant everyday conversations with friends who did not know sign. Although she continued to use a sign interpreter in the classroom to receive instruction, she began to rely increasingly on oral communication to give simple answers to her teacher, or to present show-and-tell items to her peers. Ann's use of her cochlear implant and her success in attaining language skills commensurate with her age both contributed to her ability to integrate into a regular classroom program in her neighborhood school. She has become a confident and popular member of her class and her community.

Summary

Ann's parents firmly believed in the importance of exploring options and never giving up on their goals. Their route to success with Ann took unexpected courses, but the outcomes have continued to be gratifying. Ann continues to progress with her implant and has succeeded academically in her regular elementary program with appropriate support services.

CASE 3—SARAH: CLINICAL DECISION MAKING: PLACEMENT AND COMMUNICATION MODE

The previous case illustrated the importance of objectivity and flexibility in determining the best approach for an individual child. The next case further illustrates the value of objective determination of needs before proceeding with an intervention approach.

Background Information

Sarah contracted h influenza B meningitis when she was 10 months of age. An auditory brainstem response (ABR) test conducted at a rural hospital following her illness reportedly indicated normal hearing. Sarah also had numerous bouts with otitis media during infancy. There was a documented family history of hearing loss, as well as kidney problems. Genetic assessment was recommended for Sarah and her family. When Sarah was two years, two months of age, her parents returned to an audiologist with concerns for her hearing, speech, and language. At that time, she had only a five-word vocabulary and relied primarily on gesture for communication. Behavioral results obtained with Visual Reinforcement Audiometry indicated bilateral, sensorineural hearing loss, which was moderate to severe in the right ear and moderate to profound in the left ear, as shown in Figure 11.2. Sarah was subsequently fitted with binaural amplification and FM amplification, and was referred to her school district's early-intervention program. Sarah was placed by the school district in a multi-categorical special education preschool, where she received support services from a speech-/language pathologist. The school district had limited experience with children with hearing impairment. They began implementing a total communication approach, because of Sarah's hearing loss.

Audiological Record

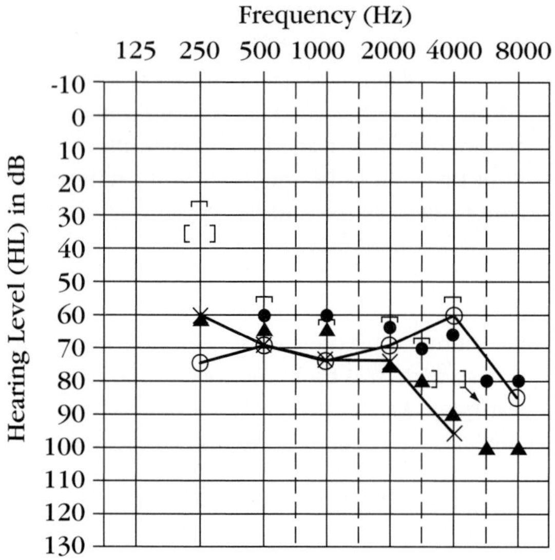

Frequency (Hz)

Key to Audiogram

	Immittance Battery	Right	Left
Tymp	Normal		
	Abnormal	X	X
Reflexes	Present		
	Absent		
	Elevated		
ETF	Vol (cc)		
	Release (daPa)		

Test

		125	250	500	750	1000	1500	2000	3000	4000	6000	8000
AC	L											
	R											
BC	L		95									
	R		95					100	95			

Effective Masking Levels to Non-Test Ear

Comments/Special Tests

SAID MY VOICE IN L-EAR AT 95DBHL
WAS TOO LOUD AND HURT HER EAR

	Ear	SRT	SAT	Level / %	Level / %	Level / %	Speech Materials
MLV X	R	55		90 / 76			PBK-50
CD ____	L	65		95 / 76	90 / 56		PBK-50
TAPE ____	SF						
	BC						

(M = masked)

Audiologic Impression:
R-MOD-SEVERE SNHL
L-MOD-PROFOUND SNHL
FAIRLY STABLE AU

Recommendations:
SEE REPORT
RE-EVAL IN 6MOS

Figure 11.2 Audiological record: Case 3—Sarah.

Assessment of Auditory Potential

When Sarah was three years, three months old, her parents attended a parent/child workshop that had been developed by a team of AR specialists for parents of children with newly identified hearing impairment. As part of that workshop, the specialists had the opportunity to involve the family in observing Sarah's responses to auditory stimulation activities. The emphasis all along in Sarah's preschool program had been primarily visual. She had been given few opportunities to rely on her residual hearing at school or at home. Formal assessment of her communicative skills identified significant delays (receptive and expressive communication skills at a 16-month level, mean length of utterance 1.3, inconsistent detection of environmental sounds and speech, very limited phonological repertoire).

Diagnostic teaching was implemented during the parent/child week. The parents and clinician set some specific goals for Sarah's listening behaviors. After only three sessions, Sarah was consistently detecting quiet voice, was discriminating simple stereotypical messages from one another, and was imitating the appropriate vowel and syllable number in modelled speech. The parents were encouraged by their daughter's responsiveness to auditory stimulation. They had not been informed that there were optional approaches to the education of their child who was hard of hearing. They had been told it was important to sign to their daughter because of her hearing loss. After seeing her succeed with auditory/oral tasks, they were convinced of the importance of raising their own expectations for her auditory performance. They were able to appreciate that Sarah may have the potential to develop a strong auditory foundation for language learning.

Auditory-Oral Training

The AR specialists and parents met with the school district to stress the positive nature of the diagnostic teaching results and their implications for Sarah's auditory language development. The AR clinician stressed the importance of a specialized rehabilitation program for Sarah, to allow her to optimize her listening skills during this critical period of language acquisition. The school district agreed to enroll Sarah in a self-contained auditory/oral preschool program for children with hearing loss. The parents discontinued the use of signs and focused on learning strategies to encourage listening and oral language behaviors at home.

Rehabilitation

Sarah made excellent progress in her auditory language skills. After one year in a specialized auditory/oral preschool program, Sarah showed evidence of "overhearing" words and concepts, and was spontaneously adding these lexical items to her language. Developmental sentence scoring completed on a language sample at four and one-half years of age yielded numerous grammatical errors and an age equivalent score of two years, six months. After two years of preschool programming (CA: six years, six months) Sarah's developmental-sentence scoring age equivalent was six years, seven months. She made few grammatical errors and showed evidence of the emergence of complex structures (e.g., "You have to wash the dishes because you are pretending to be my daughter"). At this time of formal school entry, Sarah had language skills that were within the low average to average range for her age compared to her peers with normal hearing. Furthermore, her speech was intelligible to unfamiliar listeners over 90% of the time. The school district's investment in specialized early-intervention services was efficacious. As a result of the quality of training and selection of the appropriate mode of communication, Sarah had developed the language and speech skills needed for entering the regular education setting. This case illustrates the important role of advocacy that an AR clinician may take on the educational team. Placement decisions need to be examined in light of the primary needs and capabilities of the child. In Sarah's case, modification of the placement and communication mode was necessary to allow her to fully realize her auditory potential.

CASE 4—GREG: LATE IDENTIFICATION OF A HARD OF HEARING CHILD

Children who are hard of hearing can be difficult to identify, because they respond inconsistently to sounds around them. This inconsistency confuses parents and physicians, and may delay referral for hearing testing until evidence of speech and language delays prompts referral. Once the hearing loss is identified and amplification is fitted, the child may need to embark on the process of re-learning auditory behaviors. The next case illustrates the importance of audibility in the formation of language rules by a child who is hard of hearing. In this case, the child needed to learn new ways of gaining meaning from messages around him. His auditory training program needed to focus on helping him develop productive listening and comprehension behaviors.

Background Information

Greg's parents first began to express concerns about his hearing to their pediatrician when he was two years old. He was demonstrating inconsistent responses to sound and delayed speech and language development at that time. Results of audiologic testing at a community hospital suggested borderline normal hearing sensitivity in response to speech and narrowband stimuli. One and one-half years later, the parents continued to express concern for Greg's hearing, and testing revealed at least a mild to moderate sensorineural hearing loss in the better ear. However, the audiologist reported questionable test reliability, and Greg was referred for Auditory Brainstem Response testing. Results suggested the probability of a moderate to severe sensorineural hearing loss in at least the higher frequencies, with the right ear more involved than the left. Greg was then referred to a pediatric audiologic team. A severe rising to mild hearing loss in the right ear was confirmed through behavioral testing. Left ear testing revealed responses in the mild hearing loss range, rising to within normal limits at 1 Khz, and steeply sloping to the severe hearing loss range at 2 Khz, and then rising to the mild hearing loss range in the higher frequencies. Given the unusual configuration of Greg's hearing loss (see Figure 11.3a), it was not surprising that he passed a screening evaluation that used speech and narrow bands of noise in sound field. Unfortunately, the referral for more definitive testing was delayed by the findings of the screening assessment. Medical-genetic evaluation revealed a family history of hearing loss, but etiology could not be confirmed.

Hearing-aid fitting was complex, given the unusual audiometric configuration in the left ear. However, a binaural fitting was selected, with capability for direct audio input for FM amplification. Greg was immediately referred to an AR program for the purposes of evaluating his individual communication needs and determining considerations for educational placement.

Communication Assessment

Greg demonstrated an unusual communication profile at four years of age. On standardized tests of language, his receptive language skills approximated a two and one-half–year level and his expressive language skills were equivalent to a three-year level. On many tests, his expressive performance was stronger than comprehension. Analysis of conversational interactions was useful in understanding the complexity of his receptive and expressive language problems. It was evident from the outset that Greg was having serious difficulty understanding those around him. Table 11.3 contains a segment from an interactive language sample, where Greg was conversing with an audiologic rehabilitation clinician.

A number of interesting patterns were reflected in Greg's spontaneous speech. Although most of his words were intelligible to the listener, it was difficult to understand Greg due to numerous semantic and grammatical errors in his spontaneous productions. It was suspected that Greg's unusual audiometric configuration had contributed to his formulation of unusual language rules. Spectral information he was receiving may have provided inconsistent cues about grammatical or semantic categories. For example, he frequently marked nouns with /s/, even when a morpheme was not required. He rarely inflected verbs. He was aware that words were marked with morphemes like /s/, but had no consistent basis for application of this rule. Lack

TABLE 11.3 *Conversational Exchange Between Greg and the Clinician*

E	Hi, Greg. How are you today?
C	Fours.
E	Oh, you are four years old. Well, how are you feeling?
C	Fine.
E	Greg, where's your mom?
C	My moms Greg go to the schools. The mom talk it the boats.
E	Oh. Hmmmm, you and mom came to school. Wow, I see you got a star!
C	I got stars my mom say no go outsides. Mom say do suns no go outside. Mom the all raining go put the backs the watch all raining.

C = Child   E = Examiner

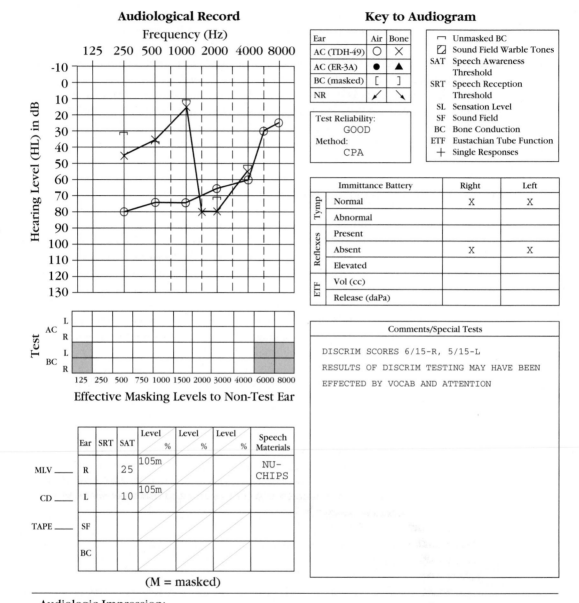

Audiological Record

Frequency (Hz)

Key to Audiogram

Ear	Air	Bone
AC (TDH-49)	○	×
AC (ER-3A)	●	▲
BC (masked)	[	]
NR	↙	↘

⌐ Unmasked BC
◪ Sound Field Warble Tones
SAT Speech Awareness Threshold
SRT Speech Reception Threshold
SL Sensation Level
SF Sound Field
BC Bone Conduction
ETF Eustachian Tube Function
+ Single Responses

Test Reliability:
GOOD
Method:
CPA

Immittance Battery		Right	Left
Tymp	Normal	X	X
	Abnormal		
Reflexes	Present		
	Absent	X	X
	Elevated		
ETF	Vol (cc)		
	Release (daPa)		

Effective Masking Levels to Non-Test Ear

Comments/Special Tests

DISCRIM SCORES 6/15-R, 5/15-L
RESULTS OF DISCRIM TESTING MAY HAVE BEEN
EFFECTED BY VOCAB AND ATTENTION

	Ear	SRT	SAT	Level %	Level %	Level %	Speech Materials
MLV ___	R		25	105m			NU-CHIPS
CD ___	L		10	105m			
TAPE ___	SF						
	BC						

(M = masked)

Audiologic Impression:

Recommendations:

Figure 11.3a Case 4—Greg: Initial audiogram.

Audiological Record

Frequency (Hz)

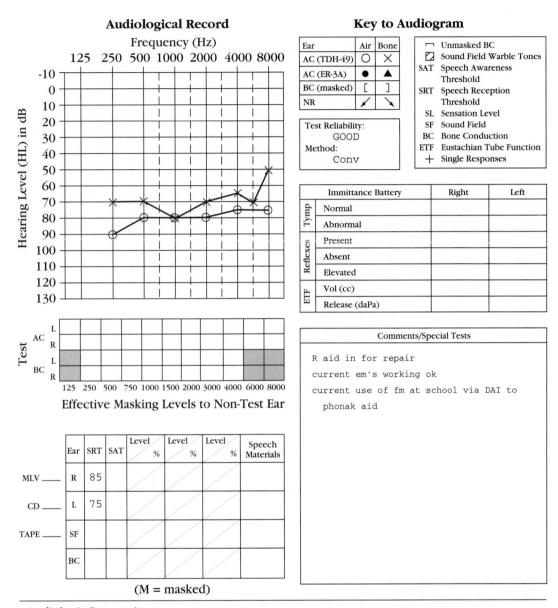

Key to Audiogram

Ear	Air	Bone
AC (TDH-49)	O	X
AC (ER-3A)	●	▲
BC (masked)	[	]
NR	↙	↘

Test Reliability:
  GOOD
Method:
  Conv

┌ Unmasked BC
◲ Sound Field Warble Tones
SAT Speech Awareness
    Threshold
SRT Speech Reception
    Threshold
SL Sensation Level
SF Sound Field
BC Bone Conduction
ETF Eustachian Tube Function
＋ Single Responses

Immittance Battery	Right	Left
Tymp — Normal		
Tymp — Abnormal		
Reflexes — Present		
Reflexes — Absent		
Reflexes — Elevated		
ETF — Vol (cc)		
ETF — Release (daPa)		

Comments/Special Tests

R aid in for repair
current em's working ok
current use of fm at school via DAI to
  phonak aid

Effective Masking Levels to Non-Test Ear

	Ear	SRT	SAT	Level %	Level %	Level %	Speech Materials
MLV —	R	85					
CD —	L	75					
TAPE —	SF						
	BC						

(M = masked)

Audiologic Impression:

Recommendations:

Figure 11.3b Case 4—Greg: Recent audiogram (following progression).

of audibility of portions of the speech spectrum may have also led to semantic confusions. Greg confused gender (*girl* vs. *boy*; *man* vs. *lady*), used nouns as verbs, used pronoun forms randomly (with confusion of *I, you, he, she,* and *we*), and had significant difficulty providing the appropriate semantic content in response to questions. Collectively, these errors appeared to be language "differences," rather than simple delays.

To understand better the nature of Greg's language problems, the AR clinician constructed probes to examine Greg's language-processing strategies. For example, she observed his responses to various questions across contexts and tasks. Greg was having such difficulty understanding others that he had developed an over-reliance on non-linguistic comprehension strategies. Chapman (1978) described young children's normal developmental use of comprehension strategies in the face of complex linguistic input. Moeller (1988) has observed that students with hearing impairment may use such comprehension "short cuts" when their comprehension is taxed well into their school years. Greg demonstrated extreme reliance on these behaviors, due to pervasive comprehension difficulties. Greg used the following strategies in his attempts to make sense of input around him:

1. Attended to key words in the message to the exclusion of other information.
2. Predicted message intention based on situational context cues.
3. Nodded his head as if he understood.
4. Selected a key, recognizable word and made comments related to that topic (without respect for the current topic of conversation).
5. Controlled the conversational topic to avoid comprehension demands.
6. Said everything known about the topic in hopes that the answer was included in the content somewhere (global response strategy).

Greg was not able to answer any types of questions with consistency. Tracking of his responses revealed correct responses in fewer than 25% of the instances. In response to commands, he failed to recognize the need for action, and would instead imitate the command or nod his head. Greg's reliance on non-linguistic strategies is evident in the discourse example provided in Table 11.4.

TABLE 11.4 *Greg's Replies to Questions about Simple Objects*

E	(*holding a boy doll*) Who is this?
C	Boy.
E	(*puts boy in helicopter*) Who is this?
C	Boy the helicopter.
E	(*holds up a mom doll*) Who is this?
C	Mom boy the helicopter.

C = Child   E = Examiner

TABLE 11.5 *Classroom Interaction Designed to Support Greg's Emerging Discourse Skills*

E	Good morning, Greg. Where's your mommy?
C	Mom Greg go go the school. My moms say Greg no go the school the rain . . .
E	Just a minute, Greg. *Listen* to the question (*focusing prompt*).
E	Where *is* mom? (*highlighting prompt*) At home? In the car? Here at school? (*multiple choice prompt*).
C	Mom right there. At school! (*points to his mother in the hall—on her way in to be room mother today*).
E	Good, Greg! You answered my question! I asked, "where's mom?" You told me . . . right there! There she is!

C = Child   *E* = Examiner
Source: Moeller, Osberger and Eccarius, 1986.

In this example, Greg showed his overdependence on context for determining what questions mean. He also demonstrated his tendency to use a global response strategy, and his assumption that "if she asks me the question again, my first response must have been wrong." The clinician observed similar behaviors from Greg in his preschool class setting. He had a "panicked" expression on his face much of the time. Greg did not appear to expect to understand. Rather, he expected to have to guess. In the classroom, he frequently produced long, confused narratives. His teacher, in an effort to be supportive, would abandon her communication agenda and follow Greg's topic to any degree possible. This was problematic, however, in that Greg needed to learn to understand and respond with semantic accuracy to classroom discourse.

Management

Communication Rehabilitation: Auditory/Linguistic Training. Once amplification was fitted, Greg was enrolled in a multi-faceted audiologic rehabilitation program. Individual auditory language therapy focused on development of productive comprehension strategies and reduction of semantic confusion through attention to appropriate auditory linguistic cues. A parent program was included, with focus on teaching the family natural ways to support Greg's comprehension. Greg had a tendency to imitate each message he heard, which interfered with processing and responding. The parents and therapist agreed to reduce emphasis on imitation and expression until success in comprehension could be increased. Further, the AR specialist provided collaborative consultation to Greg's classroom teacher. The school district provided Greg a diagnostic placement in a Language Intervention Preschool. His teacher was a speech/language pathologist. The teacher and AR specialist developed a scheme for helping Greg repair comprehension breakdowns and for helping him respond accurately in the classroom. Table 11.5 illustrates the type of teaching interaction that was implemented to scaffold or support Greg's emerging comprehension.

These classroom adaptations were successful in helping Greg begin to focus on the content of what he was hearing. As his auditory/linguistic behaviors strengthened, he began to revise language and discourse rules. His auditory language program focused specifically on helping him discriminate among linguistic elements that marked important semantic or syntactic distinctions. For example, he worked with the AR clinician in learning to distinguish pronoun forms (e.g., *I* vs. *you*), various morphological structures, and the meaning of various question forms. All intervention was incorporated in communicatively-based activities to ensure the development of pragmatically-appropriate conversational skills.

The AR clinician and teacher worked collaboratively to gradually shape in Greg productive listening and comprehension strategies. This was an essential step in helping Greg revise his expressive language behaviors. He needed to develop the confidence that he could understand and that his responses needed to be related to the conversational topic. Adjustment of Greg's approach to comprehension was necessary to prepare him for learning in a classroom environment.

Intervention Outcomes

Greg was responsive to the auditory/linguistic training program and to the supportive techniques used in the classroom to strengthen language processing. Greg continued to receive a team approach to his rehabilitation and education into his early elementary years. Although the ultimate objective was to enable him to profit from education in a regular classroom, the initial approach was conservative with emphasis on specialty services to help him develop the language foundation necessary for academic success. In this case, the conservative approach was especially fortuitous because Greg experienced progression in his sensorineural hearing loss during his early elementary years. The audiograms in Figure 11.3a/b illustrate the progression in thresholds that occurred, with the initial audiogram on the left and the final audiogram on the right. Hearing thresholds finally stabilized at a severe hearing loss level, with a bilaterally symmetrical configuration. Fortunately, optimal hearing aid fittings have been achieved (see Figure 11.4). Real-ear measures indicate that much of the speech spectrum is audible to Greg with properly fitted personal and FM amplification.

A language assessment was completed when Greg was 10 years of age. All language test scores fell solidly within the average range for his age in comparison to hearing peers. Previous comprehension and discourse problems were no longer present. In the context of a storytelling task, Greg produced complex utterances like, "The boy says that the frog should stay on the land while the rest of them sail off on a raft." Greg's expressive language was semantically and grammatically appropriate for his age. Provision of support services will continue to be important for Greg, in spite of his strong language performance. When asked if he was having any problems in school, Greg reported, "Well, it is hard sometimes because you have to be quiet to hear the teacher, but the hearing kids keep talking. Then I always have to watch what everybody's doing, and then I'll know what I'm supposed to be doing."

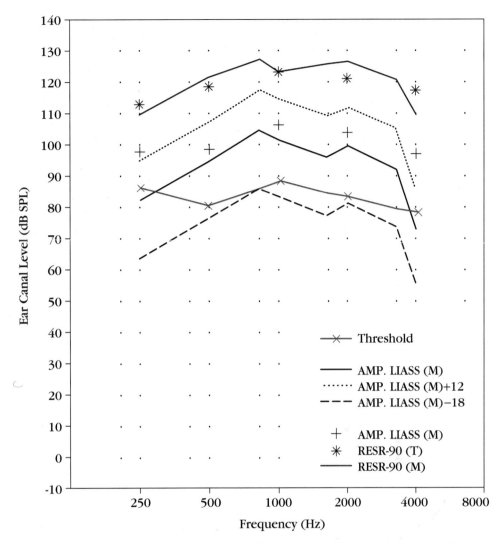

Figure 11.4 Results of real-ear measures illustrating audibility in relation to the long-term average speech spectrum.

Summary

This case has illustrated the critical importance that audibility plays in a child's language rule formation. It also underscores the importance of teamwork to address concerns in all the child's significant learning environments. With aggressive and continuous AR support, a child who is hard of hearing has an opportunity to overcome early delays. Appropriate management of amplification and auditory learning opportunities play a key role in this process.

CASE 5—STEVE: DIAGNOSTIC THERAPY: A TOOL FOR SOLVING COMPLEX INTERVENTION PROBLEMS

One of the more challenging aspects of audiologic rehabilitation is the goal of determining the most efficacious intervention approach for solving a particular problem. This requires accurate and thorough differential diagnosis of a child's problems, and design of management strategies to address the child's needs in the most effective manner. The selection of intervention priorities following thorough problem analysis is like a craft, requiring skill, theoretical preparation, and insight. It is useful for the clinician to ask: (a) if I select this goal, what difference will it make in the child's overall communicative functioning? (b) will emphasis on this goal lead to generalization or impact on other communicative behaviors? (c) is there any way to effect system-wide change with this approach?

This next case illustrates the process of differential diagnosis and discovery-oriented therapy. It is often impossible to separate assessment from management. In fact, intervention is typically guided by the constant analysis of outcomes and clinical decision making. The following case is used to illustrate this clinical decision making process.

Background Information: Assessment of Hearing Loss and Amplification

Steve's hearing loss was identified when he was 11 months of age. Audiologic results throughout his early years indicated a profound, bilateral sensorineural hearing loss, with no response to speech or tonal stimuli at the limits of the audiometric equipment. At 11 months of age he was enrolled in a comprehensive, family-centered early-intervention program (Moeller & Condon, 1994). Steve demonstrated little response to conventional amplification, and was subsequently fitted with a Tactaid II+ vibrotactile device (see Chapter 2).

Previous Rehabilitation

During early intervention, Steve's clinician documented numerous developmental concerns. Steve demonstrated hypotonia, tactile defensiveness, motor overflow, and difficulties with visual attention. His family members participated fully in the program, and became fluent and competent signers. In spite of a nurturing language environment at home, Steve was slow to develop expressive language, and was delayed in social and play skills. Steve was referred for both neurological and OT/PT assessments, due to developmental concerns. Steve passed a gross screening assessment completed by a school-based OT/PT who felt that services were unnecessary. Neurological assessment revealed physical evidence of brain damage. Psychological assessment revealed that Steve had at least average nonverbal intelligence.

Differential Diagnosis & Assessment: Communication Problems/Signing Strategies

Steve was enrolled in a self-contained preschool program for deaf children at age three, upon completion of the early-intervention program. Family members continued to participate in parent and sibling sign classes, and to demonstrate follow-through at home. In spite of aggressive efforts, Steve continued to lag behind his peers, especially in his social use of language. Steve's teachers began to make systematic observations and modifications of his curriculum in an effort to bring about better results. Steve's teacher referred him for a formal diagnostic intervention program upon discovery of motor difficulties that appeared to be affecting his sign productions. She theorized that motor problems may have been constraining his efforts at self expression. An AR specialist began to work collaboratively with the classroom teacher in attempts to understand the problem better. The teacher provided the clinician with long lists of signs that were produced incorrectly by this child, rendering many of his spontaneous language attempts unintelligible.

The audiologic rehabilitationist observed Steve in the classroom and closely examined the lists of "mispronounced signs." She began to formulate diagnostic questions on the basis of language and phonological theories and careful observations of the child's production schemes. The first question asked was: "Is there regularity to Steve's sign production errors?" Theories of phonology in spoken language suggest that children do not make random errors in production. Rather, they follow systematic rules, which have been described as developmental phonological processes (Edwards & Shriberg, 1983; Hodson, 1980). The clinician conjectured that Steve's sign production errors may also have been rule governed. If immature phonological processes were guiding his productions, this finding would impact management strategies.

The first step taken was to closely examine Steve's handshape productions on videotape. Only six primary handshapes were produced correctly, representing a restricted phonological repertoire for a four-year-old. In fact, five of the six handshapes he could produce (*I, A, L, O,* and *B*) are among those observed in the earliest developmental productions of young deaf children acquiring native signs (Battison, 1974). Steve also used the *F* handshape in substitution for several other handshapes in common signs. The clinician constructed probes to determine whether or not Steve followed consistent rules in handshape substitutions or changes. For example, the clinician gathered sets of objects that had signs representing the spectrum of handshapes needed for basic lexical use in young deaf children. She recorded Steve's responses to these stimulus items and then analyzed the results for patterns.

Motoric Limitations in Signing

All of Steve's errors clustered into five production simplification patterns or "rules." These rules were described by the clinician as follows:

1. For all signs requiring two or more fingers to be isolated and spread, Steve would substitute an *F*. Thus, on signs like *AIRPLANE, PUMPKIN, WATER*, or *THREE*, all of which have distinctive handshapes, Steve produced *F*. His counting, for example was characterized as "1, F, F, 4, 4" instead of "1, 2, 3, 4, 5." This simplification rule was having a serious effect on sign intelligibility.

2. For signs that required flexion of the hand with two fingers extended together, Steve simplified to the *B* handshape. Thus, signs with handshapes using *N, U*, or *R* became *B*.

3. When signs required distal finger flexion or extension (e.g., *Y* in *PLAY; T* in *POTTY*; or *S* in *SHOE*), Steve produced the *A* handshape.

4. Signs that required a relaxed *C* production were produced in a highly flexed and spread position, in a claw-like manner.

The clinician observed some additional patterns that were of concern and led her to ask for a second opinion from occupational therapy. Steve demonstrated reversal of the sign path in some instances. He would watch his teacher sign *WITCH* (where the dominant hand comes from the nose downward to meet the non-dominant hand) and he would sign it backwards (with his dominant hand coming up to the nose from the non-dominant hand). On a sign like *BEAR*, which requires that the hands cross midline, he failed to cross his hands, and would instead place claw-hands separately on either side of his chest. He demonstrated associated reactions, which can be indicative of immature neurological development. That is, if one hand was producing a movement pattern (e.g., signing *GIRL*), his other hand would be at his side mimicking the action of the dominant hand. Finally, Steve appeared to have poor control of his non-dominant hand, making it especially difficult for him to produce signs that required two different handshapes (e.g., *HELP, PUMPKIN*).

Overall Coordination

Following careful examination of the information to date, the clinician posed the next diagnostic question: "Are underlying motor problems influencing these simplification rules and production difficulties?" The clinician referred Steve to an occupational therapist (OT), who began serving in a consultative role with the AR team. The OT had experience with deaf children, and was sensitive to the motor production demands of signing. The OT identified the following problems:

1. Presence of Steve's asymmetric tonic neck reflex (ATNR) at age four years, reflecting an immature central nervous system. Typically, the ATNR disappears in the first few months of life in a normally developing infant (Finnie, 1975).

2. Difficulties with proprioceptive perception (e.g., knowing what position the hand is in when not looking at it) and motor planning.

3. Reduced proximal trunk stability, making skilled distal movements of the hand difficult.

4. Overflow of movement from one side of the body to another, causing associated reactions and making it hard to isolate movement on one part of the body or move one limb differently from the other.
5. Tendency to avoid crossing the midline of the body.

Management: Sign Communication Rehabilitation

The clinician made the decision to address the motor production of signs as a primary intervention target because:

1. These problems were affecting conversational initiations and communicative success. Although the child was attempting to initiate social conversation with others, his signs were often misinterpreted or misunderstood, leading to frustration and social isolation.
2. The errors appeared to have a consistent rule base, which might allow for a process-oriented intervention that could result in system-wide change. That is, if his phonological rules could be changed, several errors could be modified at the same time.

An individualized intervention was designed to address the motor sign-production problems and needs. Given the constellation of motor problems, the clinician first employed successive approximation strategies. Her goal was to implement motor changes from the easiest change to those that would require more complex motor patterns. She took her lead in developing an intervention hierarchy from tracking the child's daily progress. The therapy program implemented a phonological process approach. Rather than address each error singly, the clinician worked on clusters of phonemes to try to bring about changes in the phonological rule structure (e.g., worked on all handshapes that required flexion of the hand and two or more fingers extended and spread).

Many developmental activities were implemented to give Steve natural opportunities to explore new motor patterns. For example, play with finger puppets on several fingers helped him learned to isolate fingers while flexing the fist. Matching the clinician's handshapes in plaster of paris or in fingerpaint gave him increased proprioceptive cues about new productive forms. Playful interaction games gave him large numbers of trials with target forms (e.g., play with various vehicles and with number games gave him opportunities to practice the *3* handshape, which he later used productively as a number or as a classifier for *VEHICLE-MOVING*). Breakdown-buildup strategies were useful in helping him understand complex patterns. When a sign required him to reverse the path, the clinician would break the task down for him by positioning herself beside him, allowing him to mirror the path. He was led through successive activities until he could successfully reverse the path. Similarly, signs that required midline crossing were produced in steps. He was asked to copy the clinician holding claw-hands side by side on the table for the sign *SPIDER*. Then he copied the action of crossing, and next copied the action of moving them forward. Later in intervention, he was expected to integrate the three motor patterns involved in this action. Minimal contrasts also helped Steve modify his signing behaviors. An activity was set up where letter cards of *F* were contrasted with small bags of three stickers. When Steve wanted the three stickers, but produced F, he received the letter card. He was motivated to win the stickers and quickly adjusted his handshape to communicate his desire clearly.

The teacher, the parents and the OT were involved directly in the therapy program to ensure generalization of concepts to all intervention contexts. Through teamwork, all communication partners had the information they needed to adjust their expectations for Steve's phonological productions in sign.

Outcome Measures

Sessions were held three times weekly for a period of four months. Therapy data logs and post testing on untrained stimuli revealed the following results:

1. All target handshapes were produced accurately in spontaneous conversational contexts.
2. Changes in handshapes were maintained six months after diagnostic therapy was terminated.
3. Steve improved significantly in sign intelligibility and frequency of initiation of signed messages.
4. Bilateral coordination of signs was labored and continued to require intervention. A consultative approach to intervention in the classroom was employed to resolve remaining concerns.

Summary

The results of this case underscore the importance of professional collaboration in solving complex problems. The case further illustrates the value in implementing a diagnostic teaching approach where theory informs practice, and strategies and questions are continually modified to bring about positive results.

REFERENCES AND RECOMMENDED READINGS

Battison, R. (1978). *Lexical borrowing in American Sign Language*. Silver Spring, MD: Linstok Press.

Chapman, R. (1978). Comprehension strategies in children. In J. Kavanagh & P. Strange (Eds.), *Language and speech in the laboratory, school and clinic*. Cambridge, MA: MIT Press.

Communication and Symbolic Behavior Scales (1993). A. Wetherby & B. Prizant. Chicago, IL: Special Press, Inc.

Cross, T. (1984). Habilitating the language impaired child: Ideas from the studies of parent-child interactions. *Topics in Language Disorders*, 1–13.

Dale, P., & Thal, D. MacArthur Communicative Development Inventory (1993) (Infant and Toddler Scales used). Center for Research in Language, UCSD, San Diego, CA.

Edwards, M. L., & Shriberg, L. D. (1983). *Phonology: Applications in communicative disorders*. San Diego: College-Hill Press.

Finnie, N. R. (1975). *Handling the young cerebral palsied child at home*. New York: Dutton.

Hodson, B. W. (1980). *The assessment of phonological processes*. Danville, IL: Interstate Printers and Publishers.

Manolson, A. (1992). *It takes two to talk* (3rd ed.). Toronto, Ontario, Canada: Hanen Early Language Resource Centre.

Moeller, M. P. (1988). Combining formal and informal strategies for language assessment of hearing-impaired children [Monograph]. In R. R. Kretschmer, Jr., & L. W. Kretschmer (Eds.), *The Journal of the Academy of Rehabilitative Audiology. 21*(Suppl.), 73–101.

Moeller, M. P. & Carney, A. E. (1993). Assessment and intervention with preschool hearing-impaired children. In J. G. Alpiner & P. A. McCarthy (Eds.), *Rehabilitative audiology: Children and adults* (pp. 106–136). Baltimore: Williams & Wilkins.

Moeller, M. P. & Condon, M. C. (1994). D.E.I.P.: A collaborative problem-solving approach to early intervention. In J. Roush & N. D. Matkin (Eds.), *Infants and toddlers with hearing loss* (pp. 163-194). Baltimore: York Press, Inc.

Moeller, M. P., Coufal, K., & Hixson, P. (1990). The efficacy of speech-language intervention: Hearing impaired children. *Seminars in Speech and Language, 11*(4), 227–241.

Moeller, M. P., Osberger, M. J., & Eccarius, M. (1986). Cognitively based strategies for use with hearing-impaired students with comprehension deficits. *TLD, 6*(4), 37–50. Aspen Publishers, Inc.

Roush, J. & Matkin, N. D. (1994). *Infants and toddlers with hearing loss*. Baltimore: York Press.

Schildroth, A. M., & Hotto, S. A. (1993). Annual survey of hearing impaired children and youth: 1991-92 school year. *American Annals of the Deaf, 138*(2), 163–171.

12

Case Studies: Adults/Elderly Adults

MICHAEL A. NERBONNE
THAYNE C. SMEDLEY
CARL A. BINNIE
ALICE E. HOLMES
RONALD L. SCHOW

Contents

INTRODUCTION

The five adult/elderly cases of audiologic rehabilitation described in this chapter involve a wide range of clients with hearing impairment, in terms of both age and communication-related difficulties. While special adjustments must be considered with certain elderly patients such as those found in nursing homes (see Case 5), in general, both adult and elderly persons will most often demonstrate the same kinds of communication problems and, therefore, be candidates for similar rehabilitation strategies. Thus, we have grouped these younger and older cases together and presented them in the same chapter. Although references are made to group therapy (as detailed in Chapter 13 and in Cases 1, 3, and 4), the major emphasis with each case is on addressing the specific, unique problems with which each of these individuals is wrestling. Some of these problems relate as much to psychosocial influences as to auditory effects. Such influences need to be acknowledged in AR approaches.

Although a major goal for each case was to reduce communication-related difficulties, the specific audiologic strategies varied for each client depending on individual needs and motivation. The sampling of cases presented here ranges from involvement in hearing-aid selection and orientation/counseling to traditional and computer-assisted forms of individual and group communication rehabilitation. In addition, the pre- and post-implantation AR process for a challenging cochlear implant recipient is presented.

In the course of performing audiologic rehabilitation, the audiologist may encounter the wide range of cases described here. We hope that these cases will give some insights into the challenges and possibilities of this work. In general, the model followed here is the one detailed in the introductory chapter of this text. The model involves both assessment and management phases as part of the total audiologic rehabilitation process.

A variety of pre- and post-AR tests were used in an attempt to objectify the status of the clients during the assessment and management phases of therapy. Self-assessment tools are receiving increased emphasis in AR and several different communication assessment instruments have been used here, including both screening and diagnostic tools. Also, real-ear (probe-tube microphone) measures are used with some cases, demonstrating the utility of this tool in the rehabilitation process. No single test battery is recommended; nor is it implied that one is best for all purposes. Instead, clinicians must select the tests that will be useful for determining the exact needs of the client, assisting in specific therapy strategies, and measuring the results of management. In addition to the tests and procedures used in this chapter, the reader may refer to numerous other chapters throughout the book, particularly Chapter 13, for other relevant test and resource materials which may be useful in AR.

Even though all cases included here are based directly on real persons, minor adjustments have been made in the names used and the material presented in order to maintain the anonymity of our clients.

CASE 1—DR. M.: PROGRESSIVE HEARING LOSS

Case History

Dr. M. was a 69-year-old man who had retired four years earlier after a 40-year career as a college professor. He reported experiencing frequent difficulties in hearing, particularly at church, social functions, and plays that he and his spouse attended at the university's theater. Dr. M. had noted being aware of hearing difficulties for some time, including the last couple of years of his teaching career. The onset of his impairment was reportedly gradual and seemed to affect both ears equally.

Audiologic Rehabilitation Assessment

Figure 12.1 contains the audiometric results obtained with Dr. M. In general, he was found to possess a mild to moderate sensorineural hearing loss bilaterally. The results of speech audiometry were consistent with the pure-tone findings and indicated that Dr. M. was experiencing significant difficulty in speech perception, especially if speech stimuli were presented at a typical conversation level (50 dB HL).

The Self-Assessment of Communication (SAC) and Significant Other Assessment of Communication (SOAC) (Schow & Nerbonne, 1982) screening inventories were administered to Dr. M. and his spouse to gather further information concerning the degree of perceived hearing handicap resulting from Dr. M.'s hearing loss. Using both of these measures provides valuable information about how hearing-impaired persons view their hearing problems, as well as potentially valuable insights from the person who is communicating with the individual on a regular basis. Scores of 50 and 60% (raw scores: 30, 34) on SAC and SOAC tests presented a consistent pattern which, when evaluated according to recent research (see Table 12.1), provided further evidence that Dr. M. was experiencing considerable hearing-related difficulties (Schow, Brockett, Sturmak, & Longhurst, 1989; Sturmak, 1987).

On the basis of these test results and the patient's comments, a hearing-aid evaluation was recommended and scheduled.

Management

Hearing Aid Evaluation/Adjustment.   Prior to any testing associated with hearing aids, Dr. M. was advised about the option of utilizing behind-the-ear or in-the-ear style hearing aids. Like most individuals facing this choice, Dr. M. expressed a clear preference for the in-the-ear style. Dr. M. was also advised that, because of the severity of his hearing loss and other factors such as improved localization abilities, binaural hearing aids would be advisable.

Audiological Record

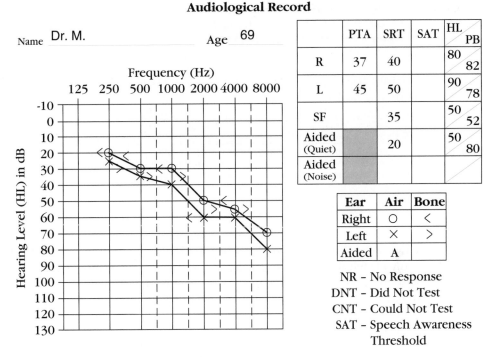

Name Dr. M.   Age 69

Frequency (Hz)

	PTA	SRT	SAT	HL / PB
R	37	40		80 / 82
L	45	50		90 / 78
SF		35		50 / 52
Aided (Quiet)		20		50 / 80
Aided (Noise)				

Ear	Air	Bone
Right	O	<
Left	×	>
Aided	A	

NR – No Response
DNT – Did Not Test
CNT – Could Not Test
SAT – Speech Awareness
          Threshold

Figure 12.1 Audiometric results for Dr. M., Case 1.

The hearing aid evaluation consisted of a series of probe-tube microphone real-ear measures with each ear, as well as soundfield speech audiometry. Data from the audiogram and real-ear measures were applied to an existing prescription approach (Libby, 1986) to determine the desired gain, frequency reponse and SSPL-90 values for the hearing aids to be fit in the right and left ears. This resulted in two ITE hearing aids being recommended with moderate gain and high-frequency emphasis. Venting of each unit was also deemed appropriate. Earmold impressions were taken and an appointment was scheduled for Dr. M. to be fit with his new aids once they were received from the manufacturer.

Dr. M. was fitted with his hearing aids at the next session and real-ear measures were taken to confirm the appropriateness of the insertion gain and SSPL-90 values for each unit. Soundfield speech audiometry was also used to evaluate further the degree of improvement provided by the binaural system. As seen in Figure 12.1, Dr. M.'s speech reception thresholds and speech recognition score improved significantly with the in-the-ear hearing aids. His comments concerning the aids were favorable and no further adjustments were made with either hearing aid. Following a thorough orientation to the operation and care of his new aids, Dr. M. was advised to return for subsequent follow-up appointments.

TABLE 12.1 *Categories and Associated Scores for Classifying Primary and Secondary Effects of Hearing Loss (Hearing Disability/Handicap) when Using the SAC and SOAC*

Category	Raw Scores	Percentage Scores
No Disability/Handicap	10–18	0–20
Slight Hearing Disability/Handicap	19–26	21–40
Mild-Moderate Hearing Disability/Handicap	27–38	41–70
Severe Hearing Disability/Handicap	39–50	71–100

Adapted from "Hearing Handicap Scores and Categories for Subjects with Normal and Impaired Hearing Sensitivity" by R. Schow and C. Tannahill, 1977, *Journal of the American Audiological Society, 3* pp.134–139. Also from *Communication Handicap Score Interpretation for Various Populations and Degrees of Hearing Impairment* by M.J. Sturmak, 1987, master's thesis, Idaho State University, and Schow, et al., 1989.

Dr. M.'s experience with his new hearing aids was, for the most part, positive. While still noting some problems hearing in group situations and at the theater, he definitely felt that the hearing aids were assisting him. Further discussion with Dr. M. regarding his hearing difficulties at the theater revealed that he had not yet tried the facility's infrared listening system. Encouraging him to do so, the audiologist explained the manner in which the system functions, as well as how Dr. M. could use the infrared receiver either with his hearing aids or as a stand-alone unit. Subsequent contact with Dr. M. revealed that he found the assistive listening device to be remarkably helpful.

While Dr. M. had adjusted well to his hearing aids and received substantial improvement as a result of their use, he did note some persistent communication difficulties. Because of this and his motivation for improvement, Dr. M. agreed to enroll in a short-term group audiologic rehabilitation program for adults.

Communication Training. Dr. M. was one of eight hearing-impaired adults who participated in the weekly group sessions. Although the activities and areas of emphasis varied somewhat as a result of the interests and needs of each group of participants, the main components of the program generally followed those outlined in Chapter 13 by Giolas. The individuals participating with Dr. M. were new hearing aid users with mild-to-moderate hearing losses. Consequently, emphasis was placed on the effective use of hearing aids, care and maintenance of the systems, and the way hearing aids can be supplemented by one or more types of assistive listening devices. Attention was also given to developing more effective listening skills and capitalizing on the visual information available in most communication situations. Interaction among the group participants was encouraged, and valuable information on a variety of topics was shared at each session.

Following the final session, Dr. M. stated that the sessions had been helpful to him. In addition to the practical information provided, such as where to buy batteries for his hearing aids and the use of hearing aids with the telephone, Dr. M. felt that a number of the communication strategies covered had been of benefit to him. The net result was that he felt much more confident when communicating with others.

Summary

It was clear from the start that Dr. M. had accepted his hearing problem and was motivated to seek out whatever assistance was available to him. His positive and cooperative behaviors, which would be categorized by Goldstein and Stephens (1981) as an example of a Type I attitude (see Chapter 9), facilitated the audiologic rehabilitation process and impacted positively on Dr. M.'s overall communication abilities. Motivation should be recognized as a key ingredient in successful audiologic rehabilitation with any individual with hearing impairment.

CASE 2—MRS. B.: HEARING-AID ORIENTATION WITH UPGRADED FITTING

Case History

Mrs. B. is a 69-year-old homemaker who previously had been referred by a local otologist for audiological services and hearing-aid consultation. Chart notes indicate a longstanding hearing loss going back several years, with reports of increased hearing difficulties during the past year. A linear circuit in-the-ear (ITE) style hearing aid had been fitted on the left ear with partial success. Mrs. B. used the hearing aid on a fairly regular basis, reported considerable benefit in most situations, but continued to complain that loud voices were bothersome, and use of the hearing aid "made her nervous." Another comment revealed, "The hearing aid does help, but speech through the hearing aid doesn't sound natural. I wear it but it nearly drives me crazy."

More recently, Mrs. B. returned to the audiologist to investigate advertised reports of improved hearing-aid technology and the possibility of acquiring a more satisfactory fitting. Patient interest focused on left-ear rehabilitation ("I think my right ear is OK"). The cost of new hearing aids, while of interest, was not a major concern in the discussion of new instruments.

Diagnostic Information

Mrs. B's audiogram is shown in Figure 12.2. Pure-tone and speech thresholds show a fairly symmetrical, bilateral mild to moderate sensorineural hearing loss. A slight conductive component shown in earlier testing had resolved by the time of the most recent examination. Speech recognition scores showed mildly impaired receptive

Audiological Record

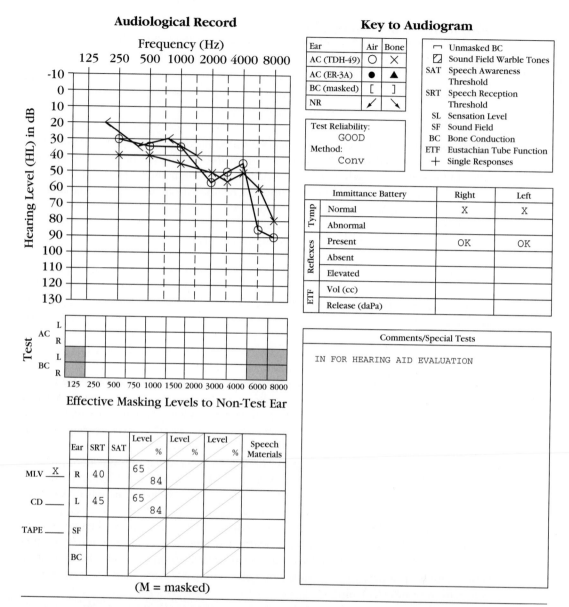

Figure 12.2 Audiogram for Mrs. B., Case 2.

communication skills. Other test data indicated elevated comfortable listening levels and a reduced dynamic range. Communication problems were quantified using the SAC and SOAC screening strategies (Schow & Nerbonne, 1982). These questionnaires revealed a high amount of communication difficulty as perceived by Mrs. B (70%; raw score of 38), and an even higher amount as reported by her husband on the SOAC (80%; raw score of 42).

Rehabilitation Assessment

Psychosocial History. Mrs. B keeps very busy with a variety of activities. She attempts to maintain a full social schedule, is active in a civic club and her church, and regularly attends recreational and entertainment events with her husband, a retired banker. However, she reports feeling constrained in her desires for full participation because of poor hearing. Hearing complaints from Mrs. B., based on both informal as well as formal assessment (SAC), included listening strain in group situations, difficulties following conversation on the telephone and at the movie theater, and reduced tolerance for loud sounds.

Management

Amplification Refitting. Her present hearing aid, while helpful, provided limited benefit. She reported that use of the hearing aid allowed her to view television at levels more acceptable to her husband, but in most other communicative situations she experienced annoyance and irritability because she did not hear well. Group listening situations caused the greatest aggravation. She expressed strong motivation for improved hearing.

Electroacoustic analysis of her existing instrument showed the hearing aid to be operating within tolerances of the original manufacturer's specifications. Further, the ANSI (coupler) gain and maximum output seemed reasonably appropriate for the degree and configuration of hearing loss, an observation confirmed with real-ear, sound-field (functional gain) measures. The client's concerns with this hearing aid seemed to have more to do with the quality than with the quantity of amplified sound.

The possibility that a different type of instrument might offer greater satisfaction was then explored with Mrs. B., including a discussion of programmable, multi-channel compression instruments in both the ITE and BTE styles. Attention was also given to a discussion of the advantages of binaural over monaural hearing. Cosmetic issues were also dealt with when she immediately objected to the prospect of the use of hearing aids larger than her present aid, especially if they were to be in both ears. With further discussion, however, the resistance diminished and Mrs. B. finally consented to a 45-day trial with new BTE hearing aids fitted to both ears. BTE aids were selected over what Mrs. B considered to be the more obtrusive ITE style. Instruments were selected which offered full dynamic-range compression, in each of two (low and high) frequency channels. The instruments also provided a variable crossover frequency which could be adjusted to shape the desirable response slope. Instrument programming was done through computer input. The hearing aids were attached to a pair of small, canal-lock type clear lucite custom ear molds with 3-mm. vents. Because the cost of the new hearing aids represented more than a four-time increase in expenditure compared with her previous hearing aid, acquisition costs were carefully reviewed with both Mrs. B and her spouse. The price of the hearing aids was not seen as a major issue, but some concerns were expressed at this point over their high cost. These concerns, however, were alleviated with a review of the office "trial" program and the contractual agreement to refund 85% of the price of the hearing aids if they were found to be unacceptable after 45 days' use.

Amplification Orientation/Counseling. At the initial fitting, following the appropriate instrument programming, Mrs. B's response to the new instruments was immediate and dramatic. After only a few moments of conversation, Mrs. B exclaimed, "These aids are wonderful! I can hear so much better, and speech sounds natural; and I sense a balance of hearing I did not have with the other hearing aid!" Cautioned against a possible Hawthorne effect, which involves being very impressed with something new, Mrs. B. was counseled regarding realistic expectations, especially in less favorable acoustic environments. Further counseling included a review of hearing-aid care and operation, battery drain (probably 30% more than with the previous aid), and telephone use. Additionally, instruction in optimizing communication strategies was provided in a brief session similar in content to a program recently described by Montgomery (1994).

At the first follow-up visit one week later, Mrs. B. continued to express enthusiasm for the new hearing aids. She reported improved hearing in virtually all situations. She also expressed appreciation for her added knowledge and skills in dealing with the more difficult situations. Noisy environments continued to be bothersome, but not to the degree reported with her previous aid. She was especially impressed that she could now hear soft voices with less strain, and loud voice levels were not objectionable. Another important observation was that her husband had also noted a dramatic change in her hearing and communication ability, as well even as an improvement in temperament. She reported that, "He says I am less irritable and more pleasant to be around. He says he thinks he's married to a different woman!"

Real-ear probe-tube microphone measures taken during the second visit verified a satisfactory fit (re NAL targets) and a functioning full-range compression system (see Figure 12.3). Mrs. B. continued to express great satisfaction with her new hearing aids over the remaining two follow-up visits and made final purchase of the instruments. SAC and SOAC self-report, re-measured at the close of the 45-day trial period, showed a significant improvement from 70% to 35% for SAC, and from 80% to 30% for SOAC, differences beyond the 95% confidence level (Short, 1982; Schow, 1995).

Summary

This case illustrates a rehabilitation strategy that focuses on hearing-aid amplification, combined with AR efforts and counseling. Many older adult hearing-aid wearers complain bitterly about their hearing aids (Smedley & Schow, 1990) and do not achieve the level of satisfaction enjoyed by users of other types of prostheses (Smedley, 1990). The audiologist needs to recognize that more recent technology, when

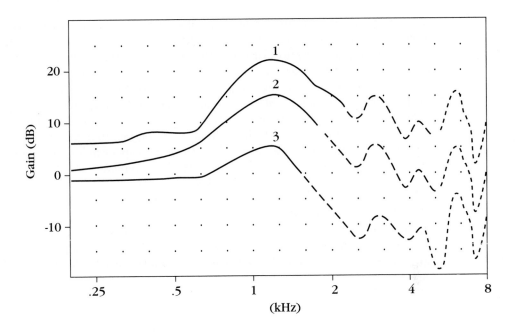

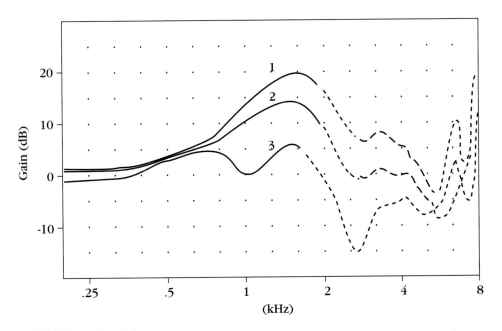

Figure 12.3 Insertion gain as a function of input SPL (1=50 dB; 2=70 dB; 3=90 dB), for right (upper) and left (lower) ears.

accompanied with effective counseling and training, may help many of these people achieve a higher level of benefit and satisfaction.

The hearing-aid features that resulted in a remarkable improvement in hearing-aid satisfaction in this case are both obvious and subtle. One obvious feature of the new instruments is the manner by which loudness is controlled. Controlling hearing-aid output so that sound is always contained within the tolerance limits of the user is viewed by Mueller and Bright (1994) as the most critical element in hearing-aid fitting. Linear amplification with peak clipping, in contrast to some form of compression, is known to have poor control over loudness, especially in sensorineural hearing loss (Dillon, 1988). A current view of the ideal amplifier is one that makes soft sounds and soft speech audible to the listener with hearing impairment; sounds and speech that are comfortably loud to the normal ear should sound comfortably loud to the amplified ear; and sounds judged as loud by the normal ear should be perceived as loud, but not uncomfortable, by the ear showing impairment (Independent Hearing Aid Fitting Forum, 1994). New compression technology provides much greater control of loudness variables and the benefits which result were evident in this case.

For a number of years, use of binaural amplification has been known to provide advantages in hearing not available through a monaural fitting (Byrne, 1980). These advantages include sound localization, binaural loudness summation, and improved speech recognition in noise. This case identifies another feature often seen clinically that relates to a sense of improved "auditory balance" when both ears are amplified.

Other acoustic aspects of hearing-aid amplification not routinely measured may provide more subtle influences on hearing-aid satisfaction. According to McCandless (1994), such influences may include differences in harmonic or other forms of distortion, damping characteristics, frequency bandwidth, or smoothness of the gain curve. Limited "headroom" (the dB difference between hearing-aid gain plus input, and saturation level) is also more of a problem in linear circuits and can contribute to poor sound quality (Preves & Newton 1989).

In conclusion, fitting new-technology hearing aids can result in a dramatic improvement in hearing-aid benefit, as illustrated in this case. However, carefully applied instrumentation needs to accompany the required hearing-aid orientation and appropriate follow-up, to ensure a favorable outcome. Further, self-report and real ear measures allow a more formal documentation of benefit (outcome measures) that go well beyond the anecdotal reports of an earlier era.

CASE 3—MRS. A.: COMPUTER-ASSISTED AUDIOLOGIC REHABILITATION

Case History

Mrs. A. is a 68-year-old female patient who was referred for individual communication training by an audiologist in private practice because of the availability of skill-building instrumentation in the form of interactive video at our facility. This patient first experienced a communication deficit in 1982 and has been wearing hearing instruments since that time. She was recently fitted with digital programmable behind-the-ear instruments, worn in a binaural arrangement. The case history interview revealed that this patient was experiencing significant communication problems in the presence of background noise. Specifically, she reported experiencing difficulty monitoring the intensity of her voice in group situations and indicated that she frequently interrupted other speakers when she failed to understand the spoken message.

Assessment Information

Results from an audiologic assessment revealed a bilateral, moderately severe sensorineural hearing loss with fair word recognition scores in quiet, and poor performance in noise, using NU Auditory Test #6 word lists presented at 20-dB sensation level (RE:SRT), which was her most comfortable level. A copy of the audiogram is shown in Figure 12.4.

This patient completed the Communication Profile for the Hearing Impaired (CPHI) (Demorest & Erdman, 1986) which indicated that she rated herself as being able to communicate effectively about 50% of the time in social, home, average and adverse communication situations. However, it also demonstrated that she felt a strong desire to communicate more effectively in these situations and experienced

Audiometric Evaluation

Name Mrs. A.

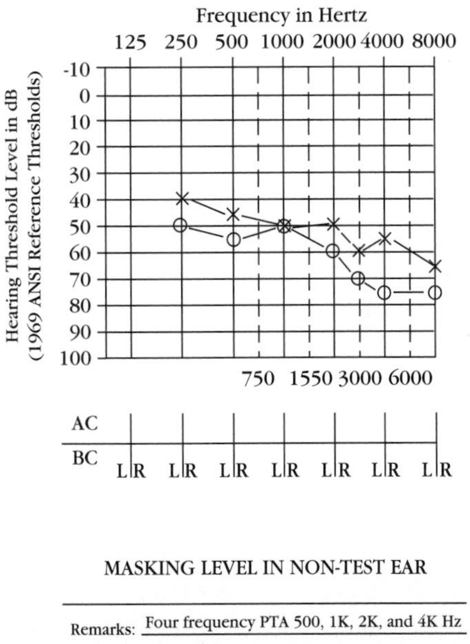

PURE TONE AVERAGE
(500 – 2000 Hz)

Ear	
Right	Left
60	50

SPEECH AUDIOMETRY

	R		L		SF	LV or Rec
SRT	55	Masking	55	Masking	50	
PB in Quiet	70 / 20	ML / SL	72 / 20	ML / SL		
PB in Noise	54 / 20	ML / +8	50 / 20	ML / S-N		
MCL	75		75			
UCL	95		95			

MASKING LEVEL IN NON-TEST EAR

Remarks: Four frequency PTA 500, 1K, 2K, and 4K Hz

Figure 12.4. Audiometric results for Mrs. A., Case 3.

feelings of depression, frustration, discouragement, inadequacy, and apathy when communication breakdowns occurred.

This patient's auditory and auditory-visual speech perception skills were evaluated in quiet and noise using the Connected Speech Test (CST) (Cox, Alexander, Gilmore, & Pusakulich, 1988) which is a laserdisc and interactive video system. Prior to completing the testing, however, the patient passed a vision screening at 20/30. A total of four paragraphs were presented while she wore her hearing instruments set at the most comfortable listening level for a 70-dB SPL signal. Scores were obtained for each of the conditions with the following results: (1) Auditory only: 97% in quiet and 56% in noise (+4 dB S/N ratio); (2) Auditory-Visual: 97% in the noise condition. This indicated an excellent visual enhancement score of approximately 40 percent. It was felt that this patient had developed excellent auditory-visual speech perception performance and that further skill-building efforts should focus on communication strategies designed to facilitate understanding in those situations when she experienced a communication breakdown. She agreed to participate in a short-term skill-building program, described below.

Audiologic Rehabilitation

Five goals were established for this patient's individual communication training program. These were:

1. Increasing the patient's overall level of assertiveness when communicating in group situations.
2. Educating the patient about the use of more effective anticipatory and repair strategies.
3. Establishing realistic communication expectations in noisy group situations in order to reduce emotional stress.
4. Reducing the intensity of her voice in group situations.
5. Decreasing the number of times she interrupted a speaker in group situations.

Several synthetically-oriented activities were employed during the skill-building portion of the communication training sessions. The first included reviewing and discussing effective ways to employ appropriate anticipatory and repair strategies. In addition, the two notions that the "gist" of the message was more critical than understanding each word in every sentence, and that complete comprehension of the spoken message was not realistic in every situation, were reinforced. To bolster the use of these techniques and to present ways to grasp the general concept being conveyed in a conversation, handouts and a book, *Coping with Hearing Loss*, by Rezen and Hausman (1985), were provided.

A second activity incorporated QUEST?AR (Erber, 1988) to provide the patient with the opportunity to practice her various repair strategies. An adverse listening environment was created by introducing speech babble along with the use of poor speaker speech behaviors (e.g., hand covering mouth, increased rate, reduced volume).

A third activity included the use of the interactive video program, CASPER (A computer-assisted system for speech-perception testing and training, A. Boothroyd, 1987). Several such programs have been developed to assist in the development of auditory-visual speech perception. Continuous discourse tracking is one method used to train speech perception. CASPER allows for the testing and training of auditory-visual presentations of paragraph material. The stimuli were presented via laserdisc controlled by a computer. In this case, the auditory stimuli were presented at her speech-detection thresholds and with full video. Verbatim responses were required and were assisted by computer-controlled feedback. Scores were calculated in percent correct and in words per minute. This patient participated in four short-term skill-building exercises with two paragraphs presented in each session. Other activities described above were interspersed into the communication training program.

Results

The results from the CASPER interactive video computer-assisted speech tracking program indicated that this patient increased her performance for the four training sessions. Percent correct scores ranged from 34% in session 1 to 61% in session 4, and word-per-minute rate increased from 21 to 28. It was felt that this interactive video approach was an excellent option to enhance auditory-visual speech performance for contextually-based stimuli.

In addition to the results from CASPER, this patient reported an increase in the use of repair strategies in group situations. It was recommended that she participate in our four-week group communication training program with her husband and several other couples so that her communication performance could be monitored. She agreed to this and demonstrated very good use of those communication skills developed in her individual skill-building program.

Summary

This case demonstrates how computerized technology can be incorporated into an overall program of audiologic rehabilitation for some adults. In this case, individualized attention directed toward enhancing auditory-visual speech perception was successfully carried out with CASPER, and this was followed up by additional communication skill building of a related nature in a short-term, group program.

CASE 4—MRS. W.: COCHLEAR IMPLANT USER

Case History

Mrs. W. was a 58-year-old office worker who had a profound sensorineural hearing loss for approximately ten years. She reported that her hearing loss was sudden in onset, with unknown etiology. She wore binaural behind-the-ear (BTE) hearing aids, which she stated helped her perceive pauses in speech, and some intonation cues. Mrs. W. indicated that her hearing loss was severely affecting her interactions with co-

Audiometric Evaluation

Name: **Mrs. W.**   Evaluator:_____

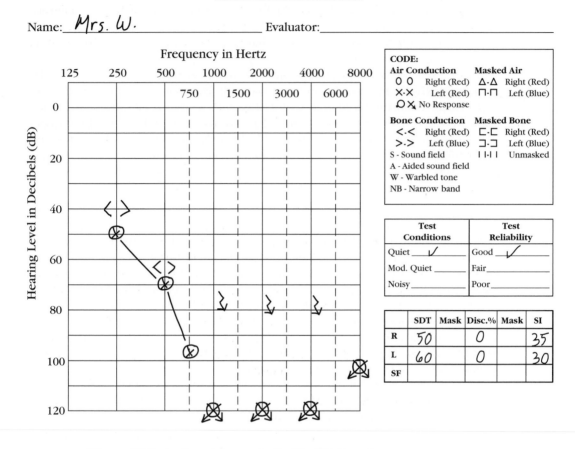

Figure 12.5 Audiometric results for Mrs. W., Case 4.

workers and supervisors in her job setting. Her speech was very intelligible and her vision and overall health were good. Mrs. W. was seen initially for an evaluation for cochlear implant (CI) candidacy and speechreading therapy. According to the otologist on the CI team, Mrs. W. was a medically suitable candidate for CI surgery.

Diagnostic Information

Audiometric evaluation revealed a bilateral sensorineural hearing loss (Figure 12.5). Pure-tone thresholds were obtained at 50 dB HL at 250 Hz, 70 dB HL at 500 Hz, and 95 dB HL at 750 Hz bilaterally. Mrs. W. was unable to respond to pure-tone stimuli at the limits of the audiometer above 750 Hz. Speech-detection thresholds were obtained at 50 and 60 dB HL in the right and left ears respectively. Her word recognition scores were 0% in both ears.

Further aided evaluation was completed with Mrs. W. using selected closed-set subsets of the Minimal Auditory Capabilities Batteries (MAC)(Owens, Kessler, Telleen, &

Schubert, 1981). She scored 42% on the Number of Syllables, 63% on the Noise/Voice, 60% on the Four Choice Spondee and 80% on the Spondee Same/Different Subtests. Using closed-set consonant and vowel recognition tasks, Mrs. W. repeated 63% of key words of the CID Everyday Sentences when using both vision and her BTE hearing aids.

Paper and pencil questionnaires were given to Mrs. W. and her husband to ascertain their expectations for a CI. Both Mr. and Mrs. W. indicated that they hoped the implant would enable Mrs. W. to use the telephone and to improve her communication abilities at home and at the office. Mrs. W. expected the implant to enable her to "hide" her hearing loss, and that after surgery most people would not suspect that she had a hearing impairment.

Pre-CI Management

Psychosocial/Counseling. Mrs. W. appeared to be a good candidate for a CI from the results of the pure-tone and speech-perception tests. However, it was apparent that she had unrealistic expectations. Extensive counseling was given to both Mr. and Mrs. W. on the limitations and benefits of the implant. They were told that the CI was designed as an aid to speechreading, not a replacement for visual cues. The CI would not give her normal hearing and she would need to inform her communication partners that she had a hearing loss. It was explained that the majority of patients with CIs need visual cues to communicate and that telephone communication would continue to be a problem with an implant. Mrs. W. was put in contact with two current CI users who answered many of her questions.

Communication Rehabilitation. It was recommended that Mrs. W. receive communication therapy prior to surgery. She attended five sessions that focused on communication repair and anticipatory strategies. Discussions on ways to modify the environment and use of nonverbal cues were also included. During these sessions, continued counseling was completed on the benefits and limitations of the implant.

Overall Coordination. Following the completion of this therapy and after CI expectations were re-evaluated, recommendations for surgery were given. Mr. and Mrs. W. demonstrated a better understanding of the benefits and long-range therapy goals for CI use. Mrs. W. was successfully implanted with a multichannel CI. All 22 electrodes were inserted with no complications.

Post-CI Management

Amplification. Five weeks after surgery, Mrs. W. returned for electrical stimulation of her CI and follow-up therapy. The protocol from the Cochlear Corporation Rehabilitation Manual (1994) was followed. Initially, Mrs. W. was seen on two consecutive days to program the CI processor and then on a weekly basis for the next three months for therapy and fine-tuning of her speech processor. Threshold and maximum comfort levels were obtained for each of her active electrodes. A speech-processing program or MAP using a feature extraction strategy was made and saved into her speech processor. Continued monitoring of her threshold and comfort levels and subsequent map modifications were made throughout her therapy sessions.

Audio-Visual Training. Therapy sessions consisted of training Mrs. W. in a hierarchy of auditory skills including sound detection, word and sentence-length discrimination and identification, pattern discrimination and identification in phrases and sentences, and identification of overlearned speech (common expressions). Drill work using consonant and vowel stimuli in auditory-only and auditory/visual modes was also used in each session. Her auditory-only vowel and consonant recognition improved from a pre-CI score of 8% to a post-CI score of 48%. Through speech tracking (DeFilippo & Scott, 1978), Mrs. W. practiced using the CI along with visual cues in understanding running speech. The use of communication strategies was stressed and practiced during the tracking exercises. Her tracking rates increased from a pre-CI score of 11.7 words per minute (wpm) to a post-CI score of 40.7 wpm. After two months of therapy, telephone use was introduced, using codes and overlearned speech. Mrs. W. found she could communicate with her husband and two other familiar individuals on the phone but for most people she needed to use codes, as described by Castle (1988). A TDD was recommended and she was taught to use a relay network, rather than her CI, for most of her telephone communications.

Counseling/Overall Coordination. Throughout the therapy sessions, Mrs. W. kept an ongoing diary of her experiences with the CI. She listed wearing times, environmental sounds heard, and communication situations. From her diary it was apparent that Mrs. W. was initially very disappointed with the CI. Even though she had tempered her expectations of the CI, she had still maintained hope that she would function as a person with normal hearing. The diary served as a focal point of behavioral counseling. Specific problems were discussed, pointing out both the benefits and limitations of the CI, along with possible strategies she might use in each situation. For example, she stated frustration with conversing in noisy places such as her car and restaurants. It was recommended that she use her external microphone in such situations to minimize the background noise. Interestingly, she did not realize how much benefit she was getting from the implant until she had some minor mechanical problems with her headset and had to go without her implant for one day. After this, her attitude towards the CI and therapy greatly improved in both her diary and in discussions. From her diary, her use of the CI went from eight hours a day, to the time she got up in the morning until the time she went to bed at night.

Her work environment continued to cause problems in communication. A detailed description of her office space revealed that the physical layout of her office prohibited speechreading. Also the acoustics of the environment (office machines, printers, etc.) were not conducive to communication for a person with hearing impairment. After discussions with her supervisor, she was able to make a lateral transfer in her department that allowed her to be in a physical environment that was more favorable to both auditory and visual communication.

Advances in cochlear implants allowed us to upgrade Mrs. W.'s speech processor to a spectral peak coding strategy three years later. She continues to successfully use the auditory cues available to her and has found the new processing strategy particularly beneficial in the presence of background noise.

Summary

Cochlear implants offer an excellent opportunity for postlingually deafened adults to receive beneficial auditory information. Many CI benefits can be seen across patients, from those who have good open-set understanding even on the telephone to those who receive minimal auditory cues. Mrs. W. is representative of an average post-lingually hearing-impaired CI patient. She was able to speechread with greater ease, could identify many more environmental sounds, and had limited telephone skills using the CI. However, she still must rely on speechreading to communicate.

Mrs. W.'s case also illustrates the importance of a full program of pre- and post-AR therapy and counseling with CI candidates and their families. Often, patients expect the CI to be a "bionic ear." Even after their expectations are tempered prior to surgery, like Mrs. W., they may be disappointed that the CI cannot provide "normal" hearing. Audio-visual training and communication strategy therapy help the patients learn to use the CI and deal with communication breakdowns. With appropriate training, the CI can improve the quality of life for an individual with profound hearing impairment.

CASE 5—MRS. E: NURSING HOME HEARING-AID USER

Case History

Mrs. E. was a 75-year-old resident of a local nursing home. She had been living in the facility for over two years, and was quite alert mentally and able to move about the facility without any special assistance. Mrs. E. was using a hearing aid at the time she was first seen by an audiologist. It was later determined that she had been a long-time hearing aid user, having had four other instruments over a period of many years. Her present hearing aid was five years old and, according to Mrs. E., did not seem to be working as well as it once had.

Diagnostic Information

Initial efforts with Mrs. E. involved air-conduction pure-tone testing and tympanometry in a quiet room within the nursing home. As seen in Figure 12.6, the client had a moderate hearing loss, which was bilaterally symmetrical. Type A tympanograms were traced bilaterally, suggesting the presence of a sensorineural disorder in each ear.

Audiologic Rehabilitation

Mrs. E. was concerned about the condition of her hearing aid, complaining that it did not seem to help her as much as it had in the past. She also appeared to be experiencing

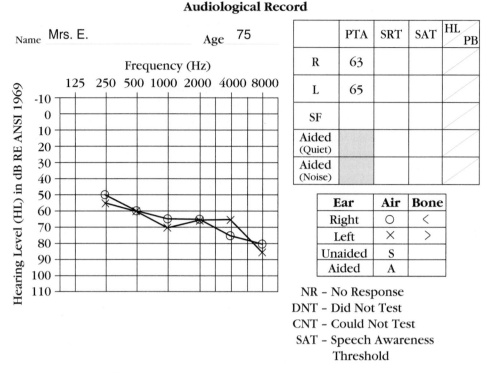

Figure 12.6. Audiometric results for Mrs. E., Case 5.

an excessive amount of acoustic feedback and reported having difficulty getting the ear-mold into her ear properly.

The hearing aid was analyzed electroacoustically by the audiologist and was found to have a reduced gain and an abnormal amount of distortion. In discussing the feasibility of purchasing a new hearing aid, it became clear that Mrs. E. was not finan-cially able to consider such a purchase. She was, therefore, advised to have her hearing aid serviced and reconditioned by the manufacturer. She was agreeable to this recommendation, and arrangements were made for this to occur.

In the course of working with Mrs. E. it became apparent that she needed a new earmold. In discussing this, Mrs. E. recalled that her current mold had also been used with her previous hearing aid. The mold was very discolored and did not appear to fit Mrs. E.'s ear canal and pinna adequately. The audiologist took an ear impression, which was sent to a laboratory for production of a new earmold.

In approximately two weeks, both the earmold and the hearing aid were returned. Mrs. E. was then fit with the reconditioned aid and her initial reaction was quite positive. She was instructed to use the aid as much as possible in the following days. A subsequent electroacoustic analysis of the instrument revealed an increase in gain and a significant improvement in the amount of distortion. Real-ear measures, taken at the nursing home with portable equipment, revealed satisfactory gain.

When she was seen again, Mrs. E. was still pleased with the help she was receiving from her hearing aid, but she indicated that she was still having difficulty inserting the earmold. Watching her attempt to do this herself made it apparent that Mrs. E. was not able to manipulate her hands sufficiently to allow her to insert the mold without great effort. It was also apparent that she was not using an efficient method when inserting the mold. To assist her, Mrs. E. was given some basic instructions on how to best insert and remove the mold. (An example of a training protocol for this purpose is found in Chapter 10.) She was encouraged to practice the procedure and was visited by the audiologist several times during the next 2 weeks to review the procedure, and to answer any questions she might have. During these visits it became apparent that Mrs. E.'s facility in placement of the mold had improved.

Along with the work done with Mrs. E. to improve the way she inserted her mold, several of the nursing home staff members working with Mrs. E. were also provided with information on how to put the earmold in properly. This allowed them to assist Mrs. E. in doing so each day. Both Mrs. E. and the staff also received helpful information on how to clean her earmold and basic instruction on the operation and use of her hearing aid.

Summary

Attempts to help Mrs. E. were successful. This is not always the case when working in a rehabilitative capacity with nursing home residents (Schow, 1982). Mrs. E.'s case illustrates one of the ways in which an audiologist can make a valuable contribution to a number of residents in a given nursing home. It is important first to identify those individuals within the facility for whom audiologic rehabilitation may be beneficial. Once this is done, the audiologist will generally work with each person individually, identifying those areas of AR that should be worked on. Individual needs must be considered, and the audiologist must be willing to devote the time necessary to accomplish the desired ends.

REFERENCES

Boothroyd, A. (1987). CASPER, computer-assisted speech perception evaluation and training. In *Proceedings of the 10th Annual Conference of the Rehabilitation Society of North America*. Washington, DC: Association for the Advancement of Rehabilitation Technology, pp. 734–736.

Byrne, D. (1980). Binaural hearing aid fitting: Research findings and clinical application. In E. Libby (Ed.), *Binaural hearing and amplification* (Vol. 2). Chicago: Zenetron, Inc.

Castle, D. (1988). *Telephone strategies: A technical and practical guide for HOH people*. Bethesda, Md: Self-Help for the HOH.

Cochlear Corporation (1994). *Rehabilitation Manual*. Englewood, CO.

Cox, R., Alexander, G., Gilmore, C., & Pusakulich, K. (1988). Use of the Connected Speech Test (CST) with hearing impaired listeners. *Ear and Hearing, 9*(4), 198–207.

DeFilippo, C., & Scott, B. (1978). A method for training and evaluating the reception of ongoing speech. *Journal of the Acoustical Society of America, 63,* 1186-1192.

Demorest, M., & Erdman, S. (1987). Development of the communication profile for the hearing impaired. *Journal of Speech and Hearing Disorders, 52,* 129-142.

Dillon, H. (1988). Compression in hearing aids. In R. Sandlin (Ed.), *Handbook of hearing aid amplification* (Vol. 1). Boston: College-Hill Press.

Erber, N. (1988). *Communication therapy for hearing impaired adults.* Melbourne, Australia: Clavis.

Goldstein, D., & Stephens, S. (1981). Audiological rehabilitation: Management model I. *Audiology, 20,* 432-452.

Independent Hearing Aid Fitting Forum (1994, August). Presentation at the 1994 Jackson Hole Rendezvous, Jackson Hole, WY.

Libby, E. (1986). The 1/3-2/3 insertion gain hearing aid selection guide. *Hearing Instruments, 37,* 27-28.

McCandless, G. (1994). Overview and rationale of threshold-based hearing aid selection procedures. In M. Valente (Ed.), *Strategies for selecting and verifying hearing aid fittings.* New York: Thieme Medical Publishers, Inc.

Montgomery, A. (1994). WATCH: A practical approach to brief auditory rehabilitation. *Hearing Journal, 47*(10), 10, 53-55.

Mueller, G., & Bright, K. (1994). Selection and verification of maximum output. In M. Valente (Ed.), *Strategies for selecting and verifying hearing aid fittings* . New York: Thieme Medical Publishers, Inc.

Owens, E., Kessler, D., Telleen, C., & Schubert, E. (1981). The minimal auditory capabilities (MAC) battery. *Hearing Journal, 34*(9), 32-34.

Preves, D., & Newton, J. (1989). The headroom problem and hearing aid performance. *Hearing Journal, 42*(10), 21.

Rezen, S., & Hausman, C. (1985). *Coping with hearing loss.* New York: Dembner.

Schow, R. L. (1982). Success of hearing aid fitting in nursing home residents. *Ear and Hearing, 3*(3), 173-177.

Schow, R. L., (1995, May). Status and future of SAC & SOAC: Psychometric studies. Presented at International Collegium of Rehabilitative Audiology, Goteborg. Sweden.

Schow, R. L., & Nerbonne, M. (1982). Communication screening profile: Use with elderly clients. *Ear and Hearing, 3*(3), 133-147.

Schow, R. L., Brockett, J., Sturmak, M., & Longhurst, T. (1989). Self assessment of hearing in rehabilitative audiology: Developments in the U.S.A. *British Journal of Audiology, 23,* 13-24.

Short, B. (1982). Communication ability assessment of an adult hard-of-hearing population. Unpublished master's thesis, Idaho State University.

Smedley, T. (1990). Self-assessed satisfaction levels in elderly hearing aid, eyeglass, and denture wearers. *Ear and Hearing, 11*(5, Suppl.), 41-47.

Smedley, T., & Schow, R. L. (1990). Frustrations with hearing aid use: Candid observations from the elderly. *Hearing Journal, 43*(6), 21-27.

13

Resource Materials

THOMAS G. GIOLAS
NANCY TYE-MURRAY
ADRIENNE KARP
OTHER COLLEAGUES

Contents

INTRODUCTION

This resource chapter brings together a set of supplementary readings from other sources and lists of materials to facilitate audiologic rehabilitation (AR) with children and adults. Several experts in AR have contributed to this chapter.

CONTRIBUTORS

"A Sample Eight-Week Rehabilitation Group Program" (page 508)

Thomas Giolas is the author of two texts on audiologic rehabilitation for adults and has had extensive experience working with adult clients. He has contributed for inclusion here an outline of an eight-week program (one meeting per week) for adult clients. While the length/content of other programs like Giolas's do vary somewhat, those who wish to provide short-term AR to an adult group will find this a useful starting point in organizing such sessions.

"Laser Videodisc Technology in the Aural Rehabilitation Setting: Good News for People with Severe and Profound Hearing Impairments" (page 516)

Nancy Tye-Murray has been a major contributor to the literature in audiologic rehabilitation in the past decade. Her article on the application of laser videodisc technology to AR has been included here to provide the student with information on how this form of instruction/therapy can be applied to work with adults with hearing loss.

"Aural Rehabilitation for the Patient with Visual and Hearing Impairment" (page 521)

Adrienne Karp has worked for many years with persons with visual impairment at the New York Association for the Blind. She has contributed an insightful piece that helps prepare the reader to work with persons with visual impairments, whether this is blindness or reduced vision acuity. Many elderly persons and others with hearing loss have limited vision. In fact, visual impairments often are associated with hearing loss; therefore, it is crucial that AR clinicians be on the alert for undetected visual impairments with any patients with hearing impairment because of the compounding effects when both disabilities are present.

"Aural Rehabilitation by ASHA Audiologists: 1980–1990" (page 529)

Ronald Schow, Navroze Balsara, Thayne Smedley, and *Curtis Whitcomb* collaborated in companion surveys at a decade interval to provide the field with insights into past and present practices in audiologic rehabilitation. Their report has identified a number of significant trends related to how practicing audiologists approach AR with their clients.

"ARA Position Statement on Au.D. Educational Standards" (page 553)

In connection with the establishment of the Doctor of Audiology (Au.D.) degree, a position statement, developed by an ad hoc committee consisting of *Michael Nerbonne* (chair), *Charles Anderson, Linda Burg, Harriet Kaplan*, and *Linda Palmer*, was approved by the membership of ARA in 1993. This statement expresses the need for programs offering the Au.D. degree to include significant academic and clinical coursework/practica in audiologic rehabilitation, and provides general direction to these academic units regarding content areas of AR in which students need to be prepared.

"ASHA Definition of and Competencies for Aural Rehabilitation" (page 555)

Over several years, the ASHA Committee on Rehabilitative Audiology updated a position statement on audiologic rehabilitation, refining the definition of and competencies required to conduct AR. Under the direction of two committee chairs, *James McCartney* and *O. T. Kenworthy*, a document was drafted and subsequently accepted by ASHA's Legislative Council in 1983. A summary of the document is reprinted here, since it should serve as a guideline for the training of all students who may use this book. It also served as a reference point in the model described in Chapter 1 and used throughout this text.

Resources and Materials Lists (children—page 556; adults—page 567)

The child and adult materials lists were prepared with input from some of our chapter authors and other colleagues. Special acknowledgment is made to these individuals for their assistance in preparing these lists.

"A SAMPLE EIGHT-WEEK REHABILITATION GROUP PROGRAM"

THOMAS G. GIOLAS

The general purpose of audiologic rehabilitation (AR) groups is to provide a dynamic setting in which the interaction among peers (persons with hearing impairment), friends and family members, and the group leader (the audiologist) generates productive discussions and, most importantly, solutions to communication problems associated with hearing loss. The focus is on communication breakdowns, where and with whom they typically occur, and what can be done about them. Below is an outline of the major components and the rationale for these groups.

Purpose. To provide supportive and substantive help to persons having communication problems associated with hearing impairment.

Goals. To analyze auditory failures and develop concrete behaviors that result in improved communication.

Process. The group process is used with the audiologist serving as the group leader.

Rationale. The group process provides a setting in which there is considerable exchange of information, mutual support, and validation of communication problems and solutions.

Role of the Group Leader. The group leader serves as the major facilitator of the discussion: by raising pertinent questions, by being a good listener, and by demonstrating continued respect for group members' comments and opinions. The group leader also serves as the expert on hearing and hearing disorders.

Session Contents. The general content of the group sessions centers, through lectures, films, and other media, on hearing and the handicapping effect of hearing impairment.

Group Members. Group participants are persons with hearing impairment and their friends or family members with whom communication is important and frequent.

Group Activities. Activities are designed to focus on (a) optimal use of auditory cues, (b) optimal use of visual cues, (c) manipulation of environment, and (d) response to auditory failures.

Sample Program

Eight 2-hour group sessions are outlined below. The contents of these sessions are offered as an example of what might be done with a group of persons with hearing impairment and their friends or family members. The outline does not represent a rigid program to be followed by all groups. A management plan for a particular group must be based on a compete assessment of participants' hearing impairments and hearing disabilities. On the other hand, it is this writer's experience that all sessions should follow a similar structure. This helps participants predict the activities to be expected from one session to another, thus minimizing confusion. Below is an outline of the general session structure followed. (The initial session will deviate slightly from this structure because of the lack of homework assignment to be discussed, and also to allow the group leader to introduce the general goals of the program.)

1. Discussion of homework assignment
2. Formal presentation of previously announced topic
3. Open discussion of issues raised in the formal presentation
4. Social break
5. Communication strategy activity
6. Homework assignment and discussion of next session's activities

First Week

1.0 Introduction
    1.1 Introduction to group members
    1.2 Setting group goals and ground rules
2.0 Formal Presentation
    2.1 Typical communication problems experienced by most persons with hearing impairment, especially those reported by the group
        2.1.1 Intensity loss
        2.1.2 Speech recognition
        2.1.3 Communication situations (use examples from self-report data)
        2.1.4 Response of the person with hearing impairment to the specific auditory failure
3.0 Open Discussion of Formal Presentation
    3.1 The major objective of this activity in the initial session is to set the stage for an atmosphere conducive to easy conversation between the group members and the leader. The nature of the content is less important at this time.
4.0 Social Break
    4.1 The group leader should circulate as much as possible during the

initial break and talk with as many of the group members as possible

5.0 Communication Strategy Activity
  5.1 Ask the group to identify difficult listening situations. Write them on the chalkboard and have the group discuss why they are difficult and identify some possible solutions.

6.0 Homework Assignment
  6.1 Each group member is asked to identify and describe two situations in which she or he had considerable difficulty during the week. Group members are to chart the situations in terms of:
    6.1.1 with whom they were talking.
    6.1.2 the environmental conditions.
    6.1.3 the purpose of the conversation.
    6.1.4 why they thought they had difficulty.
    6.1.5 what they did about it.

Second Week

1.0 Discussion of Homework Assignment
  1.1 Special note must be taken to identify early on those group members with hearing impairment who had difficulty doing the homework, so that they may receive individual responses if the difficulty continues.

2.0 Formal Presentation
  2.1 The hearing aid
    2.1.1 Hearing through a hearing aid
    2.1.2 The care and operation of a hearing aid
    2.1.3 Some tips on hearing-aid use

3.0 Open Discussion of Formal Presentation
  3.1 This discussion provides the opportunity for many problems and solutions regarding hearing-aid use to be raised. Much will be learned from the group members' listening and talking to each other. The leader should refrain from providing all the answers.

4.0 Social Break
  4.1 This break often provides a good opportunity for group members to ask specific questions concerning problems they are having with their own hearing aids. The group leader should begin noting those persons who may need to be seen for further audiological workup to assess the effectiveness of their hearing aids.

5.0 Communication Strategy Activity
  5.1 Two group members are asked to carry on a conversation in adverse listening conditions (e.g. background music). The group is asked to write down how each of the people conversing handled the difficult listening situation. A discussion is then held on what was observed.

       5.2   This activity serves as a good introduction to highlight the way responses to auditory failures help or hinder communication.

6.0   Homework Assignment

       6.1   Group members are asked to select two listening situations in which they could compare their performance with and without their hearing aids.

Third Week

1.0   Discussion of Homework Assignment

       1.1   At this point, the group leader should be encouraging discussion by those who are not participating actively. If someone is not doing the homework, a non-threatening personal conversation (perhaps during the break) is in order.

2.0   Formal Presentation

       2.1   The use of nonverbal cues

              2.1.1   The contribution of lip movements, gestures, facial expressions, and situational cues to understanding the verbal message

              2.1.2   The concept of physiologic, acoustic, and linguistic redundancy (elementary level)

              2.1.3   The benefits and limitations of speechreading

3.0   Open Discussion of Formal Presentation

       3.1   This presentation will stimulate considerable discussion, which will continue to arise in subsequent sessions. The group should be made aware that the use of nonverbal cues will be covered again later in the program.

4.0   Social Break

       4.1   This is typically the point at which some group members begin to pursue individual conferences with the group leader.

5.0   Communication Strategy Activity

       5.1   One or more of the activities described in Chapter Four, which are designed to show the advantages of nonverbal cues in general, are appropriate at this time.

6.0   Homework Assignment

       6.1   Each group is asked to bring in three to five phrases or sentences common to his or her home or work environment. They will be used in a simple lipreading activity.

Fourth Week

1.0   Discussion of Homework Assignment

       1.1   This assignment will provide the content with which to introduce a simple speechreading activity. The familiar phrases and sentences will also provide a good lead-in to the use of other communication strategies.

2.0   Formal Presentation
    2.1   Communication strategies
        2.1.1   Manipulation of the environment
        2.1.2   Constructive response to auditory failure

3.0   Open Discussion of Formal Presentation
    3.1   The group leader may begin directing the discussion toward the group's reported differential use of these strategies in social and work settings.

4.0   Social Break
    4.1   If there are some group members who are in their hearing-aid trial period or some who are considering acquiring a hearing aid, this is an appropriate time to check on their progress. They may wish to raise some questions in the group. The break provides a good opportunity to explore possible acquisition of a hearing aid with each of these members personally.

5.0   Communication Strategy Activity
    5.1   Using the ideas for speechreading activities in Chapter 4, the group leader should conduct a speechreading activity of mild difficulty to illustrate one or more of the specific speechreading strategies.
    5.2   The group members with hearing impairment should be encouraged to generalize their approach to speechreading to all communication situations.

6.0   Homework Assignment
    6.1   Each group member is asked to identify and describe several communication settings in which she had little or no difficulty. Group members should document this situation in a manner similar to that prescribed for the first week's assignment. They should pay special attention to the contribution of nonverbal cues.

Fifth Week

1.0   Discussion of Homework Assignment
    1.1   The purpose of this assignment is to help the group begin identifying strategies that members are using to facilitate communication. The discussion should include as many examples as possible to illustrate the variety of ingredients comprising a successful communication event. This discussion often becomes a turning point for many group members as they realize what others are doing to improve situations similar to those in which they have experienced difficulty.

2.0   Formal Presentation
    2.1   Continuation of Fourth Week (communication strategies)
    2.2   Promote strategies that have been identified as not being used by the group.

3.0   Open Discussion of Formal Presentation
    3.1   Continuation of the goals established for the fourth week's discussion
    3.2   It is a good idea for the group leader to review the members' self-

report responses in order to become familiar with their individual profiles. This will facilitate leading the discussion into areas relevant to all group members.

4.0 Social Break

   4.1 The best use of the group leader's time during this break is to check on the progress being made by those members considering amplification.

5.0 Communication Strategy Activity

   5.1 Six group members are seated in a circle. Every two people are paired to carry on a conversation, ignoring the other conversations. The result is three separate conversations going on simultaneously. The activity is videotaped and the group analyzes the tape in terms of how the various participants handled this difficult listening situation. The activity may be repeated with different group members.[1]

   5.2 Specific responses to auditory failure that are not being used can be emphasized.

6.0 Homework Assignment

   6.1 By this time all group members should be aware of the necessity of approaching their ability to understand what is being said. Consequently, members are asked to identify a communication setting they will encounter, develop a plan to maximize communication, use the plan, and analyze its success.

Sixth Week

1.0 Discussion of Homework Assignment

   1.1 The discussion of the various plans attempted by the group members will provide the framework for encouraging other plans specific to situations reported by group members. The group leader should use examples of situations common to all members and encourage repetition of this homework activity.

   1.2 The group may wish to devote the remaining homework assignments to this activity. It provides an opportunity for the members to receive help with specific situations especially problematic for them.

2.0 Formal Presentation

   2.1 The role of family members and close friends

      2.1.1 This topic is important because these are the people with whom the hearing-impaired spend most of their time and do most of their conversing. Significant others' understanding of the problems of persons with hearing impairment is vital so that they can contribute to improved communication conditions.

      2.1.2 Review of the options available to the person with hearing impairment.

[1] Courtesy of C. Carmen and C. Freedenberg, University of California Hearing and Speech Center, San Francisco, California.

      2.1.3   Tips on what the family member or close friend can do to facilitate communication.

3.0   Open Discussion of Formal Presentation

    3.1   The group leader should be aware that this discussion often produces an increased interaction between the person with hearing impairment and the family member or close friend attending the sessions. This interaction is important and may provide the groundwork for improved handling of communication problems.

    3.2   This discussion is also likely to produce comments that stray from the handling of communication situations. The group leader may have to remind the members of the ground-rules and goals of the group.

4.0   Social Break

    4.1   The break usually becomes an extension of the above discussion.

5.0   Communication Strategy Activity

    5.1   Repeat the activity outlined for the fourth week. The activity could be increased in difficulty to challenge the members and provide an opportunity to discuss constructive approaches to various communication situations.

6.0   Homework Assignment.

    6.1   The group members with hearing impairment should be encouraged to observe what persons with normal hearing do when they experience an auditory failure.

    6.2   Those wearing hearing aids on a trial basis should tabulate the situations in which they believe their hearing performance improved as a result of wearing a hearing aid.

Seventh Week

1.0   Discussion of Homework Assignment

    1.1   At this point, some attention should be focused on those persons considering amplification.

    1.2   The discussion of how persons with normal hearing generally handle communication breakdowns lends itself to looking at dissimilarities and similarities between their experiences and the experiences of persons with hearing impairment. The conclusion should emerge that the major difference lies in the frequency of occurrence.

2.0   Formal Presentation

    2.1   Hearing and hearing disorders

        2.1.1   Hearing disorders and audiograms

        2.1.2   Hearing disability/handicap

        2.1.3   The role of amplification

3.0   Open Discussion of Formal Presentation

    3.1   This discussion can go in a number of directions. It should provide an opportunity for the members to ask questions they have about hearing impairment in general and about their own hearing problems in particular.

3.2   In this discussion, questions may be raised about the following topics:

    3.2.1   The progressive nature of sensorineural hearing impairment.

    3.2.2   The hereditary nature of hearing impairment

    3.2.3   The destructive effects of hearing aids on residual hearing

    3.2.4   The value of one versus two hearing aids

    3.2.5   The role of surgery, vitamins, etc., in correcting sensorineural hearing impairment

4.0   Social Break

4.1   This break often becomes an extension of the above discussion

5.0   Communication Strategy Activities

5.1   Group members role-play a number of difficult listening situations and discuss how they could be handled

5.2   The use of visual, contextual, and situational cues should be stressed

5.3   Most of the suggested situations should come from the group

6.0   Homework Assignment

6.1   Group members retake the self-report inventory (the HPI), which was taken prior to the first session

Eighth Week

1.0   Discussion of Homework Assignment

1.1   This discussion can go in a number of directions. A simple lead-in question such as "How did you feel taking the test this time as opposed to when you first took it?" will start the discussion.

1.2   The goal is to help the group members crystallize any insights they believe they have gained from participating in the group and to discuss how they applied them when retaking the test.

2.0   Formal Presentation

2.1   Summary and review of program goals

3.0   Open Discussion of Formal Presentation

3.1   The group members may want to use this time to discuss how they benefitted from attending the sessions

4.0   Social Break

4.1   Because this is the last session, the break tends to be longer and more social

5.0   Communication Strategy Activity

5.1   Review a list of dos and don'ts regarding handling communication situations

5.2   Discuss and demonstrate appropriate use of a hearing aid

6.0   Homework Assignment

6.1   Each group member should be encouraged to keep a detailed log of communication situations in which difficulty occurred, to be reviewed on the individual follow-up visit approximately a month later

6.2   Appointments should be made for the follow-up visit prior to the completion of the session. This is often done by circulating a sign-up sheet with available dates and times.

Adapted from T. G. Giolas (1982), *Hearing Handicapped Adults* (pp. 109–115), Englewood Cliffs, NJ: Prentice Hall. Reprinted by permission.

"LASER VIDEODISC TECHNOLOGY IN THE AURAL REHABILITATION SETTING: GOOD NEWS FOR PEOPLE WITH SEVERE AND PROFOUND HEARING IMPAIRMENTS"

NANCY TYE-MURRAY

A few weeks ago, a friend who is the director of audiology for a Veterans Administration Hospital made an interesting observation. Whereas the advent of cochlear implants has been a momentous development in the treatment of adventitiously-deafened adults, cochlear implants seem to have diverted our attention away from hearing-aid users with severe or profound hearing impairments who are not candidates for implantation. My friend noted, "We tend to hang hearing aids on their ears and send them on their way. We need to recognize that these people are still going to have problems communicating, and start thinking about how to provide follow-up services."

There are probably few audiologists who have not wondered at some point about how to incorporate more follow-up and support services into their clinical care, particularly for the patient with severe or profound hearing impairment. Even so, traditional aural rehabilitation, which may include speechreading training, auditory training, and counseling, seems to be a rare offering in most clinical practices.

Two factors may account for the dearth of aural rehabilitation. First, many of the follow-up and support services we learned about in our training programs were described in vague terms. Few systematic procedures were suggested for implementing them. For example, we may have been instructed to encourage the patient's use of "assertive listening behaviors," but what these behaviors are and how to develop them often remained fuzzy. When it came time to provide aural rehabilitation, some of us found ourselves asking, "Now what do I do?" The second, and probably more influential factor, is that aural rehabilitation can be labor-intensive, expensive, and time-consuming. The audiologist often must devote much individualized attention to the patient during several hours, weeks, or even months. Few clinics have a large enough staff or the financial resources to provide traditional services.

Today, the field of aural rehabilitation is changing rapidly, and these two factors may soon evaporate. A number of researchers and clinicians are introducing scientific rigor into what has often been an art form. They are asking such questions as, "Which services are worth providing?", "What is the best method for providing them?", "How can we design a systematic training/counseling protocol that takes into account individual patient needs and the talents of the particular audiologist?", and finally, "How can we make these services cost-effective?"

Perhaps one of the most exciting new developments in the near future will be the introduction of laser videodisc technology into treatment programs. This technology may allow services to be evaluated rigorously, and may add more structure to many training protocols. It may also reduce the amount of clinician time required for providing rehabilitation. Thus, services may become more cost-effective. In this report, I will describe how this technology has been used in our hospital setting for providing aural rehabilitation to adults who have severe or profound hearing losses.

The Technology and Program

Laser videodisc technology emerged in the 1970s from Music Corporation of America and NV Philips (Miller, 1987). The videodisc resembles a compact disc, except that it may store video as well as audio materials. There are two features that make this technology particularly attractive for an aural rehabilitation application. First, audiovisual speech materials can be accessed from the laser videodisc rapidly, in any sequence. Second, presentation of materials can be computer-controlled, with the possibility of overlaying or interspersing computer-generated graphics and text.

A training station includes a laser videodisc player and a computer. It also includes a monitor for viewing the stimuli and audio speakers for listening. In some stations, the monitor has a touch screen so that the patient can interact with the computer by touching the monitor. Thus, the patient need not know how to type and may not even require reading skills. When the station has a touchscreen, training usually proceeds at a fast pace, and patients are not distracted or bored by a typing task.

In developing training exercises, one must develop the laser videodisc that stores the training items (such as sentences or words spoken by one or many talkers) and the computer software that determines what items are presented and when. Audiologists need not develop their own exercises from scratch because many laser videodisc materials are currently available (Sims, 1988).

When we began planning our aural rehabilitation program, we identified three services that could facilitate patients' ability to communicate verbally. These included the following: (a) training to nurture audiovisual speech-recognition abilities and increase attention to visible speech cues, (b) practice in using repair strategies, which are instructions the patient provides to a talker after not comprehending a spoken message, and communication therapy for patients' spouses and other family members. Communication therapy involves teaching relatives how to talk with appropriate speaking behaviors and repair breakdowns in communication.

After identifying the services, we developed training exercises that would assist the audiologist in providing them. The instructional materials are stored on a laser videodisc (see Appendix) and have corresponding computer software. Our training stations each include a Pioneer 6810 laser videodisc player, which is controlled by an AST or IBM AT computer. Training items are presented on an IBM Infowindow. This is a high-resolution graphics monitor (critical for presenting sentence illustrations) with built-in stereo speakers. The computer peripherals include an EGA jumper card and an EGA card for the IBM Infowindow system.

In developing the first and second services, we designed three speechreading-training programs, two of which also provide practice in using repair strategies (Tye-Murray, Tyler, Bong, & Nares, 1988; Tye-Murray, 1991; Tye-Murray, 1992). Program 1 provides analytic speechreading training, wherein patients must identify nonsense syllables, monosyllables, and words in carrier phrases. Training activities include same/different discriminations and closed-set identification tasks.

Program 2 provides practice in speechreading unrelated sentences. Patients also learn to use five different repair strategies when they cannot recognize a sentence—they learn to ask the talker to repeat the sentence, rephrase it, elaborate it, simplify it, or to indicate the topic of the sentence. In one kind of training activity, a talker appears on the touchscreen and speaks a sentence. Afterward, four pictures appear, one of which illustrates the sentence. If the patient selects the correct illustration, the sentence is repeated along with the orthographic text, and the next item is presented. If the patient selects the incorrect illustration, the five repair strategies are offered. The patient can select one, and it happens right away.

Program 3 resembles Program 2, except that sentences within an exercise relate to a common theme, such as a doctor's office or restaurant. Talkers in Program 3 occasionally speak with an inappropriate speaking behavior (for example, talking in profile or too quickly); in these instances, the patient can interact with the computer and request the talker avoid these behaviors. Every fourth sentence, the patient views a 10-second film clip (a connecting scene). Connecting scenes establish a context for speechreading the sentences and make training more interesting. (One of the most difficult challenges in developing exercises is to find ways of capturing the patient's attention. There are few certainties in speechreading training, but without a doubt, a bored patient will not benefit.) For the restaurant exercise, a group of people are (sic) shown being greeted by a hostess at the entrance. The next four sentences are spoken by the hostess. The group is then shown seated at a table, looking at menus and talking. Four sentences later, the waiter arrives with an order pad.

Our clinical experience suggests that patients who are flexible and willing to guess tend to be relatively good speechreaders. We are currently developing a fourth program that encourages patients to guess when they are unsure about a message. In instances when they understand only a few words, they are encouraged to use linguistic and environmental cues to infer the talker's message.

The speechreading-training programs offer several attractive features. First, many training items can be presented in a relatively short period of time. For instance, three adults with cochlear implants recently came to our clinic for three days of intensive aural rehabilitation. The patients practiced 1,800 training items on average (Program 1 only). Concentrated training leads to faster learning and also helps to maintain the patient's interest. Another attractive feature is that the computer software maintains a record of the patient's response during training. Thus, we can monitor a patient's performance on a daily or weekly basis, and we have a precise record of how many and which training items were included in training. Different versions of the training software are available. The level of training difficulty can be adjusted for patients who have poor language or speech recognition skills. The patient can practice speechreading many different talkers without leaving the clinic. For instance, in Program 2, 16 different talkers speak during training. Finally, the audiologist need not be present in the room throughout training, although the audiologist always allocates some time to interact with the patient. During this interaction, patient and audiologist role-play and practice using the repair strategies, and they discuss the patient's specific communication problems.

Involving the family in the aural rehabilitation process is extremely important, and will likely receive increased emphasis in future rehabilitation programs. Family members can learn to articulate clearly when speaking to the individual with hearing impairment, using appropriate speaking behaviors (such as speaking with their faces clearly visible). They can learn to repair breakdowns in communication. For instance, we encourage family members to elaborate their messages or repeat an important key word after the hearing-impaired person misunderstands them. Finally, family members can become more informed about hearing loss and the ambiguities of the visual speech signal. By understanding the difficulty of speech recognition with limited hearing, they may become more empathetic with the patient.

For the third service, communication therapy for family members, our aim was to involve the family without requiring major time or financial commitments. One of our family-training programs lasts about 45 minutes and can be completed while the patient is being fitted with a hearing aid. The family member is taken into the training station. During training, various talkers appear on the monitor and speak sentences two times each. During the first presentation, the talker speaks with an inappropriate speaking behavior, such a with a pencil end in the mouth. During the second presentation, the talker removes the pencil and speaks appropriately. Training items are presented in a vision-only condition. Immediately after each example, a brief tutorial appears on the monitor explaining why the particular behavior makes speechreading more difficult. The family member touches the computer touchscreen to see the next example. This program serves as an introduction to appropriate speaking behaviors. The audiologist provides additional counseling.

We also have a program that teaches family members to elaborate a message or repeat a key word following a communication breakdown. After completing the program, the family member is provided with pencil-and-paper activities to perform at home. One activity consists of a list of sentences. The family member's task is to circle an important key word in each sentence.

There are other applications for laser videodisc technology in the aural rehabilitation clinic that are not instructional. Researchers and clinicians are using it for testing speechreading skills with various communication aids, for assessing the need for aural rehabilitation, and for evaluating the effects of therapy intervention (e.g., Cox, Alexander, & Gilmore, 1987; Tye-Murray, 1991; Tyler, Preece, & Tye-Murray, 1986). For example, the Iowa Medial Consonant Test (Tyler, et al., 1986) presents 13 consonants in an /iCi/ context. The test can be presented in an audition-only or an audiovisual condition. The audition-only test scores indicated the need for auditory training and the audiovisual scores indicate the need for speechreading training. Consonant confusion matrices can be constructed with the patient responses. Using the computer, information transmission analysis (Miller & Nicely, 1955) can be performed to determine which speech features are being utilized for speech recognition. This information can guide the development of therapy objectives.

Laser videodisc technology is only one of many technologies available to audiologists. VHS audiovideo tapes and home VHS players, lap-top computers with built-in audio speakers, Compact Disc-Interactive (CD-I)[2], and audio-tape card machines portend a broadened array of services for individuals with severe and profound hearing impairments. For instance, with the availability of hand-held audiovideo recorders, we may soon be making custom-made speechreading VHS programs. Patients could then practice speechreading those individuals with whom they interact most, such as a spouse or friend, in the privacy of their own homes. In finding ways to integrate new technology into aural rehabilitation, we need only tap our imaginations.

Acknowledgments

This work was supported by research grant CD00242 from the National Institutes of Health/NIDCD; grant RR59 from the General Clinical Research Centers Program, Division of Research Resources, NIH; and the Iowa Lions Sight and Hearing Foundation. I thank Don Schum for discussions about content.

References

Cox, R. M., Alexander, G., & Gilmore, C. (1987). Development of the Connected Speech Test (CST). *Ear and Hearing, 8,* 1195–1265.

Miller, G. A., & Nicely, P. E. (1955). An analysis of perceptual confusions among some English consonants. *Journal of the Acoustical Society of America, 27,* 338–352.

Miller, R. L. (1987). An overview of the interactive market. In S. Lambert & J. Sallis (Eds.), *CD-I and interactive videodisc technology* (pp. 1-14). Indianapolis, IN: Howard W. Sams & Co.

Sims, D. G. (1988). Video methods for speechreading instruction. *The Volta Review, 90,* 273–288.

Tye-Murray, N. (1991). Repair strategy usage by hearing-impaired adults and changes following instruction. *Journal of Speech and Hearing Research, 34*(6), 921–928.

---

[2] CD-I players can control television equipment and play standard compact discs. CD-I capabilities include a capacity for storing a large number of still photographs, audio materials (up to 19 hours), cartoon animation, and partial-screen motion video display. Soon, full-motion video will be possible. CD-I may permit interactive speechreading training in the home, without requiring a computer, laser videodisc player, or touchscreen computer monitor. In the near future, CD-I may permit interactive speechreading training in the home, without requiring a computer, laser videodisc player, or touchscreen computer monitor. In the near future, CD-I players will be comparable in price to a standard compact disc player.

Tye-Murray, N. (1992). Preparing for communication interactions: The value of anticipatory strategies for adults with hearing impairment. *Journal of Speech and Hearing Research, 35*(6), 430–435.

Tye-Murray, N., Tyler, R. S., Bong, B., & Nares, T. (1988). Using laser videodisc technology to train speech reading and assertive listening skills. *Journal of the Academy of Rehabilitation Audiology, 21*, 143–152.

Tyler, R. S., Preece, J. P., & Tye-Murray, N. (1986). *The Iowa phoneme and sentence tests.* Iowa City, IA: University of Iowa Hospitals and Clinics.

This article first appeared in American Journal of Audiology 1(2)33–36, 1992.

"AURAL REHABILITATION FOR THE PATIENT WITH VISUAL AND HEARING IMPAIRMENT"

ADRIENNE KARP

Government surveys indicate 2.7 million Americans suffer dual vision and hearing handicaps. The largest proportion are persons who are deaf:vision-impaired, followed then by persons who are vision-impaired:hearing-impaired, persons who are blind:hearing-impaired, and persons who are deaf:blind (Hicks and Pfau, 1979). The importance of auditory skills to a person with a visual disability is well documented, and the study of hearing is included in the training curriculum of many professionals who work with persons who are blind. In comparison, few hearing-health professionals have adequate knowledge of abnormal vision. Most of us are poorly informed about eye pathologies and their functional consequences, although adequate sight is required for speechreading and interpretation of sign language. Visual impairment is also known to adversely affect a patient's adjustment of the use of a hearing aid. The purpose of this article is to provide the reader with information about functional consequences of specific eye conditions and to suggest modifications of audiologic rehabilitation techniques necessitated by abnormal visual functioning.

Loss of vision is our most feared chronic affliction, even though it is not as widespread as hearing impairment. According to a 1980 report of the National Society for the Prevention of Blindness, 11.5 million Americans have some degree of irreversible vision impairment. Only 500,000 of those are classified as legally blind, but many more are unable to see well enough to read ordinary newsprint. Approximately 100,000 people in the United States have no useful vision at all.

Legal Blindness

An individual is considered legally blind if either visual acuity or peripheral vision is worse than the following specified limits: (1) Visual acuity, the ability to see and identify objects at a distance, can be no better than 20/200 in the better eye with the use of corrective lenses. In other words, the legally blind person may distinguish only at a distance of 20 feet what a normal eye is able to see from 200 feet away. This amount of vision allows a person to travel adequately without the assistance of a cane, guide dog, or sighted guide, but severely effects the ability to read print, speechread, and see the parts of a hearing aid, for example. (2) An equally important parameter if visual functioning is the size of the patient's peripheral visual field. Normal bilateral field vision measures 180°. If a patient has peripheral vision of less than 20°, he/she may be classified as legally blind. Patients with constricted peripheral fields (also known as tunnel vision) often have adequate central visual acuity which allows them to see print and other fine detail, but they have difficulty traveling safely around their environment because of an inability to see obstacles not directly in their path.

Visual Impairment

The overall functioning of a patient with hearing impairment is significantly affected by poor vision. Because some visual impairments are not obvious to the observer, the audiologist is advised to ask each patient about visual functioning when a case history is taken. Questions contained in Appendix 13B will help determine a patient's visual capabilities. In addition, the audiologist can utilize the Snellen Chart to test visual acuity.[3]

Of all the causes for impaired vision, those resulting from refractive errors are the most widespread in our society. They occur when the structures of the eye that bend light onto the retina (cornea and lens) are not a normal shape. Since such errors can be reversed with corrective lenses, people with refractive errors are not at issue at in this article. It is the 11.5 million Americans whose vision cannot be fully restored with lenses or medical intervention to whom attention is given here.

Individuals with irreversible visual impairments who still retain a significant amount of usable sight are known as "low-vision" patients. In a sense, low vision is analogous to sensorineural hearing loss, since neither can be cured or restored completely to normal function. Refractive errors discussed in the previous paragraph could, on the other hand, be viewed as analogous to conductive hearing loss. A simple refractive adjustment can bring vision into clear focus in most cases. Although they are handicapped by their visual impairment, many low-vision patients are not legally blind since their sight may not be equal to or worse than the specified limits of 20/200 acuity or 20° peripheral vision.

Visual impairment does not always imply severe handicap. Over 90% of the low vision population retain a good deal of usable sight. The remaining 6–10%, however, have severe impairment and require the assistance of guide dogs, canes, or sighted guides for traveling purposes. With no appreciable amount of useful vision, they are dependent on tactile cues and audition for orientation and learning tasks.

Central Field vs. Peripheral Field Defects

The most common cases of non-refractive low-vision impairments (those not fully reversible with corrective lenses) treated in a general ophthalmologic practice involve conditions that affect *central visual acuity*, the ability to clearly distinguish objects directly in our path of vision. Central field defects can result in overall blurry

---

[3] Editor's Note: For a discussion on the use of the Snellen Chart for assessing far visual acuity of hearing-impaired persons, see D. Johnson and F. Caccamise, (1983). Hearing-impaired students: Options for far visual acuity screening. *American Annals of the Deaf, 128,* 402–406.

vision, as experienced by people with cataracts. Other pathologies, like macular degeneration, affect central acuity by resulting in a gray or blurry spot known as a scotoma. These patchy spots can effectively block out discrete portions of a visual image. A person is immediately aware when central vision becomes impaired because the capacity to see fine detail is affected. Such a disability has consequences for many activities of daily living that are dependent on the ability to read print, thread a needle, work at a job involving small objects, see the temperature setting on an oven, or identify the price of foods on the labels of items at supermarkets. Most people with central visual dysfunction are over age 60.

A potentially more disabling type of vision problem is that resulting in *constricted peripheral fields*. This dysfunction interferes with the ability to see obstacles not in the direct line of sight, with drastic consequences relative to the ease with which people are able to move around the environment independently. This type of visual field defect may develop so insidiously that individuals are unaware of its existence until the advanced stages. People with constricted peripheral fields find themselves tripping over obstacles and bumping into obstructions which are no longer visible. They often assume that other people are placing obstacles where they cannot be seen. It may not be until many accidents are sustained that these persons seek help from an eye specialist. A number of pathologies that cause peripheral field loss eventually affect central vision as well, thereby leading to blindness. Some of the more common etiologies resulting in peripheral field loss are glaucoma, retinitis pigmentosa, and optic nerve atrophy.

Eye Pathology and Treatment

Causes of visual disorders are numerous. Table 13.1 provides brief descriptions for some of the more familiar and prevalent etiologies of visual disorders and their recommended treatments.

In addition to conditions that cause visual dysfunction in isolation, there are numbers of systematic conditions that result in both vision and hearing impairment. Table 13.2 lists the most common of these conditions.

The interested reader can investigate several recommended references which are listed at the end of this material for more detailed information concerning the patient with visual or dual visual and hearing impairment.

Aural Rehabilitation Strategies for Central Visual Defects

When considering a program of auditory training for persons with dual disabilities, it becomes necessary for the audiologist to alter rehabilitation techniques. The patient whose central vision alone is impaired will have considerable difficulty discriminating fine visual detail. Speechreading skills may no longer be useful in compensating for the hearing impairment. Because people with central visual defects are mainly over 60 years of age, presbycusis is often the cause of their hearing loss. Consonant sounds, which are difficult for them to hear, are now difficult for them to see as well. This often leads them to believe that their visual and auditory impairments are neurologically connected and,

TABLE 13.1 Eye Pathologies Resulting in Low Vision

Eye Pathology	Etiology	Visual Dysfunction	Usual Age of Onset	Medical Treatment	Cure
Cataracts	numerous theories exist	cloudy vision due to opacity of crystaline lens of eye	usually occurs in aging eyes but can be secondary to retinitis pigmentosa and congenital rubella	surgery and lens replacement	usually good surgical success
Diabetic Retinopathy	possible consequences of diabetes	overall blurred vision due to proliferation of retinal blood vessels with hemorrhages into vitreous fluid	dependent on type, severity and age of onset of diabetic condition	laser beam treatments to cauterize blood vessels	prognosis is guarded and changes in vision may be rapid and unpredictable
Glaucoma (Open Angle)	increased intraocular fluid pressure	peripheral field loss leading to blindness if untreated	usually after 40 years of age	eye drops; laser treatments	none: condition can be arrested but damage cannot be reversed
Macular Degeneration (atrophic)	vascular insufficiency	blurred or blotched central vision	usually occurs in adults over 60 years of age	none	none
Macular Degeneration (exudative)	vascular abnormality	blurred or blotched central vision	usually occurs in adults over 60 years of age	early laser treatment in selected cases	laser treatment may arrest the progression of the condition; otherwise no known cure

TABLE 13.1 *continued*

Eye Pathology	Etiology	Visual Dysfunction	Usual Age of Onset	Medical Treatment	Cure
Optic Atrophy	too numerous to list	peripheral field loss	any age	none	none
Retinitis Pigmentosa (RP)	genetic inheritance	night blindness; progressive peripheral visual field loss which eventually leads to total blindness	late childhood	none	none
Retinopathy of Prematurity (ROP)	excessive exposure to oxygen in early life	overall cloudy vision or blindness due to proliferative retinopathy and/or tissue growth behind crystaline lens	neonatally, especially in premature and low birth weight infants	none	none
Strabismus	weakness of lateral eye muscles or disturbance in nerve innervation of those muscles	diplopia (double vision) may lead to amblyopia in one eye (functional blindness with no evidence of pathology)	at birth	surgery and/or exercise	usually good success with early intervention

TABLE 13.2 *Conditions Involving Vision and Hearing Loss*

Medical Condition	Etiology	Eye Pathology	Hearing Impairment	Usual Age of Onset
Age-related sensory impairment	aging process	several pathologies including cataracts, macular degeneration, glaucoma and diabetic retinopathy	sensorineural loss	older adulthood
Cogan's Syndrome Type I	unknown	non-syphilitic corneal inflammation (interstitial keratitis)	tinnitus, vertigo, fluctuating sensorineural loss eventually becoming severe and intractable	early adulthood; more often in males
Congenital Rubella	maternal rubella; most damaging in first trimester of pregnancy	congenital cataract and glaucoma; may be unstable	mild to profound sensorineural loss	at birth
Congenital Syphilis	maternal syphilitic condition at conception	syphilitic inflammation of the cornea (interstitial keratitis)	progressive sensorineural loss sometimes leading to deafness	adulthood
Didmoad Syndrome	genetic inheritance	peripheral field loss secondary to optic atrophy	progressive high-frequency sensorineural	early adulthood in persons with juvenile diabetes mellitus
Low birth weight; prematurity	numerous causes	overall blurred vision secondary to retinopathy of prematurity (ROP)	any type and severity	at birth
Sickle-cell anemia	genetic inheritance	overall poor vision secondary to proliferative retinopathy	severe sensorineural loss greater in low frequencies	early adulthood
Usher's Syndrome	genetic inheritance	peripheral field loss eventually leading to total blindness secondary to retinitis pigmentosa	sensorineural loss, most often congenital and profound	late childhood

as they lose one sense, they will necessarily lose the other. An explanation of the role of speechreading in compensating for a high-frequency impairment is of great assistance to these patients. A large central scotoma is also likely to interfere with a patient's capacity to see the lips or the face of the speaker, thereby negating the benefits of visual cues.

If speechreading does prove to be a viable training technique, lighting used in the therapy area is of considerable significance. Many people with vision problems, no matter what the cause or visual consequence, report glare to be one of the most debilitating conditions associated with their eye pathology. A low vision specialist, either an ophthalmologist, optometrist, or low-vision nurse, should be consulted regarding the type of lighting required to help with this problem. For more information about proper illumination, see E. Faye, *Clinical Low Vision* (see References).

Hearing-aid selection for the patient with poor central vision alone needs to be primarily concerned with help in understanding conversation. Fitting parameters (i.e., gain, output, frequency emphasis, and ear-mold style) are no different for this population than for those with normal vision. Eyeglass hearing aids are not usually the style of choice since many people with visual disabilities use different optical devices for different visual tasks. It is impractical for more than one pair of eyeglasses to house the needed hearing aids. It is important to know if a patient uses low-vision aids such as special lenses or magnifiers to see fine detail, since these devices should be utilized during hearing-aid management training.

For those patients who depend on sign language for communication purposes, interpretation ability will be affected by a central visual impairment. Hand movements must be made in that portion of the patient's field where vision is best, and signs should be slowed down to help compensate for distorted visual cues.

Aural Rehabilitation Strategies for Peripheral Field Defects and Blindness

The patient who has no usable vision or an extensive peripheral field loss requires auditory cues not only for conversation but for orientation and traveling purposes as well. Hearing aids must provide this patient both with the ability to understand and with adequate localization skills in order to compensate for inadequate vision. This, of course, requires microphone placement at the ear and necessitates binaural hearing-aid fittings for bilateral hearing loss. If the hearing loss is unilateral or asymmetrical, localization skills may be harder to achieve. CROS aids may then be considered.

BTE or ITE aids are the styles of choice. Some patients with severe hearing impairment may require a body aid or auditory trainer for conversation and classroom use, but these should be used only indoors since the microphone placement may impair localization skills needed for traveling. In order to select the proper amplification for mobility purposes, hearing aids must be tested in real-life circumstances as well as in a sound-treated testing chamber. Whether this will be on a quiet suburban street or a noisy city street will depend on where the individual patient travels.

Because of the masking effects of wind and rain, many patients with visual impairment prefer not to use their hearing aids outdoors. This problem can be partially resolved with a windscreen over the microphone.

The person with dual disabilities often uses audition to determine distance from a danger signal. Such need requires the reduction of compression amplification. The bus 5 feet away should not be made to sound like the car 50 feet away.

People with severe visual impairments that affect independent travel need low-frequency as well as high-frequency information. It is not advisable to amplify only high frequencies for speech discrimination. Hearing aids with wide-band frequency response and external tone controls should be considered. The patient can be taught to set the tone control depending on the auditory need at that moment. Microphone type is also an important issue with this population. Unidirectional microphones are recommended for conversational settings, but traveling requires an omnidirectional type. For this reason, it is advisable to fit hearing aids with dual microphone settings which the patient can manipulate depending on the listening situations.

The patient who is blind needs to rely on tactile cues rather than vision to master hearing aid management. Many patients with peripheral field defects, however, have adequate central acuity and can be taught to handle their aids using vision. For those who cannot, plastic models of ears can be useful in teaching how to insert a hearing aid. Battery insertion and manipulation of external controls can be taught by use of enlarged drawings made with felt-tip pens or through tactile cues alone.

Speechreading abilities will be contingent upon the extent of sight remaining in the patient's central field of vision. Not all peripheral defects impinge on central acuity, certainly not in their beginning stages. Many patients with tunnel vision have extensive use of their central visual areas and can learn to speechread quite effectively.

Sign-language communication requires enough adequate central vision to see hand movement. Fingerspelling will be more difficult for any patient with visual impairment to follow, but more so for those with central acuity difficulties. Tunnel vision, however, will also affect sign language interpretation because of the constriction in the area that now carries the visual image. Distance from the person with visual impairment should be determined individually to afford each patient the optimal visual field. Signs should be delivered more slowly and the magnitude of the presentations should be reduced as well (Hicks, 1979).

Summary and Conclusions

The following is a summary of recommendations that should be employed when treating a patient with dual vision and hearing impairments:

1. Determine the existence and functional consequences of any non-correctable visual disorder through case history and contact with the patient's eye-care specialist.
2. Select amplification that addresses orientation and localization needs as well as speech-reception and discrimination capabilities.
3. Design speechreading programs appropriate to the amount and type of remaining vision. Set realistic training goals accordingly.
4. Reduce glare in the therapy environment.

5. Adjust the speed, distance, and magnitude of sign-language presentations to promote better communication with the patient with visual and hearing impairment.

Patients with dual vision and hearing impairments may not be receiving the best rehabilitation available to them. They are often treated separately for their vision and hearing disorders with no dialogue between managing health-care professionals. The purpose of this article has been to acquaint audiologists with the causes and consequences of a variety of eye pathologies so that audiologic rehabilitation techniques can be modified in accordance with a patient's visual impairment.

References and Recommended Readings

Readings for Persons with Visual Impairment and Dual Hearing and Visual Impairment.

Faye, E. (1984). *Clinical low vision* (2nd ed.). Boston: Little, Brown.

Geeraets, W. (1976). *Ocular syndromes* (3rd ed.). Philadelphia: Lea and Febiger.

Hicks, W. (1979). Communication variables associated with hearing-impaired/vision-impaired persons-a pilot study. *American Annals of the Deaf, 124*, 419–422.

Hicks, W., and Pfau, G. (1979). Deaf-visually impaired persons: Incidence and services. *American Annals of the Deaf, 124*, 76–92.

Kauvar, K. (1982). *Eyes only.* Norwalk CT: Appleton-Century-Crofts.

National Society for the Prevention of Blindness (NSPB). (1977). *Understanding eye language (P607/77).* New York: NSPB.

National Society for the Prevention of Blindness (NSPB). (1980). *Vision problems in the U.S.* New York: NSPB.

Note. An earlier version of this material first appeared in the *Journal of the Academy of Rehabilitative Audiology, 16*, 1938, pp. 23-32. Used here with permission.

"AURAL REHABILITATION BY ASHA AUDIOLOGISTS: 1980–1990"

RONALD L. SCHOW
NAVROZE R. BALSARA
THAYNE C. SMEDLEY
CURTIS J. WHITCOMB

Introduction

There has been a long-standing neglect of rehabilitative services and a preference for the diagnostic aspects of audiology (Rosen, 1967; Hardick, 1977). A series of surveys extending back to 1971 concerning the state of diagnostic audiology and the large variety of diagnostic procedures available attest to the current state of affairs (Martin and Pennington, 1971, 1972; Martin and Forbis, 1978; Martin and Sides, 1985; Cherow, 1986; Martin and Morris, 1989).

To learn more about this neglected area, in 1980 at Idaho State University Whitcomb (1982) conducted a survey on the status of aural rehabilitation (AR) services provided by American Speech-Language-Hearing Association (ASHA) audiologists. Selected findings from this 1980 survey have been reported in a variety of sources (Schow, 1986; Schow and Nerbonne, 1989; Schow, 1990). Since the 1980 Whitcomb survey, a number of survey reports including those by Martin and Morris (1989), ASHA (1990, 1991) and Cranmer (1991) have provided the most recent and notable comparison data in this area. Martin and Morris (1989) performed an in-depth survey of current trends in diagnostic audiology. ASHA (1990) membership data and a limited survey (ASHA, 1991) conducted in 1989 revealed current trends in audiology. This ASHA survey was lacking in depth and contained only information on demographics of members and limited questions on diagnostic and rehabilitative clinical practices. Possibly due to the simple "yes/no" nature of most response options the percentages reported represent only rough estimates of current practices. Lastly, Cranmer (1991) surveyed dispensing audiologists employed in private practice and clinical settings about a limited number of specific issues related to hearing aid dispensing (e.g. use of real ear measures, type and number of hearing aids sold per year, promotional activities).

As helpful as these more recent surveys have been, there has been no comprehensive survey on AR since the 1980 Whitcomb survey. Therefore, the current project was undertaken to update the Whitcomb data one decade later. The primary goal was to determine from among ASHA membership the current status in AR services and trends over the past ten years.

Methodology and Procedures

Survey recipients were selected from the membership list of 8658 audiologists in ASHA as of 1990. Of this population only 6267 (74%) had designated a primary employment setting. Because this survey focused on clinically active ASHA members the aforementioned population of 6267 was periodically sampled (every sixth name) to obtain a list of 1000 for the survey group. A number of audiologists belong to professional organizations other than ASHA, such as the Academy of Dispensing Audiologists, the American Academy of Audiology, and the American Auditory Society. The sample of ASHA audiologists, however, is thought to provide a better cross-section of audiologists than could be achieved from any other professional organization.

Since the present study was a follow-up on the 1980 survey, the questionnaire was similar to the one used by Whitcomb (1982) with the following topic areas: 1) demographic information; 2) evaluation, fitting, and orientation procedures for hearing aids; 3) counseling practices; overall coordination of services; and 4) communication training (e.g. speechreading and auditory training).

Mailing and Returns. Each questionnaire was sent at the end of the 1990 calendar year, accompanied by an explanatory cover letter and a stamped pre-addressed envelope. A second mailing was sent approximately three weeks after the initial mailing to those who had not returned the questionnaire. Only questionnaires returned within three months of the initial mailing were included in the final analysis. The return rate for this survey was 54.6% (or 546). Of these 546 surveys, 8 were returned completely blank. This left 538 usable surveys which were the basis of the results in the following section and in Tables 13.3 and 13.4.

Results and Discussion

Demographics. Respondents are 76% female and trained mostly at the masters level (84%) with a smaller percentage (15%) trained at the doctoral level. Education level showed no change from the 1980 data (Whitcomb, 1982) and is reasonably consistent with ASHA demographic data of 79% with master's degrees (ASHA, 1991). However, the proportion of female respondents are (sic) greater than in the 1980 study (63%) and also greater than the proportion of female audiologists in ASHA (63%; ASHA, 1990). Thus females may be slightly over-represented in the findings that follow.

About 71% reported active involvement in clinical audiology of at least 20 hours per week. Overall, 87% of respondents are active in clinical audiology, while the remainder are administrators (3%) or supervisors (4%), or involved in non-clinical duties (9%). A majority of respondents have 6–15 years of clinical experience, reflecting added maturity of ASHA audiologists compared with 1980 (Table 13.3). Likewise, the largest age group of 1990 (53%) was between 30–39 years, compared with the largest age category (44%) of 1980, which was between 20 and 29 years.

WORK SETTINGS. Table 13.4 gives the distribution of audiologists across different employment settings. The data indicate there has been an increase in the percent of

TABLE 13.3 *Number and Percentage of Respondents Reporting Various Years of Clinical Experience*

Years of Clinical Experience	1980		1990	
	N	%	N	%
5 or less	179	48.4	81	15.1
6–10	103	27.8	156	29.1
11–15	34	9.2	148	27.6
16–20	31	8.4	87	16.2
21–25	15	4.1	38	7.1
26–30	5	1.4	12	2.2
31–35	3	0.8	9	1.7
36+	0	0.0	6	1.1
Totals	370	100.0	537	100.0

TABLE 13.4 *Number and Percentage of Respondents Indicating their Primary Employment Setting in 1980 and 1990 Idaho State University (ISU) Surveys, in 1990 ASHA Membership Data, and the 1989 Martin and Morris Survey*

Employment Setting	ISU 1980 N	ISU 1980 %	ISU 1990 N	ISU 1990 %	ASHA 1990 %	Martin and Morris 1989 %
Hospital Facility	125	33	107	20	23	28
Speech Hearing Center Clinic	37	10	30	6	6	5
Medical/Community Speech/Hearing Center		46%		46%	48.8%	55%
Government or Military Hospital						
Private MD or ENT Office	13	3	107	20	20	22
Private Practice	57	15	101	19	11	18
Public Schools	49	13	42	8	10	4
College/University Clinic	60	16	44	8	10	12
Non-Hospital Rehabilitation Setting			10	2	4	
School for the Deaf	12	3		NA	NA	NA
Other	28	7	91	17	17	12
More Than One Setting			1	NA	NA	NA
Totals	385	100	532	100	100	100

audiologists working in private practice with private medical doctors and ear, nose, and throat (ENT) specialists, but there has been little change in the percent 43 of audiologists working in medical/community centers of all types combined (46–49%). ASHA (1990) reported the percent of audiologists working in private practice was lower (11% ASHA vs. 19% current results). A more detailed analysis of specific rehabilitation practices for audiologists working in selected settings has been undertaken elsewhere (Balsara and Schow).

There were 69 respondents in this demographic section who indicated active involvement in clinical audiology within the past three years only during their formal education. Altogether with the 8 blank surveys this resulted in 77 which were unusable. These were eliminated, leaving a total of 469 completed questionnaires considered representative of clinically active ASHA audiologists during 1990. Remaining tables and analyses are based on responses from these 469.

CLIENT POPULATIONS. Most respondents (75%) report working with all age populations. At least 90% of respondents work with adults, school-age children, and pediatric populations, while slightly fewer audiologists (87%) work with the elderly. Whitcomb found about 10% more respondents in 1989 were working with school-age and pediatric populations compared with adult and elderly populations. There has been an increased emphasis on clinical work involving adults, while the smallest number of audiologists continues to work with the elderly.

Table 13.5 shows that most current respondents (78%) report providing AR services primarily to hard of hearing while also serving some deaf clients. A few (17%) serve the hard of hearing exclusively while only 4% do AR primarily or exclusively with the deaf. The level of clinical service to the deaf is tied to another item on the survey, namely signing skill. In 1980, 61% of respondents reported the ability to use some sign language, 15% indicated proficiency, less than one percent were at the interpreter level, and 23% could not use any sign language. Ten years later there is a slight drop in the number of persons indicating use of some sign language (53%) and among those indicating proficiency (12%). Only 1% of audiologists in 1990 function at the interpreter level. The number of respondents that do not use sign language has increased to 34%. In the past 10 years there appears to be a moderate decrease in the number of audiologists who can use sign language or are proficient in it while

TABLE 13.5 *Number and Percentage of Respondents Indicating the Population with Whom They Perform Aural Rehabilitation Work — 1990*

Clinical Population	N	%
Hard-of-Hearing Clients Only	75	17.3
Primarily Hard-of-Hearing		
Fewer than 10 Deaf Clients/Year	231	53.3
More than 10 Deaf Clients/Year	108	24.9
Primarily Deaf Clients	13	3.0
Deaf Clients Only	6	1.4
Totals	433	100.0

TABLE 13.6 Number and Percentage of Specific Clinical Duties

Clinical Duties	1980		Combination	1990		Entry and Combination*	
	N	%	%	N	%	N	%
Clinician	266	72.7	72.7	245	49.7	245 + 107	75.6
Clinical Supervisor	17	4.6	16.7	33	7.1	33 + 47	17.2
Administrator	14	3.8	14.5	16	3.4	16 + 51	14.4
Instructor in Audiology	29	7.9	9.6	8	1.7	8 + 29	14.2
Identification Audiometry	16	4.4	17.2	7	1.5	7 + 47	11.6
Researcher	1	0.3	3.6	7	1.5	7 + 23	6.5
School Hearing Therapist	11	3.0	7.1	5	1.2	5 + 13	3.8
Early Intervention (for children 5 years and younger who have impaired hearing)	7	1.9	9.8	5	1.1	5 + 56	13.1
Other	5	1.4	0.8	14	3.0		
Combination of Above	NA	NA		125	26.8		
Totals	366	100.0		465	100.0		

NA: Not Applicable

*Includes single entry plus combination responses including that entry.

number of audiologists who can use sign language or are proficient in it while the number of respondents at the interpreter level continues to be about 1%.

CLINICAL DUTIES. Table 13.6 shows detailed data on clinical duties. The largest number of single-entry respondents (50%) indicate "clinician" as their primary clinical duty. Many respondents (27%) also report performing a combination of duties. When these two groups of responders are added together, 76% of audiologists specify *clinician* as a main responsibility. It appears that audiologists continue to work primarily as clinicians, with sizable numbers working in a variety of other capacities.

Overall Summary of Audiologic Rehabilitation. Table 13.7 shows rehabilitation in combination with diagnostics is now more often seen as a primary clinical duty than it was in 1980. Although we were unable to analyze dispensing in this or the previous question (Table 13.4), we wonder if the explanation for increased rehabilitation may relate to greater involvement in hearing-aid sales. We will return to this question later.

A total of 440 of the 469 clinically active audiologists (94%) report doing some form of AR (Table 13.8). There is a slight increase (from 80% in 1980 to 86% in 1990) in the percentage of clinician respondents performing hearing-aid assessments.

Notable increases can be seen in use of self-assessment and tinnitus evaluations. Decreases are seen in auditory training and speechreading activities. AHSA (1991) data reported more activities of this type than reported here but the current survey separated out those who provided speechreading instruction as part of a general hearing-aid orientation (HAO) and this may account for the difference.

Since Table 13.8 has shown the percent involvement for all clinically active respondents, through the remainder of this report non responders were removed from tabular data and calculations. Thus, in each case the results reflect responses among those who indicated activity of that type rather than among all the clinically active.

Hearing-Aid Procedures. CANDIDACY. In determining candidacy for hearing aids, respondents use information from a combination of sources, including pure-tone data (99%), speech audiometry (96%), client subjective reports (94%), and case history (86%). Another 37% of audiologists indicate "all of the above," which includes the

TABLE 13.7 *Number and Percentage of Responding Audiologist's General Clinical Duties*

General Clinical Duties	1980		1990	
	N	%	N	%
Diagnostic Audiology	205	56.5	169	36.2
Rehabilitative Audiology	25	6.9	32	6.8
Both of the Above	133	36.6	265	56.8
Totals	363	100.0	466	100.0

TABLE 13.8 Total Number and Percentage of Clinically Active Respondents in 1980 and 1990 Involved in Rehabilitative Activities

Activities	1980 (N =371)		1990 (N = 469)	
	N	%	N	%
General Hearing Aid Evaluations	295	79.5	403	85.9
Hearing Aid Evaluations (with Children)	206	55.5	263	56.1
Dispensing Hearing Aids	79	21.3	**(343	73.1)
General Hearing Aid Orientation	322	86.8	414	88.3
Individual Hearing Aid Orientation	306	82.5	404	86.1
Group Hearing Aid Orientation	50	13.5	80	17.1
Self Assessment	66	17.8	155	33.0
Counseling with Family and Friends	295	79.5	403	85.9
Tinnitus Evaluation	*(97	26.1)	197	42.0
Cochlear Implant Therapy	NA	NA	55	11.7
Communication Training	142	38.3	108	23.0
Speechreading	140	37.7	87	18.6
Auditory Training	115	30.9	73	15.6
Speech/Language Training	24	6.5	51	10.9
Manual/TC	26	7.0	32	6.8
No AR Involvement	29	6.2	–	–

NA: Not Applicable

*Different emphasis in 1980

**Implied from Audiologists offering trial/rental period to hearing aid clients above practices plus use of communication or handicap questionnaires. These responses are virtually unchanged from Whitcomb's findings.

HEARING-AID SELECTION. Over half of the 1990 respondents (51%) report the selection and recommendation of the specific make and model of hearing aid as their goal during the evaluation and fitting of amplification. About 34% indicate using a combination of goals. When the single entries are added to the combination responses, 82% of audiologists select and recommend the make and model of hearing aid for purchase, 32% orient/familiarize the client with the aid(s), 12% make recommendations but don't choose a specific aid for purchase, and 10% give general recommendations only. The results from the 1980 survey were within 6% of the current findings, suggesting that little has changed with respect to the goals audiologists have for the hearing-aid evaluation/fitting.

Table 13.9 shows a summary of different approaches for hearing aid evaluation/fitting. The data show there has been a major shift away from the use of the comparative method toward prescriptive and factory selection practices today.

BINAURAL SELECTION. When considering the recommendation of binaural amplification most audiologists use audiometric data (96%), client's listening demands (93%), client's preference (92%), the developmental status of the client (84%), client's finances (80%), or "all of the above" (73%). Whitcomb found similar results in 1980.

MEASURES OF HEARING-AID PERFORMANCE. Approximately one third of audiologists in 1990 perform electroacoustic analyses about 100% of the time during the hearing-aid assessment/fitting process, up from one fourth of audiologists in 1980 (Table 13.10). There is a trend toward increased use of electroacoustic measures by ASHA audiologists. This was confirmed by Cranmer, 1991, who found that most dispensing audiologists (77%) now possess the necessary equipment to perform electroacoustic tests.

Also shown in Table 13.10, approximately one half of respondents use real-ear measures some time during the evaluation/fitting process, with a fourth of them performing such measures routinely. The ASHA (1991) survey similarly reports that 45% of audiologists perform real-ear measures as part of the hearing-aid evaluation. On the other hand, Cranmer (1991) found that 89% of dispensing audiologists use such measures during hearing-aid evaluations. Apparently dispensing audiologists are doing a lot more of this than the average ASHA audiologist. No comparable data were gathered by Whitcomb.

HEARING AID TRIAL/RENTAL. Most respondents today (81%) and in 1980 (77%) provide a trial/rental period for their hearing-aid clients. Only a small portion of respondents (n=84, 18%) charge their clients a trial/rental fee (x = $76 per aid). Twelve audiologists report a percentage of the total cost of aids as the trial/rental fee (half of these reported 15%). There were 42% of dispensing audiologists who do not indicate a trial/rental fee, which might reflect responders who are audiologists working in government settings, military hospitals, schools for the deaf, or other facilities that may not require such a fee. The percentage of audiologists providing a trial/rental provides

TABLE 13.9 Number and Percentage of Respondents Reporting Various Approaches Used in Hearing Aid Fitting and Evaluation

HAE and Fitting Approaches	1980 N	1980 %	1990 N	1990 %		Entry + Combination N	Entry + Combination %
Comparative Procedure							
with client preference	219	77.1	36	9.3	⎱ 16.8	30 + 77	29.3
with real ear or client preference	NA	NA	29	7.5	⎰	29 + 55	21.8
with master hearing aid	13	4.6	NA	NA			
Factory Selected Response/Output							
with real ear	NA	NA	11	2.8	⎱ 18.6	11 + 63	19.7
with client preference	NA	NA	61	15.8	⎰	67 + 71	34.2
Prescriptive Fitting							
with real ear	NA	NA	34	8.8	⎱ 16.1	4 + 72	27.5
with client preference	NA	NA	28	7.3	⎰	28 + 94	31.6
Client Preference	5	1.8	NA	NA			
Stimuli Recorded Through Hearing Aid	3	1.1	NA	NA			
Combination of Above	NA	NA	171	44.3			
Other	6	2.1	16	4.1			
Totals	284	100.0	386	100.0			

NA: Not Applicable
17 Nonresponders (1990)

TABLE 13.10 Number and Percentage of Respondents Reporting Frequency of Use of Electroacoustic and Real Ear Measures During Hearing Aid Evaluation/Fitting

| | Electroacoustic Analysis | | | | Real Ear Analysis | |
| | 1980 | | 1990 | | 1990 | |
Time Used	N	%	N	%	N	%
About 100%	74	25.5	131	33.2	100	25.1
About 75%	21	7.2	46	11.6	38	9.4
About 50%	21	7.2	38	9.6	31	7.8
About 25%	18	6.2	43	10.9	35	8.8
Hardly Ever	25	8.6	70	17.7	41	10.3
Never	92	31.7	67	16.9	153	38.4
Only on Hearing Aid Reevaluations	39	13.4	NA	NA	NA	NA
Totals	290	100.0	395	100.0	398	100.0

NA: Not Applicable

TABLE 13.11 *Number and Percentage of Respondents Reporting the Approximate Percentage of All Aids Recommended/Dispensed in the Past Year that are Ear-Level Hearing Aids (i.e., BTE, ITE, ITC)*

1980

Aid Type	0–5% N	%	10–25% N	%	30–50% N	%	55–75% N	%	80–95% N	%	100% N	%
BTE*	1	0.3	6	2.1	25	8.7	80	27.8	152	52.8	24	8.2
ITE**	146	54.7	70	26.2	37	13.9	11	4.1	3	1.1	0	0.0

1990

Aid Type	0–10% N	%	20–30% N	%	40–50% N	%	60–70% N	%	80–90% N	%	100% N	%
BTE	122	31.9	152	39.8	41	10.7	22	5.8	30	7.9	15	3.9
ITE	35	9.5	49	13.2	95	25.7	133	35.9	56	15.1	2	0.5
ITC	181	52.6	102	29.7	41	11.9	16	4.7	4	1.2	0	0.0

*1980, N=288
**1980, N=267

an indirect measure of those respondents dispensing hearing aids. This inferred percentage (81%) of audiologists who are dispensing is comparable to the one from the ASHA (1991) study (76%). Whitcomb found only 21% of the respondents dispensed hearing aids. Expectedly, there has been a dramatic increase in the percentage of audiologists dispensing since 1980.

HEARING-AID STYLE RECOMMENDATION. Audiologists now are recommending/dispensing many fewer BTE aids (31% of total aids recommended) and greater numbers of in-the-ear (52% of all aids recommended) and intracanal aids (just under 20% of all aids recommended) than in 1980. A further breakdown of percentages of the three styles recommended is shown in Table 13.11. This trend is well documented in other surveys (Cranmer, 1991).

The mean number of hearing aid evaluations/fittings by audiologists in 1990 is 14 per month. Whitcomb found that the largest percentage of audiologists (33%) reported conducting 6 to 10 hearing aid evaluations per month. The number of hearing-aid assessments performed by audiologists has increased somewhat in the past ten years, probably reflecting the increased numbers of audiologists dispensing and working with doctors or in private practice.

ASSISTIVE LISTENING DEVICES (ALD's). The majority of 1990 respondents (57%) routinely advise selected clients about ALDs, but only 19% regularly dispense, maintain, and display these devices. Another 17% of the respondents answer questions about these devices, only if asked, and about 7% do not deal with ALD's at all. As for why audiologists do not handle these devices, of those not involved 39% indicate they preferred to refer their clients to other sources, and 31% indicate there is no demand. Another 23% report a combination of explanations, while 4% indicate difficulty maintaining stock, and another 4% report a lack of client interest. ASHA's (1991) survey reports 63% of audiologists dispense ALD's, which is over three times the percentage found in this study. The discrepancy may relate to some audiologists who do not display these devices but do advise clients about them and dispense on demand. In any case, it appears that 24–37% of audiologists continue to give these forms of amplification little or no attention. When recommended, telephone amplifiers and FM systems are the most frequently mentioned items (Table 13.12). Only 2% of gross revenue among audiologists comes from sales of ALD's (Cranmer, 1991).

HEARING-AID RECOMMENDATIONS FOR YOUNG CHILDREN. Among respondents (n=254; 54% of all respondents) who fit hearing aids on children 2 years of age and younger (2 per month on average), eighty four percent recommended BTE aids and 13% fit either a body aid or BTE. Four percent fit body aids exclusively, and no respondents indicated fitting ITE aids. This number represents a halving of clinical audiologists recommending a body aid since 1980 (44%). Most respondents (69%) recommend 100% binaural fitting of young children.

Hearing-Aid Orientation/General Audiologic Rehabilitation. Of the 469 clinically active audiologists, 414 (88%) provide hearing-aid orientation (HAO) (Table

TABLE 13.12 *Number and Percentage of Respondents who Recommend Specific Assistive Listening Devices*

Device	1990		Entry + Combination	
	N	%	N	%
Telephone Amplifier	109	30.4	109 + 176	79.6
FM System	39	10.9	39 + 125	45.8
Infrared System	9	2.5	9 + 104	31.6
Hardwired Unit	3	0.8	3 + 39	11.7
Loop System	0	0.0	0 + 24	6.7
Other	22	6.1		
Combination of Above	176	49.2		
Totals	358	100.0		

13.8). Most ASHA (1991) survey respondents (98%) also report providing HAO. Among 397 of the current audiologists who report in more detail on the form of HAO, the majority (76%) do this in individual follow-up sessions while about 15% provide either group or combined individual/group sessions. In 1980, 20% reported some form of group work. Group activity appears to have dropped even though various HAO services continue to be performed by a large proportion of audiologists.

INDIVIDUAL HEARING-AID ORIENTATION. On average, current audiologists provide about three individual orientation sessions in connection with hearing-aid fitting or adjustment. In 1980, around 22% of the respondents offered 3 orientation sessions, while most (41%) offered 2 sessions. Apparently, audiologists are increasing the number of such sessions they offer routinely. Most audiologists spend about 30 minutes per orientation session (Table 13.13).

GROUP HEARING-AID ORIENTATION. Among a reduced group (n=78) doing group orientation sessions, the average number of clients per group was estimated to be fewer than eight by 76% of respondents. Half the members of this group (50%) conduct eight or more group sessions per year and most sessions (63%) last from 30–60 minutes. These figures were little changed from 1980. Focus of group sessions was also

TABLE 13.13 *Number and Percentage of Respondents Reporting Various Times Spent in Individual Hearing Aid Orientation Sessions*

Time spent	1980		1990	
	N	%	N	%
About 5 Minutes	7	2.3	3	0.8
10–20 Minutes	113	37.2	97	25.1
About 30 minutes	126	41.4	181	46.9
45–60 Minutes	53	17.4	97	25.1
Longer than 1 hour	5	1.6	8	2.1
Totals	304	100.0	386	100.0

unchanged from 1980 (Table 13.14) except for a slight deemphasis of auditory training and speechreading over the past decade. ALD's (unmeasured in 1980) are not stressed as much as the other four topics.

Counseling/Overall Coordination and Miscellaneous. In Table 13.8, 155 (33%) of the clinically active audiologists reported using self-assessment questionnaires. Among these 155, 76% said they used them "occasionally" or "inconsistently", while only 24% used them routinely. The most used questionnaires were the Hearing Handicap Inventory for the Elderly (HHIE), the Hearing Handicap Scale (HHS) and the Denver Scale (Table 13.15). Other sizable use patterns were shown for the Hearing Performance Inventory (HPI), the Self/Significant Other Assessment of Communication (SAC/SOAC) and the Communication Profile for the Hearing Impaired (CPHI). Of the 27 persons reporting use of "other" questionnaires, 21 indicated using a unique, informal, in-house form, two were using a questionnaire by Oticon, and one each reported use of the McCarthy-Alpiner Scale, the Kasten questionnaire, a Walter Reed scale, and a Minnesota parent assessment scale. As noted previously (Table 13.8) the number of self-assessment users among clinically active audiologists has nearly doubled in the past ten years (18–33%). There also appears to be a shift toward the use of newer handicap questionnaires such as the HHIE, SAC/SOAC, and the CPHI, as well as the older instruments such as the HHS and the Denver.

Altogether, 79% of responders made some form of counseling referral. Referrals for vocational rehabilitation or professional (social/emotional) counseling are made by 22% and 16% of audiologists respectively, or some combination of referrals (34%). There are 7% of respondents that report "other" forms of referral such as speech therapy, genetic counseling, family counseling, etc. The majority of respondents (69%) indicates recommending participation in self-help groups to their clients. Whitcomb did not inquire into referral practices in a similar manner in 1980.

Promotion/Marketing. A combination of practices are used to promote hearing-aid sales and audiologic rehabilitation (AR) services (Table 13.16). Community screening programs, newspaper ads/inserts, and direct-mail programs are the most often used methods of promotion.

A large proportion of respondents (46%; n=152) reported "other" methods of promotion such as word of mouth recommendations (n=30), medical referrals (n=25), Yellow Page ads (n=20), and one or two respondents reported using medical journal ads, newsletters, billboards, and literature left at medical doctor offices or senior citizen centers. About one-third of those responding "other" reported working in settings that did not formally promote or advertise their services (i.e. government/VA settings, or schools). Cranmer (1991) surveyed dispensing audiologists and found Yellow Page ads were the most popular form of advertising. She also found that newsletters, referral incentives, and discounts were used to promote services.

Tinnitus. As noted in Table 13.8 the percent of clinically active audiologists that indicate performing tinnitus evaluations has increased from 26% in 1980 to 42% in 1990. Among the 197 who report such activity, 191 gave additional detail. The largest

TABLE 13.14 *Number and Percentage of Respondents Indicating Percentage of Time Spent in Group Hearing Aid Orientation Sessions on Various Topics*

Percentage of Time Spent	Hearing Aids		Speechreading		Auditory Training		Communication Strategy		ALDs		Other	
	N	%	N	%	N	%	N	%	N	%	N	%
1980												
0–5%	2	4.3	10	23.8	12	27.3	2	4.4	NA		6	40.0
10–25%	23	48.9	20	47.6	20	45.5	24	53.3	NA		5	33.3
30–50%	12	25.5	9	21.4	10	22.7	17	37.8	NA		4	26.7
60–75%	7	14.9	3	7.1	2	4.5	1	2.2	NA		0	0.0
80–95%	3	6.4	0	0.0	0	0.0	1	2.2	NA		0	0.0
100%	0	0.0	0	0.0	0	0.0	0	0.0	NA		0	0.0
Totals	47	100.0	42	100.0	44	100.0	45	100.0	NA		15	100.0
1990 (N=78)												
0–10%	6	8.5	37	58.7	33	55.0	16	22.2	44	70.9	16	69.6
20–30%	32	45.1	24	38.1	23	38.3	43	59.7	13	20.9	7	30.4
40–50%	18	25.3	2	3.2	1	1.6	12	16.7	3	4.8	0	0.0
60–70%	8	11.3	0	0.0	1	1.6	1	1.4	1	1.6	0	0.0
80–90%	6	8.5	0	0.0	2	3.3	0	0.0	1	1.6	0	0.0
100%	1	1.4	0	0.0	0	0.0	0	0.0	0	0.0	0	0.0
Totals	71	100.0	63	100.0	60	100.0	72	100.0	62	100.0	23	100.0
Means	34.5		11.8		14.8		20.6		11.9		9.6	
Non Responders	(9)		(17)		(20)		(8)		(18)		(57)	

NA: Not Applicable

TABLE 13.15 Number and Percentage of Respondents Using Various Self-Assessment Questionnaires

Questionnaires	1980 N	1980 %	1990 N	1990 %	Entry + Combination N	Entry + Combination %
HHIE	NA	NA	28	20.0	28 + 22	35.7
HHS	23	34.8	15	10.7	15 + 19	24.3
Denver Scale	36	54.5	12	8.6	12 + 20	22.8
HPI	18	27.3	9	6.4	9 + 12	15.0
SAC/SOAC	NA	NA	4	2.9	4 + 15	13.6
CPHI	NA	NA	7	5.0	7 + 7	10.0
SAI	14	21.2	NA	NA		
Sander's Scale	9	13.6	NA	NA		
HMS	6	9.1	NA	NA		
SHHI	5	7.6	NA	NA		
Combination of Above	NA	NA	38	12.5		
Other	11	16.7	27	8.8		
Totals	66	100.0	140	100.0		

165 do not use these scales (1990); 241 do not use these scales (1980)

HHIE: Hearing Handicap Inventory for the Elderly; HHS: Hearing Handicap Scale; HPI: Hearing Performance Inventory; SAC: Self Assessment of Communication; SOAC: Significant Other Assessment of Communication; CPHI: Communication Profile for the Hearing Impaired; SAI: Social Adequacy Index; HMS: Hearing Measurement Scale; SHHI: Social Hearing Handicap Index

NA: Not Applicable

TABLE 13.16 *Number and Percentage of Respondents Reporting Various Promotional Practices Involving Hearing Aids and Aural Rehabilitation*

Promotional Practice	1990		Entry + Combination	
	N	%	N	%
Community Screening Program	30	9.2	30 + 85	35.2
Newspaper Ads/Inserts	20	6.1	20 + 87	32.7
Direct Mail Program	11	3.4	11 + 75	26.3
Dispenser Sponsored Open House	3	0.9	3 + 31	10.1
Manufacturer Sponsored Open House	1	0.3	1 + 21	6.7
Telemarketing	1	0.3	1 + 19	6.1
Radio Advertising	1	0.3	1 + 19	6.1
TV Advertising	3	0.9	3 + 14	5.2
Combination of Above	105	32.1		
Other	152	45.5		
Totals	327	100.0		

increase (from 23% to 39%) is in the percent performing brief evaluations. There is a slight decline in the percentage of audiologists reporting extensive assessment (8% to 5%) and in those reporting both brief plus extensive workups (8% to 6%). It appears that the percentage of audiologists performing tinnitus evaluations is on the rise, while the depth of such tests is on the decline. Tinnitus evaluations almost universally include pitch matching, while loudness matching and maskability evaluations are done to a lesser extent (Table 13.17).

As for the rationale behind tinnitus evaluations, the largest percentage (45%) indicate a combination of reasons. Medical/diagnostic purposes (22%), fitting of tinnitus maskers (15%), and patient information/curiosity (15%) were the reasons given most often by the single-entry responders. The same patterns were evident when the combination responders are included (57%, 43%, 41% respectively).

From the 1980 survey, among clinically active audiologists, 45 (12%) dispensed tinnitus maskers, and most of these 45 (n=36) recommended/dispensed one tinnitus

TABLE 13.17 *Number and Percentage of Respondents Conducting Various Tinnitus Evaluation Procedures*

Evaluation Procedures	1990		Entry + All + Combination	
	N	%	N	%
Pitch Matching Task	31	15.9	31 + 52 + 99	93.8
Loudness Evaluation	2	1.0	2 + 52 + 97	77.8
Maskability Evaluation	1	0.5	1 + 52 + 46	51.0
Residual Inhibition Test	1	0.5	1 + 52 + 11	32.9
All of the Above	52	26.8		
Other	8	4.1		
Combination	99	51.0		
Totals	194	100.0		

masker per month. Currently, 110 (23%) of the clinically active report using these devices. Of these 110, the largest number (n=50) recommend/dispense one of these devices per year and only a few (n=6) recommend six or more per year. Far fewer maskers are being distributed currently, though more audiologists are distributing these as compared to 1980.

Cochlear Implants. Of the 469 clinically active audiologists, only 67 (14%) indicated performing cochlear implant evaluations (see Table 13.8). Among this small group, the majority (67%) performs between 1 and 3 evaluations per year while another 19% perform between 4 and 6 evaluations per year. A few offered even more. As for therapy with implant patients, of the 469 respondents, only 55 (12%) provide clients with therapy. Again the majority (60%) of these 55 provide between 1 and 3 patients with therapy per year while 16% work with between four and six patients and 24% work with more than eight patients per year. Thus, very few audiologists currently appear to be involved in cochlear implant assessment and follow-up therapy. Whitcomb did not survey this item.

Communication Training. Table 13.8 shows that specific rehabilitation therapy distinct from and in addition to general HAO therapy was offered by 108 (23%) of the clinically active respondents. Based on N=469 we found 19% and 16% respectively provide speechreading and auditory training, and all of these activities are markedly reduced since 1980 (see Table 13.8). Among audiologists offering specific services (N=108), a majority offers a combination of traditional programs (Table 13.18), which is little different from the 1980 report. In general there has been a substantial decrease in the percent of audiologists providing speechreading and auditory training of a specific nature, although the recent ASHA (1991) survey which did not separate out these activities when used in HAO, gives a more favorable impression. The latter survey reveals 28% of audiologists doing speechreading and 61% auditory training. The higher percentage reporting auditory training contrasts with the trend found in our 1980 and 1990 comprehensive surveys and supports the contention that the ASHA data are heavily influenced by HAO.

In 1990, the largest proportion of audiologists (47%) who provide communication training do so in individual training sessions, while 16% of the respondents

TABLE 13.18 *Number and Percentage of Respondents Providing or Recommending Specific Rehabilitation Services Beyond Hearing Aid Orientation*

Rehabilitation Service	1990		Entry + Combination	
	N	%	N	%
Speechreading	29	27.9	29 + 58	80.6
Auditory Training	15	13.9	15 + 58	67.6
Speech/Language	3	2.8	3 + 48	47.2
Manual/Total Communication	3	2.8	3 + 29	29.6
Combination of Above	58	53.7		
Totals	108	100.0		

conduct group training sessions and 37% engage in combination group/individual therapy. Whitcomb found equal percentages provided individual therapy (46%) and combination group/individual therapy sessions (46%), with only 8% of audiologists performing group training sessions. There seems to be a trend away from combination therapy sessions and an increase in the amount of group instruction, while the amount of individual training has remained relatively unchanged since 1980.

Among the 108 reporting on combined communication training, as noted in Table 13.18, there are only 87 and 73 surveys, respectively, from respondents pertaining to specific speechreading and auditory training practices.

SPEECHREADING. A combination of tests is used to evaluate the speechreading ability of patients, with the Utley Test continuing to receive greatest usage (Table 13.19). Visual acuity may be an important variable in speechreading evaluations, but only 16% of audiologists who evaluate speechreading ability screen for visual adequacy. This was only half the 33% reported in 1980.

Regarding speechreading therapy, a unique combination of material is used by 77% of current audiologists, followed by 13% who use "other" material and 10% who use a published program. These results were almost identical to 1980 findings.

Over one half (51%) of the audiologists indicate using a combination of approaches for speechreading instruction, including in order of preference, drillwork (27%), tracking (18%), and interactive videos (5%). A majority (63%) of participating audiologists offer patients between 5 and 15 sessions, with each session lasting typically 30 minutes and involving an average 18 persons per year. No dramatic change in these percentages was noted since 1980.

AUDITORY TRAINING. Current audiologists use a broad assortment of materials when involved in auditory training (Table 13.20), among which the most popular are the Auditory Skills Curriculum, CID W-22, WIPI, NUCHIPS, and PB-K. There is also increased use of new materials such as GASP, SSI, and SPIN. The majority of audiologists (70%) use background noise in connection with auditory training, which is virtually unchanged from 1980 findings.

In Table 13.21 we see that nearly half the 1990 respondents (49%) report using a combination of the listed approaches to auditory training. Combination, unique (self-developed or unpublished), and "other" approaches were the most popular. Also used frequently were the methods of Ling, Tracking, the Erber approach, the Acoupedic method, and the Sanders and Verbotonal method.

In 1980 the majority of audiologists (95%) used personal hearing aids as the major amplification system during auditory training. Also, 21% of the respondents used FM systems, and 16% used a desk or hard wire unit either alone or in combination with personal aids. Ten years later, examination of the total (combination and single entry) respondents reveals that most (85%) still use the patients personal hearing aids. However, twice as many in 1990 use FM systems (43%) compared with 1980, while 10% fewer audiologists use desk/hard wire units. Use of induction loop amplification was similar (4% vs. 5%). Most respondents provide either 10–14 sessions per client (26%), or more than 25 sessions per client (26%), with typical sessions lasting

TABLE 13.19 Number and Percentage of Respondents Indicating Test(s) Used for Evaluating Speechreading Abilities

Test Used	1980 Combination		1990		1990 Entry + Combination	
	N	%	N	%	N	%
Utley	83	59.3	18	23.4	18 + 21	50.6
Informal Test	36	25.7	13	16.9	13 + 12	32.5
Barley	21	15.0	5	6.5	5 + 13	23.4
Self-Made Test	30	21.4	4	5.2	4 + 10	18.2
Craig	14	10.0	3	3.9	3 + 6	11.7
Modification of Standard Test	14	10.0	2	2.6	2 + 5	9.1
Keaster	6	4.3	1	1.3	1 + 2	3.9
Combination of Above	NA	NA	24	31.2		
Other	11	7.9	7	9.1		
Totals	140	100.0	77	100.0		

TABLE 13.20 Number and Percentage of Respondents Indicating Tests Used for Auditory Training Purposes

Test Used	1980 Combination		1990		1990 Entry + Combination	
	N	%	N	%	N	%
Auditory Curriculum (LA Schools)	NA	NA	6	8.5	6 + 26	45.1
CID W-22	51	45.9	5	7.0	5 + 21	36.6
WIPI	46	41.4	0	0.0	0 + 24	33.8
PB-K (Haskins)	44	39.6	0	0.0	0 + 18	25.4
NU-CHIPS	NA	NA	3	4.2	3 + 14	23.9
NU-6	25	22.5	0	0.0	0 + 13	18.3
SSI	NA	NA	1	1.4	1 + 11	16.9
GASP	NA	NA	0	0.0	0 + 11	15.5
SPIN	4	3.6	2	2.8	2 + 7	12.7
Other	33	29.7	21	29.6		
DIP	9	8.1	NA	NA		
Combination of Above	NA	NA	29	40.8		
Do Not Test	NA	NA	4	5.6		
Totals	111	100.0	71	100.0		

NA: Not Applicable

TABLE 13.21 Number and Percentage of Respondents Indicating the Auditory Training Approaches Used

Approach	1980 Combination		1990		Entry and Combination	
	N	%	N	%	N	%
Unique Approach	63	57.3	11	16.2	11 + 23	50.0
Ling	17	15.5	3	4.4	3 + 28	45.6
Tracking	NA	NA	3	4.4	3 + 15	26.5
Erber	NA	NA	1	1.5	1 + 16	25.0
Acoupedic	11	10.0	3	4.4	3 + 11	20.1
Self-Programmed Approach	NA	NA	3	4.4	3 + 5	11.8
Carhart or Modified Carhart	11	10.0	1	1.5	1 + 6	10.3
Sanders	18	16.4	1	1.5	1 + 6	10.3
Verbotonal Method	6	5.5	1	1.5	1 + 6	10.3
Interactive Audio/Video	NA	NA	0	0.0	0 + 6	8.8
Audio Flash Cards	6	5.5	NA	NA		
Other	13	11.8	8	11.8		
Combination of Above	NA	NA	33	48.5		
Totals	110	100.0	68	100.0		

NA: Not Applicable

30 minutes and involving an average of three training groups per year. These results were also similar to the 1980 survey.

Summary/Conclusions

Decade trends (1980-1990) in aural rehabilitation practices were studied from 538 responses received from 1000 mailings to 6267 ASHA audiologists. A notable finding was that 20% fewer audiologists describe their major clinical duties as diagnostic only, with a corresponding increase in those who see their job as both diagnostic and rehabilitative. A greater emphasis on rehabilitative audiology is related to increased hearing-aid dispensing on the part of audiologists and their involvement in private practice or work in MD offices where dispensing is common. Slight increases since 1980 were apparent in the percent of audiologists involved in general hearing-aid orientation, counseling, and instruction in speech/language training. Larger increases were seen in the percent of respondents involved in the dispensing of hearing aids, use of in the ear and in the canal aids, use of self-assessment questionnaires, and tinnitus evaluations. There was little change in the past 10 years in the percent of audiologists engaged in hearing-aid evaluations with children, individual and group hearing-aid orientation, and instruction in manual/total communication. Substantial decreases were found in the percent of respondents involved in specific communication training, speechreading, and auditory training.

Overall, the survey results reveal an evolved and more mature profession in which audiologists now give less emphasis to some classic forms of rehabilitative audiology (speechreading and auditory training). At the same time, they are assuming an expanded role in direct provision of rehabilitative services involving amplification and positioning themselves increasingly in MD and private practice settings.

References

ASHA—American Speech-Language-Hearing Association (1990). ASHA membership employment setting information

ASHA (1991). Results of 1989 ASHA audiology opinion survey. *Asha, 10*(1), 9-11.

Cherow, E. (1986). The practice of audiology: A national perspective. *Asha*, Sept., 31-38.

Cranmer, K. S. (1991). Hearing instrument dispensing—1991. *Hearing Instruments, 42*(6), 6-13.

Hardick, E. (1977). Aural rehabilitation programs for the aged can be successful. *Journal of Academy Rehabilitative Audiology, 10*, 51-67.

Martin, F., and Forbis, N. (1978). The present status of audiometric practice: A follow-up study. *Asha, 20*, 531-541.

Martin, F., and Pennington, C. (1971). Current trends in audiometric practice. *Asha, 13*, 671-677.

Martin, F., and Pennington, C. (1972). ASHA audiologists: Professional background information. *Asha, 15*, 255-256.

Martin, F., and Sides, D. G. (1985). Survey of current audiometric practice. *Asha*, *27*, 29–36.

Martin, F., and Morris, L. J. (1989). Current audiological practice in the United States. *Hearing Journal*, April, 25–42.

Rosen, J. (1967). Distortions in the training of audiologists. *Asha*, *9*, 171–174.

Schow, R. L. (1986). Rehabilitating the elderly hearing impaired, audiologists as hearing aid dispensers. *Corti's Organ*, *11*(1), 2–9.

Schow, R. L., and Nerbonne, M. A. (1989). *Introduction to Aural Rehabilitation* (2nd ed.). Needham Heights, MA: Allyn and Bacon.

Schow, R. L. (1990). Status of aural rehabilitation in the USA. *British Journal of Audiology*, *24*, 258–260.

This article first appeared in American Journal of Audiology 2(3)28-37. Used here with permission.

"ARA POSITION STATEMENT ON Au.D. EDUCATIONAL STANDARDS"

Background

Over an extended period of time there has been a growing realization that the scope of practice in audiology has expanded to such an extent that the master's degree no longer is well-suited to prepare audiologists adequately enough to meet the challenges of today's workplace. Concern for the quality of education received by individuals entering the practice of audiology, coupled with other related issues, led the Academy of Dispensing Audiologists (ADA) to hold a Conference on Professional Education in Audiology in 1988. A recommendation emerged from the conference to establish a professional doctorate in audiology, the Au.D. degree, which would replace the master's degree as the entry-level degree for the practice of audiology.

While the Au.D. proposal has been a major topic of discussion since then and the source of some controversy, it generally has received strong support from rank-and-file audiologists and numerous professional organizations at the state and national levels, including the Academy of Rehabilitative Audiology (ARA). In 1989 the Executive Committee of ARA approved the following position statement:

> The Executive Committee of the Academy of Rehabilitative Audiology supports efforts to implement the concept of the professional doctorate degree to be designated as a doctor of audiology. In addition the Executive Committee encourages a coalition of audiology organizations to support and advance efforts to develop the professional doctorate in audiology and seeks Academy of Rehabilitative Audiology representation on the educational foundation being established to advance these goals.

Since 1988 major efforts have been made at a growing number of universities to develop professional doctorate programs in audiology. While no Au.D. programs presently are in place, significant progress toward this end has occurred, and it is anticipated that several universities will implement programs for the Doctor of Audiology in the near future.

Areas of Preparation in Aural Rehabilitation

While universities electing to establish their own Au.D. will retain autonomy with respect to all aspects of the degree, some general guidelines have been developed related to key features of the proposed professional doctorate, especially with respect to curriculum. Both the ADA (1988) and the American Academy of Audiology (1991) have outlined guidelines which specify the courses/areas of study which ought to be included in the curriculum for the Au.D. Because the intent of the professional doctorate is to prepare highly skilled practitioners, these curricular guidelines are comprehensive and include an emphasis in both the diagnostic and rehabilitative aspects of audiology (Lesner, Flexer, and Goldstein, 1991).

As universities continue to develop their own requirements for the Au.D., it is crucial that emphasis be placed on providing the necessary coursework and clinical practicum experiences in *each* of these two major areas of audiology. Toward this end, it is the position of the Academy of Rehabilitative Audiology that while the degree to which they are emphasized may vary from program to program, knowledge in the following areas of aural rehabilitation and related topics is considered essential for the practice of audiology and should be incorporated into the academic and clinical practicum experiences of any program offering a Doctor of Audiology degree:

General
Normative developmental models

Speech acoustics/perception

Assessment of communication status (hearing, vision, speech-language, etc.)

Amplification and Related Devices
Hearing aids

Assistive devices/systems

Cochlear implants/tactile aids

Electroacoustic characteristics of amplifying devices

Methods of evaluation/fitting/orientation

Dispensing practices/issues

Aural Rehabilitation Treatment
Auditory training/Auditory learning

Speechreading

Communication strategies

Manual communication/ASL

Speech/language of the HI

Psychosocial aspects of HI

Early intervention

Educational management/issues

Audiologic counseling

Multimodal communication

Related Competencies

Deaf culture

Interdisciplinary programs/issues

Legislation/consumerism

References

AAA. (1991). Position paper: The American Academy of Audiology and the professional doctorate (Au.D.). *Audiology Today, 3*(4), 10-12.

ADA. (1988, October). *Proceedings; Academy of Dispensing Audiologists Conference on Professional Education.* Chicago.

ARA. (1989, July). The professional doctorate in audiology. *President's Newsletter.*

Lesner, S. A., Flexer, C., and Goldstein, D. P. (1991). Diagnostics and rehabilitation = Au.D.: Equation for a Unified Profession. *Journal of the Academy of Rehabilitative Audiology, 24,* 113-120.

This article first appeared in September, 1993 *ARA Newsletter.*

"ASHA DEFINITION OF AND COMPETENCIES FOR AURAL REHABILITATION (POSITION STATEMENT)"

I.   Identification and Evaluation of Sensory Capabilities
    A.   Identification and evaluation of the extent of the impairment, including assessment, periodic monitoring, and re-evaluation of auditory abilities.
    B.   Monitoring of other sensory capabilities as they relate to receptive and expressive communication.
    C.   Evaluation, fitting, and monitoring of auditory aids and monitoring of other sensory aids.
    D.   Evaluation and monitoring of the acoustic characteristics of the communicative environments confronted by the hearing-impaired person.
II. Interpretation of Results, Counseling, and Referral
    A.   Interpretation of audiologic findings to the client, family, employer, teachers and significant others involved in communication with the hearing-impaired person.

    B.   Guidance and counseling for the client, family, employer, caregiver, teach-
         ers, and significant others concerning the educational, psychosocial, and
         communicative effects of hearing impairment.
    C.   Guidance and counseling for the parent/caregiver regarding:
         1.   educational options available:
         2.   selection of educational programs; and
         3.   facilitation of communicative and cognitive development.
    D.   Individual and/or family counseling regarding:
         1.   acceptance and understanding of hearing impairment;
         2.   functioning within difficult listening situations;
         3.   facilitation of effective strategies and attitudes toward commu-
              nication;
         4.   modification of communicative behavior in keeping with those strate-
              gies and attitudes; and
    5.   Promotion of independent management of communication-related problems.
    E.   Referral for additional services.
III. Intervention for Communicative Difficulties
    A.   Development and provision of an intervention program to facilitate
         expressive and receptive communication.
    B.   Provision of hearing and speech conservation programming.
    C.   Service as a liaison between the client, family, and other agencies con-
         cerned with the management of communicative disorders related to hear-
         ing impairment.
IV.   Re-evaluation of the Client's Status
V.   Evaluation and Modification of the Intervention Program
Excerpts from: Position Statement (1984). Asha, 26, 37-41.

RESOURCES AND MATERIALS LIST—CHILDREN

The following list of materials is not intended to be exhaustive. The list provides
samples of materials and protocols that are useful for pre- and post-audiologic rehabilitation evaluations and for management. Because of the individuality of each client,
clinicians must often modify existing materials or develop new ones. This list of materials may be helpful as a guide.

Language Assessment Tools

Parent Questionnaires
    Ecoscales Manual. J. McDonald, Y. Gillette, and T. Hutchinson (1989). San Antonio,
        TX: Special Press.
    The Rosetti Infant-Toddler Language Scale (1990). East Moline, IL:
        Linguisystems.

Diagnostic Tests

Assessment of Children's Language Comprehension. R. Foster, J. Stark, and J. Giddon (1972). Consulting Psychologists Press Inc., 577 College Avenue, Palo Alto, CA 94306. (3+ years).

Assessing language production in children. J. Miller (1981). Austin, TX: Pro-Ed.

Carrow Elicited Language Inventory. E. Carrow, et al. (1974). Teaching Resources Corporation, 100 Boylston Street, Boston, MA 02116. (3–7 years).

Expressive One Word Picture Vocabulary Test. M. Gardner (1979). Novato, CA: Academic Therapy Productions.

Grammatical Analysis of Elicited Language. J. Moog, V. Kozak, and A. Geers (1983). St. Louis, MO: Central Institute for the Deaf Press.

Kretschmer Spontaneous Language Analysis Procedure. R. Kretschmer and L. Kretschmer (1978). In *Language development and intervention with the hearing impaired.* Austin, TX: Pro-Ed.

Preschool Language Assessment Instrument (PLAI). (1978). Grune and Stratton, Inc., 111 Fifth Avenue, New York, NY 10003.

Reynell Development Language Scale. J. Reynell (1977). Windsor, Ontario: NFER Publishing.

Sequenced Inventory of Communicative Disorders. D. L. Hedrick, E. Prather, and A. Tobin (1975). University of Washington Press, Seattle, WA 98105. (4 months–4 years)

Teacher Assessment of Grammatical Structure. J. Moog and V. Kozak (1983). Central Institute for the Deaf, 818 S. Euclid Ave., St. Louis, MO.

Test of Expressive Language Ability. G. Bunch (1981). Toronto, Ontario: G. B. Services.

Test of Receptive Language Ability. G. Bunch (1981). Toronto, Ontario: G. B. Services.

Test of Syntactic Ability. S. Quigley, M. Steinkamp, D. Power, and B. Jones (1978). Dormac Inc., Beaverton, OR 97006.

Written Language Syntax Test. S. Berry (1981). Washington, DC: Gallaudet College Press.

Developmental Profiles

Criterion References. P. Tesauro and C. Takeshita (1975). Speech and Hearing, State Health Department, 2450 South Vine, Denver, CO 80210. (0–5 years)

MacArthur Communicative Development Inventory. P. Dale and D. Thal (1989). San Diego, CA: Center for Research in Language.

Scales of early communication skills for hearing impaired children. J.S. Moog and A. Geers (1975). Central Institute for the Deaf, 818 South Euclid Avenue, St. Louis, MO 63110.

Schedules of Development in Audition, Speech, Language, Communication for Hearing Impaired Infants and Their Parents. D. Ling (1977). Alexander Graham Bell Association for the Deaf, 3417 Volta Place NW, Washington, DC 20007.

SKI-HI Language Development Scale. S. Watkins (1979). Home Oriented Program Essentials (HOPE Inc.), 809 North 800 East, Logan, UT 84321.

Communication/Language Stimulation Programs

Child Oriented

Appletree. J. Caniglia, N. J. Cole, W. Howard, E. Krohn, and M. Rice (1972). Dormac Inc., P.O. Box 752, Beaverton, OR 97005.

Baby Talk—The Art of Communicating with Infants and Toddlers. M. Devine (1991). Plenum Press, 233 Spring St., New York, NY 10013.

Becoming Partners with Children from Play to Conversation. J. MacDonald (1989). San Antonio, TX: Special Press.

Blueprint for Developing Conversational Competence: A Planning/Instruction Model with Detailed Scenarios. P. Stone (1988). Tucker-Maxon Oral School. Director, Alexander Graham Bell Association for the Deaf, 3417 Volta Place, NW, WAshington DC 20007.

Curriculum Guide—Hearing Impaired Children. W. Northcott (1972). UNISTAPS, University of Minnesota, State Department of Education, Minneapolis, MN 55455.

Developmental Language Centered Curriculum for Hearing Impaired Children. Texas Education Agency (1982). Statewide Project for the Deaf, P.O. Box 35358, Austin, TX 78764.

Developmental Syntax Program (2nd ed.). L. Coughran and B. Liles. Teaching Resources Corporation, 100 Boylston Street, Boston, MA 02116.

How to Talk so Kids Will Listen and Listen so Kids Will Talk. A. Faber, and E. Mazlish (1982). Avon Books, New York, NY.

It Takes Two to Talk (3rd ed.). A. Manolsen (1992). Hanen Early Language Resource Centre, sold by Imaginart in Bisbee, AZ. (800) 828-1376.

Language, Learning and Deafness. A. H. Strong, R. R. Kretschmer, and L. W. Kretschmer (1978). Grune and Stratton, 111 Fifth Avenue, New York, NY 10003.

Learning staircase. L. Coughran and M. Goff. Teaching Resources Corporation, 100 Boylston Street, Boston, MA 02116.

Learning to Talk is Child's Play: Helping Preschoolers Develop Language. Communication Skill Builders, Inc., 3130 North Dodge Blvd., PO Box 42050, Tuscon, AZ 85733, (602) 323-7500.

Lessons in Syntax. J. E. McCan (1973). Dormac Inc., P.O. Box 752, Beaverton, OR 97005.

Listen, Talk, Do Activity Cards. (1975). Department of Head Start Training, Tennessee State University, Intersect, 1101 17th Avenue South, Nashville, TN 37203. (HI)

MWM Program for Developing Language Abilities. E. Minskoff and D. Wiseman (1972). Ridgefield, NJ: Educational Performance Associates.

Natural Language Processing Program. M. M. Ernst and H. M. Wallace (1982). Denver, CO: Educational Audiology Programs.

Peabody Language Development Kits. 1968. American Guidance Service Inc., Publishers Building, Circle Pines, MN 55014.

Read with me. Schick, B., Dougherty, F., & Moeller, M. P. (1995). Boys Town Press: 13603 Flanagan Blvd., Boys Ton, NE 68010 (800-282-6657).

Sentences and Other Systems. P. O. Blackwell, E. Engen, J. E. Fischgrund, and C. Zarcadoolas (1978). Alexander Graham Bell Association for the Deaf, 3417 Volta Place NW, Washington, DC 20007.

Structured Tasks for English. E. Costello, L. G. Lane, S. D. Lopez, C. S. Melman, and I. B. Pittle (1981). Gallaudet College, Division of Public Services, Florida Avenue at 7th Street NE, Washington, DC 20002.

Structured Tasks for English Practice. I. B. Pittle (1984). Washington, DC: Kendall Publications.

Teaching communication skills to preschool hearing impaired child. M. Whitehurst (1975). Alexander Graham Bell Association for the Deaf, 3417 Volta Place NW, Washington, DC 20007.

Things to do with Toddlers and Twos. K. Miller (1984). Telshare Publishing Co., Inc., P.O. Box 679, Marshfield, MA 02050.

TSA Syntax Program. S. Quigley and D. Powers (1979). Dormac, Inc., P.O. Box 752, Beaverton, OR 97005.

Parent/Family Oriented

An activity-based approach to early intervention. D. Bricker and J. Cripe (1992). Baltimore: Paul H. Brookes Publishing.

Becoming partners with children: From play to conversation. J. MacDonald (1989). San Antonio, TX: Special Press.

Chats with Johnny's parents. A. Simmons-Martin (1975). Alexander Graham Bell Association for the Deaf, 3417 Volta Place NW, Washington, DC 20007.

Early Intervention Series: Promoting Early Communication I and II. Infant and Hearing Resource (1993). Portland, OR.

Educational strategies for the youngest hearing impaired children 0-5. (1977). Alexander Graham Bell Association for the Deaf, 3417 Volta Place NW, Washington, DC 20002.

Experiences, our worlds, our words. 1976. Bill Wilkerson Hearing and Speech Center, 1114 19th Avenue South, Nashville, TN 37212.

The John Tracy Correspondence Course. 1983. John Tracy Clinic, 806 West Adams Boulevard, Los Angeles, CA 90007.

Karnes early language activities. 1975. Generators of Educational Materials Enterprises, P.O. Box 2339, Station A, Champaign, IL 68120.

Learning Language at Home. M. Karnes (1977). Council for Exceptional Children, Publication Sales, 120 Association Drive, Reston, VA 22091.

Parents and teachers: Partners in language development. A. Simmons-Martin and K. Rossi (1990). Washington, DC: Alexander Graham Bell Association for the Deaf.

SKI-HI Resource Manual: Family-Centered Home-Based Programming for Infants, Toddlers, and Preschool-Aged Children with Hearing Impairment. T. Clark and S. Watkins (1993). Logan, UT: Hope, Inc.

Auditory Processing/Skills Assessment

Auditory Continuous Performance Test. R. Keith (1978). The Psychological Corporation, San Antonio, TX.

Auditory Duration Pattern Test. F. Musiek, J. Baran, and M. Pinheiro (1990). Duration patters recognition in normal subjects and patients with cerebral and cochlear lesions. *Audiology*, 29:304-313.

Children's Auditory Processing Performace Scale. W. Smoski, M. Brunt, and C. Tannahill (1992). *Language, speech and hearing services in the schools*, 23:145-152.

Dichotic Digits. F. Musiek, N. Geurkink, S. Keitel (1982). Test battery assessment of auditory perceptual dysfunction in children. *Larynoscope*, 92:251-257.

Five-Sound Test. D. Ling (1978). Auditory coding and recoding. An analysis of auditory training procedures for hearing impaired children. In M. Ross and T. Giolas (Eds.), *Auditory management of hearing-impaired children* (pp. 181–218). Austin, TX: Pro-Ed.

Flowers-Costello Test of Central Auditory Abilities. A. Flowers and R. Costello (1970). Perception Learning Systems, Deaborn, MI.

Glendonald Auditory Screening Procedure. N. Erber (1982). Alexander Graham Bell Association for the Deaf, 3417 Volta Place, NW, Washington, DC 20007.

Northwestern University children's perception of speech. I. Elliott and D. Katz (1980). Auditec of St. Louis, 2515 S. Big Bend Blvd., St. Louis, MO 63143-2105.

PB-K's. H. Haskins (1949). Auditec, 2515 S. Big Bend Blvd, St. Louis, MO 63143.

Pediatric Speech Intelligibility Test. S. Jerger (1983). Auditec of St. Louis, 2515 S. Big Bend Blvd., St. Louis, MO 63143.

Pitch Pattern Sequence. M. Pinheiro (1977). Tests of central auditory function in children with learning disabilities. In R. Keith (ed.), *Central auditory dysfunction*. New Yok: Grune and Stratton.

SCAN. A Screening Test for Auditory Processing Disorders. R. Keith (1986). The Psychological Corporation. San Antonio, TX: Harcourt Brace.

SCAN A. A Test for Auditory Processing Disorders in Adolescents and Adults. R. Keith (1994). San Antonio, TX: The Psychological Corp., Harcourt Brace.

Selective Auditory Attention Test. R. Cherry (198). Auditec of St. Louis, St. Louis, MO.

Staggered Spondaic Word Test. J. Katz (1962). Precision Acoustics, Vancounver, WA.

Test of Auditory Comprehension. 1976. C. Farrar, et al. Foreworks, Box 7947, North Hollywood, CA.

Willeford Test Battery. J. Willeford (1980). Auditec of St. Louis, 2515 S. Big Bend Blvd., St. Louis, MO 63143.

Word Intelligibility by Picture Identification. M. Ross and I. W. Lerman (1971). Auditec of St. Louis, 2515 S. Big Bend Blvd., St. Louis, MO 63143.

Auditory Stimulation and Management Programs

Auditory Skills Curriculum. D. Stein, G. Benner, G. Hoversten, M. McGinnis, and T. Thies (1978). Foreworks, Box 7947, North Hollywood, CA, 91609.

Auditory Skills Instructional Planning System. 1979. (Los Angeles County Schools.) Foreworks, 7112 Teesdale Avenue, North Hollywood, CA 91605.

Auditory training. N. P. Erber (1982). Alexander Graham Bell Association for the Deaf, 3417 Volta Place, NW, Washington, DC 20007.

Curriculum guide: Hearing-impaired children and their parents. W. Northcott (1977). Alexander Graham Bell Association for the Deaf, 3417 Volta Place NW, Washington, DC 20007.

Developmental Approach to Successful Listening II. G. Goldberg Stout and J. Van Ert Windle (1992). Resource Point, Inc., 61 Inverness Dr. East, Suite 200, Englewood, CO 80112.

Educational audiology for the limited-hearing infant and preschooler. D. Pollack (1985). Fellendorf Associates Inc., 1300 Ruppert Road, Silver Spring, MD 20903.

Facilitating hearing and listening in young children. C. Flexer (1994). Alexander Graham Bell Association for the Deaf, 3417 Volta Place NW, Washington, DC 20007.

I heard that. W. Northcott (1978). Alexander Graham Bell Association for the Deaf, 3417 Volta Place, NW, Washington, DC 20007.

Listening Games—Building Listening Skills with Instructional Games. G. Wagner, M. Hosier, and M. Blackman (1972). Teachers Publishing, Division of the Macmillan Company, New York, NY 10022

Miami Cochlear Implant, Auditory, and Tactile Skills Curriculum (CHATS). K.C. Vergara, L. Miskiel, B. Lewis, K. Chiarello, M. Chonjnicki, P. Donovan, and T. Punch (1994). Miami, FL: Intelligent Hearing Systems. (305) 595-9170.

The joy of listening. J. Light (1978). Alexander Graham Bell Association for the Deaf, 3417 Volta Place, NW, Washington, DC 20007.

Play it by ear. E. Lowell and M. Stoner (1960). Wolfer Publishing Company, John Tracy Clinic, 806 West Adams Boulevard, Los Angeles, CA 90007.

Speechreading Tests

Children's Speechreading Test. D. Butt (1968). *Volta Review, 70,* 225–244.

Craig Lipreading Inventory. W. N. Craig (1964). Englewood, CO: Resource Point.

How well can you read lips? J. Utley (1946). *Journal of Speech Disorders, 11,* 109–116.

Resources on Speech Disorders

Foundations of spoken language for hearing impaired children. D. Ling (1989). Alexander Graham Bell Association for the Deaf, 3417 Volta Place NW, Washington, DC 20007.

Parent's Guide to Speech and Deafness. D. R. Calvert (1984). Alexander Graham Bell Association for the Deaf, 3417 Volta Place, NW, Washington, DC 20007.

Speech and deafness. D. R. Calvert and S. Silverman (1975). Alexander Graham Bell Association for the Deaf, 3417 Volta Place NW, Washington, DC 20007.

Speech and the hearing impaired child: Theory and practice. D. Ling (1976). Alexander Graham Bell Association for the Deaf, 3417 Volta Place, NW, Washington, DC 20007.

Speech assessment and speech improvement for the hearing impaired. J. Subtelny (1980). Alexander Graham Bell Association for the Deaf, 3417 Volta Place, NW, Washington, DC 20007.

Speech for the hearing impaired child. D. Stovall (1982). Charles C. Thomas, 301-327 East Lawrence Ave., Springfield, IL.

Speech of the hearing impaired. I. Hochberg, H. Levitt, and M. J. Osberger (1983). Austin, TX: Pro-Ed.

Speech production in hearing impaired children and youth: Theory and practice [Monograph]. R. Stoker and D. Ling (Eds.) (1992) *Volta Review*, November, Vol. 94.

Teacher/Clinician Planbook and Guide to the Development of Speech Skills and Cumulative Record of Speech Skill Acquisition. D. Ling (1978). Alexander Graham Bell Association for the Deaf, 3417 Volta Place, NW, Washington, DC 20007.

Understanding speech intelligibility in the hearing impaired. A. Carney (1992). *Topics in Language Development*, 6(3), 47–59.

Resources on Total Communication

Come sign with us. J. Hafer and R. Wilson (1990). Washington DC: Gallaudet University Press.

Early intervention for hearing impaired children: Total communication options. D. Ling (1984). College-Hill Press, 4284 41st Street, San Diego, CA 92105.

Manual communication: Implications for education. H. Bornstein (Ed.) (1990). Washington, DC: Gallaudet University Press.

Signing exact english. G. Gustason and E. Zawolkow (1993). Los Altimos, CA: Modern Signs Press.

Signs of the times. E. Shroyer (1982). Washington, DC: Gallaudet University Press.

SKI-HI Total Communication Video Program and Sign Language for the Family: A Total Communication Picture Reference Book to Accompany the SKI-HI Total Communication Video Program. S. Watkins (Ed.). Logan, UT: Hope, Inc.

The signed English schoolbook. H. Bornstein and K. Saulnier (1987). Washington, DC: Kendall Green Publications.

Total communication. J. Pahz and C. Pahz (1978). Springfield, IL: Charles C. Thomas.

Total communication structure and strategy. L. Evans (1983). Washington, DC: Gallaudet University Press.

Various Total Communication games, flashcards, children's storybooks, songbooks, instructional books, etc., available from (1) The National Association of the Deaf, 814 Thayer Avenue, Silver Spring, MD 20910, and (2) Sign Language Sotre, 8753 Shirley, P.O. Box 4440, Northridge, CA 91328.

Resources on American Sign Language, Deaf Culture, and Bilingualism

Bowe, F. (1986). *Changing the rules.* Silver Spring, MD:T. J. Publishers.

Humphries, T., and Padden, C. (1992). *Learning American Sign Language.* Englewood Cliffs, NJ: Prentice Hall.

Jacobs, J. M. (1989). *A deaf adult speaks out* (3rd ed.). Washington, DC: Gallaudet University Press.

Lentz, E. M., Mikos, K., and Smith, C. (1988). *Signing naturally: Teacher's curriculum guide.* Berkeley, CA: Dawn Sign Press.

Padden, C. (1988). *Deaf in America: Voices from a culture.* Cambridge, MA: Harvard University Press.

Robinette, D. (1990). *Hometown heroes: Successful deaf youth in America.* Washington, DC: Kendall Green Publications.

Sacks, O. (1989). *Seeing voices: A journey into the world of the deaf.* Berkeley, CA: University of California Press.

Schick, B., and Moeller, M.P. (Eds.). *Issues in language and deafness: The use of sign language in educational settings: Current concepts and controversies.* Omaha, NE: Boys Town National Research Hospital.

Sign Enhancers, Inc. (1992). *Bravo* videotape series (15 videotapes). Salem, OR: Sign Enhancers.

Stokoe, W. C. (Ed). (1980). *Sign and culture: A reader for students of American Sign Language.* Silver Spring, MD: Linstok Press.

Various materials and guidebooks on Deaf Mentor Programming (Early Home-Based Bilingual-Bicultural Programming). SKI-HI Institute, 809 North 800 East, Logan, UT 84321.

Wilcox, S (Ed). (1989) *American deaf culture: An anthology.* T. J. Publishers, Inc. (800) 999-1168

Williams, K. W. and Schick, B. (1995) *Educational Interpreter Performance Appraisal (EIPA).* Boys Town National Research Hospital, 555 North 30th St., Omaha, NE 68131. (402) 498-6765.

Technical Information for Parents and Teachers on Rehabilitation Aspects of Hearing Loss, Amplification, and Audiology

Auslander, M., Beauchaine, K., Larson, L., Lewis, D., Markley, S. Nelson, N., Rines, D., and Stelmachowicz, P. *Hearing aids adjustment for children*. Boys Town National Research Hospital. (402) 498-6511.

Auslander, M., Beauchaine K., Larson, L., Lewis, D., Markley, S. Nelson, N., Rines, D., and Stelmachowicz, P. *Hearing aids and how they work*. Boys Town National Research Hospital. (402) 498-6511.

Bess, F. H., Freeman, B.A., and Sinclair, J. S. (Eds.). (1981). *Amplification in education*. Alexander Graham Bell Association for the Deaf, 3417 Volta Place, NW, Washington, DC 20007.

Bess, F. H., and McConnell, F. E. (1981). *Audiology, education and the hearing impaired*. St. Louis, MO: C.V. Mosby.

Clark, T. C., and Watkins, S. (Eds.). (1993). *SKI-HI resource manual: Family-centered, home-based programming for infants, toddlers, and preschool-aged children with hearing impairment*. Logan, UT: HOPE, Inc.

Davis, J. M., and Hardick, E. J. (1981). *Rehabilitative audiology for children and adults.* New York: John Wiley and Sons.

Hasenstab, M. S., and Homer, J. S. (1982). *Comprehensive intervention with hearing impaired infants and preschool children*. Rockville, MD: Aspen Publications.

Eiten, L., and Beauchaine, K. (1995). *Parents and choices*. (videotape). Boys Town Press: 13603 Flanagan Blvd., Boys Town, NE 68010 (800) 282-6657.

Fewel, R. R., and Vadasy, P. F. (1983). *Learning through play: A resource manual for teachers and parents—birth to three years*. Teaching Resources Corporation, 50 Pond Park Rd., Hingham MA 02043.

Hall, E. (1982). *Is it catching? A book for children with hearing-impaired sisters or brothers*. Ellen Hall, P.O. Box 8005, Suite 192, Boulder, CO 80306-8005.

James, J., and Cherry, F. (1988). *The grief recovery handbook*. Harper & Row. 10 E. 53rd St., New York, NY 10022.

Lamore, G. S. (1986). *Now I understand—A book about hearing impairment*. Kendall Green Publications, Galludet University PRess, 800 Florida Ave., NW, Washington DC, 20002, (202) 651-5454 (V/TDD).

Ling, D., and Ling, A. H. (1978). *Aural habilitation*. Alexander Graham Bell Association for the Deaf, 3417 Volta Place, NW, Washington, DC 20007.

Luterman, D. (1987). *Deafness in the family*. Austin, TX: Pro-Ed.

McGonigel, M. J., Kaufman, R. K. and Johnson, B. H. (Eds) (1991). *Guidelines and recommended practices for the individualized family service plan*. (2nd ed.) National Early Childhood Technical Assistance System and Association for the Care of Children's Health, 7910 Woodmont Ave., Ste 300, Bethesda, MD 20814.

Meadow, K. (1980). *Deafness and child development*. Berkeley, CA: University of California Press.

Moeller, M. P., and Schick, B. (1993, 1994). *Sign with me: A family sign program*. BoysTown Press: 13603 Flanagan Blvd., BoysTown, NE 68010, (800) 282-6657.

Panara, R., and Panara, J. (1981) *Great deaf americans*.T.J. Publishers, Inc., 817 Silver Spring Ave., 305-D, Silver Spring, MD 20910.

Parent to Parent (1990). Parent Resource Library, House Ear Institute, 256 South Lake St., Los Angeles, CA 90057, (213) 483-4431, or TDD (213) 484-2642.

Paul, P., and Quigley, S. (1990). *Education and deafness*. New York: Longman.

Pollack, M. (1988). *Amplification for the hearing impaired*. New York: Grune and Stratton.

Quigley, S. P., and Kretschmer, R. E. (1982). *Education of deaf children*. Austin, TX: Pro-Ed.

Roeser, R. J., and Downs, M. P. (1988). *Auditory disorders on school children*. Thieme-Stratton Inc., 381 Park Avenue South, New York, NY 10016.

Sanders, D. A. (1982). *Aural rehabilitation*. Englewood Cliffs, NJ: Prentice Hall.

Schwartz, S. (1987). *Choices in deafness: A parents guide*. Woodbine House, Inc., 10400 Connecticut Avenue, Kensington, MD 20895.

Simons, R. (187). *After the tears*. Harcourt Brace Jovanovich Publishers, 1250 Sixth Avenue, San Diego, CA 92101.

Staab, W. (1991). *Hearing aids: A user's guide*. 512 E. Canterbury Lane, Phoenix, AZ 85022.

Tye-Murray, N. (1993). *Communication training for hearing-impaired children and teenagers*. Austin, TX: Pro-Ed.

What about me? (1990). Brothers and sisters of children with disabilities. Video and manual. Eduacational Productions, 4925 SW Humphrey Park Crest, Portland, OR, 97221.

What can my child hear? Videotape. House Ear Institute, 256 South Lake St., Los Angeles, CA, 90057, (213) 483-4431, or TDD (213) 484-2642.

What do I do now? Videotape. House Ear Institute, 256 South Lake St., Los Angeles, CA, 90057, (213) 483-4431, or TDD (213) 484-2642.

General Books for Parents and Clinicians about Hearing Impairment

Advances in cognition, education, and deafness. D. Martin (Ed.) (1991). Washington, DC: Gallaudet University Press.

Broken ears, wounded hearts. G. A. Harris (1983). Washington, DC: Gallaudet University Press.

Can't your child hear: A guide for those who care about deaf children. R. D. Freeman, C. F. Carbin, and R. J. Boese (1981). Austin, TX: Pro-Ed.

Choices in deafness: A parent's guide. S. Schwartz (1987). Woodbine House, Inc.

Dancing without music: Deafness in America. B. L. Benderly (1980). Garden City, NY: Anchor Press/Doubleday.

Deaf like me. T. S. Sprodley and J. P. Sprodley (1978). Random Books.

Deafness in the family. D. Luterman (1987). San Diego: College-Hill.

Educating the deaf. D. Moores (1987). Boston, MA: Houghton Mifflin.

Educational and developmental aspects of deafness. D. Moores and K. Meadows-Orlans (1990). Washington, DC: Gallaudet University Press.

Effectively educating students with hearing impairments. B. Luetke-Stahlman and J. Luckner (1991). White Plains, NY: Longman.

Getting the most out of your hearing aid. (1981). Alexander Graham Bell Association for the Deaf, 3417 Volta Place, NW, Washington, DC 20007.

Family to family. B. F. Griffin (1980). Alexander Graham Bell Association for the Deaf, 3417 Volta Place, NW, Washington, DC 20007.

Hearing impairments in young children. A. Boothroyd (1982). Englewood Cliffs, NJ: Prentice Hall.

Hearing loss help. A. Combs (1986). Alpenglow Press, P.O. Box 1841, Santa Maria, CA 93456.

I am going to have a hearing test: What will happen to me? E. Hall (1984). Fellendorf Associates Inc., 1300 Ruppert Rd., Silver Spring, MD 20903.

Infants and toddlers with hearing loss: Family centered assessment and intervention. Baltimore: York Press.

Learning to communicate: Implications for the hearing impaired. R. Truax and J. Shultz (1983). Alexander Graham Bell Association for the Deaf, 3417 Volta Place, NW, Washington, DC 20007.

Legal rights: The guide for deaf and hard of hearing people. Washington, DC: Gallaudet University Press.

Looking back—looking forward: Living with deafness. A. Griffith and D. Scott (1985). Fellendorf Associates Inc., 1300 Ruppert Road, Silver Spring, MD 20903.

Promoting social and emotional development in deaf children: The PATHS project. M. Greenberg and C. Kusche (1993). Seattle, WA: University of Washington Press.

Raising your hearing-impaired child: A guide for parents. S. McArthur (1982). Alexander Graham Bell Association for the Deaf, 3417 Volta Place NW, Washington, DC 20007.

Signs unseen, sounds unheard. C. Norris (1981). Alinda Press, Box 553, Eureka, CA 95503.

Talk with me. E. Altman (1988). Alexander Graham Bell Association for the Deaf, 3417 Volta Place NW, Washington DC, 20007.

The Hispanic deaf: Issues and challenges for bilingual special education. G. Delgado (1984). Washington, DC: Gallaudet University Press.

The rights of hearing impaired children. G. Nix (Ed.) (1977). Alexander Graham Bell Association for the Deaf, 3417 Volta Place, NW, Washington, DC 20007.

The silent garden. P. Ogden and S. Lipsett (1982). St. Martin's Press.

When your child is deaf: A guide for parents. D. Lutermann and M. Ross (1991). Alexander Graham Bell Association for the Deaf, 3417 Volta Place, NW, Washington, DC 20007.

You and your hearing-impaired child: A self-instructional guide for parents. Washington, DC: Gallaudet University Press.

Books for Parents by Parents

Featherstone, H. (1980). *A difference in the family: Life with a disabled child.* London: Basic Books.

Ferris, C. (1985). *A hug just isn't enough.* Washington, DC: Gallaudet University Press.

Fletcher, L. (1987). *Ben's story: A deaf child's right to sign.* Washington, DC: Gallaudet University Press.

Forecki, M. C. (1985). *Speak to me.* Washington, DC: Gallaudet University Press.

Glick, F. P., and Pellman, D. R. (1982). *Breaking silence.* Scottdale, PA: Herald.

Harris, G. A. (1983). *Broken ears, wounded hearts.* Washington, DC: Gallaudet University Press.

Simons, R. (1987). *After the tears: Parents talk about raising a child with a disability.* New York: Harcourt Brace Jovanovich.

Spiegle, J. A., and van den Pol, R. A. (1993). *Making changes: Family voices on living with disability.* Cambridge, MA: Brookline Books.

Spradley, T. S., and Spradley, J. P. (1985). *Deaf like me* (2nd ed.). Washington, DC: Gallaudet University Press.

Turnbull, H. R., and Turnbull, A. P. (1985). *Parents speak out: Then and now.* New York: Macmillan Publishing.

Parent-Professional Partnerships

Duffy, S., Phillips, S., Davis, S., Maloney, T., Tromnes, J., Miller, B., Colling, K., and Larsen, K. (1994). *We're all in this together so let's talk.* Missoula, MT: University of Montana, Dynamic Communication Process Project, Rural Institute on Disabilities.

Edelman, L., Greenland, B., and Mills, B. L. (1993). *Building parent/professional collaboration.* St. Paul, MN: Pathfinder Resources.

Mulik, J. A., and Pueschel, S. M. (1983). *Parent-professional partnerships in developmental disability services.* Washington, DC: Academic Guild Publishers.

Rosin, P., Whitehead, A., Tuchman, L., Jesien, G., and Begun, A. (1993). *Partnerships in early intervention.* Madison, WI: University of Wisconsin—Madison.

Seligman, M. (Ed.). (1991). *The family with a handicapped child* (2nd ed.). Needham Heights, MA: Allyn and Bacon.

Speigle-Mariska, J., and Harper-Whalen, S. (1993). *Forging partnerships with families.* Missoula, MT: University of Montana, Co-Teach Programs Division of Educational Research and Service, School of Education.

Turnbull, A. P., and Turnbull, H. R. (1990). *Families, professionals, and exceptionality: A special partnership* (2nd ed.). Columbus, OH: Merrill.

RESOURCES AND MATERIALS LIST—ADULTS/ELDERLY

The following list of materials is not intended to be exhaustive. The list provides samples of materials and protocols that are useful for pre- and post-audiologic rehabilitation and for therapy. Because of the individuality of each client, clinicians must often modify existing materials or develop new ones. This list may be helpful as a guide.

Stimulus Materials

Phonemes

CONSONANTS.
Miller, G., and Nicely, P. (1955). An analysis of perceptual confusions among some English consonants. *Journal of the Acoustical Society of America, 27,* 338–352.

> Provides confusion matrices of auditory perception among English consonants. Useful for developing materials of varying degrees of difficulty for auditory training.

Owens, E., and Schubert, E. (1977). Development of the California Consonant Test. *Journal of Speech and Hearing Disorders, 20,* 463–474.

> Yields an in-depth summary of consonant-discrimination abilities.

Tannahill, J. C., and McReynolds, L. V. (1972). Consonant discrimination as a function of distinctive feature differences. *Journal of Auditory Research, 12,* 101–108.

> Provides pairs of consonants for "same-different" tasks. Pairs are arranged in order of difficulty for auditory discrimination.

Woodward, M. F., and Barber, C. G. (1960). Phoneme perception in lipreading. *Journal of Speech and Hearing Research, 3,* 212–222.

> Provides a rank-order of consonant pairs based on visual differences. Useful for developing materials of varying degrees of speechreading ability.

Words

VISUAL IDENTIFICATION WORD LIST.
Brannon, J. (1961). Speechreading of various speech materials. *Journal of Speech and Hearing, 26,* 348–353.

> Provides relative difficulty of visual identification of 50 words.

PAL PB-50 WORDS.
Egan, J. P. (1948). Articulation testing methods. *Laryngoscope, 58,* 955–991.

> PAL PB-50 word lists provide several lists of single-syllable words. These lists contain less familiar words than CID W-22 and are more difficult.

HIGH-FREQUENCY CONSONANT WORD LIST.
Gardner, N. J. 1971. Application of a high-frequency consonant discrimination word list in hearing-aid evaluation. *Journal of Speech and Hearing Disorders, 36,* 354–355.

Lists of single-syllable words that are loaded with high-frequency consonants. Useful as a difficult auditory test and for demonstrating the value of vision plus audition.

CID W-22, CID W-1.
Hirsh, I. J., Davis, H., Silverman, S. R., Reynolds, E., Eldert, E., and Benson, R. W. (1952). Development of materials for speech audiometry. *Journal of Speech and Hearing Disorders, 17,* 321-337.

CID W-22 word lists provide several lists of single-syllable words. These words represent an easier visual or auditory discrimination task compared with single-syllable words.

HUTTON SEMI-DIAGNOSTIC.
Hutton, C., Curry, E. T., and Armstrong, M. B. (1959). Semi-diagnostic test material for aural rehabilitation. *Journal of Speech and Hearing Disorders, 24,* 319-239.

Single-syllable words, multiple-choice test designed to evaluate auditory-only, visual-only, and combined modes of reception.

CCTs.
Owens, E., and Schubert, E. (1977). Development of the California Consonant Test. *Journal of Speech and Hearing Research, 20,* 463–474.

Monosyllabic word lists containing difficult-to-perceive consonants.

Sentences

CID EVERYDAY SENTENCES.
Davis, H., and Silverman, S. R. (1970). *Hearing and deafness.* New York: Holt, Rinehart and Winston.

CID Everyday Sentences provide several lists of common sentences, 10 sentences per list.

SPIN.
Kalikow, D., Stevens, K., and Elliott, L. (1977). Development of a test of speech intelligibility in noise using sentence materials with controlled word predictability. *Journal of the Acoustical Society of America, 61,* 1337-1351.

Speech intelligibility in noise (SPIN) provides information on a listener's use of contextual information.

Iᴏᴡᴀ Sᴇɴᴛᴇɴᴄᴇs Wɪᴛʜᴏᴜᴛ Cᴏɴᴛᴇxᴛ.
Tyler, R., Preece, J., and Lowder, M. (1983). The Iowa Cochlear Implant Tests. Iowa City, IA: U. of Iowa.

Uᴛʟᴇʏ Sᴇɴᴛᴇɴᴄᴇ Tᴇsᴛ.
Utley, J. (1946). A test of lipreading ability. *Journal of Speech Disorders*, *11*, 109–116.

Sentence portion of the speechreading test provides common, everyday sentences. As a speechreading test it is considered fairly difficult.

Hearing Aid, Hearing Disability/Handicap, and Communication Self-Assessment Questionnaires

These scales are useful for obtaining self-estimates of hearing-aid performance, hearing-handicap and communication problems. Results can be used to supplement other information in determining need for and measuring the effect of audiologic rehabilitation. (See Appendices in Chapters 9 and 10.)

Abbreviated Profile of Hearing Aid Benefit. R. Cox and G. Alexander. (April, 1994). Abbreviated profile of hearing aid benefit. Presented at annual convention of American Academy of Audiology, Richmond, VA.

Communication Assessment Profile. R. Schow and M. Nerbonne (1982). Communication screening profile: Use with elderly clients. *Ear and Hearing, 3*, 135–147. (SAC and SOAC; see Chapter 9.)

Communication Profile for the Hearing Impaired. M. Demorest and S. Erdman (1987). *Journal of Speech and Hearing Disorders, 52*, 143–155.

Denver Scale of Communication Function. Alpiner, J. G., Cheverette, W., Clascoe, G., Metz, M., and Olsen, B., unpublished study (1974). See J. Alpiner and P. McCarthy (Eds.) (1993). *Rehabilitative audiology: Children and adults.* Baltimore: Williams and Wilkins. (Also see Quantified Denver Scale, Chapter 9.)

Denver Scale of Communication Function for Senior Citizens Living in Retirement Centers. J. Zarnoch and J. Alpiner, unpublished study (1977). See J. Alpiner and P. McCarthy (Eds.) (1993). *Rehabilitative audiology: Children and adults.* Baltimore: Williams and Wilkins.

Hearing Aid Performance Inventory. B. Walden, M. Demorest, and E. Hepler (1984). Self-report approach to assessing benefit from amplification. *Journal of Speech and Hearing Research, 27*, 49–56.

Hearing Handicap Inventory for Adults. C. Newman, B. Weinstein, G. Jacobson, and G. Hug (1991). Test-retest of the Hearing Handicap Inventory for Adults. *Ear and Hearing, 12*, 355–357.

Hearing Handicap Inventory for the Elderly. I. Ventry and B. Weinstein (1982). The Hearing Handicap Inventory for the elderly: A new tool. *Ear and Hearing, 3*, 128–134. (See Chapter 10.)

Hearing Handicap Scale. W. High, G. Fairbanks, and A. Glorig (1964). Scale for self-assessment of hearing handicap. *Journal of Speech and Hearing Disorders, 29*, 215–230. (See Chapter 9.)

Hearing Measurement Scale. W. Noble and G. Atherley (1970). The hearing measurement scale: A questionnaire for the assessment of auditory disability. *Journal of Auditory Research, 10,* 229-250.

Hearing Performance Inventory (Revised). S. Lamb, E. Owens, and E. Schubert (1983). The revised form of the hearing performance inventory. *Ear and Hearing, 4,* 152-157.

McCarthy-Alpiner Scale of Hearing Handicap. P. McCarthy and J. Alpiner (1983). An assessment scale of hearing handicap for use in family counseling. *Journal of the Academy of Rehabilitative Audiology, 10,* 2-12. (See Chapter 9.)

Nursing Home Hearing Handicap Index (NHHI). R. Schow and M. Nerbonne (1977). Assessment of hearing handicap by nursing home residents and staff. *Journal of the Academy of Rehabilitative Audiology, 10,* 2-12. (See Chapter 10.)

Profile Questionnaire for Rating Communicative Performance in a Home Environment. D. Sanders (1988). Hearing and orientation and counseling. In M. Pollack (Ed.), *Amplification for the hearing impaired.* New York: Grune and Stratton.

Self-Assessment of Communication/Significant Other Assessment of Communication (SAC/SOAC). R. Schow and M. Nerbonne (1982). Communication Screening Profile: Use with Elderly Clients. *Ear and Hearing, 3,* 135-147. (See Chapter 9)

Computer-Assisted Hearing Aid Assessment and Fitting

Berger Hearing Aid Prescription. K. W. Berger, Herald Publishing House, 647 Longmeere Dr., Kent, OH 44240, (216)673-5654.

Comprehensive Hearing Aid Selection and Evaluation System (CHASE). L. Humes (1992). Beyond insertion gain. *Hearing Instruments, 43*(2), 32-35.

Desired Sensation Level (DSL). R. Seewald (1991). The desired sensation level method for fitting children. Version 3.0. *Hearing Journal, 45*(4), 36-41.

Hearing Aid Selection and Evaluation (CID). G. Popelka and A. Engelbretson (1983). A computer-based system for hearing aid assessment. *Hearing Instruments, 34*(7), 6-9, 44. Central Institute for the Deaf, 818 South Euclid, St. Louis, MO 63110, (314)652-3200.

Hearing Aid Manager (HAM). G. J. Glascoe, Parrot Software, 190 Sandy Ridge Road, State College, PA 16803, (814)237-7282.

Select a Hearing Aid (SELECT). G. J. Glascoe, Parrot Software, 190 Sandy Ridge Road, State College, PA 16803, (814)237-7282.

Select an Aid. R. de Jonge, Department of Speech Pathology and Audiology, Central Missouri State University, Warrensburg, MO 64093.

Systematic Hearing Aid Prescriptions (SHAP). D. Moomaw (1984). San Diego: College-Hill.

Evaluation of Cochlear Implant Performance

Iowa cochlear implant tests. R. Tyler, R. Preece, and M. Lowder (1983; addendum, 1985). The Iowa Cochlear Implant Tests. Iowa City: University of Iowa.

Minimum Auditory Capabilities (MAC) battery. E. Owens, D. Kessler, C. Telleen, and E. Schubert (1981). The Minimum Auditory Capabilities (MAC) battery. *Hearing Aid Journal, 9,* 32–34.

Technical Information on Rehabilitation Aspects of Hearing Loss, Amplification, and Audiology

Alpiner, J., and McCarthy, P. (Eds). (1993). *Rehabilitative audiology: Children and adults.* Baltimore: Williams and Wilkins.

Beck, L. B., and Preves, D. A. (1987). Update on real ear measures of hearing aid performance. *Ear and Hearing, 8*(5, Suppl., Special Issue), 59–126.

Castle, D. L. (1980). *Telephone training for the deaf.* Rochester, NY: National Technical Institute for the Deaf.

Cooper, H. (Ed). (1991). *Cochlear implants: A practical guide.* London: Whurr.

DeFilippo, C., and Scott, B. (1978). A method for training and evaluating the reception of ongoing speech. *Journal of the Acoustical Society of America, 63,* 1186–1192.

Erickson, J. G. (1978). *Speech reading: An aid to communication.* Interstate Printers and Publishers, Inc., Danville, IL 61832.

Fleming, M. (1972). A total approach to communication therapy. *Journal of the Academy of Rehabilitative Audiology, 5,* 28–31.

Gagne, J.-P., and Tye-Murray, N. (Eds.). (1994). Research in audiological rehabilitation: Current trends and future directions [Monograph]. *Journal of the Academy of Rehabilitative Audiology, 27.*

Garstecki, D. (1981). Audio-visual training paradigm for hearing impaired adults. *Journal of the Academy of Rehabilitative Audiology, 14,* 223–228.

Giolas, T. (1982). *Hearing handicapped adults.* Englewood Cliffs, NJ: Prentice Hall.

Hull, R. (1994). Assisting the older client. In J. Katz (Ed.), *Handbook of clinical audiology* (3rd ed). Baltimore: Williams and Wilkins.

Hutchinson, K. (1981). *Listening and speechreading.* National Technical Institute for the Deaf, Rochester, NY 14623.

Jacobs, M. (1981). *Associational cues.* National Technical Institute for the Deaf, Rochester, NY 14623.

Jacobs-Condit, L. (1984). *Gerontology and communication disorders.* Rockville, MD: American Speech-Language-Hearing Association.

Kaplan, J., Bally, S., and Garretson, S. (1985). *Speechreading: A way to improve understanding.* Washington, DC: Gallaudet College Press.

Montgomery, A. (1994). WATCH: A practical approach to brief auditory rehabilitation. *Hearing Journal, 47*(10), 10, 53–55.

Mueller, G., Hawkins, D., and Northern, J. (1992). *Probe microphone measurements*. San Diego: Singular.

Sanders, D. (1993). *Management of Hearing Handicap* (3rd ed.). Englewood Cliffs, NJ: Prentice Hall.

Shadden, B. B. (1988). *Communication behavior and aging: A sourcebook for clinicians*. Baltimore: Williams and Wilkins.

Smith, C., and Fay, T. (1977). A program of auditory rehabilitation for aged persons in a chronic disease hospital. *Asha, 19*, 417–420.

Traynor, R., and Smaldino, J. (1986). *Computerized adult aural rehabilitation (CARR)*. San Diego, CA: College-Hill.

Valente, M. (Ed). (1994). *Strategies for selecting and verifying hearing aid fittings*. New York: Thieme.

Walden, B., Erdman, J., Montgomery, A., Schwartz, D., and Prosak, R. (1981). Some effects of training on speech recognition by hearing impaired adults. *Journal of Speech and Hearing Research, 24*, 207–216.

General Books for Adults about Hearing Impairment

Carmen, R. (1977). *Our endangered hearing: Understanding and coping with hearing loss*. Emmaus, PA: Rodale.

Combs, A. (1986). *Hearing loss help*. Santa Maria, CA: Alpenglow.

Fritz, G., and Smith, N. (1985). *The hearing impaired employee: An untapped resource*. Austin, TX: Pro-Ed.

House, M. D. (1985). *Questions and answers about the cochlear implant*. House Ear Institute, 256 S. Lake St., Los Angeles, CA 90057.

Orleans, H. (1985). *Adjustment to adult hearing loss*. San Diego, CA: College-Hill.

Staab, W. (1991). *Hearing aids: A user's guide*. Phoenix, AZ: Wayne Staab, Ph.D.

Zazone, P. (1993). *When the phone rings, my bed shakes (Memoirs of a deaf doctor)*. Washington, DC: Gallaudet University Press.

General Resource Groups

Academy of Rehabilitative Audiology, P.O. Box 26532, Minneapolis, MN 55426

Alexander Graham Bell Association for the Deaf, 3417 Volta Place, NW, Washington, DC 20007, (202)337-5220 (Voice or TTY)

American Academy of Audiology (AAA), 1735 N. Lyon St, Suite 950, Arlington, Virginia 22209-2022

American Association of Retired Persons (AARP), 1909 K St., NW, Washington, DC 20049, (202)872-4700

American Auditory Society, 1966 Inwood Rd., Dallas, TX 75235

American Coalition of Citizens with Disabilities (ACCD), 1012 14th St., NW #901, Washington, DC 20005, (202)628-3470

American Hearing Research Foundation, 55 E. Washington Street, Suite #2105, Chicago, IL 60602, (312)726-9670

American Speech-Language-Hearing Association, 10801 Rockville Pike, Rockville, MD 20852, (800)424-8576

American Tinnitus Association, P.O. Box 5, Portland, OR 97207, (503)248-9985

Better Hearing Institute, 1430 K St., NW, Suite 200, Washington, DC 20005, (800)424-8576

Center for Childhood Deafness, Boys Town National Research Hospital, 555 North 30th St., Omaha, NE 68131, (402)498-6521 (voice or TDD)

Consumer Organization for the Hearing Impaired, P.O. Box 8188, Silver Spring, MD 20907, (301)647-4333

Greater Los Angeles Council on Deafness, Inc. (GLAD), 616 So. Westmoreland Ave., Los Angeles, CA 90005, (213)383-2220

House Ear Institute, 256 South Lake St., Los Angeles, CA 90057

National Association of the Deaf (NAD), 814 Thayer Avenue, Silver Spring, MD 20910, (301)587-1788

National Association for Hearing and Speech Action (NAHSA), 10801 Rockville Pike, Box L, Rockville, MD 20852, (800)638-8255

Self-Help for Hard of Hearing People (SHHH), 7800 Wisconsin Ave., Bethesda, MD 20814

Information about Assistive Devices

AT&T Special Needs Center, (800)233-1222, (800)833-3232 (TDD)

Council on Assistive Devices and Listening Systems (COADLS, Inc.), c/o Fellendorf and Associates, Inc., P.O. Box 32227, Washington, DC 20007, (301)593-1636

General Telephone, (800)352-7437

Hearing Aid Consumer Protection Hotline (hearing-aid complaints), (800) 572-3270 (voice or TDD)

International Hearing Dog, Inc., 5901 E. 89th Avenue, Henderson, CO 80640, (303)287-3277 (voice or TDD)

National Captioning Institute (NCI), 5203 Leesburg Pike, Suite 1500, Falls Church, VA 22041, (703) 998-2400 (voice or TTY)

The National Information Center on Deafness, Gallaudet University, 800 Florida Avenue, NE, Washington, DC 20002

The National Hearing Aid Society, 20361 Middlebelt Road, Livonia, MI 48152, (800)521-5247

Organization for Use of the Telephone, Inc. (OUT), P.O. Box 175, Owings Mills, MD 23117-0175, (301)655-1827

Pacific Telephone, (800)772-3140 (TDD)

Self-Help for Hard of Hearing People, Inc. (SHHH), 7800 Wisconsin Avenue, Bethesda, MD 20814, (301)657-2248 (voice), (301)675-2249 (TTY)

The Washington Area Group for the Hard of Hearing (WAG-HOH), P.O. Box 6283, Silver Spring, MD 20906, (301)942-7612

Author Index

Subject Index